Integrated Drug Discovery Technologies

Integrated Drug Discovery Technologies

edited by

Houng-Yau Mei

Rubicon Genomics, Inc.
Ann Arbor, Michigan

Anthony W. Czarnik

Sensors for Medicine and Science, Inc.
Germantown, Maryland

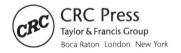

CRC Press
Taylor & Francis Group
Boca Raton London New York

CRC Press is an imprint of the
Taylor & Francis Group, an **informa** business

CRC Press
Taylor & Francis Group
6000 Broken Sound Parkway NW, Suite 300
Boca Raton, FL 33487-2742

First issued in paperback 2019

© 2002 by Taylor & Francis Group, LLC
CRC Press is an imprint of Taylor & Francis Group, an Informa business

ISBN-13: 978-0-8247-0649-4 (hbk)
ISBN-13: 978-0-367-39626-8 (pbk)

Visit the Taylor & Francis Web site at
http://www.taylorandfrancis.com

and the CRC Press Web site at
http://www.crcpress.com

Preface

We scientists in the drug discovery business are not so different from alchemists of old: "Convert this lead into gold and I shall share my wealth with you." Or perhaps, "Convert this lead into gold or else!" You've no doubt felt motivation from both the carrot and the stick during your career, but it probably sounded more like this: "If you can make a better COX-2 inhibitor, the company's stock will triple!" Or, "If we don't fill our pipeline quickly, someone is going to buy us!" Whether then or now, the risk/reward ratio is literally a step function, not a continuum, dependent on a scientist accomplishing a mission his analytical conscience cannot guarantee.

Now, as in earlier times, we try anything that makes sense in the discovery process. Because no one method has provided a "lock" on discovery, scientists have room for style and intuition. "I know the value of computer-aided drug design." "The more times you're up at bat, the more often you'll hit a home run— so screen." "Drug discovery requires a genomic/proteomic/metabolic pathway approach." "Start with someone else's drug and synthesize around the patent." Who's right? It begins to sound like a debate of the merits of one religion versus another. But science is about quantitation; why can't we simply calculate which approach is the best? Perhaps because no one does "outcomes research" on the drug discovery process. I think instead it is because science is ultimately a human endeavor, and each person espousing a discovery philosophy is motivated to make that choice look like the right one. In the marketplace of ideas, steak sells, and sizzle sells.

This book is about steak. If you hear a little sizzle as well, it's because the authors believe passionately in their technology and the philosophy that accompanies it. "Lead into gold," each plaintively wails. Lead, gold, carrots, sticks, steak, sizzle, and drugs. Let the games begin.

Anthony W. Czarnik

Contents

Contents

Contributors

Lee Amon   MarketQwest Associates, Fremont, California

Tony J. Beugelsdijk, Ph.D.   Los Alamos National Laboratory, Los Alamos, New Mexico

James A. Blackledge   Department of Discovery Technologies, Pfizer Global Research and Development, Ann Arbor, Michigan

Mark Bradley, Ph.D.   Department of Chemistry, University of Southampton, Southampton, United Kingdom

Jocelyn W. Burke, Ph.D.   Department of BioChipventures, Packard Bio-Science, Meriden, Connecticut

Hong Cai   BioScience Division, Los Alamos National Laboratory, Los Alamos, New Mexico

Peter J. Coassin   Department of Instrumentation Research and Development, Aurora Biosciences Corporation, San Diego, California

Andrew P. Combs, Ph.D.   Directed Parallel Synthesis Group, Bristol-Myers Squibb Company, Wilmington, Delaware

Anthony W. Czarnik, Ph.D.   Chief Scientific Officer, Sensors for Medicine and Science, Inc., Germantown, Maryland

John P. Devlin, Ph.D.   MicroSource Discovery Systems, Inc., Gaylordsville, Connecticut

Ping Du   Department of Discovery Technologies, Pfizer Global Research and Development, Ann Arbor, Michigan

Christophe Fromont, Ph.D.   Ribo Targets Ltd., Cambridge, United Kingdom

Kenneth A. Giuliano, Ph.D.   Department of Assay Development, Cellomics, Inc., Pittsburgh, Pennsylvania

Tasir S. Haque, Ph.D.   Directed Parallel Synthesis Group, Bristol-Myers Squibb Company, Wilmington, Delaware

Betty Howard, M.S.   Microplate Detection Systems, Packard BioScience, Downers Grove, Illinois

Ravi Kapur, Ph.D.   CellChip Department, Cellomics, Inc., Pittsburgh, Pennsylvania

Paul A. Keifer, Ph.D.   CST Associates, Omaha, Nebraska

Greg W. Kilby   Department of Discovery Technologies, Pfizer Global Research and Development, Ann Arbor, Michigan

David A. Kniaz, B.S., M.B.A.   Product Development, SciQuest Inc., Newton Square, Pennsylvania

Michal Lebl, Ph.D., D.Sc.   High Throughput Synthesis Department, Illumina, Inc., San Diego, California

Robert A. Lepley, Ph.D.*   Department of Discovery Technologies, Pfizer Global Research and Development, Ann Arbor, Michigan

Albert P. Li, Ph.D.   In Vitro Technologies, Inc., Baltimore, Maryland

Joseph A. Loo, Ph.D.   Department of Discovery Technologies, Pfizer Global Research and Development, Ann Arbor, Michigan

Current affiliation: TIS Group, Minneapolis, Minnesota

Rachel R. Ogorzalek Loo, Ph.D.   Department of Discovery Technologies, Pfizer Global Research and Development, Ann Arbor, Michigan

Joseph Macri, Ph.D.*   Department of Discovery Technologies, Pfizer Global Research and Development, Ann Arbor, Michigan

Gerard Mathis   Department of Research and Development, Division of In Vitro Technologies, CIS Bio International, Bagnols sur Céze, France

Gary McMaster, Ph.D.   Target Discovery Research, Eli Lilly and Company, Indianapolis, Indiana

Houng-Yau Mei, Ph.D., M.B.A.   Department of Operations, Rubicon Genomics, Inc., Ann Arbor, Michigan

Tina S. Morris, Ph.D.   Department of Protein Development, Human Genome Sciences, Inc., Rockville, Maryland

Walter D. Niles, Ph.D.   Department of Biophysics and Instrumentation, Aurora Biosciences Corporation, San Diego, California

John P. Nolan, Ph.D.   BioScience Division, Los Alamos National Laboratory, Los Alamos, New Mexico

David O'Hagan, Ph.D.   Streamline Proteomics, Ann Arbor, Michigan

Keith R. Olson, Ph.D.   Cellomics, Inc., Pittsburgh, Pennsylvania

Vincent Pomel, Ph.D.   Department of Chemistry, Serono Pharmaceutical Research Institute, Grand-Lancy, Switzerland

Stephen T. Rapundalo, Ph.D.   Department of Cardiovascular Molecular Sciences, Pfizer Global Research and Development, Ann Arbor, Michigan

Christian Rohlff, Ph.D.   Department of Biology, Oxford GlycoSciences, Abingdon, United Kingdom

Cornelia Rufenach, Ph.D.   Department of Sales and Marketing, Evotec BioSystems AG, Hamburg, Germany

---

Current affiliation: McMaster University, Hamilton, Ontario, Canada

Andreas Scheel   Department of Screening Operations, Evotec BioSystems AG, Hamburg, Germany

Sylvia Sterrer   Evotec BioSystems AG, Hamburg, Germany

Tracy I. Stevenson   Department of Discovery Technologies, Pfizer Global Research and Development, Ann Arbor, Michigan

Lorin A. Thompson, Ph.D.   Directed Parallel Synthesis Group, Bristol-Myers Squibb Company, Wilmington, Delaware

Rodney Turner   Evotec BioSystems AG, Hamburg, Germany

Loraine V. Upham   Microplate Detection Systems, Packard BioScience, Downers Grove, Illinois

Chandrasekaran Vasudevan, Ph.D.   Cellomics, Inc., Pittsburgh, Pennsylvania

Jian Wang, Ph.D.   Cellomics, Inc., Pittsburgh, Pennsylvania

P. Scott White   BioScience Division, Los Alamos National Laboratory, Los Alamos, New Mexico

Wendell Wierenga, Ph.D.   Syrrx, Inc., San Diego, California

Elizabeth S. Woo, Ph.D.   Marketing Department, Cellomics, Inc., Pittsburgh, Pennsylvania

1
The Motivation: A Top-Down View

Wendell Wierenga
Syrrx, Inc.
San Diego, California

If one were to start the process of drug discovery de novo one would probably not begin; it is an incredibly daunting task. If you look at what one is up against in terms of discovering and developing a drug, the challenges are almost overwhelming. There is a veritable physiological labyrinth for determining drug efficacy and safety. What does a pharmacological agent, whether it is a large or small molecule, have to go through to be of some benefit to an individual with some pathologic state? It must survive gastric pH and gastrointestinal enzymes if it is an orally administered drug. Absorption is a key issue: it has to get to the systemic circulation. There is also the problem of enterohepatic recycling. There are barriers—lymphatic barriers, endothelial barriers, blood–brain barriers, and blood–retina barriers—blocking the movement of the molecule to the appropriate site of action or pathology. All of these are very important challenges for a potential new drug. Many of these barriers do not have good laboratory models at the present time. And this doesn't even take into account what the body likes to do with xenobiotics, namely, to metabolize, conjugate, excrete, and eliminate them. Eventually, some of the drug must get to the right organ, cell type, and molecular target (enzyme, receptor) to effect a beneficial response. In so doing, it must have sufficient selectivity relative to potentially deleterious effects on normal tissue to yield an acceptable benefit/risk. This physiological labyrinth often takes more than a decade of research time for a single drug to traverse, while, in parallel, many more drugs fail.

There are yet other prerequisites for a drug. It has to be stable, of course. It has to have a decent shelf life, but not only as the bulk material on large scale under a variety of conditions; the formulation also must be stable and compatible with human life. There has to be an economical source because in the end if one cannot produce the drug in a reasonably cost-effective manner, it is not going to be

1

available to the marketplace. Lastly, one must have the necessary analytical tools for determining the various physical and chemical properties of the molecule and its presence in various biological fluids. All these tools need to be made available for one eventually to have something called a drug.

How did we discover drugs? Figure 1 divides drug discovery into five categories. The two that are highlighted—modifying the structure of known drugs and screening inventories of natural products (primarily)—represent the history of drug discovery in the 1950s, 1960s, and 1970s. The others—proteins as therapeutics, modifying the structure of natural substrates, and structure-based, computer-aided drug design—emerged in the past 15 years or so, and are only today really beginning to make an impact. Let's review each of these categories of approaches to drug discovery.

Figure 2 shows a few examples of drugs created by modification of known drugs. There are certainly many more, but these are a few examples from the Parke-Davis research laboratories of building on past leads and establishing improvements in a molecule based on a previously known drug: angiotensin-converting enzyme (ACE) inhibitors, quinolone antibiotics, cephalosporins, κ agonists, and 3-hydroxy-3-methylglutaryl coenzyme A (HMG-CoA) reductase inhibitors. In some cases, these examples were very successfully marketed; other cases were not commercially successful but resulted in the creation of effective drugs. Nonetheless, modification of known drugs is a successful paradigm for drug discovery and represents the vast majority of the research investment in the 1960s and 1970s in drug discovery.

In many ways this approach was predated by natural products. Many of our early drugs came from plant sources or, later on, from *Streptomyces* or other microorganisms. Figure 3 is a nonexhaustive but representative list of natural products that were sources of drugs, discovered using a screening paradigm. In some cases, the knowledge of "traditional medicines" and folklore contributed significantly to the nonrandom sourcing for the eventual isolation and purification

- Modify Structure of Known Drugs

- Screen Inventories of Natural Products in Laboratory Models of Diseases

- Proteins as Therapeutics/Vaccines

- Modify Structure of Natural Substrate of Enzyme or Receptor

- Structure-based Design/CADD

Figure 1   How did we discover drugs?

Building on Past Leads
SAR Profile

- ACE Inhibitors

- Quinolone Antibiotics

- Cephalosporin Antibiotics

- Kappa Agonist Analgesics

- HMG-CoA Reductase Inhibitors

Figure 2 Modify structure of known drugs.

- - Antibiotics
    * Macrolides
    * β-Lactams
    * Aminoglycosides
    * Tetracyclins

  - Antifungals
    * Amphotericin
    * Griseofulvin

  - Atherosclerosis
    * Mevinolin

  - Hypertension/Angina
    * Digoxin

- Anticancers
    * Vinca Alkaloids
    * Anthracyclines
    * Etoposide
    * Mitomycin
    * Taxol

  - Neurologics
    * Atropine
    * Cocaine

  - Immunosuppressives
    * Cyclosporin
    * FK 506

Figure 3 Screening: extensive history of natural products and microbial secondary metabolites.

of the natural product. These secondary metabolites are still having a significant impact on medical therapy today. There are anti-infective products (antibiotics and antifungals), as well as products for the treatment of atherosclerosis. Mevinolin (also known as lovastatin) is a paradigm for very important treatments of dyslipidemias and atherosclerosis, i.e., HMG-CoA reductase inhibitors. There are also treatments for hypertension and angina. There is an expanding group of anticancer drugs, many of them based on original plant- or microorganism-derived secondary metabolites that exhibited cytotoxic activity in a number of tumor cell assays. Finally, there are neurologics and immunosuppressives. The category of drugs comprising natural products and derivatives is extensive.

This sourcing of drugs from natural products has changed over the past 5–10 years, with increasing numbers of drugs coming from chemical libraries rather than from natural products. The reason for this is that over the last 30 or 40 years pharmaceutical companies and chemical companies have established significant inventories of small molecules. These inventories were not being exploited as potential sources of drugs because of the absence of broad-based, automated screening methods and biologically relevant assays. This has changed dramatically in the last decade. Today one can come up with an extensive list of potential drug candidates coming from the screening of chemical libraries (Fig. 4), and this has become the basis for significant new technologies in the area of high-throughput screening and combinatorial chemistry. So how did one discover drugs in the past? To recapitulate, in large part, one did it by modifying the structure of known drugs or screening inventories of natural products.

With the advent of molecular biology in the late 1970s, proteins as therapeutics came on the scene. While the list of protein-based drugs is not yet long, it is growing, and it represents a very important drug category (Fig. 5). These drugs are important not only from the point of view of medical therapy but also because of their economic impact. This particular list of seven proteins represents currently over $7 billion in sales annually. These proteins are having a dramatic impact on our industry, and they are having a dramatic impact on patient therapy.

The fourth approach to drug discovery, the modification of natural substrates, has had less success in yielding new drugs. Figure 6 lists examples taken from our laboratory research efforts at Parke-Davis. These include adenosine deaminase inhibitors, renin inhibitors, angiotensin receptor antagonists (a very large area of investment for many pharmaceutical research laboratories over the past 10 years), and cholecystokinin B (CCK-B) receptor antagonists. While this is another valid approach for drug discovery, one subset of this approach—peptidomimetics as drugs—continues to be characterized by poor pharmacokinetics and delivery-related challenges.

There was an interesting statement in the May 1991 issue of *Business Week:* "The old way—screening thousands of chemicals in a hit or miss search—is inefficient and wastes time. That is why it can now cost more than $200 million to

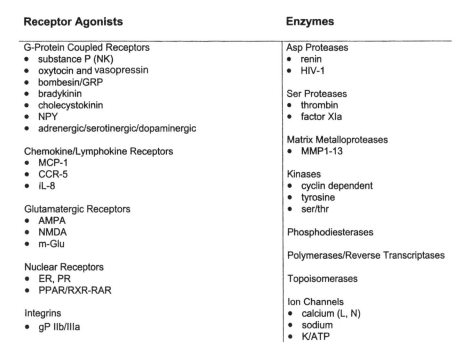

Receptor Agonists	Enzymes
G-Protein Coupled Receptors • substance P (NK) • oxytocin and vasopressin • bombesin/GRP • bradykinin • cholecystokinin • NPY • adrenergic/serotinergic/dopaminergic	Asp Proteases • renin • HIV-1 Ser Proteases • thrombin • factor XIa Matrix Metalloproteases • MMP1-13
Chemokine/Lymphokine Receptors • MCP-1 • CCR-5 • IL-8	Kinases • cyclin dependent • tyrosine • ser/thr
Glutamatergic Receptors • AMPA • NMDA • m-Glu	Phosphodiesterases Polymerases/Reverse Transcriptases
Nuclear Receptors • ER, PR • PPAR/RXR-RAR	Topoisomerases
Integrins • gP IIb/IIIa	Ion Channels • calcium (L, N) • sodium • K/ATP

Figure 4   Screening: a more recent history of the chemical library.

bring one drug to market." One can debate that statement, but it is still the case that "Boger and others like him are carrying the flag for a new wave of research and development, often called rational drug design." While rational drug design includes the approach of modifying natural substrates, it is most often thought of as structure-based and computer-aided drug design. This approach to drug discovery started in the early 1980s and is now a significant skill set in many pharmaceutical companies.

The factor that drives this approach is specificity. The driving force for many in drug discovery is to find agents that are more specific for a particular molecular target because that should enhance efficacy, reduce side effects, and yield an agent that is unique to a particular pathology. However, the task is very daunting, as one can see by going down the list of molecular targets in Figure 7 and thinking about the implications. For instance, we are good at finding specific inhibitors of enzymes, but there are multiple classes, and even within classes there are isozymes. Similarly, with receptors, there are isoforms. Receptors are found not only in the plasma membrane but in the cytoplasm and nucleus as well. Ion channels have multiple subunits. The complications go on and on. There is, in each one of these cat-

- Human Growth Hormone   (Growth)
- tPA   (Thrombolysis)
- Interferon-α, β   (Cancer, Viral Diseases, Multiple Sclerosis)
- Insulin   (Diabetes)
- Erythropoietin   (Anemia)
- G-CSF and GM-CSF   (Leukopenia)
- r-hepatitis B vaccine   (Hepatitis B)
- IL-2   (Cancer)
- rec antihemophilic factors
- PDGF gel   (Diabetic Foot Ulcers)
- α-glucocerebrosidase   (Gaucher's Disease)
- TNF receptor/binding protein   (Rheumatoid Arthritis)
- Ab-EGF receptor   (Cancer)
- DNAse   (Cystic Fibrosis)
- Ab-gpIIb/IIIa   (Thromboembolism/unstable angina)
- Ab-CD20 B cells   (Lymphoma)

Figure 5   Biologicals (r-DNA based).

- Adenosine Deaminase Inhibitors

- Renin Inhibitors

- Angiotensin Receptor Antagonists

- CCK-B Receptor Antagonists

Figure 6   Modify natural substrates.

egories of potential molecular targets, a multiplicity of targets with, in many cases, a lot of similarity between those targets in terms of binding sites for the putative antagonist or modulator. There can be active sites and allosteric binding sites. Also, one must not forget other important carriers or modifiers to drugs in the biological milieu: serum proteins, P450 modification, glucuronidation, and sulfation, to name a few. These all represent important factors in this aspect of specificity, and they must be taken into account in the area of rational drug design.

- Enzymes: Multiple Classes, Isozymes

- Receptors: Multiple Classes, Isoforms

- Ion Channels: Multiple Subunits and Classes

- Intracellular Transducers: Kinases, Phosphatases, G-proteins, Lipases, Prenylases, Ion-binding Proteins

- Transcription Factors

- DNA: Nucleus, Mitochondria, Coding/Non-coding, Binding Proteins, Repair Enzymes

- RNA: Cytosolic (r-RNA), Nuclear (t-, m-RNA)

  Serum Proteins, p450s, Glucuronidation/Sulfation

Figure 7   Specificity, The Holy Grail.

How, then, does one achieve specificity? Specificity is fundamentally molecular information. One builds in specificity by understanding the "rules of recognition" between one molecule and another through the use of hydrogen bonds, ionic interactions, hydrophobic interactions, and, of course, the overall three-dimensional structure. If one analyzes our success in drug discovery so far, one can derive a "specificity scale" (shown in Fig. 8) relating the complexity of molecular targets to the amount of information one can incorporate into a potential inhibitor or binding agent. We have been most successful with enzymes in terms of specificity. On the other hand, transcription complexes, including transcription factors, activators, repressors, often seven to nine components along with DNA in the milieu, represent a much more daunting challenge. They may very well represent the most complicated state so far for targets of drug discovery. In the middle tier are nucleic acids, antibodies, dimeric domain recognition kinds of targets, signaling proteins, and receptors. If one reviews the past decade of drug discovery progress, it parallels the specificity scale.

The challenge, then, is to build specificity into our drugs through the use of molecular information. Using proteins as drugs is one way of enhancing specificity (Fig. 9). By definition, you can build a lot of information into a large molecule, even if it has repeating units of amide bonds or, with an oligonucleotide, repeating units of phosphodiester bonds. There are related approaches to enhance specificity that have yielded to drug discovery in the last 10 years, such as antisense and ribozymes targeting RNA or DNA in the nucleus or the cytosol, having exquisite specificity for a particular sequence. Thus, structure-based drug design is increasing in importance as an approach to drug discovery by enhancing drug specificity.

- Molecular Information

  - H-bonds

  - Ionic Bonds

  - Hydrophobic Interactions (van der Waals' forces)

  - 3-D Structure

- Specificity Scale

  | Multimeric Complexes (e.g., TFs)
  | Nucleic Acids
  | Antibodies
  | Dimeric/Domain Recognition (e.g., signaling proteins, receptors)
  ▼Enzymes

Figure 8   Specificity equals information.

- Proteins (IFN, IL, CSF, EPO, HGH, Insulin)

- Peptides (ANP, LHRH)

- Antibodies

- Antisense

- Ribozymes

- Structure-based Drug Design

Figure 9   Approaches to enhance drug specificity.

However, one should not forget that nature has already shown us that small molecules can have sufficient information built into them to achieve specificity as drugs. Consider steroids, leukotrienes, nucleosides, mononucleotides, catecholamines, excitatory amino acids, or even something as simple as acetylcholine (Fig. 10). These are small-molecule messengers acting extra- or intracellularly, or both, and represent drugs with legitimate specificity in terms of their molecular targets. One does not necessarily need a molecular weight of 3000 in a drug to achieve appropriate selectivity or specificity. This provides continuing impetus that small molecules can, through various approaches, yield the degree of selectivity necessary to achieve the goal of being a drug for a particular disease.

In spite of the efficacy of some of these newer approaches, however, one cannot forget screening because screening has advanced in speed, quality, and in diversity of sources and targets. At Parke-Davis in 1991 we initiated an effort aimed at high-throughput screening, which has become a very key component of drug discovery for us, as in many companies. Over the past several years, the industry has moved from high throughput to ultrahigh throughput. Today one can set up a screen and go through a library of 100,000 compounds in a day, even with a cell-based screen. Rapid, automated, high-volume techniques and instrumentation, as well as novel sources for diversity, biological as well as chemical, and the generation of molecular targets through biotechnology, have revolutionized screening as an important paradigm in drug discovery.

In a parallel fashion, another translational technology for enhancing screening as a drug discovery tool is the explosion in diversity of screening sources, namely, through combinatorial libraries. Many libraries have been generated, including those for peptides, monoclonal antibodies, oligosaccharides, and oligonucleotides. Over the past several years, an additional focus on small mole-

- Steroids

- Leukotrienes

- Mononucleotides (cAMP, ADP)

- Catecholamines

- Acetylcholine

- Excitatory Amino Acids

Figure 10 Small molecule messengers.

cule combinatorial chemistry has generated multiple additions of low molecular weight "organic" compound libraries for high-throughput screening. Rapid generation of libraries is becoming routine. Indeed, we are finding certain chemotypes recurring as frequent "hits" (Fig. 11).

The power of this technology has been brought to bear, together with modification of natural substrate or structure-based drug design in this decade. If one looks back to 1990, one can find hardly any small molecules that bound to G-protein-coupled receptors (GPCRs) and demonstrated appropriate agonist or antagonist activity. Within the past few years, this field has exploded, in large part because of these technologies. For example, some early work from the Smith Kline Beecham (SKB) Laboratories used ligand-based modification to generate cyclopeptides based on the natural ligand vasopressin, and SKB scientists were able to generate nanomolar level antagonists targeting the V1 receptor [1]. Concomitantly, scientists at Otsuka Pharmaceuticals in Japan were actually screening a chemical library for V1 antagonists and came up with a compound with lower molecular weight than the cyclopeptide on which the SKB scientists had been working [2]. (Scientists at Yamanouchi had a parallel effort.) This represented an early example of a small molecule derived via screening that could act as an appropriate antagonist with reasonable selectivity, in comparison with the rather complicated natural ligand vasopressin or the cyclopeptides from SKB.

In a similar fashion, discoveries were made regarding the related receptor, oxytocin (OT). It had been shown that meperidine bound the OT receptor extremely weakly, but by modifying the structure, scientists generated a small molecule, where the natural ligand was a cyclopeptide for the OT receptor and, again, exhibited quite high selectivity [3]. A natural product that had high selectivity for the OT receptor was found by screening natural product libraries in parallel research efforts at Merck [4].

- Steroids   • Sugars

- Tricyclics   • Macrolides

- Benzodiazepines   • Cyclopeptides

- Phenylpiperidines

- β-Hydroxyalkylamines

Figure 11   Promiscuous scaffolds or chemotypes.

The relatively huge investment in angiotensin (AT) receptor antagonists really began from an initial disclosure of a Takeda Pharmaceutical's patent on a small molecule that was based on a two-amino-acid component structure of angiotensin. From this came a plethora of AT1 receptor antagonists from many laboratories. At Parke-Davis we were screening using a different receptor as it turned out (we didn't know it at the time) and found that a structurally unrelated low molecular weight compound was quite specific for the AT2 receptor. In fact, this has turned out to be an interesting lead in terms of understanding the pharmacology of the AT2 receptor relative to AT1. Again, the screening of small molecules in combination with structure-based design approaches generated interesting potential drug candidates.

In our laboratories, we took a reductionist approach to looking for low molecular weight compounds that would act as agonists or antagonists at the CCK receptors. This approach led to the conclusion that trp-phe were the two key recognition sites in a portion of the natural ligand for binding to the CCK-B receptor. Our scientists were able to generate a 2 nM level antagonist at the CCK-B receptor; this agent eventually went into clinical trials [5,6] (Fig. 12). This agent has a molecular weight of about 600, which is, of course, much smaller than the natural ligand itself. This is an approach exemplifying structure-based ligand modification to generate a drug candidate. In a parallel fashion, drug discovery efforts generated low molecular weight (benzodiazepine-like) CCK-B antagonists at several other pharmaceutical companies. These molecules came out of a screening

	CCK-B Binding (Ki)
asp-tyr(SO₃H)-met-gly-trp-met-asp-phe (CCK 26-33)	3 nM
trp-met-asp-phe (CCK 30-33)	3 nM
Boc-trp-phe	70 μM
Boc-αMe-trp-phe	6 μM

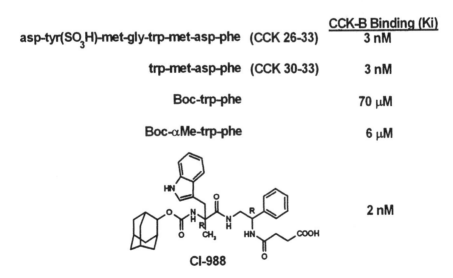

CI-988

2 nM

Figure 12   Peptidomimetic cholecystokinin antagonists.

approach based on finding a natural product, asperlicin, that exhibited high binding to the CCK-B receptor. So, a combination of approaches yielded potential drugs that were evaluated in the clinic against several disease states.

Structure-based, computer-aided drug design, the last category of the five, is an area of increasing investment for many groups in drug discovery. Figure 13 lists four examples from our own laboratories. These approaches illustrate the increasing importance of structure-based drug design in the area of drug discovery. The HIV-1 aspartyl protease and its dimeric structure has really become the first major success story of this approach. We learned much in the early 1980s about inhibitors of a related aspartyl protease, renin, and applied this science to the first generation of inhibitors of HIV-1 protease. The industry now has five inhibitors that are approved, on the market, and being used, representing a significant advance in the treatment of HIV-positive individuals. They all share a key element, which is a hydroxy group that is involved in the binding site to water and aspartic acid in the recognition site of the dimeric aspartyl protease. They are elongated peptide-like structures and represent a challenge to achieving acceptable bioavailability and drug–drug interactions.

Second-generation agents (Fig. 14) are under clinical evaluation and represent smaller versions of the first-generation molecules, or even radically modified or divergent forms. The drug PNU 140690 was recently disclosed from Pharmacia and Upjohn, and has little structural relationship to the other inhibitors. It does have a close structural relationship to a series discovered through parallel research in our laboratories. These compounds represent the combination of structure-based drug design with an iterative cycle of modeling, synthesis, testing, and crystallography to come up with improvements in specificity, selectivity, and bioavailability.

In early 1992 we found through screening our compound library that a particular pyrone, shown in Figure 15, was a very modest, but nonetheless reproducible, inhibitor of HIV-1 protease. It was selective for HIV protease over other aspartyl proteases and related families. An iterative design cycle was begun, consisting of the structure determination (using x-ray crystallography, cocrystallization, and soaking experiments with additional inhibitors), modeling, additional

- HIV-1 Protease Inhibitors

- Thymidylate Synthetase Inhibitors

- M$_1$ Selective Muscarinic Agonists

- Purine Nucleoside Phosphorylase Inhibitors

Figure 13 Examples of structure-based, computer-aided drug design.

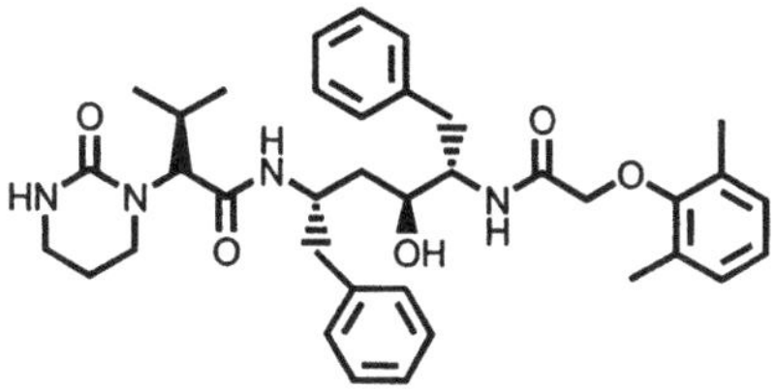

ABT 378

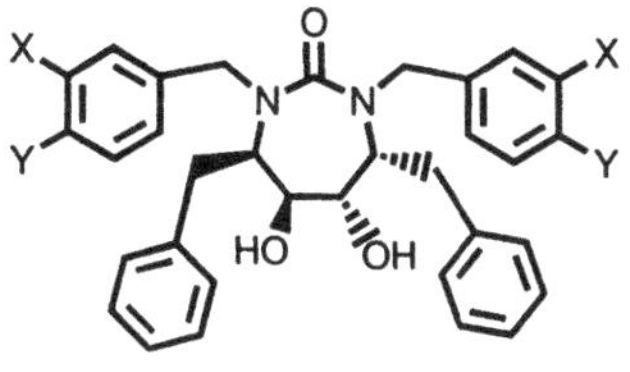

DMP323 X=H, Y=CH₂OH
DMP450 X=NH₂, Y=H

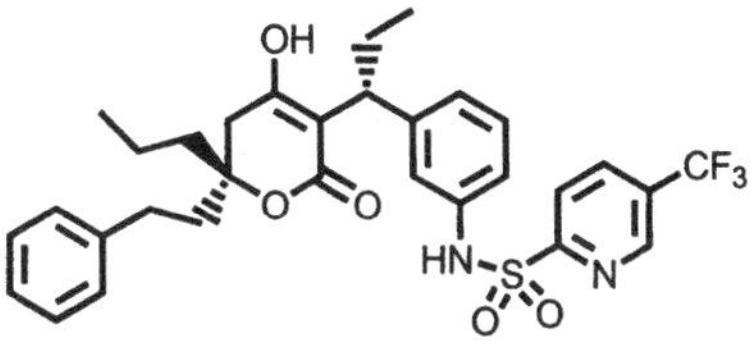

Tipranavir
PNU140690

Figure 14 Second generation HIV-1 protease inhibitors.

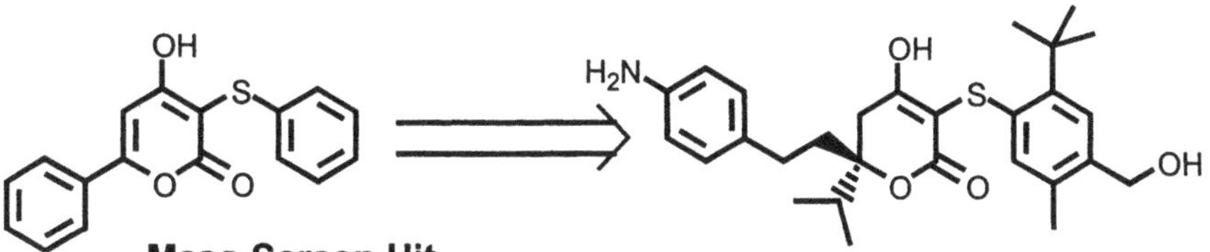

Mass Screen Hit
Ki = 11,700 nM

PD0178390
Ki = 0.028 nM
>410,000 Fold Increase

Figure 15 Third generation, non-peptidic HIV protease inhibitors.

chemistry to modify the structure based on what we had learned from modeling, and looking at the requisite biochemistry and enzymology of the agents. This cycle was repeated to determine the appropriate binding of these molecules in the three-dimensional structure using structure-based drug design.

We were able to alter this relatively simple pyrone with a series of modifications, principally in the P2 and P2-prime sites, which very rapidly led to nanomolar level inhibitors and represented legitimate advances in non-peptide based HIV protease inhibitors. This has now been extended to an interesting molecule whose IC_{50} is 5 nm. It has a different structure, but nonetheless binds in the active site, does not use water within the binding site, and is quite different from the first- and second-generation inhibitors [7]. This demonstrates the power of structure-based drug design, coming originally from a screening approach, to yield a drug candidate lead.

In the muscarinic area, quite a different approach was taken. We had determined that there was a three-point pharmacophore based on a series of agonists that to bind to the M1 receptor; however, the pharmacophore analysis had gotten bogged down at that point. As we modeled this within the GPCR model, we thought about where it was binding and looked at the other muscarinic receptors (M2 or M5) in terms of differences in the transmembrane region. We hypothesized that, not unlike retinal binding to rhodopsin, if this very small agonist was binding in the transmembrane region, we could elongate this simple pharmacophore (much like retinal is extended) to generate something that would have greater specificity. In fact, we were able to extend the basic pharmacophore to produce a molecule that has much greater specificity for the central versus the peripheral muscarinic receptors. This compound is now under investigation in clinical studies targeting the treatment of patients with Alzheimer's disease. Thus, this original idea of molecular modeling and pharmacophore analysis is in fact a validated approach to drug discovery.

How will we discover drugs in the future? While I believe that all five categories will be used, modification of known drugs (validated chemotypes) will probably be of decreasing interest over time. The integration of the other four approaches will become more important in the future application of drug discovery. The targets are manifold. Figure 4 is a highly simplistic representation of the source of molecular targets that we currently spend so much time identifying and finding antagonists or agonists for. They can be extracellular, membrane-based receptors, nuclear receptors, or cytosolic signaling receptors. There is a growing list of targets such as serine/threonine kinases, tyrosine kinases, and phosphatases, as well as a significant interest in the cell cycle and understanding the regulatory enzymes involved in the cycle. Probably the newest frontier is transcription factors, where many are working on ways of finding agents that would regulate gene expression and affect some particular pathological state.

The technological foci for drug discovery, shown in Figure 16, are organized for a specific reason. The technologies of high-throughput screening, and biomolecular structure determination, molecular modeling, and combinatorial chemistry are having a dramatic impact on drug discovery today and will continue to become even more important in the future. However, they are very dependent on finding the molecular targets. A veritable avalanche of new targets will be coming via genomics and proteomics. Concomitantly, there is the critical aspect of managing the plethora of data that emerge as a result of these data-rich approaches, and

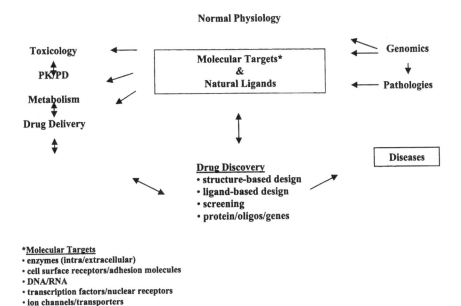

Figure 16 New drug discovery paradigm.

understanding from those data which are the truths that are important in the drug discovery process.

Genomics is a simple word, but it envelops many components that are more than simply the genetic map, or the physical map, or even the gene sequence. The advances made in these three areas during the last 3 or 4 years alone have been striking, and much more rapid than any of us would have imagined. In many ways, gene sequencing, as well as the maps, will probably be well in hand for a number of genomes in the next couple of years. However, gene function and gene regulation represent a formidable challenge for drug discovery and the molecular sciences. Genetic functional analysis has a number of tools already available, and there will undoubtedly be more to come. Transgenics, knock-outs, and gene replacement are very powerful technologies in our understanding of gene function. Antisense is already available, and of course the two-hybrid technique is being exploited in many laboratories investigating gene function. Synteny, differential display, and single-nucleotide polymorphism (SNP) analyses are additional tools. Nonetheless, this is a bottleneck, and improvements are needed before we can move forward from sequence to function and understand regulation. The challenges in this field will include sequencing, informatics, multiple species, and the fact that it is not only the natural state that we are interested in but the pathological state as well. We need to understand function and mutations relevant to the pathological state. The output is the genetic footprint. Disease phenotype is what we are interested in. It has implications for diagnostics as well as for drug discovery, and it has implications down the road for preventive medicine and gene therapy.

Proteomics is also an important area. In fact, this is here and now, not in the future. Two-dimensional gel electrophoresis, together with matrix-assisted laser desorption/ionization (MALDI) mass spectrometry and image analysis, is used to determine the output of genomics. This is an area of intense investment in many laboratories that must be included in the bioinformatics database that is being generated. This database will be used to help determine which targets are the appropriate ones for drug discovery or for diagnostics.

Lastly, there are some important components for which tools are slowly evolving. We need to optimize a drug candidate, not only for selectivity but for bioavailability, toxicity, target organ selectivity, stability, and scalability. These are all legitimate and important components. We have drug class issues in drug discovery and development that act as guides for us, but nonetheless there are going to be discoveries unique to particular drug candidates. Small molecules continue to present difficulties with toxicity and bioavailability. Proteins have associated cost and delivery issues. Peptides have stability and bioavailability issues. Oligonucleotides often have the same class issues as proteins and peptides. Gene therapy certainly has to face the safety, delivery, and duration-of-effect issues.

What, then, are the future issues for drug discovery and development, given all of these technological foci? Determining the importance of the molecular targets is one such issue. For the next few years, we will continue to operate with a pretty tenuous linkage of molecular target to disease. In many cases, our molecular targets are hypothesized to be linked to a particular disease; we don't really determine this until we find inhibitors and take them to the clinic to see if they work. Also, the diseases we are facing today and tomorrow are more challenging than those that confronted us yesterday and the day before. Many are chronic diseases with multiple etiologic factors and will probably require combination therapy—another complication to drug development. Of course, we will have novel toxicities. Finally, as we move further into the area of gene regulation, nuclear targets will represent additional complexities. The opportunities and the challenges will yield new drugs, combination therapies, and patient-specific treatments during the next decade.

REFERENCES

1. Ruffolo RR, et al. Drug News Persp, May 1991. p. 217–222.
2. Ogawa H, et al. J Med Chem, 1993; 36:2011–2017.
3. Evans BF, et al. J Med Chem, 1993; 36:3993–4055.

4. Salituro GM, et al. Bioorg Med Lett 1993; 3:337–340.
5. Hughes J, Boden P, Costall B, Domeney A, Kelly E, Horwell DC, Hunter JC, Pinnock RD, Woodruff GN. Development of a class of selective cholecytstokinin type B receptor antagonists having potent anxiolytic activity. Proc Nat Acad Sci USA 1990; 87: 6728–6732.
6. Horwell DC, Birchmore B, Boden PR, Higginbottom M, Ping Ho Y, Hughes J, Hunter JC, Richardson RS. Alpha-methyl tryptophanylphenylalanines and their arylethylamine "dipeptoid" analogues of the tetrapeptide cholecystokinin [30–33]. Eur J Med Chem 1990; 25:53–60.
7. Vara Prasad JVN, Boyer FE, Domagala JM, Ellsworth EL, Gajda C, Hagen SE, Markoski LJ, Tait BD, Lunney EA, Tummino PJ, Ferguson D, Holler T, Hupe D, Nouhan C, Gracheck SJ, VanderRoest S, Saunders J, Iyer K, Sinz M, Brodfuehrer J. Bioorg Med Chem Lett 1999; 9:1481–1486.

2

Target Identification and Validation: Coupling Genotype to Phenotype

Gary McMaster
Eli Lilly and Company
Indianapolis, Indiana

I. INTRODUCTION

There are three basic components necessary for drug discovery and lead identification: (1) targets, (2) screens and (3) compounds. Each of these plays a pivotal role in the drug discovery process and ultimately the success of clinical trials. During the past 50 years there has been a paradigm shift in drug discovery (Fig. 1), closely bound to the development of technology [1]. Initially, companies focused on the effects of putative therapeutics on whole-animal models to study pharmacology and efficacy. Later, tissue and cell cultures led to a refinement in pharmacological studies and in the number of screenings performed. More recent progress has involved advanced purification and molecular biology technologies, which in the past 10 years has lead to a wholesale move toward selecting molecular targets to screen. Most recent, there has been an explosion of genomics, proteomics, bioinformatics, and information technologies, which will significantly increase the potential to identify and validate novel disease genes and their corresponding pathways, representing enormous value to the pharmaceutical industry. Of the approximately 80,000–150,000 human genes, there may be as many as 10,000 potential "drugable" targets, i.e., amenable to low molecular weight molecules (e.g., enzymes, receptors, ion channels, hormone receptors, etc.) for treatment of the most common multifactorial diseases [2].

In addition to these novel disease targets, there are a significant number of partially validated targets associated with major human diseases, such as nuclear receptors and G-protein-coupled receptors [3–6]. These targets, combined with

Paradigm Shift in Drug Discovery

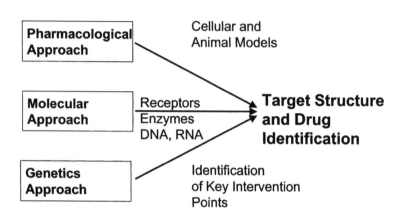

Figure 1   There has been a paradigm shift in the drug discovery process during the past 50 years. The pharmacological approach has used whole-animal and cellular models to discover drugs. Later, molecular targets were employed to screen for drugs. Most recently, genetics and genomics opened up a whole new approach to discover disease genes and pathways, creating enormous potential value to the pharmaceutical industry.

genomic technologies (including genetics, bioinformatics, data mining, structural informatics) and compounds, offer potential for very selective drugs of the future. The best example of these are the so-called SERMs (selective estrogen receptor modulators), where a compound can be agonist in one cell type and an antagonist in another. In addition, one needs to consider that multifactorial diseases themselves have overlap (e.g., diabetes and obesity) and that single genes (e.g., chloride transporter) can be involved in the etiology of multiple diseases (e.g., cystic fibrosis, asthma, pancreatitis, and male infertility).

The process "gene to drug" will accelerate with the ever-increasing volumes of new genetic information, with increased biological understanding of how the pathways are connected, and with the technologies that make it possible for each step of the process to be completed more quickly and efficiently. The purpose of this chapter is to demonstrate to the reader which technologies can be used to identify gene targets and validate them to speed up the quality of drug discovery by providing an increased number of better validated targets.

II. TARGET IDENTIFICATION/VALIDATION

A. Genomics

Thomas Roderick [7] coined the term "genomics" in 1986. Genomics describes the study of a genome by molecular means distinct from traditional genetic approaches. The term is derived from *genome,* a fusion of the words *gene* and *chromosome* to describe the complete collection of genes possessed by an organism [8].

Genomics as currently practiced can be categorized as follows:

1. Structural genomics
2. Functional genomics
3. Pharmacogenomics

Genomics technologies, which are already more or less impacting drug discovery identification and validation, are as follows:

- Positional cloning and association genetics
- Genome sequencing (humans, animals, and pathogens)
- Expressed sequence tag (EST) sequencing
- Derivation of full-length cDNAs and their sequences (gene families)
- Microarrays of oligonucleotides and cDNAs (chips)
- Subtractive hybridization
- Differential display
- Antisense
- In situ hybridization
- Serial amplification of gene expression (SAGE)
- Taq-Man/quantitative polymerase chain reaction (PCR)
- Protein–protein interactions using yeast 2 hybrid
- Reporter genes (e.g., green fluorescent proteins, GFPs)
- Transgenic/knockout animals (especially mice)
- Model organisms (e.g., yeast, *C. elegans, Drosophila,* zebrafish, mouse, rat)
- Two-dimensional gel electrophoresis
- Databases (bioinformatics, structural informatics)

Presently, this collection of genomics technologies for drug discovery are used in variations or combinations of two approaches:

1. The "top-down" approach, which uses positional cloning and association genetics to identify disease-related genes.
2. The "bottom-up" approach, which predominately focuses on the random sequencing of cDNA and an inference of the protein product's function based on sequence similarity to well-characterized genes and proteins.

In the future emerging technologies will further impact drug discovery target identification and validation. These are:

- Integrated databases (structure to function)
- Single-nucleotide polymorphism (SNP) identification/scoring in high-throughput modus
- Second-generation solid-phase DNA arrays
- Single-cell PCR
- Laser capture
- Protein–protein and protein–compound interactions
- In solution RNA profiling technologies (liquid arrays)
- Phage display libraries (antibodies)
- Genetic suppressor elements (GSEs)
- Zinc finger proteins
- Conditional knockout mice (Cre/lox)
- Inducible promoters in vitro and in vivo (e.g., tetracycline on/off systems)
- Gene trapping
- Biochips
- Microfluidics
- In vitro and in vivo imaging
- Fiberoptics
- Structures of membrane-bound proteins (e.g., G-protein-coupled receptors)
- RNA as targets for infectious diseases

The approach is to first describe the existing technologies and their impact on target identification and validation and then to turn to many of the emerging technologies to predict their potential impact on drug discovery.

1. Genetic Mapping and Positional Cloning

One of the objectives of the Human Genome Project was to advance genetic mapping from the restriction fragment length polymorphisms (RFLPs) used initially to microsatellite markers [9]. The accent now is on biallelic marker systems using SNPs, which are very prevalent within the genome [10–12]. This has allowed the cloning of many single genes causing human diseases inherited in a simple Mendelian fashion. Some of the most important genes controlling hypertension have been found by studying the molecular genetics of blood pressure variation in this way [13,14]. Recently, the ATP-binding cassette transporter 1 (ABC-1) was positionally cloned using Tangiers patients [15]. The ABC-1 transporter is involved in cholesterol efflux and linked to low levels of high-density lipoprotein (HDL) and coronary heart disease (CHD). Furthermore, the implication of potassium channels in long-QT syndrome and epilepsy by their positional cloning [16] simply reinforces the power of genetics for biochemical understanding and for providing a genetic validation of a biological hypothesis [17,18]. It also illustrates that the comprehensive study of a gene family (e.g., potassium or sodium channels) by using data mining and genomics approaches in concert with genetic mapping is a paradigm for the study of more complex traits. It may also be a rapid way to find new "genetically validated targets" for drug intervention [19]. Unfortunately, until now the unraveling of the biochemical pathology of common diseases in humans based on an understanding of complex, polygenic disease traits by cloning of relevant genes has been somewhat disappointing. A number of linkages have been made for several diseases such as diabetes, obesity, asthma, and cognition, but very few of the genes have been uncovered [22–24].

Positional cloning has also been used to isolate mouse genes, which cause Mendelian diseases in this species. Several of these genes have been instructive regarding similar human syndromes [20]. One of the best studied is leptin and the leptin receptor for obesity derived from analysis of ob/db mice [21]. The mouse has certainly become one of the most useful models of polygenic models of human disorders. Often, the phenotypic characteristics are strikingly similar to that for the analogous human disorder [25]. Generally, the predicted amino acid sequence homology ranges from approximately 80% to near identity. Therefore, in some cases it is likely that drugs that interact with these gene targets using mouse as the model will have similar physiological effects in humans, although the downstream signaling (e.g, the interleukin-4 receptor) may not be identical in mouse and human. However, the mouse can be "humanized," i.e., the mouse gene exchanged for the human in a knock-out/knock-in approach [25].

In addition, there has been conserved organization of the gene order and relative position in the genomes of human and mouse for large chromosomal regions. This is known as *synteny*, and the ability to jump between human and mouse genetic information based on synteny is of great advantage in gene identification and localization [26]. The fundamental approach is to use conserved synteny to determine if the same genomic region is functionally involved in a disease phenotype in both human populations and the mouse [27]. If the same chromosomal region is involved, then it is generally easier to identify the gene in the mouse than in humans, and one can use mutation detection/analysis to determine if the same gene is involved in human polygenic disease. "Although several textbooks and other reference works give a correct definition, the term *synteny* nowadays is often used to refer to gene loci in different organisms located on a chromosomal region of common evolutionary ancestry," as just described [28]. Originally, the term synteny (or syntenic) refers to gene loci on the same chromosome regardless of whether or not they are genetically linked by classical linkage analysis. However, molecular biologists (including myself) inappropriately use the original definition of synteny and its etymological derivation, especially as this term is still needed to refer to genes located on the same chromosome. "Correct terms exist: 'paralogous' for genes that arose from a common ancestor gene within one species and 'orthologous' for the same gene in different species" [28]. To make a long story short, the process described above as synteny should be described as orthologous. None the less, the approach is very powerful. Gene mapping of complex disorders has resulted in the identification of a number of cases that one clearly orthologous between human and the mouse [29,28]. Furthermore, the similarity in gene structure between mouse and human is very high. This homology extends from the exon–intron organization of many genes to the predicted amino acid sequence of the gene products [22].

One of the best examples of the power of genetics has been provided by studies on Alzheimer's disease. All of the genes known to be involved unequivocally were found by positional cloning or by association genetics: amyloid precursor protein (APP), presenilin genes (PS1 and PS2), and ApoE4 [30]. There is unlikely to be a pharmaceutical or biotechnology company investigating Alzheimer's disease, which does not have a drug discovery program, based on one or other of these genes. It is also worth mentioning that access to transgenic animals is still an important component of the drug discovery process (see Sec. II. A. 4 below). In Alzheimer's disease, for example, various transgenic mice strains have been used to examine amyloid deposition. Genetic crosses have shown that ApoE4 and transforming growth factor β_1 (TGF-β_1) influence amyloid deposition and that the presenilins act synergistically with APP in the development of the pathology. Some of these animals may become models for the disease, with utility for finding compounds that modify the pathology of plaque formation [31]. None of this would have been possible without having the genes in hand. The lesson is simple: genetics is the key to mechanism; mechanism is the key to therapeutic discovery; and therefore genetics is the key to therapeutic discovery.

2. Genome Sequencing

At present, the greatest impact of genomic research has come from DNA sequencing projects [32]. One of the first applications of genomics to drug discovery was through the development of EST (expressed sequence tag) sequencing and the creation of large gene sequence databases [22]. This approach to generating large-scale DNA sequence information was carried out by Craig Venter at TIGR and by Human Genome Sciences. These initiatives and the development of commercial EST sequence databases and data-mining tools by companies such as Human Genome Sciences and Incyte have had a rapid effect on drug discovery by giving pharmaceutical companies access to potentially new targets related to previously known ones. The best (and most obvious) examples are targets such as G-protein-coupled receptors, steroid hormone receptors, ion channels, proteases, and enzymes. The value from this approach is considerable although it is not always clear what disease a relative of a known target might be useful for without further validation. Any antagonist or agonist of such a target however can be used in animals to rationalize or validate the protein as a target for intervention in a particular disease. A reasonable example would be the development of novel serotonin receptor of active small molecules working via a new receptor [33]. Evidence of the anticipated impact on drug discovery of such sequence databases is clear from the rapid take-up of subscriptions to the Incyte (ESTs) and Celera (genomic) databases by many of the major pharmaceutical companies.

Nowhere has comprehensive genome sequencing had more effect than in bacterial genetics. The sequences of well over 20 different bacterial genomes are now available [34–36]. The information derived from the comparisons of these sequences within and between microorganisms and with eukaryotic sequences is truly changing microbiology. The greatest benefit from these approaches comes from being able to examine homologies and gene organization across whole genomes at once. For target identification this has obvious benefits because if the potential target is conserved among target organisms but not in the host then it may be a reasonable target. This is not new thinking; the development of dihydrofolate reductase inhibitors and some antifungal drugs followed exactly the same rationale. In the bacterial studies, procedures such as "signature-tagged mutagenesis" and in vivo expression methods are tying together genomic and biological data to reveal genes permissive for virulence and pathogenicity [37,38]. Recently, the smallest of all genomes, *Mycoplasma genitalium,* which has only 517 genes, was sequenced at Celera. The big surprise was that only 300 of the 517 genes are essential for life of the organism and 103 of these 300 essential genes are of unknown function [39]. This tells us what is in store for the future when we consider that the human genome is estimated to have some 80,000–150,000 genes. Still, this approach will be valid for higher eukaryotes, too, once the genomes of mouse and human have been fully sequenced and assembled [40].

Genomics is made possible through the large-scale DNA sequencing efforts of many public and private organizations, including the Human Genome Project, which has provided major impetus to the discovery of the genome and information technologies [9]. This international program is well underway to determine the complete DNA sequence (3000 million bases). As of October 1999, 30% of the sequence is available in the public domain (see *http://www.nhgri.nih.gov/HGP/*).

By 2002 a comprehensive working draft (90% of the genome) is expected, and by 2003 the entire sequence is projected for completion [41]. Recently, chromosome 22 (*http://www./genome/guide/HsChr22.shtml*) has been completely sequenced as part of the Human Genome Project. Chromosome 22 is especially rich in genes. While sequencing the 33 million base pair chromosome, Dunham et al. [42] identified 679 genes, 55% of which were previously unknown. Approximately 35 diseases have been linked to mutations in chromosome 22. These include immune system diseases, congenital heart disease, and schizophrenia, among others.

The purpose of structural genomics is to discover, map, and sequence genetic elements. Annotation of the sequence with the gene structures is achieved by a combination of computational analysis (predictive and homology-based; see:

http://compbio.ornl.gov/structure/) and experimental confirmation by cDNA sequencing (see *http://genome.ornl.gov/GCat/species.shtml*). Recently, a web site entitled the "Genome Channel" (see *http://compbio.ornl.gov/channel*) has offered a road atlas for finding genes by zooming in from chromosomes to annotated DNA sequences. Furthermore, the site links the user to sequencing centers for 24 organisms, including humans, mice, and *Escherichia coli,* to name a few. Detecting homologies between newly defined gene products and proteins of known function helps to postulate biochemical functions for them, which can then be tested. Establishing the association of specific genes with disease phenotypes by mutation screening, particularly for monogenic/single disorders, provides further assistance in defining the functions of some gene products, as well as helping to establish the cause of the disease. As our knowledge of gene sequences and sequence variation (see Sec. II.C) in populations increases, we will pinpoint more and more of the genes and proteins that are important in common, complex diseases [41]. In addition, by comparing corresponding genomic sequences (comparative genomics) in different species (man, mouse, chicken and zebrafish, *Drosophila, Caenorhabditis elegans,* yeast, *E. coli*) regions that have been highly conserved during evolution can be identified, many of which reflect conserved functions, such as gene regulation. These approaches promise to greatly accelerate our interpretation of the human genome sequence [43]. In the future it will be possible to understand how specific sequences regulate the expression of genes in the genome.

3. Functional Genomics

Complete sequencing of the human genome is really only the beginning. As the geneticist Eric Lander has characterized, "Molecular and cell biologists are still only approaching a phase of development of their discipline reached by chemists 100 years ago, when the periodic table was first described" [44]. We still need to link the genetic makeup of an organism (its genotype) to its form and function (its phenotype) and how the environment effects them. To that end, whereas structural genomics seeks to discover, map, and sequence these genetic elements, functional genomics is the discipline that seeks to assign function to genetic elements. A more detailed understanding of the function of the human genome will be achieved as we identify sequences that control gene expression. In recent years, our knowledge of gene sequence has increased massively, principally due to large-scale cDNA and genome sequencing programs [41]. The availability of this information resource has fueled efforts to develop ways of analyzing gene expression systematically, and as a result there are a range of approaches available that allow parallel analysis of a large number of genes. These tools can provide a comprehensive view of the genes expressed in samples of tissue and even individual cells, and in so doing will advance our understanding of biochemical pathways and the functional roles of novel genes. Most important, genome sequences will provide the foundation for a new era of experimental and computational biology, providing the essential resources for future study.

Genes are sections of genomic DNA that encode proteins. They are copied into messenger RNA (transcribed) and it is this mRNA that carries the genetic code from the nucleus to the cytoplasm to direct protein synthesis. It is thought that there are 80,000–150,000 genes in the genome of man and other mammals. In each cell only a portion of these genes is active at any one time, thought to be in the region of 10,000–15,000. The expression of these genes instructs the protein synthetic machinery to produce a specific set of proteins that are required for the cell to perform its normal functional role. Certain genes are expressed in all cells all of the time and encode so-called housekeeping proteins, whereas others are expressed only in certain cell types and/or at certain times. It is these latter proteins that give a cell its unique structural and functional characteristics and ultimately make one cell different from another. However, the complement of genes expressed by a cell is not a fixed entity, and there are many genes whose expression can be induced or reduced as required. This provides the flexibility in biological systems to respond and adapt to different stimuli, whether they are part of the normal development and homeostatic processes, or a response to injury, disease, or drug treatment. As the transcription status of a biological system reflects its physiological status, the ability to study the complement of genes expressing its "signature" and the abundance of their mRNAs in a tissue or cell will ultimately provide a powerful insight into their biochemistry and function [45].

However, there are certain inherent difficulties in the study of gene expression. Unlike DNA, which is essentially the same in all cells of an individual, there can be enormous variation in abundance and distribution of a particular mRNA species between cells. Some genes are highly expressed, i.e., their mRNA is abundant (>1000 copies per cell), whereas other genes are weakly expressed, with their transcripts present at only a few copies per cell. In addition, because most tissues are composed of distinct cell populations, an mRNA, which is only present in one of those cell types, perhaps already at low levels, becomes even rarer when the RNA is extracted from that tissue as it is diluted in the RNA derived from nonexpressing cells. It is also becoming increasingly apparent that for many genes the transcripts can exist in different forms, so-called alternative splice variants. These splice variants allow an even greater diversity in the complement of proteins that can be generated from the genetic code, but adds another level of complexity to the analysis of gene expression. Furthermore, these mutations of splice sites can lead to reduction of a biological function (e.g., sodium channels [19]).

Knowledge of a novel gene's sequence alone usually provides few clues as to the functional role of the protein that it encodes. However, sequence information can be used for further characterization of the gene and is a good starting point in defining its expression. If a gene's expression is limited to certain tissues or cell types or is changed during disease, then we can begin to postulate and focus in on those sites. Likewise, if other genes' expression maps to the same cells, we can begin to understand which protein complex or biochemical pathway the gene product might interact with [45].

The other major goal of RNA expression profiling has always been the identification of genes that are expressed at different levels between one system or experimental paradigm and another. Knowledge of these genes not only sheds light on the biochemical events underlying the change but in some cases also provides a list of potentially interesting genes, such as which genes are expressed in malignant but not in normal cells. For these reasons, expression profiling will help in our understanding gene function and the biology of complex systems, as well as in many aspects of the drug discovery process [45].

The past several years have witnessed the development of a plethora of new methodologies to study gene expression:

1. Subtractive hybridization [46]
2. Subtractive PCR ([47] and *http://www.clontech.com*)
3. Differential display [48]
4. In situ PCR [49,50]
5. Single-cell PCR [51,52]
6. Serial analysis of gene expression, "SAGE" ([53] and *http://www.genzyme.com*)
7. DNA chips ([54] and *http://www.Affymetrix.com*)
8. Microarrays ([55] and *http://www.synteni.com*)

These all can provide insights into the complement of genes expressed in a particular system. However, what really makes the difference and ultimately determines how widely they are used in the future is the detail of how they work and quality of data they yield. We also need to distinguish what is important in (1) discovery of novel genes (e.g., subtractive hybridization, subtractive PCR, SAGE), (2) large-volume RNA profiling of known genes (e.g., PCR, DNA chips, microarrays), and (3) if the expression of genes in a subcellular region of a tissue (in situ hybridization, in situ PCR).

The main issues in expression profiling are therefore as follows:

- Novel versus known genes—Is the objective to discover novel genes or to evaluate known genes in a high-throughput mode?
- Localization within a tissue—Can the technology distinguishes expression at the cellular level within a tissue?
- Sensitivity—Can the method detect low-abundance sequences and how much starting material (mRNA) is required?
- Specificity—Is the assay highly specific for the transcript of interest?
- Quantification—How accurately can it measure mRNA abundance?
- Reproducibility—How robust is the methodology?

- Coverage—How many transcripts can be analyzed at once and does the approach have the ability to detect previously uncharacterized genes?
- Redundancy—How often is each transcript sampled? (Some systems have the potential to analyze the same mRNA a number of times, therefore increasing the complexity of the data.)
- False positives—How often do things appear to be differentially expressed but turn out not to be?
- Scale of analysis—Is the approach amenable to high-throughput screening data output and does the assay give results that are easy to interpret?
- Cost—How much does it cost for the initial investment and cost/gene/ assay?

Depending on the question the experimenter is asking, one or a combination of these technologies will be needed. This is outlined in Figure 2, which illustrates that any one RNA sample may require use of one of these technologies (e.g., SAGE) to detect novel and known genes at low throughput and thereafter require use of DNA chips or arrays for high-volume throughput and reproducibility testing. In situ hybridization, in situ PCR, and/or single-cell PCR would test the most important genes identified and validated by chips and arrays.

As mentioned above, though the methodologies have been widely used in the research environment, not all are applicable for high-throughput, routine analysis of gene expression. However, one approach above all others shows most promise in this respect and is now driving the field of expression profiling: DNA chips and microarrays. Although there are some important differences between DNA chips and microarrays, both work by a similar mechanism, i.e., hybridization of complex mixtures of DNA or RNA to complementary DNA probes immobilized on a solid surface. DNA chips are presently available through one company, Affymetrix [54]. This approach was pioneered by Affymetrix, which makes microchips of overlapping oligonucleotides ("oligos") available, representing sequences from thousands of genes. These chips can also be used to measure sequence variation and for detection of SNPs. One of the perceived disadvantages of the Affymetrix format is its lack of flexibility.

Other chips are available from Synteni and elsewhere that comprise cDNAs or oligos [56] covalently attached to a solid phase. Oligos have an advantage over cDNAs in that oligos can detect splice variants, which can make very interesting drug targets. These chips can be interrogated by using fluorescently labeled hybridization probes and the results displayed by color integration. By far the most impressive use of such chips has been carried out in Pat Brown's laboratory at Stanford. Two elegant experiments have been done. The first compared the pattern of yeast gene expression during sporulation [55], and the second looked at the expression of a subset of the genes expressed in fibroblasts after serum starvation and activation. The take-home messages from these beautiful experiments are as

Honing in on Genes

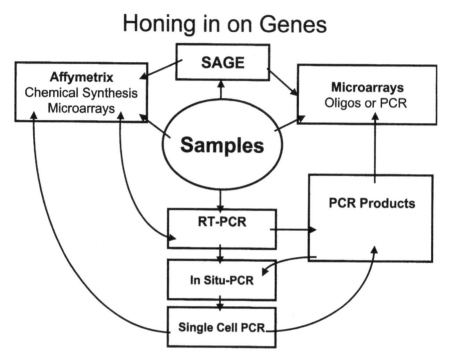

Figure 2 Numerous RNA profiling technologies are available, which are interdependent. Depending on the question posed, the experimenter may choose to use a specific combination of technologies. SAGE provides the best approach to discover and quanitate novel and known genes. However, the throughput is lower than that of Affymetrix DNA chips or microarrays. Affymetrix chips are convenient to use, but cost more than microarrays and are less flexible for following up on genes of interest in a high-throughput mode. PCR microarrays are more sensitive than oligomicroarrays; however, PCR microarrays cannot detect splice variants like oligomicroarrays.

follows: the reproducibility of the biology of the system is crucial for consistent results; (2) the need for sophisticated pattern matching is absolutely essential for data interpretation [57,58]. Function of an unknown gene based on its pattern of expression under different conditions is compared to a known dataset. From the experiments reported above, the functions of many "unknown" yeast and human genes were suggested based on their expression characteristics relative to known sets such as cell cycle genes or genes involved in DNA replication. Now that the *C. elegans* and *Drosophila* genomes are completely sequenced [59], it will not be long before worm and fly gene chips are available for the same kind of experiments. In fact, first signs are here; White et al. [60] recently published an elegant paper on the microarray analysis of *Drosophila* development during metamorphosis, where both known and novel pathways were assigned to metamorphosis.

So what role will RNA profiling have in the future of drug discovery? High-throughput RNA expression profiling is still in its infancy, and clearly much remains to be done to apply it for a maximum impact on drug discovery. We have yet to identify all human genes and, to an even greater extent, those of the model organisms, mouse and rat. There is also considerable room for improvement on the basic technologies and methodology. Judging by the number of recent small start-up companies and new emerging industries (Motorola, HP, Corning, IBM), one of the most active areas of genomics is the use of microarrays for large-scale measurement of gene expression [61]. In addition, second-generation technologies (e.g., Corning, Third Wave Technologies, Luminex, Curagen, QuantumDot) are underway. These second-generation technologies are expected to (1) design better surfaces, (2) produce more sensitive dyes (QuantumDot *http://www.qdots.com*), and (3) develop totally new approaches such as the in-solution assays (liquid arrays), e.g., "Invader" technology (see *http://www.twt.com*) or by exploiting electronics by designing digital micromirrors [62].

The ability to examine the expression of all or a large number of genes at once will provide new insights into the biology of disease, such as in the identification of the differences between normal and cancerous cells [63], as well as gene expression during aging [64] or during HIV infection [65]. Undoubtedly, there must be gene products that play a crucial role in metastasis that could be targeted by drug treatment. However, working out which those are, which cancers they are active in, and their specificity to tumor cells should now be possible. Recently, Golub et al. [63] demonstrated that molecular classification of cancer types could be predicted by gene expression profiling. Furthermore, this information can be integrated into the genetics of cancer and histopathology building a 3D model [66]. Companies such as LifeSpan (*www.lsbio.com*) provide disease and normal tissue banks of more than 1,000,0000 samples or a "customized approach" to genomics. In addition, Velculescu et al. [67] released approximately 3.5 million SAGE transcript tags from normal and diseased tissues.

Indeed, expression profiling is a powerful research tool for analyzing the differences between tumor types and for distinguishing between tumors, which up to now have been classified based on their morphological characteristics and presence of a few markers. The just recently developed technology "Laser Capture" should also help to better define tumor types in vivo in combination with chips [68] and how they relate to mouse xenografts, not to forget just defining differences or reliable markers in tumor cell lines for in vivo studies. Another example is the case of genetic disorders that have a complex multigenic basis but that can be mapped back to so-called quantitative trait loci (QTLs). It has been recently demonstrated how microarrays can be used alongside classical genetic approaches to identify the genes underlying the defect [69].

Genome-wide arrays also have more direct application in drug discovery. It is possible to use them to profile the effect of various drugs or compounds on gene expression so as to assess their potential efficacy or side effects [70]. It is also possible to compare the profile of genes expressed in a deletion mutant compared to wild type. If the deletion mutant has a "desirable" phenotype it may be possible to phenocopy the deletion by finding a chemical inhibitor of the protein product or the deleted gene using whole-scale gene expression screening. In addition, the gene's expression can be induced or repressed in vitro or in vivo, and then its responsiveness characterized by RNA profiling. Such examples are (1) tetracycline on/off [71]; (2) genetic suppressor elements [72,73]; (3) zinc finger proteins [74]; (4) gene trapping [8]; (5) correcting the mutation using chimeric RNA-DNA oligonucleotides [75–83].

Still, one of the major problems with the simultaneous analysis of the expression of thousands of genes is the shear weight of data generated (see sec. II.D). Not only is it essential to link the result from each DNA probe back to the parent sequence; it is also necessary to decide which result is significant and then generate a list of 'interesting genes." If, say, 300 genes change in a given experimental paradigm, due to experimental error, which ones are interesting and worthy of follow-up and what do they tell us about what is really happening in the system under investigation? How also can one store and integrate this enormous amount of data over years of experimentation and even compare data generated by different labs? These problems will undoubtedly remain for sometime; however, too much data is better than not enough. While clearly there is much to do on many fronts, it is almost certainly true to say that expression profiling will help revolutionize the way in which we perform biological investigations in the future. RNA profiling, together with the many other genomic technologies, promises to have a big impact on the process of drug discovery [45].

Recently, three new approaches to validate target genes have been developed:

1. Genetic suppressor Element (GSEs')
2. Zinc finger proteins
3. Gene trapping

(1) *Genetic suppressor element* (GSE; retroviral based) is a unique technology to rapidly discover and validate novel pharmaceutical targets, as well as design therapeutic agents that regulate the function of these targets in specific disease processes [72,73]. Presently, there are four start-up biotechs dominating the field: Arcaris Inc. (formerly Ventana), Rigel Pharmaceuticals Inc., Genetica Inc., and PPD Inc. GSE technology is based on the rapid creation of high-titer helper-free recombinant retroviruses capable of infecting nearly any higher eukaryotic cell type [84]. Novel in its conception and application, this technology facilitates both target and drug discovery in diseases previously resistant to standard approaches. Unlike traditional small-molecule screening approaches, which can

underrepresent a given library, the GSE technology delivers highly complex "expression libraries" into target cells where each cell contains unique information. This information is decoded to synthesize a single peptide or anitisense RNA, which interacts with potential targets within the cell. By examining the specific physiological effect of the introduced molecule, the peptide or antisense RNA capable of changing cellular physiology in a desired manner is obtained and the essential link to identifying a target is made [85–87]. To date these studies have been primarily in oncology and virology [88,89]. Other fields of immediate potential use include antimicrobials, neurosciences, immunology and transplantation, cardiovascular and metabolic diseases.

(2) Zinc finger proteins are DNA-binding proteins that mediate the expression, replication, modification, and repair of genes. Pabo and Pavletich [74] solved and published the first crystal structure of a zinc finger protein bound to its cognate DNA sequence,—perhaps the seminal publication in the field of zinc finger protein rational design. The discovery of zinc finger DNA-binding proteins and the rules by which they recognize their cognate genetic sequences (up to 18 base pairs) has made possible the rational design of novel transcription factors that can recognize any gene or DNA sequence. The start-up biotech company Sangamo has combined these protein–DNA recognition rules with powerful selection methods to allow the rapid generation of proteins that recognize and bind to target DNA sequences (see *http://www.sangamo.com*). Sangamo can rationally design zinc finger proteins that selectively up or down regulate the expression of target genes and that in vitro or in vivo.

(3) Traditional gene-trapping approaches, in which genes are randomly disrupted with DNA elements inserted throughout the genome, have been used to generate large numbers of mutant organisms for genetic analysis. Recent modifications of gene trapping methods and their increased use in mammalian systems are likely to result in a wealth of new information on gene function. Various trapping strategies allow genes to be segregated based on criteria such as the specific subcellular location of an encoded protein, the tissue expression profile, or responsiveness to specific stimuli. Genome-wide gene trapping strategies, which integrate gene discovery and expression profiling, can be applied in a massively parallel format to produce living assays for drug discovery [8]. Gene trapping was originally described in bacteria [90,91]. Since then it has been used in many other organisms, including plants [92], *C. elegans* [93], *Drosophila* [94], mouse embryonic stem cells [95], zebrafish [96], and yeast [97].

Gene trapping provides another approach to help validate targets for modern drug discovery efforts, including bioassays to sort through the large number of potentially active compounds. The need for an integrated technology platform to discover genes, pathways, and corresponding drug candidates drives the development of novel approaches, termed "gene-to-screen genomics." Gene trapping/tagging strategies may provide such a link to drug discovery [98].

4. Model Organisms (Yeast, *C. elegans, Drosophila,* Mouse, Rat)

"Connecting genotype to phenotype is not always straightforward" [99]. Thus, the power of less complex organisms for understanding the function of unknown human genes derives from the essential homology of many genes from different organisms [22]. Examples are transcription factors, neurotransmitters and their receptors, growth factors, signaling molecules, apoptosis factors, G-protein-coupled receptors, membrane trafficking and secretion factors, etc. [100,101]. During the past several years, a great deal of work, much of it in yeast, has identified a network of proteins, constituting "checkpoints" of cell cycle regulation. One has been linked to the hereditary disease Li–Fraumeni syndrome, which leaves patients prone to develop multiple forms of cancer [102]. Yeast genetic screening has also been used to identify mammalian nonreceptor modulators of G-protein signaling [103]. Recently, yeast screening resulted in identification of novel biochemical pathways based on a biochemical genomics approach to identify genes by the activity of their products [104]. The authors of Ref. 4 took the global approach by developing an array of 6144 individual yeast strains, each containing a different yeast open reading frame (ORF) fused to a reporter gene/purification tool, glutatione *S*-transferase (GST), as originally described by Simonsen and Lodish [105]. The strains were grown in defined pools, GST-ORFs purified, and activities of each strain identified after deconvoluting. This approach yielded three novel enzyme activities.

The nematode *C. elegans* is a principal organism for the analysis of the development and function of the nervous system. This is because it is especially amenable to molecular genetic analysis [106]. Its complete cell lineage and nervous system connectivity have been mapped [107]. *C. elegans* is the first animal for which the complete genome has been sequenced [59]. Since the *C. elegans* genome was sequenced, an enormous amount of novel functions have been discovered and linked to more complex organisms, including humans [106,108–111]. For example, presenilins and APP of *C. elegans* are particularly attractive given the ease of making animals lacking the function of a single gene either genetically or by using RNA interference [108]. Subsequently, suppressor mutations are selected in genes in the same pathway and their DNA sequence is determined. One of the most impressive examples of this approach is in studies of apoptosis where the major components of apoptosis pathway are conserved in *C. elegans* and mammalian cells [112]. Another example is the identification that p66 shc expands life by enhancing resistance to environmental stresses such as UV light and reactive oxygen species [113]. Recently, p66 shc knockout mice show the same phenotype as the worms [114]. Taking a global two-hybrid approach, Walhout et al. [115] have functionally annotated 100 uncharacterized gene products starting with 27 proteins of known function. The most striking set of interactions involves the Rb tumor suppressor protein complex, which regulates gene expression during the cell cycle. The screens yielded 10 interacting proteins, comprising 3 known interactors and 7 known to interact with other proteins of the complex. This publication showed that by having the total sequence of *C. elegans,* it is now possible on a genome-wide scale to map the interacting proteins and enhance our understanding of molecular mechanisms both in this organism and in humans. The model organism *Drosophila* has also provided insights into mammalian signaling pathways and their importance in development [116] and will continue to, especially since its genome has been recently sequenced [117]. Both yeast and *C. elegans* are used for drug screening both at the expression level using chips and at the organism level and by creating strains designed (by phenotype and genotype) for screening compounds against a particular biochemical step or pathway [22,118]. Recently, Andretic et al. [119] demonstrated that cocaine sensitization could be demonstrated in 'Drosophila'. Cocaine sensitization was absent in all but the mutant fly strains missing the timeless gene. This implication of a subset of the circadian clock genes in drug responsiveness echoes recent suggestions that at least some of these genes may act in more places and in more functions than just the brain's clock [120].

Over the past 40 years, the mouse has certainly become one of the most useful models of human genetic disease. Multiple single-gene and polygenic models of human disorders have been characterized in the mouse. Often the phenotypic characteristics are strikingly similar to that for the analogous human disorder [121–126]. The mouse has many advantages over other model organisms for these kinds of studies:

1. The relatively short generation time facilitates breeding approaches for genetic linkage studies and accelerates the development of genetic models [25].
2. The genetic understanding and characterization of the genome in the mouse is second only to humans in depth and breadth among mammalian species. The ability to genetically map in the mouse *(http://www.jax.org)* and then clone single-gene disorders rapidly with the "emerging technologies" will allow the economical identification of the polygenes controlling quantitative traits [27,127,128]. There are numerous examples of single-gene mutations in the mouse having virtually identical phenotypes in human, and cloning of the mouse gene has led to cloning of the human homologue [129].
3. The sequence/structural homology between human and mouse is quite good. The mouse can be used in parallel with human studies for gene discovery and target identification. This parallel approach can be used for the identification of disease genes (and putative targets or pathways involved in pathogenesis) as well for as phenotypic characterization. As described above (see Sec. II.A.I), the fundamental approach is to use conserved "synteny" (or orthology) to determine if the same genomic region is functionally involved in a disease phenotype in both human populations and the mouse. If the same chromosomal region is

involved, then it is generally easier to identify the gene in the mouse than in humans, and one can use mutation detection/analysis to determine if the same gene is involved in human polygenic disease.

4. The ability to make transgenic and gene-targeted deletions or substitutions both classical and conditional is now a mature technology for the mouse ([121,122,130,131] and Biomed Net Knockout database: *http://www.biomednet.com/db/mkmd*).

5. The ability to phenotype the mouse is becoming more precise and achievable despite the small size of the animal (e.g., MRI imaging [132–134]). The ability to phenotype is of utmost importance. This is why obesity was one of the first therapeutic indications tackled. Many obesity genes have been identified in the mouse during the past 7 years [135–138]. Therefore, the mouse is emerging as one of the premier models for disease gene discovery and utility in the drug discovery process.

The premise of genomics in drug discovery and validation is that genes found to be associated with disease are prevalidated. If mutations in these genes affect the disease risk or phenotype, then we know that these genes are likely to be important in the disease process [25]. However, the identification of an association between a gene mutation or sequence variant and a disease trait does not necessarily imply that the gene, or its protein product, is a "drugable" target. In addition, one must not forget the role of environment even in well-controlled genetic backgrounds. Recently, Crabbe et al. [139] demonstrated that subtle environmental differences between laboratories could have a significant effect on behavioral measures in inbred and mutant mouse strains, not to mention nongemomic transmission across generations of maternal behavior and stress responses found recently in rats [140]. Thus, these genes may simply be important players in the disease process, and an understanding of their role may serve to provide access to the pathways involved in disease and ultimately the appropriate targets for therapeutic intervention. Still, the utility of the mouse extends beyond being just a gene discovery tool to provide prevalidated targets. It can also be used for the development of animal models, and the testing of compounds in specifically constructed transgenic and knockout strains to further define the target and pathway of a therapeutic compound [25].

B. Proteomics

The *proteome* of an organism is the complete set of proteins that it can produce. *Proteomics* is the study of the proteome of cells, tissues, or organisms, including the interaction of the proteome with the environment, where the proteomic signature is the subset of proteins whose alteration in expression is characteristic of a response to a defined condition or genetic change [141]. Besides genomics there is also a great interest in working at the genome level with polypeptides or proteomics. In fact, proteomics is one of the most important "postgenomic" approaches to understanding gene function. Given that the mRNA concentration in any cell and the amount of cognate protein are not always correlated (owning to the differential kinetics of both types of molecule), there may be a good deal of new information to be found by studying proteins in this way. Thus is especially interesting because posttranscriptional regulation of gene expression is a common phenomenon in higher organisms [142].

Presently, proteomics primarily uses two-dimensional gel electrophoresis to profile gene expression and cell responses at the protein level. Protein spots are identified by matrix-assisted laser desorption/ionization (MALDI) and tandem MS/MS techniques, using proteomics for target identification, mechanism of action studies, and for comparing compounds based on the similarity of proteomic signatures they elicit. Probably the most advanced organization taking the global approach to proteomics, especially in higher eukaryotes, is Oxford GlycoSciences *(http://www.ogs.com),* which recently announced, along with Incyte, that they had launched an integrated proteomics database that includes information about how mRNA expression levels correlated to protein expression levels. Large Scale Biology Inc. has focused on establishing databases of hundreds of compounds, effects on rat liver and Proteome Inc. *(http://www.prteome.com)* has established excellent yeast (C. albicans) and *C. elegans* protein databases. To date, the bottleneck with the two-dimensional gel approach has not been running the gels but rather sensitivity, the quantitative detection of spots, as well as the time needed to "gel-gaze," (i.e., to image the gel so as to identify differences from gel to gel). To that end, Genomic Solutions *(http://www.genomicsolutions.com)* has assembled and developed a rather complete suite of technologies and systems for protein characterization–based electrophoretic separation, which includes a fairly sophisticated and proven imaging technology that permits the identification, quantification, and comparison of two-dimensional separations. Other companies, such as Amersham/NycoMed, are developing second-generation dyes and stains to increase the sensitivity of the detection of the spots in the two-dimensional gels. Ruedi Abersold at the University of Washington is developing an approach where by he is miniaturizing classical electrophoresis technologies in a way that is compatible with automation [143].

As described in a recent *Nature* survey [143] on the prospects of proteomics, the now well-established two-dimensional gel approach has many limitations. Still, development of the more advanced technologies (e.g. protein chip, antibody, and protein array) that may deliver fast and parallel quantitative analyses of protein distributions has a way to go (e.g., see below Phylos, Ciphergen, CAT, Morphosys, etc.).

One such technology that is further advanced comes from Ciphergen Biosystems. The ProteinChip system that Ciphergen uses is the patented SELDI

(Surface-Enhanced Laser Desorption/Ionization) ProteinChip technology to rapidly perform the separation, detection, and analysis of proteins at the femtomole level directly from biological samples. The ProteinChip System can replace and complement a wide range of traditional analytical methods, which not only are more time consuming but require specialized scientific expertise (see *http://www.chihergen.com*). Ciphergen's ProteinChip arrays allow the researcher to affinity-capture minute quantities of proteins via specific surface chemistries. Each aluminum chip contains eight individual, chemically treated spots for sample application; this setup facilitates simultaneous analysis of multiple samples. A colored, hydrophobic coating retains samples on the spots and simultaneously allows for quick identification of chip type. Typically, a few microliters of sample applied on the ProteinChip array yields sufficient protein for analysis with the ProteinChip Reader. Designed with proprietary technology, the Reader takes advantage of modern time-of-flight (TOF) mass spectrometry to determine the precise molecular weight of multiple proteins from a native biological sample. To enhance the appearance and facilitate interpretation of the protein mass data collected, ProteinChip software offers various presentation formats or "data views." Recently, Garvin et al. [144] employed MALDI-TOF to detect mutations in gene products by tagging a PCR fragment after in vitro transcription and translation. The process can be multiplexed and is amenable to automation, providing an efficient, high-throughput means for mutation discovery and genetic profiling.

To bring functional genomics to the protein arena, Phylos (*http://www.phylos.com*) has pioneered PROfusion technology whereby proteins are covalently tagged to the mRNA [145]. Using this technology, both synthetic and natural libraries (representing the repertoire of proteins naturally expressed in a given cell type or tissue source) have been constructed. Due to the in vitro nature of library construction, Phylos libraries are the largest described to date, up to 10^{14} in size. From a library of such molecules one can select for a protein function of choice, with the benefit that the genetic material is linked to the protein for subsequent PCR amplification, enrichment, and, ultimately, identification [146]. The key to the Phylos technology is in the development of a puromycin-containing DNA linker that is ligated to RNA prior to translation. Puromycin is an antibiotic that mimics the aminoacyl end of tRNA and acts as a translation inhibitor by entering the ribosomal A site and accepting the nascent peptide, a process catalyzed by the peptidyltransferase activity of the ribosome. To accomplish this, puromycin is chemically protected and attached to controlled-pore glass for automated synthesis of a DNA linker consisting of 5'- dA27dCdC-P (P = puromycin). The PROfusion molecule represents a very unique entity with characteristics that can be utilized for the production of protein chips. The presence of the RNA tail offers a convenient appendage for anchoring the antibody mimic onto a microarray similar to a DNA chip. Since the technical aspects of chemical attachment of nucleic acids to a chip surface have been well worked out, one can take advantage of this reagent and convert an existing DNA chip to a protein chip through the hybridization of a pool of PROfusion molecules. Because the PROfusion molecule has a unique genetic tag associated with it, specific capture probes can be designed and a specific DNA chip produced for the pool of molecules. Upon hybridization of the PROfusion molecule to the DNA chip, the surface now displays the covalently attached peptide or protein portion of the PROfusion molecule [145]. Furthermore, by using a drug or protein physically anchored either to a solid support or to a chemical ligand (e.g., biotin), the PROfusion cellular library is passed over the target and the interacting proteins eluted and amplified for the next round. Such a methodology brings with it a number of significant advantages. Direct selection of interacting proteins from a cellular PROfusion library through rounds of selection and amplification allows for the identification of both low-abundance and low-affinity targets [145].

Other approaches to identifying interactions of chemical entities with target peptide libraries are described by Kay et al. [147]. These libraries can be generated on pins, beads, or in solution, expressed in bacteria attached to phage or synthesized in vitro off of polysomes. However, the complexities only range from 10^8 to 10^{10}. Recently, a method of quantitative analysis of complex protein mixtures using isotope-coded affinity tags was reported by Gygi et al. [148]. The method is based on a class of new chemical regents, termed isotope-coded affinity tags (ICATs), and tandem mass spectrometry. The first successful attempt using this technology was comparing yeast using various sources of carbon to grow on. The future will show if this technology can be used to quantitatively compare global protein expression in other cell types and tissues.

Another protein chip approach was recently demonstrated by Bieri et al. [149] by which they were able to develop a novel assay of G-protein-coupled receptor (GPCR) activity that employs immobilized receptors on a solid surface and in a functional form. To achieve this, the authors used a specific labeling procedure to biotinylate the carbohydrate located in the glycosylated extracellular domain region of the rhodopsin receptor, a GPCR responsible for dim light detection in animals. This in turn reacts with the surface on the chip using lithography. Rhodopsin interacts with a specific Gα subunit, transducin, to activate cyclic GMP phosphodiesterase and thus can activate the immobilized rhodopsin on the sensor chip with the flash of light, which is monitored by receptor activation through the release of transducin from the chip surface.

Monoclonal antibodies raised against purified, native protein have typically been used as the optimal reagent for many research purposes. However, creation of this type of reagent is both costly and time consuming. A more rapid and cost-effective alternative, but one that is less attractive, is the use of polyclonal antibodies to the target protein or peptides derived from the target. These reagents are generally inferior to monoclonal antibodies with respect to affinity of binding, specificity of reactivity, and utility. An attractive alternative to these approaches is phage display antibody technology (see) Cambridge Antibody Technologies (CAT), Cambridge, UK; Morphosys, Munich, Germany; Dyax, Cambridge, MA; and UbiSys, Netherlands). Phage display antibodies are at least equal, and in most cases superior, to monoclonal and polyclonal antibody approaches with regard to affinity of interaction, selectivity of reactivity, utility in a variety of applications, speed of antibody generation, and numbers of antibodies that can be generated. Moreover, single-chain variable regions with affinities and selectivity equal to monoclonal antibodies can be generated in a period of weeks (as opposed to months). As a result, it is possible to generate much larger numbers of antibodies in the same period of time. It has become clear that there is a critical need for potent and selective antibodies for target identification and validation.

C. Pharmacogenetics and Pharmacogenomics

The intimate connection between drug discovery and genetic information has only become widely recognized in recent years, primarily due to the fact that the two disciplines were perceived to have nothing in common. The discovery of single-Nucleotide Polymorphisms (SNPs) has united the two fields [150,151]. SNPs are the predominant basis of genetic variability in the human population. SNPs will provide the genetic markers for the next era in human genetics [41]. Particular advantages of using SNPs over other types of genetic marker include the relative ease of automating SNP typing assays for cheap, robust, large-scale genotyping, and the abundance of SNPs throughout the genome. Comparisons of the DNA sequence between two individuals reveals on average one nucleotide difference for every 1000 base pairs [152]. This frequency increases as more samples are included in the comparison [153,154]. The majority of changes are single-base substitutions, termed SNPs, although deletions and insertions of one or more bases are also observed. Heritable sequence variations arise as a result of a copying error, or damage and misrepair of DNA that results in alteration of the genomic sequence in germ cells. As a result, the changes are passed on in subsequent generations, and the two or more alternatives at a particular position, or locus, become established in the population. Further diversity arises as a result of recombination between homologous segments of chromosomes during meiosis [41,155].

By 2001 a comprehensive working draft of the human genome is expected and possibly the entire three billion base pairs may be completed. "The Human Pharmaco SNP Consortium" will also identify approximately 300,000 common sequence variants (SNPs) during this time. In addition, private companies are assembling SNP databases (e.g., Celera, Curagen, Genset, Orchid, Phenogenex, etc.) in partnership with larger pharmaceutical companies. In the interim, pharmaceutical companies are limiting their analysis of SNPs to selected candidate genes (pharmacogenetics) to identify associations between polymorphism and drug [41].

The goals for pharmacogenetics/pharmacogenomics are to associate human sequence polymorphisms with drug metabolism, adverse events, and therapeutic efficacy. Defining such associations will help decrease drug development costs, optimize selection of clinical trial participants, and increase patient benefit. Retrospective analysis and rescue of nonconclusive studies as well as determination of the genetic causality of disease are also possible. In addition, the ascertainment of DNA samples from clinical trial patients will facilitate the discovery and validation of targets using linkage disequilibrium and association methods. Candidate genes identified by positional cloning in the mouse can be followed up by using the appropriate patient's DNA to confirm the gene's (or genes') importance in disease [156].

Pharmacogenetics covers a new aspect of drug development, which will apply to discovery, development, and marketed programs. To date, benchmarking-type information is not available. However, it is expected to play an important role in the near future for many pharmaceutical companies. To associate polymorphism with drug effects, DNA samples are obtained from both drug- and placebo-treated patients. To associate polymorphism with disease risk (i.e., target discovery/validation), DNA from patients affected by a specific disease should be compared with DNA from patients unaffected by that disease. The latter group may be affected with other disease states; hence, patient DNA samples from one trial may serve as controls in another, provided that they have been obtained from a population of comparable ethnic composition. In effect, supplementary DNA collection will not be necessary to effect properly controlled pharmacogenetic and target validation studies. Moreover, power simulations suggest that sample sizes obtained during standard clinical trials are sufficient to detect genetic association, given that the genetic effect is of sufficient magnitude and the allele is not rare [157]. Drugs can be more accurately profiled for drug–drug interactions by looking at the metabolism of the compound by the known enzymes and variants thereof. If a drug is found to have limited efficacy but virtually no (or very mild) side effects, then it may also be possible to subtype the patients by genotype so as to distinguish responders from nonresponders. Similarly, if a compound has a potentially severe but very rare side effect (but good efficacy), then genotyping may be used to identify patients in whom a side effect is more likely.

Polymorphisms in coding, regulatory, intronic, untranslated, and other regions can all cause variation in gene activity. Cytochrome P450 gene 2d6 is an example of a coding polymorphism that modulates the activity of the gene and can thereby have a sheat influence on the rate of drug metabolism. Finally, there is growing activity in profiling compounds for toxicity by using SNP and expression chip "signatures" [158]. Good examples of genotyping currently being done in clinical trials include measuring ApoE4 genotypes for Alzheimer's disease and measuring polymorphism in various cytochrome P450 genes. As the general population to be treated is genetically diverse the statistical considerations of these approaches are complex. However, recent examples show that in outbred populations, linkage disequilibrium can be regularly observed at distances of 25 kb from causative polymorphism. Hence, a useful genome-wide SNP map will be composed of 300,000 evenly distributed SNPs localized to specific points in the genome [159]. Given the sample sizes available in clinical trials, the rare allele in a biallelic SNP must be present in a population at a frequency greater than 15%. The Holy Grail is undoubtedly a genome-wide "SNP" map by which correlation of SNP haplotypes with drug–person phenotypes will be made. From a commercial perspective, there will be a trade-off between marketing a drug in a subset of the population and prescribing it for everyone with the disease. Diagnostics will go hand in hand with pharmacogenetic/pharmacogenomic testing [22]. Presently, there are numerous start-up companies developing technologies to score SNPs in a very high-throughput mode to meet the needs of pharmacogenetics and, in the future, pharmacogenomics. These technologies include mass spectrometry and DNA arrays to fiberoptic arrays [159]. For more information, see the web sites of the following companies: Third Wave Technologies, Kiva Genetics, Hexagen, CuraGen, GeneTrace, Sequenom, Orchid, PE, RapidGene/Chiroscience, Affymetrix, Nanogen, Illumina, Renaissance Pharmaceuticals, Varigenics, Celera, PPGx, Sangamo, and others. It is safe to say that profiling humans by genotyping will become part of drug development in the future; it is simply a question of when [22].

D. Bioinformatics/Structural Informatics/Chemi-informatics

Bioinformatics encompasses the acquisition, storage, and analysis of information obtained from biological systems. The information is derived primarily from genomics (genomic and EST DNA sequences, RNA profiling, proteomics) and high-throughput screening [160]. Structural informatics refers to the acquisition, storage, and analysis of structural genomics data, especially that from whole genomes, i.e., genomes that have been totally sequenced (e.g., microbes, yeast, *C. elegans*) [161,162]. "High level protein expression systems, robotic crystallization, cryogenic crystal handling, X-ray area detectors, high field NMR spectrometers, tunable synchrotron radiation sources and high performance computing have together catapulted structural biology from an esoteric niche to biological mainstream" [162]. The next step is to integrate the bioinformatics and structural informatics data. There are both private (Inpharmatica) and public (Structural Research Consortium, *http://proteome.bnl.gov/*) initiatives underway. As described above in the introduction, defining SERMs by using the three-dimensional structure of the estrogen receptor, combining expression profiling (chips) to specific cell types (both in vitro and in vivo), and linking there data to chemi-informatics will be most fruitful for drug discovery in the future.

Many pharmaceutical and biotech organizations have expressed the desire to create a means for tying together structural genomics and chemical information.

A GenChem Database would map gene sequence (actually, protein sequence) to chemical structure in a multidimensional matrix. Two dimensions would be the sequence and the chemical compounds, where each dimension could be examined for similar or dissimilar sequence or chemistry (technology for both exists). The additional dimensions are the different ways to fill in the two-dimensional chemistry versus sequence matrix. A simple way that has some predictability is to score sequences against chemicals for binding ability. You would then find, for example, that proteases cluster by sequence similarity and by inhibitor similarity. Another way to map the sequence-to-chemical matrix would be in terms of whether the chemical compound up-regulates or down-regulates the gene expression.

What is expected to happen in the next 5 years is that research will be done to populate the multidimensional matrix with different types of data (ligand binding affinities, expression changes, etc.). In addition, so-called digital organisms are already on the horizon. These are computer programs that self-replicate, mutate, and adapt by natural selection [163]. The availability of these comprehensive datasets will fundamentally change biomedical research and health care practices. Bioinformatics, structural informatics, and chemi-informatics seek to lead the industry into this new era by bringing genomic information to bear on drug discovery, development, and therapy (Fig. 3 and *http://www.bme.jhu.edu/ccmb*).

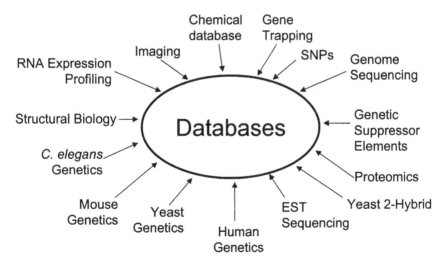

Figure 3 To capitalize on genomics, the most important task is the integration of databases. The plea is for better visualization and data-mining tools as well as better interface of databases.

However, in the "postgenomics" thinking world, everyone has realized that bottlenecks exist in the measurement and analysis of data. participants at the Genome V session held on October 6–10, 1999 [164] discussed strategies for the systematic information gathering on genes and proteins, how to improve pattern recognition algorithms, and ways of analyzing large datasets efficiently without the need for supercomputers.

Genomic studies have shown that many genes in mammals are present in four copies relative to metazoan genomes [165]. Individual members of these gene families have, in many cases, evolved to take on new functions. Nonetheless, there are numerous cases of functional redundancy in mammalian genomes. Therefore, drugs that target single proteins may induce the activity compensatory proteins that cancel the drug's effect. Using sequence similarity algorithms, bioinformatics may identify targets likely to have functionally redundant gene relatives. Reports of multifunctional proteins have become increasingly common; for example, signal transduction pathways have proteins that act on multiple substrates. Drugs that inhibit multifunctional proteins may induce unwanted effects. Gene expression (RNA profiling) and protein expression (proteomics) tools reveal patterns that characterize the response of a cell or tissue to compounds [160]. When correlated to efficacy, toxicity, and biological mechanism, these patterns become powerful tools for generating testable hypotheses. In the future, when the databases are large and robust enough, such patterns will be diagnostic and will not require further experimental validation.

A common problem in large, multidimensional datasets is variable data quality. It is seldom possible to apply weighting factors in genomic datasets, and therefore early genomic datasets will be noisy. Key in identifying important signals in this background are larger experiments (increased sampling frequencies) and the creation of novel algorithms tuned to identify biologically significant patterns. A typical array experiment generates thousands of data points and creates serious challenges for storing and processing data. Informatics can include both "tools" and "analyzers." Tools include software that operate arraying devices and perform image analysis of data from the readers, databases to hold and link information, and software to link data from individual clones to web databases. Pat Brown's laboratory at Stanford has made available software for operating custom built arrayers (*http://cmgm.stanford.edu/pbrown/mguide/software.html*).

The quality of image analysis programs is crucial for the accurate interpretation of signals for slides (chips) and filters. Yidong Chen (NHGRI) has developed a software image analysis package for slides and filters called "deArray" that is available but not supported (*www.nhgri.nih.gov/DIR/LCG/15K/HTML*). Mark Boguski and colleagues have developed software to analyze and link databases such as Entrez and UniGene [58], which can be downloaded at *www.nhgri.nih.gov/DIR/LCG/15K/HTML/*. Software packages for commercial arrayers and chips are also available:

1. Synteni (Gem Tools)
2. Genomic Solutions (Visage Suite)
3. Silicon Genetics/Affymetrix (GeneSpring)
4. Additional development of algorithms for pattern recognition and cluster analysis of complex genomic datasets is key to the successful completion and integration of the complex datasets [164].

Most EST databases and all gene expression technologies are tuned to detect genes expressed at moderate to high levels (100 transcripts per cell or better). Genomic sequence, subtracted normalized cDNA libraries, and gene-finding sequence analysis algorithms will all help to identify genes expressed at low levels. Tools for highly parallel measurement of mRNA levels will require significant improvements before gene expression changes for rare transcripts can be reliably measured. Similar gains in technology will be requisite to approach comprehensive sampling of the proteome and molecular identification of its constituents. Presuming adequate quality control, genomic databases (sequence, polymorphism, gene expression, and proteomic) all increase in value as more data are deposited. To maximize the investment in genomics and bioinformatics, data must be stored in a series of central databases. These databases must be made available for browsing/mining to scientists and those interested in multiple therapeutic areas. Moreover, links between databases will facilitate the integration of information from multiple types of experiments and data. A current common theme in the pharmaceutical industry is the importance of information technology as a key support factor in drug discovery and development.

III. CONCLUSION

As the reader can see, there are two major approaches using numerous technologies to identify and validate targets: "top-down" and "bottom-up." Choice of approach depends on the knowledge of the disease indication at hand, and in some cases both approaches may apply. Irrelevant of the approach or approaches, key is information technologies. Pharmaceutical companies' biggest concern in terms of drug discovery in the postgenomic era is data integration, particularly as it relates to target validation. The plea is for better visualization and data mining tools as well as better interface of databases [166]. At present, there is no quick way to validate a target. Indeed, there is no universal definition of what a validated target is. All of the data being generated on a genome-wide scale must be captured and integrated with other data and with information derived by classical, hypothesis-driven biological experimentation to provide the picture from which completely new targets will emerge. This is a daunting bioinformatics challenge [167]. However, one thing is clear: target validation has become a term that is often used but not rigorously applied. The evolution of truly validated targets is a much slower process than target identification. At present, even large drug discovery organizations in the biggest pharmaceutical companies are not capable of producing more than a handful of well-validated targets each year [2]. Thus, the technologies described in this chapter must be applied such that the number of disease gene targets identified is rigorously validated to improve the quality of drug discovery while providing an increased number of better validated targets because even the best validated target doesn't guarantee lead compounds for development. Targets are only truly validated when a successful drug (not compound), working through that mechanism, has been found.

REFERENCES

1. Drews J. Research and development. Basic science and pharmaceutical innovation. Nat Biotechnol 1999 May;17(5):406.
2. Editorial: Drews J. Drug discovery today—and tomorrow. Drug Disc Today 2000 Jan;5(1)2–4.
3. Wilson S, Bergsma DJ, Chambers JK, Muir AI, Fantom KG, Ellis C, Murdock PR, Herrity NC, Stadel JM. Orphan G-protein-coupled receptors: the next generation of drug targets? Br J Pharmacol 1998 Dec;125(7):1387–1392.
4. Bikker JA, Trumpp-Kallmeyer S, Humblet C. G-Protein coupled receptors: models, mutagenesis, and drug design. J Med Chem 1998 Jul 30;41(16):2911–2927.
5. Valdenaire O, Giller T, Breu V, Ardati A, Schweizer A, Richards JG. A new family of orphan G protein-coupled receptors predominantly expressed in the brain. FEBS Lett 1998 Mar 13;424(3):193–196.
6. Hinuma S, Onda H, Fujino M. The quest for novel bioactive peptides utilizing orphan seven-transmembrane-domain receptors. J Mol Med 1999 Jun;77(6):495–504.
7. McKusick VA. Genomics: structural and functional studies of genomes. Genomics 1997 Oct 15;45(2):244–249.
8. Durick K, Mendlein J, Xanthopoulos KG. Hunting with traps: genome-wide strategies for gene discovery and functional analysis. Genome Res 1999 Nov;9(11):1019–1025.
9. Collins FS. Shattuck lecture—medical and societal consequences of the Human Genome Project. N Engl J Med 1999 Jul 1;341(1):28–37.
10. Kruglyak L. Prospects for whole-genome linkage disequilibrium mapping of common disease genes. Nat Genet 1999 Jun;22(2):139–144.
11. Winzeler EA, Richards DR, Conway AR, Goldstein AL, Kalman S, McCullough MJ, McCusker JH, Stevens DA, Wodicka L, Lockhart DJ, Davis RW. Direct allelic variation scanning of the yeast genome. Science 1998 Aug 21;281(5380):1194–1197.
12. Cargill M, Altshuler D, Ireland J, Sklar P, Ardlie K, Patil N, Lane CR, Lim EP, Kalayanaraman N, Nemesh J, Ziaugra L, Friedland L, Rolfe A, Warrington J, Lipshutz R, Daley GQ, Lander ES. Characterization of single-nucleotide polymorphisms in coding regions of human genes. Nat Genet 1999 Jul;22(3):231–238.
13. Lifton RP. Molecular genetics of human blood pressure variation. Science 1996 May 3;272(5262):676–680.

14. Halushka MK, Fan JB, Bentley K, Hsie L, Shen N, Weder A, Cooper R, Lipshutz R, Chakravarti A. Patterns of single-nucleotide polymorphisms in candidate genes for blood-pressure homeostasis. Nat Genet 1999 Jul;22(3):239–247.

15. Rust S, Rosier M, Funke H, Real J, Amoura Z, Piette JC, Deleuze JF, Brewer HB, Duverger N, Denefle P, Assmann G. Tangier disease is caused by mutations in the gene encoding ATP-binding cassette transporter 1. Nat Genet 1999 Aug;22(4): 352–355.

16. Curran ME. Potassium ion channels and human disease: phenotypes to drug targets? Curr Opin Biotechnol 1998 Dec;9(6):565–572.

17. Burmeister M. Basic concepts in the study of diseases with complex genetics. Biol Psychiatry 1999 Mar 1;45(5):522–532.

18. Wright AF, Carothers AD, Pirastu M. Population choice in mapping genes for complex diseases. Nat Genet 1999 Dec;23(4):397–404.

19. Chen Q, Kirsch GE, Zhang D, Brugada R, Brugada J, Brugada P, Potenza D, Moya A, Borggrefe M, Breithardt G, Ortiz-Lopez R, Wang Z, Antzelevitch C, O'Brien RE, Schulze-Bahr E, Keating MT, Towbin JA, Wang Q. Genetic basis and molecular mechanism for idiopathic ventricular fibrillation. Nature 1998 Mar 19;392(6673): 293–296.

20. Puranam RS, McNamara JO. Stargazing nets new calcium channel subunit. Nat Genet 1998 Aug;19(4):313–314.

21. Friedman JM, Halaas JL. Leptin and the regulation of body weight in mammals. Nature 1998 Oct 22;395(6704):763–770.

22. Harris T. Genetics, genomics and drug discovery. Med Res Rev. 2000; 20(3):203–211.

23. Chagnon YC, Perusse L, Bouchard C. Familial aggregation of obesity, candidate genes and quantitative trait loci. Curr Opin Lipidol 1997 Aug;8(4):205–211.

24. Plomin R. Genetics and general cognitive ability. Nature 1999 Dec 2;402(6761 Suppl):C25–29.

25. West DB, Iakougova O, Olsson C, Ross D, Ohmen J, Chatterjee A. Mouse genetics/genomics: an effective approach for drug target discovery and validation. Med Res Rev. 2000; 20(3):216–230.

26. Carver EA, Stubbs L. Zooming in on the human-mouse comparative map: genome conservation re-examined on a high-resolution scale. Genome Res 1997 Dec;7(12): 1123–1137.

27. Castellani LW, Weinreb A, Bodnar J, Goto AM, Doolittle M, Mehrabian M, Demant P, Lusis AJ. Mapping a gene for combined hyperlipidaemia in a mutant mouse strain. Nat Genet 1998 Apr;18(4):374–377.

28. Passarge E, Horsthemke B, Farber RA. Incorrect use of the term synteny. Nat Genet 1999 Dec;23(4):387.

29. Lembertas AV, Perusse L, Chagnon YC, Fisler JS, Warden CH, Purcell-Huynh DA, Dionne FT, Gagnon J, Nadeau A, Lusis AJ, Bouchard C. Identification of an obesity quantitative trait locus on mouse chromosome 2 and evidence of linkage to body fat and insulin on the human homologous region 20q. J Clin Invest 1997 Sep 1;100(5):1240–1247.

30. Roses AD. Alzheimer diseases: a model of gene mutations and susceptibility polymorphisms for complex psychiatric diseases. Am J Med Genet 1998 Feb 7;81(1): 49–57.

31. Duff K. Recent work on Alzheimer's disease transgenics. Curr Opin Biotechnol 1998 Dec;9(6):561–564.

32. Brent R. Genomic biology. Cell 2000 Jan 7;100(1):169–183.

33. Martin GR, Eglen RM, Hamblin MW, Hoyer D, Yocca F. The structure and signalling properties of 5-HT receptors: an endless diversity? Trends Pharmacol Sci 1998 Jan;19(1):2–4.

34. Strauss EJ, Falkow S. Microbial pathogenesis: genomics and beyond. Science 1997 May 2;276(5313):707–712.

35. Blattner FR, Plunkett G 3rd, Bloch CA, Perna NT, Burland V, Riley M, Collado-Vides J, Glasner JD, Rode CK, Mayhew GF, Gregor J, Davis NW, Kirkpatrick HA, Goeden MA, Rose DJ, Mau B, Shao Y. The complete genome sequence of Escherichia coli K-12. Science 1997 Sep 5;277(5331):1453–1474.

36. Snel B, Bork P, Huynen MA. Genome phylogeny based on gene content. Nat Genet 1999 Jan;21(1):108–110.

37. Allsop AE. Bacterial genome sequencing and drug discovery. Curr Opin Biotechnol 1998 Dec;9(6):637–642.

38. Saunders NJ, Moxon ER. Implications of sequencing bacterial genomes for pathogenesis and vaccine development. Curr Opin Biotechnol 1998 Dec;9(6):618–623.

39. Garber K. Venter announces new celera timetables for producing sequence data, SNP targets. Bioinform 2000 Jan;4(1):4–6.

40. Battey J, Jordan E, Cox D, Dove W. An action plan for mouse genomics. Nat Genet 1999 Jan;21(1):73–75.

41. Bentley DR. The human genome project—an overview. Med Res Rev. 2000; 20(3): 189–196.

42. Dunham I, Shimizu N, Roe BA, Chissoe S, Hunt AR, Collins JE, Bruskiewich R, Beare DM, Clamp M, Smink LJ, Ainscough R, Almeida JP, Babbage A, Bagguley C, Bailey J, Barlow K, Bates KN, Beasley O, Bird CP, Blakey S, Bridgeman AM, Buck D, Burgess J, Burrill WD, O'Brien KP, et al. The DNA sequence of human chromosome 22. Nature 1999 Dec 2;402(6761):489–495.

43. O'Brien SJ, Menotti-Raymond M, Murphy WJ, Nash WG, Wienberg J, Stanyon R, Copeland NG, Jenkins NA, Womack JE, Marshall Graves JA. The promise of comparative genomics in mammals. Science 1999 Oct 15;286(5439):458–62; 479–481.

44. Campbell P. Tales of the expected. Nature Suppl, Dec 2, 1999;402(6761)C7–C9.

45. Freeman T. High throughput gene expression screening; its emerging role in drug discovery. Med Res Rev. 2000; 20(3):197–202.

46. Watson JB, Margulies JE. Differential cDNA screening strategies to identify novel stage-specific proteins in the developing mammalian brain. Dev Neurosci 1993;15(2):77–86.

47. Diatchenko L, Lau YF, Campbell AP, Chenchik A, Moqadam F, Huang B, Lukyanov S, Lukyanov K, Gurskaya N, Sverdlov ED, Siebert PD. Suppression subtractive hybridization: a method for generating differentially regulated or tissue-specific cDNA probes and libraries. Proc Natl Acad Sci USA 1996 Jun 11;93(12):6025–6030.

48. Liang P, Pardee AB. Differential display of eukaryotic messenger RNA by means of the polymerase chain reaction. Science 1992 Aug 14;257(5072):967–971.

49. Nakai M, Kawamata T, Taniguchi T, Maeda K, Tanaka C. Expression of apolipoprotein E mRNA in rat microglia. Neurosci Lett 1996 Jun 14;211(1):41–44.

50. Ohtaka-Maruyama C, Hanaoka F, Chepelinsky AB. A novel alternative spliced variant of the transcription factor AP2alpha is expressed in the murine ocular lens. Dev Biol 1998 Oct 1;202(1):125–135.

51. Eberwine J, Yeh H, Miyashiro K, Cao Y, Nair S, Finnell R, Zettel M, Coleman P. Analysis of gene expression in single live neurons. Proc Natl Acad Sci USA 1992 Apr 1;89(7):3010–3014.

52. Dixon AK, Richardson PJ, Lee K, Carter NP, Freeman TC. Expression profiling of single cells using 3 prime end amplification (TPEA) PCR. Nucleic Acids Res 1998 Oct 1;26(19):4426–4431.

53. Velculescu VE, Zhang L, Vogelstein B, Kinzler KW. Serial analysis of gene expression. Science 1995 Oct 20;270(5235):484–487.

54. Fodor S, Read JL, Pirrung MC, Stryer L, Tsai Lu, A and Solas D. Light-directed, spatially addressable parallel chemical synthesis. Science 1991;251:767–773.

55. Chu S, DeRisi J, Eisen M, Mulholland J, Botstein D, Brown PO, Herskowitz I. The transcriptional program of sporulation in budding yeast. Science 1998 Oct 23;282(5389):699–705.

56. Editorial: Getting hip to the chip. Nat Genet 1998 Mar;18(3):195–197.

57. Eisen MB, Spellman PT, Brown PO, Botstein D. Cluster analysis and display of genome-wide expression patterns. Proc Natl Acad Sci USA 1998 Dec 8;95(25): 14863–14868.

58. Ermolaeva O, Rastogi M, Pruitt KD, Schuler GD, Bittner ML, Chen Y, Simon R, Meltzer P, Trent JM, Boguski MS. Data management and analysis for gene expression arrays. Nat Genet 1998 Sep;20(1):19–23.

59. Review: Genome sequence of the nematode *C. elegans:* a platform for investigating biology. The *C. elegans* Sequencing Consortium. Science 1998 Dec 11;282(5396): 2012–2018.

60. White KP, Rifkin SA, Hurban P, Hogness DS. Microarray analysis of *Drosophila* development during metamorphosis. Science 1999 Dec 10;286(5447):2179–2184.

61. Butler D. IBM promises scientists 500-fold leap in supercomputing power . . . and a chance to tackle protein structure. Nature 1999 Dec 16;402(6763):705–706.

62. Singh-Gasson S, Green RD, Yue Y, Nelson C, Blattner F, Sussman MR, Cerrina F. Maskless fabrication of light-directed oligonucleotide microarrays using a digital micromirror array. Nat Biotechnol 1999 Oct;17(10):974–978.

63. Golub TR, Slonim DK, Tamayo P, Huard C, Gaasenbeek M, Mesirov JP, Coller H, Loh ML, Downing JR, Caligiuri MA, Bloomfield CD, Lander ES. Molecular classification of cancer: class discovery and class prediction by gene expression monitoring. Science. 1999 Oct 15;286(5439):531–537.

64. Lee CK, Klopp RG, Weindruch R, Prolla TA. Gene expression profile of aging and its retardation by caloric restriction. Science 1999 Aug 27;285(5432):1390–1393.

65. Geiss GK, Bumgarner RE, An MC, Agy MB, van't Wout AB, Hammersmark E, Carter VS, Upchurch D, Mullins JI, Katze MG. Large-scale monitoring of host cell gene expression during HIV-1 infection using cDNA microarrays. Virology 2000 Jan 5;266(1):8–16.

66. Cole KA, Krizman DB, Emmert-Buck MR. The genetics of cancer—a 3D model. Nat Genet 1999 Jan;21(1 Suppl):38–41.

67.　Velculescu VE, Madden SL, Zhang L, Lash AE, Yu J, Rago C, Lal A, Wang CJ, Beaudry GA, Ciriello KM, Cook BP, Dufault MR, Ferguson AT, Gao Y, He TC, Hermeking H, Hiraldo SK, Hwang PM, Lopez MA, Luderer HF, Mathews B, Petroziello JM, Polyak K, Zawel L, Kinzler KW, et al. Analysis of human transcriptomes. Nat Genet 1999 Dec;23(4):387–388.

68.　Luo L, Salunga RC, Guo H, Bittner A, Joy KC, Galindo JE, Xiao H, Rogers KE, Wan JS, Jackson MR, Erlander MG. Gene expression profiles of laser-captured adjacent neuronal subtypes. Nat Med 1999 Jan;5(1):117–122.

69.　Naggert JK, Fricker LD, Varlamov O, Nishina PM, Rouille Y, Steiner DF, Carroll RJ, Paigen BJ, Leiter EH. Hyperproinsulinaemia in obese fat/fat mice associated with a carboxypeptidase E mutation which reduces enzyme activity. Nat Genet 1995 Jun;10(2):135–142.

70.　Marton MJ, DeRisi JL, Bennett HA, Iyer VR, Meyer MR, Roberts CJ, Stoughton R, Burchard J, Slade D, Dai H, Bassett DE Jr, Hartwell LH, Brown PO, Friend SH. Drug target validation and identification of secondary drug target effects using DNA microarrays. Nat Med 1998 Nov;4(11):1293–1301.

71.　Berns A. Turning on tumors to study cancer progression. Nat Med 1999 Sep;5(9):989–990.

72.　Longman R. Racing Biotech's commoditization clocck. In Vivo 1999 April:1–8.

73.　Dvorin J. Validated target discovery: letting nature do the work. Technol Strat 1999 June:34–41.

74.　Pavletich NP, Pabo CO. Zinc finger-DNA recognition: crystal structure of a Zif268-DNA complex at 2.1 A. Science 1991 May 10;252(5007):809–817.

75.　Yoon K, Cole-Strauss A, Kmiec EB. Targeted gene correction of episomal DNA in mammalian cells mediated by a chimeric RNA.DNA oligonucleotide. Proc Natl Acad Sci USA 1996 Mar 5;93(5):2071–2076.

76.　Cole-Strauss A, Yoon K, Xiang Y, Byrne BC, Rice MC, Gryn J, Holloman WK, Kmiec EB. Correction of the mutation responsible for sickle cell anemia by an RNA-DNA oligonucleotide. Science 1996 Sep 6;273(5280):1386–1389.

77.　Xiang Y, Cole-Strauss A, Yoon K, Gryn J, Kmiec EB. Targeted gene conversion in a mammalian CD34+-enriched cell population using a chimeric RNA/DNA oligonucleotide. J Mol Med 1997 Nov–Dec;75(11–12):829–835.

78.　Kren BT, Cole-Strauss A, Kmiec EB, Steer CJ. Targeted nucleotide exchange in the alkaline phosphatase gene of HuH-7 cells mediated by a chimeric RNA/DNA oligonucleotide. Hepatology 1997 Jun;25(6):1462–1668.

79.　Kren BT, Bandyopadhyay P, Steer CJ. In vivo site-directed mutagenesis of the factor IX gene by chimeric RNA/DNA oligonucleotides. Nat Med 1998 Mar;4(3):285–290.

80.　Alexeev V, Yoon K. Stable and inheritable changes in genotype and phenotype of albino melanocytes induced by an RNA-DNA oligonucleotide. Nat Biotechnol 1998 Dec;16(13):1343–1346.

81.　Santana E, Peritz AE, Iyer S, Uitto J, Yoon K. Different frequency of gene targeting events by the RNA-DNA oligonucleotide among epithelial cells. J Invest Dermatol 1998 Dec;111(6):1172–1177.

82.　Yoon, K. Single-base conversion of mammalian genes by an RNA-DNA oligonucleotide. 1999 Biog Amines 15:137–167.

83. Vitali T, Sossi V, Tiziano F, Zappata S, Giuli A, Paravatou-Petsotas M, Neri G, Brahe C. Detection of the survival motor neuron (SMN) genes by FISH: further evidence for a role for SMN2 in the modulation of disease severity in SMA patients. Hum Mol Genet 1999 Dec;8(13):2525–2532.

84. Pear W, Scott M, Nolan GP. Generation of high titre, helper-free retroviruses by transient transfection. In: Methods in Molecular Medicine: Gene Therapy Protocols. Totowa, NJ: Humana Press, 1997:41–57.

85. Holzmayer TA, Pestov DG, Roninson IB. Isolation of dominant negative mutants and inhibitory antisense RNA sequences by expression selection of random DNA fragments. Nucleic Acids Res 1992 Feb 25;20(4):711–717.

86. Gudkov AV, Kazarov AR, Thimmapaya R, Axenovich SA, Mazo IA, Roninson IB. Cloning mammalian genes by expression selection of genetic suppressor elements: association of kinesin with drug resistance and cell immortalization. Proc Natl Acad Sci USA 1994 Apr 26;91(9):3744–3748.

87. Onishi M, Kinoshita S, Morikawa Y, Shibuya A, Phillips J, Lanier LL, Gorman DM, Nolan GP, Miyajima A, Kitamura T. Applications of retrovirus-mediated expression cloning. Exp Hematol 1996 Feb;24(2):324–329.

88. Roninson IB, Levenson VV, Lausch E, Schott B, Kirschling DJ, Zuhn DL, Tarasewicz D, Kandel ES, Iraj ES, Fedosova V, Zhu H, Chen C-J, Salov S, Gudkov AV. Molecular determinants of drug response: a genetic suppressor element analysis. Anti-Cancer Drugs 1996;7(3)83–91.

89. Kinoshita S, Chen BK, Kaneshima H, Nolan GP. Host control of HIV-1 parasitism in T cells by the nuclear factor of activated T cells. Cell 1998 Nov 25;95(5):595–604.

90. Casadaban MJ, Cohen SN. Lactose genes fused to exogenous promoters in one step using a Mu-lac bacteriophage: in vivo probe for transcriptional control sequences. Proc Natl Acad Sci USA 1979 Sep;76(9):4530–4533.

91. Bellofatto V, Shapiro L, Hodgson DA. Generation of a Tn5 promoter probe and its use in the study of gene expression in *Caulobacter crescentus*. Proc Natl Acad Sci USA 1984 Feb;81(4):1035–1039.

92. Schell J. Transgenic plants as tools to study the molecular organization of plant genes. Science 1987;237:1176–1183.

93. Hope IA. "Promoter trapping" in *Caenorhabditis elegans*. Development 1991 Oct;113(2):399–408.

94. O'Kane CJ, Gehring WJ. Detection in situ of genomic regulatory elements in *Drosophila*. Proc Natl Acad Sci USA 1987 Dec;84(24):9123–9127.

95. Zambrowicz BP, Friedrich GA, Buxton EC, Lilleberg SL, Person C, Sands AT. Disruption and sequence identification of 2,000 genes in mouse embryonic stem cells. Nature 1998 Apr 9;392(6676):608–611.

96. Amsterdam A, Burgess S, Golling G, Chen W, Sun Z, Townsend K, Farrington S, Haldi M, Hopkins N. A large-scale insertional mutagenesis screen in zebrafish. Genes Dev 1999 Oct 15;13(20):2713–2724.

97. Ross-Macdonald P, Coelho PS, Roemer T, Agarwal S, Kumar A, Jansen R, Cheung KH, Sheehan A, Symoniatis D, Umansky L, Heidtman M, Nelson FK, Iwasaki H, Hager K, Gerstein M, Miller P, Roeder GS, Snyder M. Large-scale analysis of the yeast genome by transposon tagging and gene disruption. Nature 1999 Nov 25;402(6760):413–418.

98. Whitney M, Rockenstein E, Cantin G, Knapp T, Zlokarnik G, Sanders P, Durick K, Craig FF, Negulescu PA. A genome-wide functional assay of signal transduction in living mammalian cells. Nat Biotechnol 1998 Dec;16(13):1329–1333.

99. Morris SC. Evolution: bringing molecules into the fold. Cell 2000 Jan 7;100(1):1–11.

100. Hodgkin J, Herman RK. Changing styles in *C. elegans* genetics. Trends Genet 1998 Sep;14(9):352–357.

101. Plasterk RH. Hershey heaven and *Caenorhabditis elegans*. Nat Genet 1999 Jan;21(1):63–64.

102. Bell DW, Varley JM, Szydlo TE, Kang DH, Wahrer DC, Shannon KE, Lubratovich M, Verselis SJ, Isselbacher KJ, Fraumeni JF, Birch JM, Li FP, Garber JE, Haber DA. Heterozygous germ line hCHK2 mutations in Li–Fraumeni syndrome. Science 1999 Dec 24;286(5449):2528–2531.

103. Cismowski MJ, Takesono A, Ma C, Lizano JS, Xie X, Fuernkranz H, Lanier SM, Duzic. E. Genetic screens in yeast to identify mammalian nonreceptor modulators of G-protein signaling. Nat Biotechnol 1999 Sep;17(9):878–883.

104. Martzen MR, McCraith SM, Spinelli SL, Torres FM, Fields S, Grayhack EJ, Phizicky EM. A biochemical genomics approach for identifying genes by the activity of their products. Science 1999 Nov 5;286(5442):1153–1155.

105. Simonsen H, Lodish HF. Cloning by function: expression cloning in mammalian cells. Trends Pharmacol Sci 1994 Dec;15(12):437–441.

106. Goodwin SF. Molecular neurogenetics of sexual differentiation and behaviour. Curr Opin Neurobiol 1999 Dec;9(6):759–765.

107. Bargmann CI. Neurobiology of the *Caenorhabditis elegans* genome. Science 1998 Dec 11;282(5396):2028–2033.

108. Fire A, Xu S, Montgomery MK, Kostas SA, Driver SE, Mello CC. Potent and specific genetic interference by double-stranded RNA in *Caenorhabditis elegans*. Nature 1998 Feb 19;391(6669):806–811.

109. Zheng Y, Brockie PJ, Mellem JE, Madsen DM, Maricq AV. Neuronal control of locomotion in *C. elegans* is modified by a dominant mutation in the GLR-1 ionotropic glutamate receptor. Neuron 1999 Oct;24(2):347–361.

110. Zhen M, Jin Y. The liprin protein SYD-2 regulates the differentiation of presynaptic termini in *C. elegans*. Nature 1999 Sep 23;401(6751):371–375.

111. Tabara H, Sarkissian M, Kelly WG, Fleenor J, Grishok A, Timmons L, Fire A, Mello CC. The rde-1 gene, RNA interference, and transposon silencing in *C. elegans*. Cell 1999 Oct 15;99(2):123–132.

112. Metzstein MM, Stanfield GM, Horvitz HR. Genetics of programmed cell death in *C. elegans:* past, present and future. Trends Genet 1998 Oct;14(10):410–416.

113. Martin GM, Austad SN, Johnson TE. Genetic analysis of ageing: role of oxidative damage and environmental stresses. Nat Genet. 1996 May;13(1):25–34.

114. Migliaccio E, Giorgio M, Mele S, Pelicci G, Reboldi P, Pandolfi PP, Lanfrancone L, Pelicci PG. The p66shc adaptor protein controls oxidative stress response and life span in mammals.

115. Walhout AJ, Sordella R, Lu X, Hartley JL, Temple GF, Brasch MA, Thierry-Mieg N, Vidal M. Protein interaction mapping in *C. elegans* using proteins involved in vulval development. Science 2000 Jan 7;287(5450):116–122.

116. Mathey-Prevot B, Perrimon N. Mammalian and *Drosophila* blood: JAK of all trades? Cell 1998 Mar 20;92(6):697–700.

117. Review: The compleat fly. Science 1999 Sept 17;285(5435):1829.

118. Schafer WR. How do antidepressants work? Prospects for genetic analysis of drug mechanisms. Cell 1999 Sep 3;98(5):551–554.

119. Andretic R, Chaney S, Hirsh J. Requirement of circadian genes for cocaine sensitization in *Drosophila*. Science 1999 Aug 13;285(5430):1066–1068.

120. Editorial: Cocaine and clocks. Science 1999 Aug 13;285(5430):981.

121. Bedell MA, Jenkins NA, Copeland NG. Mouse models of human disease. I. Techniques and resources for genetic analysis in mice. Genes Dev 1997 Jan 1;11(1): 1–10.

122. Bedell MA, Largaespada DA, Jenkins NA, Copeland NG. Mouse models of human disease. II. Recent progress and future directions. Genes Dev 1997 Jan 1;11(1): 11–43.

123. Copeland NG, Jenkins NA, Gilbert DJ, Eppig JT, Maltais LJ, Miller JC, Dietrich WF, Weaver A, Lincoln SE, Steen RG, Stein LD, Nadeau JH, Lander ES. A genetic linkage map of the mouse: current applications and future prospects. Science 1993 Oct 1;262(5130):57–66.

124. Crabbe JC, Belknap JK, Buck KJ. Genetic animal models of alcohol and drug abuse. Science 1994 Jun 17;264(5166):1715–1723.

125. Frankel WN. Taking stock of complex trait genetics in mice. Trends Genet 1995 Dec;11(12):471–477.

126. Purcell-Huynh DA, Weinreb A, Castellani LW, Mehrabian M, Doolittle MH, Lusis AJ. Genetic factors in lipoprotein metabolism. Analysis of a genetic cross between inbred mouse strains NZB/BINJ and SM/J using a complete linkage map approach. J Clin Invest 1995 Oct;96(4):1845–1858.

127. Mogil JS, Wilson SG, Bon K, Lee SE, Chung K, Raber P, Pieper JO, Hain HS, Belknap JK, Hubert L, Elmer GI, Chung JM, Devor M. Heritability of nociception II. "Types" of nociception revealed by genetic correlation analysis. Pain 1999 Mar;80(1–2):83–93.

128. Spearow JL, Doemeny P, Sera R, Leffler R, Barkley M. Genetic variation in susceptibility to endocrine disruption by estrogen in mice. Science 1999 Aug 20;285(5431):1259–1261.

129. Ahmad W, Faiyaz ul Haque M, Brancolini V, Tsou HC, ul Haque S, Lam H, Aita VM, Owen J, deBlaquiere M, Frank J, Cserhalmi-Friedman PB, Leask A, McGrath JA, Peacocke M, Ahmad M, Ott J, Christiano AM. Alopecia universalis associated with a mutation in the human hairless gene. Science 1998 Jan 30;279(5351): 720–724.

130. Chemelli RM, Willie JT, Sinton CM, Elmquist JK, Scammell T, Lee C, Richardson JA, Williams SC, Xiong Y, Kisanuki Y, Fitch TE, Nakazato M, Hammer RE, Saper CB, Yanagisawa M. Narcolepsy in orexin knockout mice: molecular genetics of sleep regulation. Cell 1999 Aug 20;98(4):437–451.

131. Mohn AR, Gainetdinov RR, Caron MG, Koller BH. Mice with reduced NMDA receptor expression display behaviors related to schizophrenia. Cell 1999 Aug 20;98(4):427–436.

132. Sadelain M, Blasberg RG. Imaging transgene expression for gene therapy. J Clin Pharmacol 1999 Aug;Suppl:34S–39S.

133. Stokstad E. Humane science finds sharper and kinder tools. Science 1999 Nov 5;286(5442):1068–1071.

134. Tsodyks M, Kenet T, Grinvald A, Arieli A. Linking spontaneous activity of single cortical neurons and the underlying functional architecture. Science 1999 Dec 3;286(5446):1943–1946.

135. Bultman SJ, Michaud EJ, Woychik RP. Molecular characterization of the mouse agouti locus. Cell 1992 Dec 24;71(7):1195–1204.

136. Zhang Y, Proenca R, Maffei M, Barone M, Leopold L, Friedman JM. Positional cloning of the mouse obese gene and its human homologue. Nature 1994 Dec 1;372(6505):425–432.

137. Tartaglia LA, Dembski M, Weng X, Deng N, Culpepper J, Devos R, Richards GJ, Campfield LA, Clark FT, Deeds J, et al. Identification and expression cloning of a leptin receptor, OB-R. Cell 1995 Dec 29;83(7):1263–1271.

138. Noben-Trauth K, Naggert JK, North MA, Nishina PM. A candidate gene for the mouse mutation tubby. Nature 1996 Apr 11;380(6574):534–538.

139. Crabbe JC, Wahlsten D, Dudek BC. Genetics of mouse behavior: interactions with laboratory environment. Science 1999 Jun 4;284(5420):1670–1672.

140. Francis D, Diorio J, Liu D, Meaney MJ. Nongenomic transmission across generations of maternal behavior and stress responses in the rat. Science 1999 Nov 5;286(5442):1155–1158.

141. Abbott A. A post-genomic challenge: learning to read patterns of protein synthesis. Nature 1999 Dec 16;402(6763):715–720.

142. Anderson L, Seilhamer J. A comparison of selected mRNA and protein abundances in human liver. Electrophoresis 1997 Mar–Apr;18(3–4):533–537.

143. Editoral: The promise of proteomics. Nature 1999 Dec 16;402(6763):703.

144. Garvin AM, Parker KC, Haff L. MALDI-TOF based mutation detection using tagged in vitro synthesized peptides. Nat Biotechnol 2000 Jan;18(1):95–97.

145. Kreider BL. PROfusions: genetically tagged-proteins for functional proteomics and beyond. Med Res Rev. In press.

146. Roberts RW, Szostak JW. RNA-peptide fusions for the in vitro selection of peptides and proteins. Proc Natl Acad Sci USA 1997 Nov 11;94(23):12297–12302.

147. Kay BK, Kurakin AV, Hyde-DeRuyscher R. From peptides to drugs via phage display. DDT 1998 Aug;3(8):370–378.

148. Gygi SP, Rist B, Gerber SA, Turecek F, Gelb MH, Aebersold R. Quantitative analysis of complex protein mixtures using isotope-coded affinity tags. Nat Biotechnol 1999 Oct;17(10):994–999.

149. Bieri C, Ernst OP, Heyse S, Hofmann KP, Vogel H. Micropatterned immobilization of a G protein–coupled receptor and direct detection of G protein activation. Nat Biotechnol 1999 Nov;17(11):1105–1108.

150. Chakravarti A. Population genetics—making sense out of sequence. Nat Genet 1999 Jan;21(1 Suppl):56–60.

151. Fikes BJ. SNP Research, Another step towards deciphering the human genome. Bioventure View 1999 Nov;14(11):1–4.

152. Taillon-Miller P, Gu Z, Li Q, Hillier L, Kwok PY. Overlapping genomic sequences: a treasure trove of single-nucleotide polymorphisms. Genome Res 1998 Jul;8(7):748–754.

153. Wang DG, Fan JB, Siao CJ, Berno A, Young P, Sapolsky R, Ghandour G, Perkins N, Winchester E, Spencer J, Kruglyak L, Stein L, Hsie L, Topaloglou T, Hubbell E, Robinson E, Mittmann M, Morris MS, Shen N, Kilburn D, Rioux J, Nusbaum C, Rozen S, Hudson TJ, Lander ES, et al. Large-Scale identification, mapping, and genotyping of single-nucleotide polymorphisms in the human genome. Science 1998 May 15;280(5366):1077–1082.

154. Nickerson DA, Taylor SL, Weiss KM, Clark AG, Hutchinson RG, Stengard J, Salomaa V, Vartiainen E, Boerwinkle E, Sing CF. DNA sequence diversity in a 9.7-kb region of the human lipoprotein lipase gene. Nat Genet 1998 Jul;19(3):233–240.

155. Chakravarti A. It's raining SNPs, hallelujah? Nat Genet 1998 Jul;19(3):216–2177.

156. Housman D, Ledley FD. Why pharmacogenomics? Why now? Nat Biotechnol 1998 Jun;16(6):492–493.

157. Sherry ST, Ward M and Sirotkin K. dbSNP—Database for single nucleotide polymorphisms and other classes of minor genetic variation. Genome Res 1999 Aug;9(8):677–679.

158. Lipshutz RJ, Fodor SP, Gingeras TR, Lockhart DJ. High density synthetic oligonucleotide arrays. Nat Genet 1999 Jan;21(1 Suppl):20–24.

159. Steemers FJ, Ferguson JA, Walt DR. Screening unlabeled DNA targets with randomly ordered fiber-optic gene arrays. Nat Biotechnol 2000 Jan;18(1):91–94.

160. Bowtell DD. Options available—from start to finish—for obtaining expression data by microarray. Nat Genet 1999 Jan;21(1 Suppl):25–32.

161. Chervitz SA, Aravind L, Sherlock G, Ball CA, Koonin EV, Dwight SS, Harris MA, Dolinski K, Mohr S, Smith T, Weng S, Cherry JM, Botstein D. Comparison of the complete protein sets of worm and yeast: orthology and divergence. Science 1998 Dec 11;282(5396):2022–2028.

162. Burley SK, Almo SC, Bonanno JB, Capel M, Chance MR, Gaasterland T, Lin D, Sali A, Studier FW, Swaminathan S. Structural genomics: beyond the human genome project. Nat Genet 1999 Oct;23(2):151–157.

163. Lenski RE, Ofria C, Collier TC, Adami C. Genome complexity, robustness and genetic interactions in digital organisms. Nature 1999 Aug 12;400(6745):661–664.

164. Editorial: Connecting the dots. Nat Genet 1999 (23)249–252.

165. Pennisi E. Sifting through and making sense of genome sequences. Science 1998 Jun 12;280(5370):1692–1693.

166. Editorial: Shaw I. Information overflow from discovery to development. Pharm Sci Technol Today 1999 Sept;2(9)345–347.

167. Gelbart WM. Databases in genomic research. Science 1998 Oct 23; 282(5389): 659–661.

3
Functional Genomics

David O'Hagan
Streamline Proteomics
Ann Arbor, Michigan

I. INTRODUCTION

A well-known paradigm in biology is that the function of a biological entity is closely linked to its physical structure. Based on this principal, predictions of biological function have been made by analyzing the structure of the organic molecules on which cells are constructed, such as DNA, RNA, and proteins (Fig. 1). Since proteins provide the raw materials by which the superstructures of cells are constructed, it is reasonable to conclude that the amount, kind, and state of proteins found within a cell can be used to predict how a cell or organism will respond to chemicals, drugs, and the environment. Due to the hierarchical nature of genetic information, i.e., DNA to RNA to protein, it has been possible to approximate the structure and function of proteins by studying the information contained within the primary sequence and abundance of DNA and RNA, respectively. The massively parallel research methods used to determine the sequence and abundance of DNA and RNA are collectively called genomics. Functional genomics is the study of the DNA and RNA component of gene expression, coupled with biological and biochemical experimental data, to approximate the structure and function of proteins [6].

Since it is with proteins that drugs primarily interact, investigating the properties of proteins may lead to innovations in the treatment of human disease [21]. Nevertheless, due to the public resources now available through the efforts of the Human Genome Project, it is the study of the DNA and RNA component of gene expression that is most immediately available. For this reason, genomic methodologies allowing for the parallel characterization of DNA and RNA are now available and routinely practiced. Functional genomics now serves as a tool by which

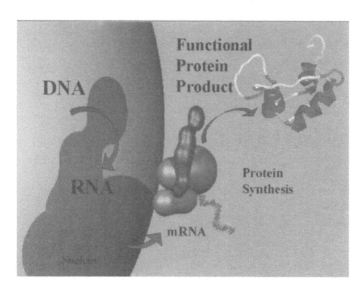

Figure 1   Hierarchy of genetic information.

predictions of cellular function and potential drug–cell interaction can be made. Moreover, given the complexity of cellular signaling and regulatory pathways, numerous simultaneous measurements of the interdependent changes occurring during biological processes can be used to predict how drugs will affect these pathways [22]. The following chapter is designed to highlight the primary considerations given to the use of functional genomics as an approach to drug discovery. These are (1) functional characterization of proteins, (2) the molecular pathways by which proteins provide complex cellular function, and (3) the use of genomic technologies to determine function and find drug targets.

II.   PROTEINS: STRUCTURE AND FUNCTION

All proteins rely on a linear arrangement of 20 amino acids to create the complicated structures that serve a cell or organism with such properties as locomotion, exchange of raw materials, and procreation. Although there are as many as 10.24 trillion combinations of these 20 amino acids for every 10 residues, based on the proteins sequenced to date many of the same sequences are observed. This observation suggests that very few protein sequences translate into proteins that can perform some function. In the hope of better understanding how certain protein sequences are selected over others we must explore the way in which proteins originate and improve the cell's or organism's reproductive strength, its evolutionary history.

The term "molecular evolution" suggests that just as species are selected based on their reproductive advantage, that proteins are selected based on their ability to improve the health and well-being of a cell at the molecular level. The origin of all proteins starts with the production of an open reading frame (ORF) through genetic alterations introduced by such events as point mutations, chromosomal rearrangements, and transposable elements. Therefore, it is the environment that provides the physical and functional constraint by which proteins are selected through the evolving genomes of the world. By relying on the form and fit of proteins to the molecules of the cellular microenvironment, such as nucleic acids, ions, and other proteins, a subset of all possible protein sequences have been selected and modified to produce the diversified adaptations observed in nature [4,11,16]. Moreover, it is this connectivity between sequence and function that provides biologists with the primer for unraveling the cellular role of proteins with unknown function ("orphans"). By observing the conservation of sequence elements, the profile of protein expression and the effects of mutations, a crude approximation of the function of an orphan protein can be ascertained [5,9,12,15,17,18].

A. Molecular Evolution

Since it is the function of the protein that keeps it from being lost during evolutionary selection, it is reasonable to conclude that any segment of a protein that has not been altered in sequence over great evolutionary distances must be performing some role in the health of the organism. The most abundant and extensively characterized class of proteins, first observed in prokaryotes, appears to be selected to perform a series of functions related to the maintenance of the cellular microenvironment, i.e., housekeeping genes. These consist mostly of proteins involved in energy metabolism, biosynthesis of required amino and nucleic acids, transcription/translation, and the replication of the cell's genome (Fig. 2). [10].

These fundamental requirements of all cells provide the backbone on which subsequent protein adaptations are made during evolution. As a consequence of speciation, many proteins are composites of functional units acquired during the fusion or rearrangement of ancestral genes. These small segments of protein sequence are called domains or modules [2,8,12]. These modules are made up of independent segments (motifs), which provide the module with important contact and energetic attributes, allowing the module to perform a task. It has been suggested that during molecular evolution the exons containing these functional units are partially responsible for the shuffling of modules to create alternative composite proteins [7–9,12]. Many environmental changes occur over small periods of evolutionary time and therefore require adaptations on behalf of the organism to survive. Due to this immediate need in the production of proteins required to compensate for the environmental change, it is easy to see how the coordinated rearrangement of functional domains within a genome would arise. By using

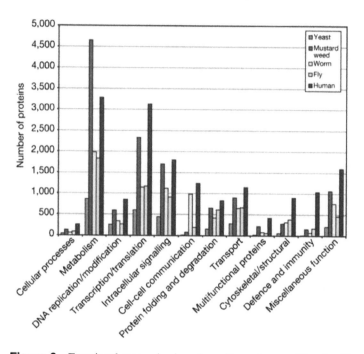

Figure 2 Functional categories in eukaryotic proteomes. The classification categories were derived from functional classification systems, including the top-level biological function category of the Gene Ontology Project (GO; see *http://www.geneontology.org*). Initial sequencing and analysis of the human genome. International Human Genome Sequencing Consortium. Nature. Feb 15, 2001; 409(6822): 860–921.

bioinformatic sequence alignment tools it has been possible to group these modules into classes and demonstrate the conservation and expansion of shared modules during the course of evolution (Table 1).

Ancestral proteins of prokaryotic origin have given rise to eukaryotic proteins with new functions, such as the suspected transition of the bacterial FtsZ to the eukaryotic tubulin protein [4], as well as immunological proteins restricted to multicellular organisms. It is the molecular evolution of these ancestral genes that have given rise to a multitude of proteins that have diverse function yet can be categorized into families on the basis of their relatedness.

In addition, through genetic and biochemical experimentation of proteins with similar motifs and domains, the functions of these sequences are being identified and will provide us with even more information about proteins with undefined function. By the association of sequence and biochemical/biological data, the suggestion of biological function for proteins is possible.

Table 1 Domain Sharing and Order Conservation Within Human and Between Human and Other Eukaryotes

Human versus	Domain sharing					Identical domain arrangements			
	No. of proteins sharing domains	No. of cases				Total no. of domains in a protein	No. of identical arrangements/no. of human proteins		
		No. of domain types					No of domain types*		
		1	2	3	>3		2	3	>3
Human	2	214	194	73	61	1	-	-	-
	3	147	88	25	18	2	141/656	-	-
	4	123	38	17	5	3	57/208	21/62	-
	5	67	17	5	3	4	53/188	18/63	4/10
	6	56	19	5	0	5	44/173	11/27	5/16
	>6	377	79	20	5	>5	150/605	66/172	34/78
Fly	1	143	129	32	23	1	-	-	-
	2	134	65	14	12	2	119/337	-	-
	3	97	47	11	5	3	35/98	10/18	-
	4	83	19	7	0	4	28/65	10/24	1/1
	5	51	9	2	2	5	25/74	8/17	5/13
	>5	359	65	14	2	>5	58/137	11/19	12/16
Worm	1	136	92	27	9	1	-	-	-
	2	124	56	11	12	2	89/307	-	-
	3	94	38	9	7	3	28/118	10/24	-
	4	84	17	5	2	4	16/39	6/20	0/0
	5	46	8	2	2	5	16/60	3/8	3/6
	>5	355	61	11	1	>5	43/118	8/16	9/13
Yeast	1	135	51	8	2	1	-	-	-
	2	91	27	5	0	2	51/199	-	-
	3	64	18	2	0	3	9/20	4/12	-
	4	58	5	0	0	4	4/7	3/3	0/0
	5	41	3	0	0	5	3/6	1/2	1/1
	>5	260	24	4	1	>5	36/16	1/3	0/0
Fly, worm and yeast	1	75	24	4	1	1	-	-	-
	2	78	16	3	0	2	26/145	-	-
	3	49	12	1	0	3	**4/10**	1/3	-
	4	48	3	0	0	4	3/5	0/0	0/0
	5	33	2	0	0	5	3/6	0/0	1/1
	>5	249	21	3	1	>5	7/18	0/0	0/0

*Number of unique domain arrangements/number of human proteins in which these arrangements are found. The second number is larger than the first because many proteins may share the same arrangement. For example, in the case 4/10 (bold numbers) there are four unique arrangements of three-domain proteins with two domain types (for example, the arrangement A-B-A has three domains but only two domain types: A and B) that have been conserved among human, fly, worm, and yeast: In human there are 10 such proteins.

B. Sequence and Protein Families

As stated previously, the proteins selected by molecular evolution are a subset of all possible proteins and can be categorized into families (Table 2). It is the sequence similarity of DNA, as well as the protein, that serves as the measure of evolutionary distance and perhaps suggests altered or new protein function.

Table 2 The Largest Protein Families[a]

Family	Source	Modules in SwissProt	Found where?
C2H2 zinc fingers	PF00096	1826	Eukaryotes, archaea
Immunoglobulin module	F000471	351	Animals
Protein (Ser/Thr/Tyr) kinases	PF00069	928	All kingdoms
EGF-like domain	PF00008	854	Animals
EF-hand (Ca binding)	PF00036	790	Animals
Globins	PF00042	699	Eukaryotes, bacteria
GPCR-rhodopsin	PF00001	597	Animals
Fibronectin type III	PF00041	514	Eukaryotes, bacteria
Chymotrypsins	PR00722	464	Eukaryotes, bacteria
Homeodomain	PF00046	453	Eukaryotes
ABC cassette	PF00005	373	All kingdoms
Sushi domain	PF00084	343	Animals
RNA-binding domain	PF00076	331	Eukaryotes
Ankrin repeat	PF00023	330	Eukaryotes
RuBisCo large subunit	PF00016	319	Plants, bacteria
LDL receptor A	PF00057	309	Animals

[a]The sources for there numbers of modules are Pfam (PE) or Prints (PR).
GPCR, G-protein-coupled receptor; EGF, epidermal growth factor; ABC, xxxxx; LDL, low-density lipoprotein.

Through the use of bioinformatic tools, as well as the extensive amount of sequence data available in public databases, it is now becoming a common practice to investigate the relationships between the protein sequence of a gene and to classify it in a specific protein family. Comparing the protein and DNA sequence of novel proteins with other proteins of known function and similar structure, we are able to predict biochemical or biological properties based on previously collected data on these family members [2,3,5,7–9,12]. An important caveat and difficulty with this process is that many proteins in higher organisms have evolved through fusion of the functional domains of existing proteins and are a composite of more than one protein ancestral family (Fig. 3).

The homeodomain family of transcription factors serves as the best example of this modular design. Since many transcription factors rely on a DNA binding domain as well as an additional domain that allows for the activation of the transcription factor, multiple protein sequences will align and cluster under these separate domains. Therefore, insight into the biological function of these new proteins from its family association can be misleading. Nevertheless, these bioinformatic techniques are expected to provide a wealth of detailed information to the

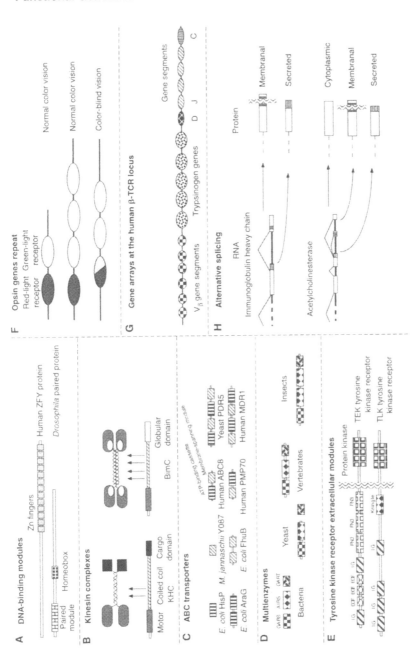

Figure 3 A comparison of protein families in which the sequence conservation during molecular evolution has given rise to proteins of similar yet distinct function.

biologist searching for clues as to how the orphan protein of interest is involved with the model under investigation [13]. Table 2 is a short list of the largest protein families and where they can be found [2].

As a consequence, the DNA sequence similarity of most proteins is highly conserved between protein families as well as species in regions of functional importance. The most common observation is that the portion of the protein that is responsible for the interaction of that protein with other molecules has at least a weak similarity in protein sequence and is the focus of family categorization.

III. MOLECULAR PATHWAYS

Through large-scale analysis of human genes and the proteins they produce, a detailed map of the human body will provide a blueprint of molecular pathways, which will describe how the complicated interactions of proteins support our existence. A blueprint of this interdependent network is vital to the development of drugs that will be used to influence the quality of life through pharmaceutical intervention. Figure 4 represents a common molecular pathway that helps illustrate the dependency on many factors to respond to the extracellular signal provided by platelet-derived growth factor (PDGF). The final response to the envi-

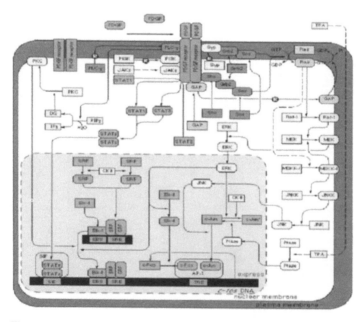

Figure 4   The platelet-derived growth factor molecular pathway.

ronmental signal is largely dependent on the abundance and state of the proteins the pathway. The lack of expression or the inactivation of the downstream proteins can lead to a breakdown in the communication of the signal or the diversion of the signal toward an alternative pathway.

Drug discovery is based on determining which compounds are best suited for the systemic, or tissue-specific, manipulation of biological function for the long-term chemical compensation of patients with a weak genetic background or the temporary modulation of life-sustaining systems threatened as a result of injury [6,20–22]. Functional genomics promises to provide researchers with detailed feedback on the effectiveness, as well as negative consequences, of this intervention at the molecular level. In order to produce drugs that manipulate biological function but do not produce side effects that prohibit its use, it will become commonplace to incorporate large-scale genomic methods that reveal shortcomings of the drug being tested.

A. Signal Transduction

The foundation of most drug discovery projects relies on the ability of cells within a tissue to be influenced by the local environment. This response is due to the presence of proteins on the surface of the cell, like the PDGF receptor, that sense the environmental changes and transduce this signal into the cell and alter its biochemical state. By altering the behavior of even a subset of cells within a tissue, the function of whole organs can be altered, leading to the adjustment of life-sustaining parameters necessary to maintain higher order functions. *Signal transduction* is made possible by networks of interacting proteins working in concert to achieve changes in cellular function. The state of the cell is defined by parameters such as the complement of proteins being synthesized and processed, their enzymatic activity, and their location within the cell, as well as changes in the equilibrium of ions across intracellular and extracellular membranes. The state of the cell determines how it will respond to the environment [1]. For instance, will it secrete specific humoral factors, such as insulin, or contract upon neuronal stimulus like muscle cells? The presence of receptors that are inserted into the cell membrane allow for the interaction of signaling molecules, called *ligands,* on the outside of the cell to influence the function of cells by altering the state of protein networks within the cell.

B. Protein–Protein Interaction

The cellular signaling mechanism responds to perceived signals from receptors through networks of proteins that come in direct contact with one another. This protein–protein interaction serves as one criteria for protein domain conservation during molecular evolution [11,16] and can be recognized by the massively parallel collection of sequence and expression data offered by genomic technologies. Sequence alignment of protein family members across many species, in conjunction with biologically relevant experimentation, provides important insight into the function of these conserved sequence elements and therefore must be carefully considered during the assignment of function of any one protein.

C. Tertiary Structure and Convergence

In some cases the functions of two proteins separated by great evolutionary distances converge. In these cases, it is common to have very little similarity in protein sequence yet similar function (Fig. 5) [16]. By viewing the tertiary structure of two proteins that share a similar function, general similarities can be seen. The tools for comparing the three-dimensional conformation of proteins in order to understand function are still in their infancy. Therefore, it is necessary to rely on the information contained within the primary sequence of the two proteins to investigate the rules that control the ability of that protein to perform its function. Determining what structural characteristics allow proteins to interact with the rest of its molecular pathway will make it possible to more accurately predict the consequences of their individual contribution to that pathway. For example, it is well known that defined mutations within the homeodomain of certain transcription factors will specifically alter the sequence specificity on which the transcription factor binds, required for the induction or repression of gene transcription. Moreover, a better understanding of there structural characteristics would allow for the logical design of small molecules to modulate specific components of that path-

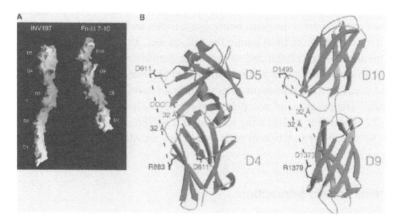

Figure 5 **A:** Note the structural similarities between the invasin extracellular region and the fibronectin type III domain. **B:** A ribbon diagram illustrating the tertiary structure with only 20% sequence identity.

way, potentially translating into drugs with higher fidelity, fewer side effects, and increasing the number of targets on which drugs are designed.

D. Gene Expression and Protein Kinetics

Proteins function at the molecular level and are governed by the laws of probability and molecular kinetics. If the concentration of a protein is increased beyond some critical value, the probability that that protein will come into contact with its correct partner is increased. Yet, as a consequence of its increased rate of interaction with all molecules in the cell, interactions with inappropriate branches of the intracellular regulatory network become common. This altered protein function is similar to the altered specificity of drugs that have been given at high doses to achieve an effect but cause unwanted side effects. By monitoring the normal concentration of regulatory proteins in the cell, it may be possible to recognize patterns of expression that are associated with disease, as well as define the correct abundance ranges of proteins to achieve stability and avoidance from a pathological state. Figure 6 represents data collected through the use of microarray technology in which mRNA from patients with the premature aging disorder progeria is compared with that of "normals" of differing age groups. These data provide an example of similarities in the abundance of proteins expressed within these two groups and suggests that these proteins are somehow involved in progeria.

Techniques that provide information on the abundance of proteins in cells will be crucial to understanding how the many molecular pathways coordinate the maintenance of the intracellular environment. It is also well known that cells of multicellular organisms do not express all available proteins in every cell. By expressing specific proteins at a particular abundance, alternate cell types are available to the organism. To understand biological function, it is necessary to determine which protein complements are required for any one specific cellular contribution to the organism.

Another possibility for the use of this kind of information is that it may make it possible to treat one cell type so that it may carry out the function of another. By modifying the abundance of a subset of proteins required to compensate for the loss of that cell type, pharmaceutical intervention may allow for the compensation of diseases in which cells of a particular type have been destroyed. Potential targets for such treatment are found in diabetic patients where the loss of insulin-producing pancreatic islet cells has been effected through an autoimmune response, as well as dopamine-producing cells of the central nervous system involved in Parkinson's disease. The ability to control cell identity is dependent on being able to determine which signaling molecules are necessary to achieve changes in protein expression, thereby mimicking the cell that has been destroyed. For this, the expression profile of that cell must serve as the defining characteristic to be achieved by pharmaceutical intervention.

Middle Age

Cell Cycle Control Proteins

Acc.#	FoldΔ	Gene Name
X13293	-4.8	B-myb
U74612	-3.3	Hepatocyte nuclear factor-3/fork head homolog 11A (HFH-11A)
Z36714	-12.5	Cyclin F
X51688	-5.4	Cyclin A
M25753	-2.9	Cyclin B
U01038	-2.8	pLK
U05340	-2.9	p55CDC

Chromosomal Processing and Assembly

Acc.#	FoldΔ	Gene Name
U30872	-2.6	Mitosin (CENP-F)
X67155	-3.5	Mitotic kinesin-like protein-1
U37436	-3.6	Kinesin-like spindle protein (HKSP)
X14850	-2.2	Histone (H2A.X)
U14518	-3.3	Centromere protein-A (CENP-A)
U63743	-2.8	Mitotic centromere-associated kinesin
X13546	-2.0	Non-histone chromosomal protein HMG-17

Protein Processing

Acc.#	FoldΔ	Gene Name
U73379	-2.3	Cyclin-selective ubiquitin carrier protein

Old Age

Cell Cycle Control Proteins

Acc.#	FoldΔ	Gene Name
X13293	-4.9	B-myb
U74612	-9.0	Hepatocyte nuclear factor-3/fork head homolog 11A (HFH-11A)
Z36714	-13.1	Cyclin F
X51688	-5.8	Cyclin A
M25753	-5.2	Cyclin B
U01038	-3.0	pLK
U05340	-4.3	p55CDC
S78187	-7.6	CDC25B
U56816	-8.7	Kinase Myt1 (Myt1)
X54941	-2.6	Clks1 Cks1 protein homologue
M30448	-2.2	Casein kinase II beta subunit
U37002	-4.0	Cyclin-dependent kinase 4 (CDK4)
U49844	-3.0	FRAP-related protein (ATR, ATM)
X74008	-3.0	Protein phosphatase 1 gamma

Chromosomal Processing and Assembly

Acc.#	FoldΔ	Gene Name
U30872	-2.6	Mitosin (CENP-F)
X67155	-3.5	Mitotic kinesin-like protein-1
U37436	-3.6	Kinesin-like spindle protein (HKSP)
X14850	-2.2	Histone (H2A.X)
U14518	-3.3	Centromere protein-A (CENP-A)
U63743	-2.8	Mitotic centromere-associated kinesin
X13546	-2.0	Non-histone chromosomal protein HMG-17
M97856	-3.0	Histone binding protein
D38076	-2.9	RanBP1 (Ran-binding protein 1)
X62534	-4.3	HMG-2
Y08612	-4.1	Nup88 protein
L4363	-2.5	Scaffold attachment factor (SAF-B)
U33286	-3.6	Chromosomal segregation gene homolog CAS
D26361	-4.3	KIAA042 (Centromere protein-E)
M37583	-3.0	Histone (H2A.2)
U72342	-2.3	Platelet activating factor acetylhydrolase (45 Kda subunit LIS1)
D43948	-2.6	KIA00097 (36% similar to yeast Suppressor of tubulin STU2)

Protein Processing

Acc.#	FoldΔ	Gene Name
U73379	-3.5	Cyclin-selective ubiquitin carrier protein
AB003102	-2.7	26S proteasome subunit p44.5
AB003103	-3.7	Proteasome subunit p55
D00760	-2.6	Proteasome subunit HC3
D00762	-3.2	Proteasome subunit HC8
D11094	-3.2	MSS1 (26S proteasome subunit)
D78275	-2.4	Proteasome subunit p42

Progeria

Cell Cycle Control Proteins

Acc.#	FoldΔ	Gene Name
X13293	-7.0	B-myb
U74612	-8.7	Hepatocyte nuclear factor-3/fork head homolog 11A (HFH-11A)
Z36714	-8.7	Cyclin F
S78187	-3.4	CDC25B
U56816	-11.3	Kinase Myt1 (Myt1)
X54941	-4.5	Clshs1 Cks1 protein homologue
M30448	-2.0	Casein kinase II beta subunit
L08246	-2.2	Myeloid cell differentiation protein (MCL1)

Chromosomal Processing and Assembly

Acc.#	FoldΔ	Gene Name
X14850	-6.1	Histone H2A.X
U14518	-4.3	Centromere protein-A (CENP-A)
U63743	-4.8	Mitotic centromere-associated kinesin
X13546	-3.0	Non-histone chromosomal protein HMG 17
M97856	-2.9	Histone binding protein
D38076	-2.7	RanBP1 (Ran-binding protein 1)
X62534	-4.4	HMG-2
Y08612	-3.5	Nup88 protein
L4363	-3.2	Scaffold attachment factor (SAF-B)
U35451	-2.5	Heterochromatin protein p25

Figure 6   Data collected through the use of microarray technology in which mRNA from patience with the premature aging disorder progeria are compared to "normals" of differing age groups.

E. Autoregulation of Gene Expression

The state of a cell is regulated by the activity as well as the complement and abundance of proteins. Therefore, it is common to have immediate changes in cellular function without any change in the expression of proteins. It is this immediate early response that allows for quick adaptation and compensation to environmental conditions. The presence of phosphate on proteins that alter their specificity or enzymatic rates, is a prime example of changes of state that lead to rapid cellular responses, as is subcellular localization. To use genomic techniques for the characterization of novel drugs that are designed to influence these sort of immediate early responses it is necessary to identify changes in protein activity. This is classically performed through the addition of radioactive phosphate that identifies proteins that have incorporated or lost these molecular markers. The purpose of this experimental approach is to ascertain if a regulatory pathway has been altered. Since genomic approaches rely on the measurement of mRNA and only approximate protein abundance, immediate early responses are not easily recognized. Nevertheless, the induction of early response mechanisms can lead to secondary effects on the abundance of proteins through transcriptional modulation. Transcription factors that regulate their own expression have been observed, and it is this autoregulation that allows inference of changes in regulatory pathways by levels of protein expression [14]. It is the change in gene expression observed at times later than the initial treatment of cells that can be used to better understand the way in which a drug has influenced the cells' state. Functional genomics is a tool, and all of the limitations must be recognized when inferring functions onto proteins, cells, and drugs based on changes in gene expression. Nevertheless, the power of large-scale experimentation may provide the information necessary for the informed selection of efficacious drugs.

IV. GENOMICS TECHNIQUES

Genomic methodologies, like microarrays, have been recently implemented to supplant techniques like Northern and Southern blot analyses because, in general, they provide the same type of information with regard to the kind and abundance of proteins in cells [23–26]. Northern blot analysis serves as a measure of the steady-state abundance of mRNA for a transcript of interest, and this is used to approximate the abundance of protein, since for most genes the mRNA abundance in the cell is at least proportional to the amount of protein. The primary difference between genomic and blotting techniques is that many simultaneous approximations of the protein complement of a cell or tissue can be obtained in a fraction of the time. Furthermore, simultaneous measurement of experimental conditions reduces the many false assumptions made from experimental data accumulated over great periods of time. This section will survey and explain a few genomic techniques so that the relevance of the techniques may become obvious.

A. High-Throughput Screening

The term *high-throughput screening* (HTS) relates to the parallel or serial processing of many individual samples in an attempt to obtain a large dataset by which subsets will be identified through selection criteria of many forms. Like looking for the proverbial needle in a hay stack, the elementary question raised by HTS is whether or not a particular "straw" matches your selection criteria. Unlike the more traditional one-straw-at-a-time approach of a sequential search, HTS is characterized by performing massively parallel searches. That is, it tries to look at large numbers of "straws" simultaneously, with each one assessed for the same criteria. As simplistic as it may seem, it is the most direct method by which one evaluates a sample and decide whether it is involved with one's model or not, and the rate at which one proceeds depends greatly on how quickly and accurately the screening takes place. Microarrays are glass slides on which DNA of many different types is placed in an array format. This substrate serves as a methodological platform to identify and measure the level of expressed genes. By placing either of these substrates in direct contact with labeled cDNA, a fluorescent copy of the cell's expressed genes, a measure of gene expression can be made. The question of whether gene A is on or gene B is off can be answered in parallel. If the question is when gene A gets turned on, a million samples may have to run in series before the answer is yes, and therefore making high-throughput screening a necessity (Fig. 7).

B. Microarrays

Microarrays and other solid substrates can augment the progression of genetic analysis. The early to mid-1960s saw the beginning of a genetic revolution, which

MICRO ARRAYS (GENE CHIPS)

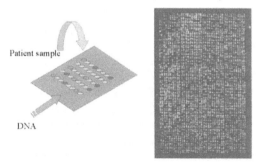

Figure 7   Microarrays (Gene Chips). (Reprinted with permission of Genomic Solutions Inc.)

led to discoveries that until then had not previously been thought possible. Regularly, such journals as *Cell, Science,* and *Nature* were publishing articles pertaining to the cloning and characterization of novel genes. As technology progressed, it became clear that the regulation of the newly found genes was complicated and interlaced with environmental influences, as well as intercellular communication pathways. To make any headway into the analysis of such a complicated network of gene regulation, a fast and effective protocol for looking at the expression of these genes would be critical. Microarray technologies were developed to help researchers investigate the complex nature of gene expression and continue to be utilized on an enormous scale. To better understand the full scope of microarray and other technologies, it is helpful to be introduced to the applications in which the genomic tools are used.

C. Single-Nucleotide Polymorphism Detection

Polymorphism is the property of taking on many forms, and it is used to describe the natural changes in the DNA sequence of a gene relative to other alleles. Microarrays and new techniques can quickly and reliably screen for single-base-pair changes in the DNA code for an entire gene (polymorphism) by using the sequence by hybridization method [26]. Sequencing through the hybridization of a target molecule to a known array of oligonucleotides has been performed successfully and will be used extensively for the monitoring of changes related to disease [26]. With the help of genomic technologies, or by knowing the sequence of a gene associated with a disease, the diagnoses of patients with a higher degree of confidence is predicted to mature [20–23]. Since the sequence of a gene can identify phenotypic characteristics that are associated with many metabolic processes, the technique may also make it possible to use this information in deciding the proper course of treatment for patients when the ailment is known; this is called *pharmacogenomics.* It is well known that patients with varying genetic backgrounds respond to treatments of disease to varying degrees. Through the sequencing of particular genes related to drug-metabolizing enzymes and genes as yet unknown, we may obtain a rationale for drug therapy and design [23].

Single-nucleotide polymorphism (SNP) detection will be very similar to the sequencing of a whole gene, but there will only be representatives of known polymorphisms. An example of this kind of approach to diagnostics was presented by Loyd Smith et al. in 1994. He used polymerase chain reaction (PCR) to produce a defined probe. He hybridized this probe to a matrix of known oligonucleotides representing exon 4 (the coding component of messenger RNA) of the human tyrosinase gene, and then scored and assessed the presence of polymorphisms. Another example of this kind of approach was performed by Kathrine W. Klinger et al. whereby a complex, defined PCR probe was used to assess the presence of polymorphisms in the genes involved in cystic fibrosis, β-thalassemia, sickle cell anemia, Tay-Sachs disease, Gaucher's disease, Canavan's disease, Fanconi's anemia, and breast cancer.

D. Deletion Detection

Microarray and others analysis may also be performed to characterize a deletion, insertion, or mutation in genes that have been correlated to disease, such as the *p53* gene to cancer. If it is suspected that a gene is mutated, clinicians will isolate DNA from the patient, use this DNA to create a probe, and then hybridize this probe to an array that can identify mutations in that gene.

E. Differential Display by Hybridization

Use of microarrays and other substrates for hybridization with cDNA produced from cells or tissue will make possible the identification of regulatory genes involved in the control of human disease [23]. There are models for cellular differentiation and diseases in which cDNA probes can be obtained for the purpose of hybridization to microarrays and others. The genes identified by differential hybridization to these substrates can be used as candidates in the characterization of human disease and, once identified, confirm the involvement of these candidate genes in disease. If this approach is successful, these disease genes can be used as a target for the production of drugs that influence the expression of the genes. Figure 8 represents an example of this approach. Prostate cancer cells were treated with a chemopreventive agent to determine its involvement in prostate cancer. The observation that make this example important is that the cells were cultured under two different conditions but, of the 5000 genes that were screened, all but a few were differentially expressed. This suggests that the change induced by the treatment may be minor and understandable. These sorts of experiments, in conjunction with additional supporting data, will provide candidates that can be screened for their usefulness as drug targets.

One of the most important questions asked by today's research scientists is, what is different between two cell types (e.g., disease vs. normal, treated vs. untreated)? The only methods available for this kind of query are differential display, representational difference analysis (RDA), subtractive hybridization, serial analysis of gene expression (SAGE), and differential hybridization to cDNA libraries. An exceptional example of this approach was performed by Bertrand R. Jordan, who implemented microarrays in his hunt for genes that define the existence of three cell types in the murine thymus. By creating a 3' complex probe and hybridizing this to a microarray, he found novel genes that were differentially expressed between the three cell types. This methodology can be implemented for other models of disease as well and may lead researchers to rational therapies for the devastating medical disorders that plague our society.

Figure 8 Prostate cancer cells were treated with a chemopreventive agent to determine its involvement in prostate cancer. (Reproduced with permission of Dr. Fazul Sarkar, Department of Pathology, and David O'Hagan, Center of Molecular Medicine and Genetics, Wayne State University.)

F. Expression Monitoring

Expression monitoring is another approach that takes advantage of the large databases of sequenced cDNAs. By designing arrays that contain representatives of the most important genes that control the cell cycle and involve cellular regulation, an evaluation of cellular and tissue state is possible. The power of new bioinformatics software will improve the usefulness of this method, and such software is frequently used. Another possible application that has been discussed is the diagnosis of disease by association of a pattern of hybridization with that disease, as compared to positive and negative controls. In other words, does a tissue resemble a specific expression pattern as a consequence of disease?

With the recent advances in bioinformatics technology and the development of microarrays and tools that contain the number of probes necessary for the analysis of gene expression, it is now possible to confront the daunting task of human genetic analysis. Moreover, some pathological conditions caused by environmental insults instigate a cascade of changes in gene expression that can have drastic outcomes, as experienced by patients with the autoimmune disorder rheumatoid arthritis. Given the complexity of cellular signaling and regulatory pathways a cell, it has been impossible to address these numerous interdependent changes occurring during biological process, be it pathological or normal. This allows physicians and scientists to address the needs of the cell, clearly a substantial contribution to the reduction of human morbidity.

G. Finding Targets for Drug Development

As mentioned previously, most drugs are small organic molecules that are ingested and introduced into the circulatory system, whereupon they bind to receptors on the surface of cells whose function is to be influenced. There are approximately 30,000–35,000 genes in the human genome producing an even greater number of proteins through alternative splicing and differences in post-translational modification. Unfortunately, only a handful of these proteins serve as targets for pharmaceutical intervention [21]. To increase the range of influence available to clinicians through drug treatment, it will be necessary to broaden the scope of protein targets used during drug development. Yet, before drugs can be specified for the treatment of clinical symptoms, a clear picture of the physiological and molecular pathways involved with the disease or pathological process must be assessed. To understand the function of any system, all the components of that system as well as their interactions must be known. It is not enough merely to catalog all of the proteins expressed in a cell type. The interrelationships of expressed proteins must be determined through careful planning of experimental models that have defined measurable physiological or molecular changes. The extent to which the model has been characterized can synergistically increase the amount and value of the conclusions drawn from the individual experiment. Like a jigsaw puzzle, the next piece of data must be based on the existing framework.

In order to increase the rate of discovery, experimental data must be gathered in parallel. This has been made possible through the advent of molecular techniques such as that associated with microarray technology. The probability of success in any experimental fishing expedition is the size and quality of the net used. With microarrays, the expression of approximately 10,000 genes can be monitored from as little as 5 µg of total mRNA. Since there are many experimental models that have distinct physiological or molecular changes associated with a defined cell type, a wealth of data can be acquired in parallel. Nevertheless, the quality of the data rests in the hands of the individuals who are responsible for the sample handling and tracking. As there are so many data to be analyzed, a small error in sample tracking can lead to devastating errors in the conclusions drawn from experiments. Sample tracking is a crucial component of the data collection and review process. In this case, the old adage "Garbage in, garbage out" rings true. If the acquisition and storage of highly parallel data can be performed with some degree of confidence, then the sky is the limit. Similarities and differences, or the correlation of expressed genes with changes in responses of cells to their environment, will expand our understanding of the human machine at rates not thought of 10 years ago.

V. SUMMARY

Functional genomics is a term used to describe the assembly of data to better understand the form and function of the cell. Much is already known about the mechanisms that govern a cell's interaction with its environment, and it is this base of knowledge that will act as the primer for solving the puzzles of biology. DNA, RNA, and proteins act together to maintain the integrity of cellular environment, and how they interact with each other is the information accessible through many newly developed high-throughput technologies. By applying high-throughput technologies to the information already known about how cells respond to their environment (functional genomics), the development of efficacious drugs with few side effects through intelligent design will be possible.

REFERENCES

1. Henikoff S, Greene EA, Pietrokovski S, Bork P, Attwood TK, Hood L. Gene families: the taxonomy of protein paralogs and chimeras. Science 1997; 278:5338 (609–614).
2. Davies DE, Djukanovic R, Holgate ST. Application of functional genomics to study of inflammatory airways disease. Thorax Jan 1999; 54(1):79–81.
3. Clayton RA, White O, Ketchum KA, Venter JC. First genome from the third domain of life. Nature May 29, 1997; 387(6632):459–462.
4. Desai A, Mitchison TJ. Tubulin and FtsZ structures: functional and therapeutic implications Bioessays Jul 1998; 20(7):523–527. Review.
5. Tatusov RL, Koonin EV, Lipman DJ, A genomic perspective on protein families. Science Oct 24 1997; 278(5338):631–637. Review
6. Hieter P, Boguski M. Functional genomics: it's all how you read it. Science Oct 24, 1997; 278(5338):601–602.
7. Aravind L, Dixit VM, Koonin EV. Apoptotic molecular machinery: vastly increased complexity in vertebrates revealed by genome comparisons. Science Feb 16, 2001; 291(5507):1279–1284.
8. Patthy L. Evolution of the proteases of blood coagulation and fibrinolysis by assembly from modules. Cell Jul 1985; 41(3):657–663. Review.
9. Green P, Lipman D, Hillier L, Waterston R, States D, Claverie JM. Ancient conserved regions in new gene sequences and the protein databases. Science Mar 19, 1993; 259(5102):1711–1716.
10. Lander ES, Linton LM, Birren B, Nusbaum C, Zody MC, Baldwin J, Devon K, Dewar K, Doyle M, FitzHugh W, Funke R, Gage D, Harris K, Heaford A, Howland J, Kann L, Lehoczky J, LeVine R, McEwan P, McKernan K, Meldrim J, Mesirov JP, Miranda C, Morris W, Naylor J, Raymond C, Rosetti M, Santos R, Sheridan A, Sougnez C, Stange-Thomann N, Stojanovic N, Subramanian A, Wyman D, Rogers J, Sulston J, Ainscough R, Beck S, Bentley D, Burton J, Clee C, Carter N, Coulson A, Deadman R, Deloukas P, Dunham A, Dunham I, Durbin R, French L, Grafham D, Gregory S, Hubbard T, Humphray S, Hunt A, Jones M, Lloyd C, McMurray A, Matthews L, Mercer S, Milne S, Mullikin JC, Mungall A, Plumb R, Ross M, Shownkeen R, Sims S, Waterston RH, Wilson RK, Hillier LW, McPherson JD, Marra MA, Mardis ER, Fulton LA, Chinwalla AT, Pepin KH, Gish WR, Chissoe SL, Wendl MC, Delehaunty KD, Miner TL, Delehaunty A, Kramer JB, Cook LL, Fulton RS, Johnson DL, Minx PJ, Clifton SW, Hawkins T, Branscomb E, Predki P, Richardson P, Wen-

ning S, Slezak T, Doggett N, Cheng JF, Olsen A, Lucas S, Elkin C, Uberbacher E, Frazier M, Gibbs RA, Muzny DM, Scherer SE, Bouck JB, Sodergren EJ, Worley KC, Rives CM, Gorrell JH, Metzker ML, Naylor SL, Kucherlapati RS, Nelson DL, Weinstock GM, Sakaki Y, Fujiyama A, Hattori M, Yada T, Toyoda A, Itoh T, Kawagoe C, Watanabe H, Totoki Y, Taylor T, Weissenbach J, Heilig R, Saurin W, Artiguenave F, Brottier P, Bruls T, Pelletier E, Robert C, Wincker P, Smith DR, Doucette-Stamm L, Rubenfield M, Weinstock K, Lee HM, Dubois J, Rosenthal A, Platzer M, Nyakatura G, Taudien S, Rump A, Yang H, Yu J, Wang J, Huang G, Gu J, Hood L, Rowen L, Madan A, Qin S, Davis RW, Federspiel NA, Abola AP, Proctor MJ, Myers RM, Schmutz J, Dickson M, Grimwood J, Cox DR, Olson MV, Kaul R, Raymond C, Shimizu N, Kawasaki K, Minoshima S, Evans GA, Athanasiou M, Schultz R, Roe BA, Chen FP. Initial sequencing and analysis of the human genome. International Human Genome Sequencing Consortium. Nature Feb 15, 2001; 409(6822):860–921.

11.   Lockless SW, Ranganathan R. Evolutionarily conserved pathways of energetic connectivity in protein families. Science Oct 8, 1999; 286(5438):295–299.

12.   Courseaux A, Nahon JL. Birth of two chimeric genes in the hominidae lineage. Science Feb 16, 2001; 291(5507):1293–1297.

13.   Nicholas HB, Deerfield DW, Ropelewski AJ. Strategies for searching sequence databases. Biotechniques Jun 2000; 28(6):1174–1178, 1180, 1182 passim.

14.   Arnone MI, Davidson EH. The hardwiring of development: organization and function of genomic regulatory systems. Development May 1997; 124(10):1851–1864. Review.

15.   Tupler R, Perini G, Green MR. Expressing the human genome. Nature Feb 15, 2001; 409(6822):832–833.

16.   Hamburger ZA, Brown MS, Isberg RR, Bjorkman PJ. Crystal structure of invasin: a bacterial integrin-binding protein. Science Oct 8, 1999; 286(5438):291–295.

17.   Weinstein JN, Myers TG, O'Connor PM, Friend SH, Fornace AJ, Kohn KW, Fojo T, Bates SE, Rubinstein LV, Anderson NL, Buolamwini JK, van Osdol WW, Monks AP, Scudiero DA, Sausville EA, Zaharevitz DW, Bunow B, Viswanadhan VN, Johnson GS, Wittes RE, Paull KD. An information-intensive approach to the molecular pharmacology of cancer. Science Jan 17, 1997; 275(5298):343–349.

18.   Caron H, Schaik Bv B, Mee Mv M, Baas F, Riggins G, Sluis Pv P, Hermus MC, Asperen Rv R, Boon K, Voute PA, Heisterkamp S, Kampen Av A, Versteeg R. The human transcriptome map: clustering of highly expressed genes in chromosomal domains. Science Feb 16, 2001; 291(5507):1289–1292.

19.   Chee M, Yang R, Hubbell E, Berno A, Huang XC, Stern D, Winkler J, Lockhart DJ, Morris MS, Fodor SP. Accessing genetic information with high-density DNA arrays. Science Oct 25, 1996; 274(5287):610–614.

20.   Friend SH. Oliff A. Emerging uses for genomic information in drug discovery. N Engl J Med Jul 6, 1998; 338(1):125–126.

21.   Drews J. Drug discovery: a historical perspective. Mar 17, 2000; 287(5460): 1960–1964.

22.   Evans WE, Relling MV. Pharmacogenomics: translating functional genomics into rational therapeutics. Science Oct 15, 1999; 286(5439):487–491. Review.

23.   Heller RA, Schena M, Chai A, Shalon D, Bedilion T, Gilmore J, Woolley DE, Davis RW. Discovery and analysis of inflammatory disease-related genes using cDNA microarrays. Proc Natl Acad Sci USA Mar 18, 1997; 94(6):2150–2155.

24. Marx J. Genetics. Chipping away at the causes of aging. Science Mar 31, 2000; 287(5462):2390.

25. Schena M, Shalon D, Davis RW, Brown PO. Quantitative monitoring of gene expression patterns with a complementary DNA microarray. Science Oct 20, 1995; 270(5235):467–470.

26. Lipshutz RJ, Morris D, Chee M, Hubbell E, Kozal MJ, Shah N, Shen N, Yang R, Fodor SP. Using oligonucleotide probe arrays to access genetic diversity. Biotechniques Sep 1995; 19(3):442–447. Review.

4
Integrated Proteomics Technologies

Joseph A. Loo, James A. Blackledge, Ping Du, Greg W. Kilby, Robert A. Lepley,* Joseph Macri,† Rachel R. Ogorzalek Loo, Stephen T. Rapundalo, and Tracy I. Stevenson
Pfizer Global Research and Development
Ann Arbor, Michigan

I. INTRODUCTION

Proteomics is a powerful approach for integration into drug discovery because it allows the examination of the cellular target of drugs, namely, proteins. Understanding how drugs affect protein expression is a key goal of proteomics in a drug discovery program. Mapping of proteomes, the protein complements to genomes, from tissues and organisms has been used for development of high-throughput screens, for validation and forwarding of new protein targets, for SAR development and for exploring mechanisms of action or toxicology of compounds, and for identification of protein biomarkers in disease. For example, Arnot and coworkers describe an integrated proteomics approach to identify proteins differing in expression levels in phenylephrine-induced hypertrophy of cardiac muscle cells (myocytes) [1]. Once a proteome is established and expressed proteins are linked to their respective genes, then the proteome becomes a powerful means to examine global changes in protein levels and expression under changing environmental conditions. The proteome becomes a reference for future comparison across cell types and species. It is expected that proteomics will lead to important new insights into disease mechanisms and improved drug discovery strategies to produce novel therapeutics.

Current affiliations: *TIS Group, Minneapolis, Minnesota
†McMaster University, Hamilton, Ontario, Canada

The application of proteomics to the study of biochemical pathways and the identification of potentially important gene products as targets for drug discovery is well established in the literature [2–4]. Celis et al. are exploring the possibility of using proteome expression profiles of fresh bladder tumors to search for protein markers that may form the basis for diagnosis, prognosis, and treatment [5]. Ultimately, the goal in these studies is to identify signaling pathways and components that are affected at various stages of bladder cancer progression and that may provide novel leads in drug discovery. The explosive growth of the proteomics arena is illustrated by the rapid increase in the number of publications in the past few years (Fig. 1). Studying individual proteins in the context of other cellular proteins is complementary to the information gathered from a genomics-based approach.

In order to increase the capacity and throughput of the information flow derived from a proteomics-based research program, several newly developed technologies must be highly integrated to yield a complete and efficient proteomics-based methodology [6,7]. The traditional approach involves the separation of the highly complex protein mixture, with two-dimensional electrophoresis (2-DE, or 2-D PAGE for two-dimensional polyacrylamide gel electrophoresis)—the most popular method because of its high sample capacity and separation efficiency. Associated with 2-DE are the necessary means to analyze and store the gel images for protein correlation and data tracking. A major component of the proteomics assembly is bioinformatics, including methods that correlate changes observed in the gel patterns (attributed to changes in the environment) and software that identifies proteins from genomic and protein sequences.

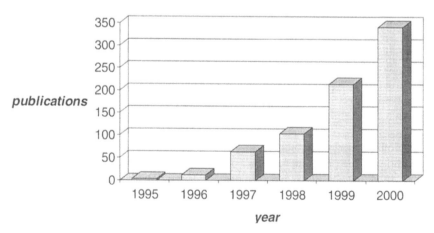

Figure 1 "Proteomics" literature publications as a function of publication year. The literature search was accomplished through the SciFinder program (American Chemical Society).

A proteomics-based approach has been practiced for many years, to monitor differential protein expression. However, at the time the term "proteomics" was coined [8], the technology presented by new mass spectrometric methods was developed to make the identification of proteins separated by PAGE more amenable, and it has greatly expanded the range of applications to which proteomics can contribute. Mass spectrometry provides a robust method for protein identification (provided the genome or protein sequences are known and available) and is being applied in many labs worldwide. The method can be automated, thereby greatly increasing the throughput of the analysis if many proteins need to be identified. The virtues of mass spectrometry have played an important role in honing the burgeoning field of proteomics, and mass spectrometry will continue to support these escalating efforts. This chapter serves to outline the major technologies associated with a proteomics-based approach to drug discovery.

II. GEL ELECTROPHORESIS

A. Two-Dimensional Gel Electrophoresis

Since its inception, 2-DE has provided researchers with a powerful tool that is capable of resolving a complex protein mixture into its individual components [9]. As implied by its descriptive nomenclature, two-dimensional electrophoresis, 2-DE systems separate proteins on the basis of distinct properties in each of two dimensions. In each dimension, the chosen property of the individual proteins within the mixture defines the mobility of individual proteins within an electrical field. As defined in this chapter, the term 2-DE describes a technique that separates proteins in the first electrophoretic dimension on the basis of their charge and in the second electrophoretic dimension on the basis of their molecular mass. While 2-DE separations of protein mixtures can theoretically be carried out in free, aqueous solvent systems, the resultant separations are of little practical value due principally to thermal convection and diffusion effects. Thermal effects caused by joule heating during the separation and the effects of diffusion following the separation will serve to severely limit protein separation and, ultimately, protein resolution. To minimize these effects, 2-DE is carried out in a polyacrylamide support medium. The utility of polymerizing acrylamide monomers into an electrophoretic support matrix capable of reproducibly separating complex protein mixtures was recognized long before the advent of 2-DE systems [10,11]. While either electrophoretic dimension alone can independently resolve 100–200 individual proteins, the combined separation properties resident in 2-DE systems offer investigators the ability to resolve up to 10,000 individual proteins [12]. The route to this level of understanding of how 2-DE systems can facilitate our understanding of the proteome has been a scientifically arduous evolution.

Protein separation in the first dimension is based on the isoelectric point (pI) of individual proteins. Isoelectric focusing (IEF) depends on the formation of a continuous pH gradient through which a protein migrates under the influence of an electrical field. The net charge on the protein varies with the pH but approaches zero at its pI. At a pH equivalent to its pI, movement of the protein in the electrical field ceases, and the protein is "isoelectrically focused." In practical terms, IEF is achieved using either carrier ampholyte gels or immobilized pH gradient (IPG) gels. Carrier ampholytes are oligoamino and oligocarboxylic acid derivatives with molecular weights ranging from 600 to 900 D. By blending many carrier ampholyte species together, highly reproducible continuous pH gradients between pH 3 and 10 can be formed in a polyacrylamide support matrix. Typically, the first-dimension pH gradient and polyacrylamide support matrix are cast in a tube gel format that conforms to the physical measurements of the second-dimension gel system. Carrier ampholyte IEF tube gels possess several advantages over IPG strip gels. First, they are easily prepared and do not require specialized gradient-forming instrumentation. Second, carrier ampholyte IEF gels can be experimentally tailored to generate linear or nonlinear pH gradients in broad or very narrow ranges [13]. Disadvantages of carrier ampholyte use include (1) lot-to-lot variation in the ampholytes themselves attributable to complicated organic synthetic methods and (2) the physical chemical effect termed "cathodic drift" that prevents a truly stable pH equilibrium state from being obtained in the first-dimension gel system. The tangible effect of cathodic drift is a progressive deterioration of the basic side of the pH gradient that can be compensated for by addressing factors such as the time and power requirements [14].

Immobilized pH gradient gel chemistry is based on Pharmacia Immobiline acrylamido buffers [15]. These chemical entities are bifunctional. The general chemical structure $CH_2=CH—CO—NH—R$ defines one end of the molecule, designated R, as the titrant moiety where a weak carboxyl or amino group provides an ionizable buffer capacity that defines the range of the continuous pH gradient. At the other end of the molecule, the $CH_2=CH—$ moiety provides an acrylic double bond that copolymerizes into the polyacrylamide support matrix. It is the polymerization of the Immobiline buffers into the polyacrylamide support matrix that provides an immobilized pH gradient. Because the Immobiline molecules themselves are rather simple chemical entities, the discrete molecules can be produced in a very reproducible manner with minimal lot-to-lot variation. This eliminates a principal concern associated with carrier ampholytes. IPG gradient gels also offer the prospect of increased sample loading over the carrier ampholytes. Carrier ampholyte tube gels can routinely accommodate up to 100 µg of protein and in certain instances several hundred micrograms of protein. In comparison, IPG gels offer higher protein loading potentials that can accommodate up to and in certain instances more than 1000 µg of protein [16]. Another benefit associated with IPG gels is the virtual elimination of cathodic drift that permits basic proteins to be resolved [17]. While both carrier ampholyte and IPG gels offer similar pI resolution, IPG gels have been viewed as providing less reliable positional focusing for discrete protein species than carrier ampholyte gels [13]. Although casting procedures for IPG gels require specialized gradient forming instrumentation, the increased commercial availability of IPG gels from several manufacturers minimizes this potential disadvantage.

Sample preparation presents a problem that must be considered in the context of the first-dimension IEF chemistry [18]. The first-dimension IEF chemistries that produce the desired continuous pH gradient depend on protein charge to effect zonal concentration of discrete protein species. Consequently, the introduction of charged species, especially detergents, with the sample must be minimized. This constraint makes sample preparation for 2-DE analysis a daunting task. To maximize protein representation with the sample and simultaneously retain a fixed linear relationship with respect to the original material being sampled necessitates that (1) the starting material be handled appropriately to minimize modification to the protein due to degradation and spurious posttranslational covalent modification, (2) the disruption and solubilization of proteins that participate in intermolecular interactions be ensured, (3) highly charged species such as nucleic acids are removed, (4) intra- and intermolecular disulfide bonds are disrupted, and (5) transmembrane proteins are solubilized and removed. To accomplish this task basic 2-DE sample preparation buffers employ high concentrations of a chaotropic agent such as urea, employ nonionic or zwitterionic detergents, use nucleases, and depend on reductants such as dithiothreitol in the presence of alkylating agents to disrupt disulfide bonds. Consideration must also be given to post-first-dimension buffer exchanges that facilitate the egress of proteins from the first-dimension gel and permit efficient penetration of the second-dimension gel matrix. An excellent compendium of recent procedures that address protein solubilization concerns associated with specific organisms and specific protein classes has been provided in a text edited by Link [19].

Protein separation in the second dimension is based on the molecular size of individual proteins. Many variations exist as to the composition of the second dimension. Specific applications have been designed that optimize protein separation under denaturing or nondenaturing conditions, reducing or nonreducing conditions, linear or nonlinear polyacrylamide support matrixes, and numerous buffer compositions. The most frequently used second-dimension buffer systems are based on the pioneering work of Laemmli [20]. In the Laemmli system, the polyacrylamide support matrix is used to sieve proteins that have been subject to denaturation in the presence of sodium dodecyl sulfate (SDS). This crucial step is based on the premise that SDS binds uniformly to denatured macromolecules with a fixed stoichiometry and in so doing forces them to assume a prolate ellipsoid shape. Theoretically, all protein species assume the same shape and migrate through the polyacrylamide support matrix with rates that are dependent on only their hydrodynamic radius. Consequently, the position to which a protein species migrates during a fixed time is correlated to its molecular size. This fact offers investigators the opportunity to move to dimensionally larger gel formats to increase protein loading and subsequently resolution. A larger 2-DE gel system can accommodate more protein. This increases the likelihood that low-abundance proteins will be detected and that these can be separated from other proteins in the gel. An alternative approach to this problem is present in so-called zoom gels. Zoom gel systems run the same sample on narrow first-dimension pH gradients and separate on as large a second-dimension gel as possible. The broadest pH range and most extensive molecular weight range can then be reassembled into a single composite image by visual means or attempted using specialized software applications. In practice, this is very difficult to accomplish.

B. Staining Methods in 2-DE

As is the case for most technologies in which there are numerous acceptable methods, there is no single method that is universally used to detect proteins separated by 2-DE. Various stains are widely available to visualize proteins [21]. A number of parameters need to be evaluated before a stain or dye can be chosen for a particular application. The weight of each parameter in the decision making process is a function of the goals of the study. The sensitivity, dynamic range, compatibility with analytical techniques associated with protein identification, as well as the cost are all important considerations that must be addressed in order to select the most appropriate visualization agent.

1. Coomassie Stains

The Coomassie blue stains have been the most widely used for proteins separated by 2-DE. Two forms of the Coomassie blue stain are available, namely, Coomassie blue G-250 and Coomassie blue R-250. First used by Meyer and Lambert to stain salivary proteins, Coomassie blue stains can be used to detect as little as 200 ng of protein/mm^2 on a 2-D gel [22]. The mechanism of binding between stain and protein occurs through several different interactions, including the binding between basic amino acids and the acid dyes, as well as by hydrogen bonding, van der Waals attraction, and hydrophobic interactions between protein and dye [22]. A common Coomassie blue staining protocol utilizes 0.1% Coomassie blue R-250 dissolved in water/methanol/glacial acetic acid (5:4:1). The duration of gel staining increases with the thickness of gel and decreases as a function of temperature. Gels that are 1.5 mm thick are generally stained overnight at room temperature. The quickest way to remove excess stain from the gel is by destaining in a solution containing 30% methanol/10% acetic acid. An alternative method dissolves the stain in trichloroacetic acid (TCA). The relative insolubility of Coomassie stain in TCA results in the preferential formation of protein–dye complexes. The result is the rapid staining of a 2-D gel with little destaining required [22].

The major disadvantages with use of Coomassie stains are the inability to accurately quantify proteins and the relative insensitivity of the stain. Despite these drawbacks, Coomassie blue stains have a number of advantages that will ensure their continued utility for visualizing proteins separated by 2-DE. There are many instances in which a high degree of sensitivity is not required. The proteins of interest may be in high abundance either naturally or through manipulation of the sample preparation using affinity chromatography. In addition, the inherent pH stability of the immobilized pH gradients strips allows the application of milligram quantities of protein to the first dimension [23], dramatically increasing the abundance of protein spots present in the SDS-PAGE gel. Most importantly, unlike silver stain, proteins stained with Coomassie blue can easily be processed with analytical procedures used in protein identification. Finally, Coomassie stains are inexpensive and reusable, making them attractive to laboratories with low budgets.

2. Silver Staining

The use of silver stain to visualize electrophoretically separated proteins was proposed in 1979 by Switzer and coworkers [24]. With a sensitivity approximately 100 times that of Coomassie blue, silver stain offers the ability to detect as little as 1 ng of protein. Numerous studies have focused on optimizing the various steps in the silver staining protocol (reviewed in [25]). The majority of methods conducted have utilized either silver diammine (alkaline method) or silver nitrate (acidic) as the silvering agent. The acidic methods can be further categorized into lengthy procedures, which require greater than 5 hr, and the less sensitive, rapid methods whereby staining can be completed in less time. A comparative study conducted by Rabilloud determined protocols utilizing silver diammine as well as glutaraldehyde as an enhancing agent (discussed below) to be the most sensitive staining methods [26]. Although somewhat laborious, the silver staining of 2-DE gels is a relatively straightforward procedure. The initial step of the silver stain procedure involves the immersion of the gels in a fixative solution. This solution (generally containing acetic acid and either methanol or ethanol) functions to precipitate the proteins within the gel matrix as well as remove interfering substances such as detergents, reducing agents, and buffer constituents such as Tris [25]. The second step is aimed at enhancing the subsequent image formation. Enhancement can be achieved through increasing the silver binding (referred to as *amplification*) to the proteins through the use of aromatic sulfonates or dyes such as Coomassie blue. The process of minimizing the formation of a background image through the use of oxidizing agents (permanganate or dichromate) is known as *contrastization* and is usually used only in the acidic methods. A third major enhancement technique (*sensitization*) involves increasing the rate at which silver reduction occurs on the proteins. Sensitization can be accomplished using sulfiding agents (thiourea) and/or reducing agents (e.g., dithiothreitol, DTT). Many of the existing staining protocols contain a combination of enhancement techniques to improve the subsequent image formation. Following silver impregnation, image development is accomplished through the reduction of Ag^+ to metallic Ag. Development solutions used with silver nitrate generally contain formaldehyde, carbonate, and thiosulfate while those methods utilizing silver diammine are composed of formaldehyde and citric acid [27].

Despite the high sensitivity of silver stain, there are a number of major drawbacks and limitations associated with this technique. The routine use of silver stain is relatively expensive due the high price of reagents as well as the cost of disposal of hazardous waste. In addition, poor images may result from high background, often resulting from the use of poor water quality. A recent study investigating the contributing factors of background silver staining also suggested the involvement of a redox initiator system like APS (ammonium persulfate), and amine, such as TEMED (N,N,N',N'-Tetramethyl-ethylenediamine [27]. There is also a significant protein-to-protein variability relative to the extent of silver deposited on the protein. Some proteins do not stain at all or are detected as negatively stained in contrast to a dark background [28]. The polypeptide sequence and the degree of glycosylation function to influence the intensity and color of the resulting stained proteins. Silver stain is not exclusive for proteins, since DNA as well as lipopolysaccharides may be stained also. Other limitations of silver staining include poor linearity to protein concentration [29] and relative incompatibility with subsequent analytical techniques. A recent study by Gharahdaghi and coworkers demonstrated improvement in the use of mass spectrometry to identify proteins from silver-stained gels by destaining with Farmer's reducer prior to enzymatic digestion and analysis [30]. The ability to routinely identify silver-stained proteins using mass spectrometric analysis would be a significant advancement in the field of proteomics.

3. Fluorescent Stains

One of the most promising new developments in the area of visualizing proteins on 2-DE gels has been the recent commercial availability of reliable fluorescent stains. A widely used fluorescent stain is the Sypro line, available from Molecular Probes (Eugene, OR). Stains such as Sypro ruby have a number of distinct of advantages over both Coomassie and silver stains. Several of these advantages are a function of the binding that occurs between the proteins and the stain. Rather than binding to specific functional groups or portions of the polypeptide backbone, the Sypro stains actually bind to the SDS molecules coating the protein [31]. This type of interaction minimizes the protein-to-protein signal variation and allows quantitative comparison between proteins. In addition, the noncovalent binding of stain to protein–SDS complexes does not mask antigenic sites permitting Western blot analysis when the gels are processed using a nonfixative staining procedure [31]. The dynamic range of the fluorescent stains is 5–10 times higher than either Coomassie or silver stains, which allows for accurate determination of protein expression levels. Equally impressive is the fact that many of the new fluorescent stains have sensitivities equal to or greater than silver stain. In addition, the protocol for fluorescent staining is very simple, requiring only a brief incubation (30 min) in a fixative solution followed by incubation in the dye from 90 min to overnight. The fluorescently labeled proteins can be visualized using an ultraviolet (UV) transilluminator, a blue-light transilluminator, or a laser scanning instrument with documentation being achieved through the use black-and-white print film, charge-coupled device (CCD) camera, or laser scanning instrument. Several of the newer stains, such as Sypro ruby, are completely compatible with mass spectrometry and microsequencing [31]. Despite all of the positive attributes of fluorescent stains, the major drawback is the cost of the stain, which can be prohibitive to most laboratories running large-format 2-D gels.

Fluorescent dyes such as the cyanine dyes have also been used to detect proteins separated by 2-DE [32]. The major advantage of fluorescent dyes is the ability to detect protein differences between samples using a single gel. The technique employed is referred to as difference gel electrophoresis (DIGE). DIGE involves labeling the samples of interest with different dyes, combining the samples into a single sample that is then subjected to 2-DE. The fluorescence images obtained from the different dyes are then superimposed to detect protein differences between samples. The use of a single gel eliminates the gel-to-gel variability associated with 2-DE as well the difficulties associated with matching spots between gels [32]. The success of DIGE is based on identical proteins labeled with different dyes having the same electrophoretic mobility. Similar to the case of fluorescent stains, the high cost associated with fluorescent dyes is the major drawback, along with the fact that many are not readily available as consumables.

The needs of a study are critical determinants when choosing a staining approach. Many factors need to be considered prior to initiating 2-DE including the need to quantify protein abundance or changes in protein expression levels, the amount of protein sample available, the number of samples involved, and the need for protein identification. Most proteomic-based studies are relatively large undertakings requiring substantial time and effort. The use of methods to visualize and detect proteins of interest consistently and to a required degree of sensitivity will ensure the success of those projects.

C. Imaging and Image Analysis

Rigorous attention to detail from sample preparation to image analysis is necessary if the 2-DE project is designed to generate valid comparative and numerical data. While precisely determining how much protein is loaded on the first-dimension gel determines the validity of subsequent image analysis, the type of 2-DE image is in large part determined by the nature of the sample itself. Autoradiographic images derived from isotopically labeled samples can be collected on film or phosphor imaging systems. Difficulties associated with film response to weak β-emitting isotopes and a modest linear dynamic range of 300:1 have led most investigators to employ phosphor imaging devices. Phosphor imaging systems have linear dynamic ranges that span up to five orders of magnitude and are as much as 250 times more intrinsically sensitive to radiolabeled proteins than film [33]. Other advantages of phosphor imaging systems include fast imaging times, acquisition of digitized data ready for computational analysis, and chemical development of films is not required. A significant drawback to phosphor imaging systems is their cost and the requirement that different screens be used to measure specific radioisotopes. A particularly attractive use of phosphor imaging technology is the application of double-label analysis. Experimental samples can be prepared with two different radiolabels. Phosphor images can be acquired that track two different biochemical processes within the same sample and from the same gel by imposing selective shielding between the source and the target following the initial image. This approach circumvents problems associated with intergel reproducibility. Nonradiolabeled samples can be imaged using chromogenic or chemiluminescent immunological methods [34,35] or conventional stains or dyes. Current methods for 2-DE image acquisition depend primarily on CCD camera systems and document scanning devices [36,37]. CCD camera systems employ CCD devices in lieu of conventional film to acquire the image. The characteristic emission spectrum and stability of the light source as well as a uniform diffusion of the light across the 2-DE gel surface is important to ensure that optimized, consistent images are obtained over time. The CCD chip image map can be readily converted to digital form and downloaded to a computer for subsequent analysis. Document scanners acquire 2-DE image information through an array of photodetectors that are moved across a 2-DE gel illuminated by a white or filtered light source. For 2-DE gel applications it is important that the scanner obtain and record a uniform image map across the length and width of the gel. Document scanning features that change gain settings to optimize text contrast during image acquisition should be disabled to ensure that a uniform image is obtained for subsequent analysis. During image acquisition any changes in the relationship between the image CCD device or scanner must be noted. A gray scale step tablet should be used initially to calibrate and to recalibrate the system following any changes.

All steps of the 2-DE process culminate in the generation of an image and establish its analytical value. The central tenet of 2-DE image analysis, i.e., to provide a comparative means to detect and measure changes, has changed little since the QUEST system was designed and developed by Garrels et al. about 25 years ago [38]. The specific intent for the QUEST system was to develop a system for quantitative 2-DE that was exemplary in gel electrophoresis, image processing, and data management. Although advances in computer computational speed and power have made more complex analyses possible by more sophisticated algorithms in less time, these principle goals remain. Currently several 2-DE image analysis software systems are available commercially; among them are Melanie II and PDQUEST (BioRad Laboratories, Hercules, CA), BioImage (Genomic Solutions, Ann Arbor, MI), and Phoretix 2D Advanced (Phoretix International, Newcastle upon Tyne, UK). While each software system possesses unique features, the basic approach to 2-DE gel analysis is quite similar. The process of image analysis begins with spot picking and image editing. Spot-picking algorithms are effective but they frequently miss spots, fail to resolve multiple spots, or identify artifacts as spots. These occurrences must be visually identified and corrected by the investigator. Once edited, reference spots are identified that appear consistently and are well resolved on each gel in a project. These are used to register the individual gels across a project. Matching individual spots across all gels in a project follows the gel registration process. This process is arduous and time consuming. For each hour spent producing a 2-DE gel, 4–6 hr may be spent in image editing and analysis. Once the imaged spots have been matched, statistical processes can be applied that detect and define significant differences between spots across respective groups within a project. At this point, data management and data visualization tools are required.

Data management and data visualization are critical concerns in the evolution of a 2-DE project. Although all investigators confront these issues when a 2-DE project is completed, an integrated approach that considers data management and visualization during the planning stages of a 2-DE project offers the best opportunity to optimize the process and achieve intended project goals. A clear understanding of the specific aim of the project at its onset can define several important strategic concerns. How will the 2-DE data be analyzed and what level of validation is needed? Is visual examination of the 2-DE gel data sufficient or are statistical methods required? Is the experimental design appropriate and are sample numbers adequate to ensure that the experimental outcomes can be determined without ambiguity? What form of raw data must be harvested from the 2-DE images and by what analytical method? Does this project stand alone or will data be integrated into a larger ongoing project? Will data be added to a database? If so, what annotation will be necessary to ensure continuity with existing data? Will important spots be excised from the gel for subsequent identification? In simple terms, the outcome of a 2-DE project is determined by careful planning. If visual inspection of the 2-DE gel data is sufficient to achieve project-specific aims, then 2-DE images must be evaluated in a consistent manner and the results crosschecked and agreed on by several observers. If statistical methods are to be used, then the type of raw data that will be used in the analysis determines the output of the image analysis system. The statistical analysis can be performed at a single level with an analysis that employs *t* tests or can be multilevel with each successive level dependent on the previous analysis. The type of assay that is used is an important determinant of whether the final 2-DE data represent a completed project or become a covariant in a larger model that includes data from other sources. Preliminary statistical analysis of the spot data can be accomplished using a straightforward *t*-test procedure based on individual spot intensity values or integrated spot intensity values. Mapping statistically changed spot matches onto the 2-DE gel images can provide a visual signature that is characteristic of a treatment, organism, or pathologic process. Signature patterns can be visualized on gels or by more complex statistical methods that cluster data and create strong visual links between related and disparate statistical data. There are many alternative approaches to the visualization of complex computational datasets [39]. In the absence of established standards, investigators should be guided by a desire to present data graphically with simplicity, clarity, precision, and efficiency [40].

D. Protein Spot Excision

The excision of protein spots from a 2-DE gel can fulfill a tactical objective or be a component of a more strategic objective. Fundamentally, spots are excised from 2-DE gels to provide a source of material that can be used to identify the protein(s) resident in the spot. From a tactical perspective, a 2-DE project can represent a completed experimental objective. In this context, the identification of important spots derived from analytical means applied completes the project. In contrast, a 2-DE project can be a component of a much larger, ongoing project. In this circumstance, exhaustive protein spot excision that accounts for all spots in a 2-DE gel may be used to establish a repository of information that can be stored and drawn on at a later date. Regardless of the intent, protein spot excision requires that spots be precisely removed, and that protein(s) present in the spot be abundant with respect to the detection limit of the identification technology and be stained in a manner that does not interfere with identification technology. Several approaches to protein spot removal should be considered. With respect to protein spots, the 2-DE gel is quite variable with respect to spot density. Consequently, picking methods that remove defined sections of the 2-DE gel in a grid pattern are inefficient in some regions of the gel and prone to cross-contamination from multiple spots in others. Conversely, a picking method that punches specific spots performs equally across the gel but requires considerable investigator skill and time. An alternative is the application of a spot excision robot to the process. This is feasible only if large numbers of protein spots are to be excised from many gels over time due to the fact that robotic systems are costly and have only recently become commercially available (e.g., Genomic Solutions), suggesting that performance and reliability remain largely unknown. Many wide-bore needles can be beveled flat and used as spot excision devises for the price of an automated robotic system. In regions of high density, great accuracy must be used to remove only the spot intended without contaminating the target spot or affecting the ability to excise proximal spots. To accomplish this manually or through automation requires that the excision device be precisely centered on the spot and have a diameter that does not exceed the diameter of the spot. The flip side of this is that in instances where a large spot needs to be excised in its entirety, a larger punching device or multiple punches must be taken. Given the present state of robotic systems this is much easier to accomplish manually. Another factor should be considered in the sampling of low-abundance protein spots. First, staining is not necessarily linearly correlated to spot intensity. If multiple spots are to be pooled to increase the apparent abundance of protein, a point of diminishing returns may be reached where excision from multiple 2-DE gels fails to increase the protein extracted from the gel above the detection limit of the detection device. In this instance, preparative sample loading on a fresh 2-DE gel is often the better solution. Keratin contamination is a major concern during spot excision. Keratin proteins from many sources must be assumed to be present in the laboratory environment unless specific and heroic measures are taken to ensure and guarantee its absence. Precaution against keratin contamination must be taken at all steps of the 2-DE gel process to avoid contamination of the sample, gel chemistry components, and the surface of the gel. During spot excision the investigator should wear protective clothing, gloves, hair net, and a mask. If a robotic system is used, careful maintenance, cleaning, and use of an enclosure system will greatly reduce potential keratin contamination.

III. PROTEIN IDENTIFICATION

A. General Concepts

Proteins are separated first by high-resolution two-dimensional PAGE and then stained. At this point, to identify an individual or set of protein spots, several options can be considered by the researcher, depending on availability of techniques. For protein spots that appear to be relatively abundant, e.g., more than 1 pmol (10^{-12} mol), traditional protein characterization methods may be employed. Specifically, methods such as amino acid analysis and Edman sequencing can be used to provide necessary protein identification information. With 2-DE, approximate molecular weight and isoelectric point characteristics are provided. Augmented with information on amino acid composition and/or amino terminal sequence, accurate identification can be achieved [6,41,42].

However, most of the emphasis the last few years has focused on employing mass spectrometry (MS)–based methods. The sensitivity gains of using MS allows for the identification of proteins below the 1-pmol level and in many cases in the femtomole (fmol, 10^{-15} mol) regime. More confident protein identifications can be made with the mass accuracy of the MS molecular mass measurement. For peptide fragments less than 3000 D, a mass accuracy of better than 100 ppm can be obtained. For example, for a peptide of molecular mass 1500 D, the accuracy of the MS measurement can be ±0.075 D (50 ppm). Moreover, MS is highly amenable to automation, as steps from sample preparation, sample injection, data acquisition, to data interpretation can be performed unattended. Automation is an important concept as capacities increase. It can reduce sources of sample contamination as well as sample handling errors. A general approach employing MS for protein identification is shown in Figure 2. Great strides have been made toward the automation of these procedures, and many more improvements will become evident in the near future. The rapid increase in proteomic sample throughput arising from constant improvements in the automation of sample preparation and data acquisition have resulted in ongoing generation of an overwhelming amount of data that must be mined for significant results. This has necessitated the parallel development of increasingly efficient computer-based data searching strategies, which can rapidly provide protein identifications from experimentally derived polypeptide molecular masses and sequences. With these clear advantages of using an MS-based approach, proteomics research has embraced MS with enthusiastic support.

B. Automated Proteolytic Digestion

For the application of MS for protein identification, the protein bands/spots from a 2-D gel are excised and are exposed to a highly specific enzymatic cleavage reagent (e.g., trypsin cleaves on the C-terminal side of arginine and lysine residues). The resulting tryptic fragments are extracted from the gel slice and are then subjected to MS methods. One of the major barriers to high throughput in the proteomic approach to protein identification is the "in-gel" proteolytic digestion and subsequent extraction of the proteolytic peptides from the gel. Common protocols for this process are often long and labor intensive. An example of an in-gel digest and extraction protocol [43] routinely used by our laboratory is as follows:

1. Wash and dehydrate gel
    a. Add 100 μl of a 1:1 mixture of 100 mM NH_4HCO_3/CH_3CN to each tube containing a gel piece and let stand for 15 min.
    b. Remove supernatant and dehydrate with 25 μl CH_3CN for 10 min.
    c. Remove supernatant and dry by vacuum centrifugation for 5 min.
2. Reduction and alkylation of protein
    a. Add 10 μl of 10 mM dithiothreitol in 100 mM NH_4HCO_3 and let stand for 60 min at 56°C.
    b. Allow to cool, then add 10 μl of 100 mM fresh iodoacetic acid in 100 mM NH_4HCO_3 and let stand for 45 min at 45°C in the dark.

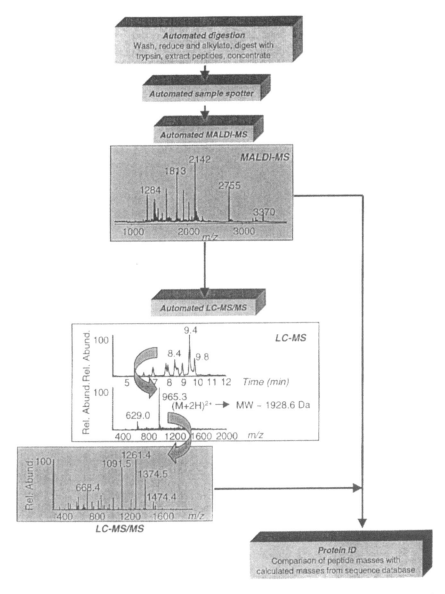

Figure 2 A general scheme for protein identification utilizing an MS-based approach applied in the authors' laboratory.

3. Wash and dehydrate gel
   a. Add 50 µl of 100 mM NH_4HCO_3 and let stand for 10 min, then remove supernatant.
   b. Add 25 µl of CH_3CN; let stand for 10 min, then remove supernatant.
   c. Repeat steps a and b.
   d. Dry by vacuum centrifugation for 5 min.
4. Trypsin digestion
   a. Swell the gel disk in 15 µl of 50 mM NH_4HCO_3 containing 10 ng/µl TPCK-modified trypsin in an ice bath for 45 min.
   b. Add 15 µl 50 mM NH_4HCO_3 and digest overnight at 37°C in the dark.
5. Extraction of tryptic peptides from gel
   a. Extract with 30 µl of 50% CH_3CN containing 1% trifluoroacetic acid (TFA) three times for 10 min each.
   b. Combine the supernatant for each of the three extractions and dry by vacuum centrifugation.
   c. Resuspend peptides in 5 µl of 30% CH_3CN containing 1% TFA and store at −80°C.

Using the above protocol, a scientist can comfortably digest and extract 25 samples in less than 36 hr, which limits throughput to approximately 100 in-gel digests and extractions per week. (In our experience, significant human error can be introduced over time while manually processing more than 25 samples per day.) Reducing the digest time from overnight to 2–3 hr can improve the throughput, but not significantly. However, a 2-D gel of a cell lysate can contain literally thousands of unique proteins, seen as stained spots. Even if the spots are excised from the gel manually, hundreds of samples requiring digestion and extraction can be generated per day. Setting aside the fact that in a proteomics project it is rare that each experiment would require every single spot from the gel to be identified, it is obvious that many more samples can be generated per week per scientist than digested and extracted manually.

A welcome alternative to the lengthy and laborious manual digest and extraction process are several automated digest and extraction robots that recently became commercially available [44–46]. The most useful of these robotic systems have the following features in common: some form of computer control, temperature control, options for allowing digestion with multiple enzymes, and the ability to digest gel pieces and extract the subsequent proteolytic peptides in a 96-well plate format, allowing parallel sample processing of 96 samples at a time. This will increase throughput to approximately 400 samples per week per robot using the above protocol, and potentially far more using a shorter digestion period.

Commercial units from Genomic Solutions (ProGest) and AbiMed (Digest-Pro) incorporate a particularly ingenious mechanism for overcoming possible sample contamination issues arising from the liquid handling syringe system. The syringe never touches the solutions in the wells. Instead, it pressurizes the wells such that the liquid flows from two small holes laser drilled into the bottom sides of each of the wells in the 96-well polymerase chain reaction (PCR) plate. The robot slides the reaction PCR 96-well plate over either a waste position for adding and discarding reaction reagents or a sample collection position for the extraction of proteolytic peptides. This methodology also decreases the opportunities for sample loss to adsorptive surfaces, although this remains a significant issue for low-level samples.

C. Peptide Mapping by MALDI-MS

A mass spectrum of the resulting digest products produces a "peptide map" or a "peptide fingerprint"; the measured masses can be compared to theoretical peptide maps derived from database sequences for identification. There are a few choices of mass analysis that can be selected from this point, depending on available instrumentation and other factors. The resulting peptide fragments can be subjected to matrix-assisted laser desorption/ionization (MALDI) [47] and/or electrospray ionization (ESI)–MS [48] analysis.

MALDI-MS is a tool that has rapidly grown in popularity in the area of bioanalytical mass spectrometry. This is due to recent improvements in time-of-flight (TOF) technology through enhancements in resolution and subsequently mass accuracy, which have increased the usefulness of MALDI-MS data. Currently, the TOF analyzer is the most common system for MALDI. Improvements such as the reflectron analyzer and time lag focusing (delayed extraction) have greatly improved the quality of MALDI-MS data [49]. Automation has also played an important role in the increased use of MALDI-MS as a tool for proteome analysis by allowing automated acquisition of data, followed by fully automated database searching of protein sequence databases such as SWISS-PROT and NCBI [2,50,51].

To better understand the reasons for the popularity of MALDI-MS, one must first understand the simplicity and speed of the approach. The peptide analyte of interest is cocrystallized on the MALDI target plate with an appropriate matrix (i.e., 4-hydroxy-α-cyanocinnamic acid or 3,5-dimethoxy-4-hydroxycinnamic acid (sinapinic acid)), which are small, highly conjugated organic molecules which strongly absorb energy at 337 nm. In most MALDI devices, 337 nm irradiation is provided by a nitrogen (N_2) laser. Although other lasers operating at different wavelengths can be used, size, cost, and ease of operation have made the nitrogen laser the most popular choice. The target plate is then inserted into the high-vacuum region of the source and the sample is irradiated with a laser pulse. The matrix absorbs the laser energy and transfers energy to the analyte molecule. The molecules are desorbed and ionized during this stage of the process. The ions are then accelerated under constant kinetic energy (V) down the flight tube of the TOF instrument by using acceleration potentials up to 30 kV. This acceleration potential imparts the ions with nearly the same kinetic energy and they each obtain a characteristic flight time (t) based on their mass-to-charge (m/z) ratio and total flight distance (L).

$$t = L \sqrt{(m/z)(1/2V)}$$

As a result, ions of different masses are separated as they travel down the field-free region of the flight tube of the mass spectrometer (lighter ions travel faster than larger ions), then strike the detector and are registered by the data system, which converts the flight times to masses. A photograph of a MALDI mass spectrometry is detailed in Figure 3.

A MALDI-TOF mass spectrometer consists of six major sections:

1. Laser system: Device capable of supplying an appropriate wavelength of energy sufficient to desorb and ionize matrix and analyte from the target surface.

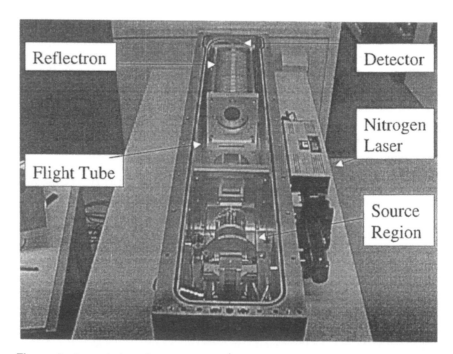

Figure 3 Internal view of a Micromass TofSpec 2E MALDI time-of-flight mass spectrometer (Beverly, MA).

2. Source: Section of instrument that contains the target plate that holds the matrix and analyte of interest. Ions generated in the source region are accelerated down the flight tube.
3. Flight tube: A field-free region of the mass spectrometer where separation of the ions based on their characteristic mass-to-charge ratio occurs.
4. Detector: Device that detects and measures ions.
5. Data system: Computer that converts detector output into an easily interpreted form (mass spectrum) and allows storage of the spectral data.
6. Vacuum system: Components necessary to evacuate the source and free-flight region, creating pressures in the 10^{-6}–10^{-7} torr range.

To obtain the best mass accuracy possible, MALDI-MS instrumentation equipped with a reflectron and time-lag focusing is commonly employed [49]. A reflectron is used to compensate for the initial energy spread that the ions may have following desorption off the sample target plate. Ions of the same mass-to-charge ratio, which have slightly different energy, have different final velocities and therefore arrive at the detector at slightly different times, resulting in loss of resolution. To compensate for this effect, an ion mirror or reflection is used to focus the ions by creating a flight distance gradient; ions with higher kinetic energy penetrate more deeply and thus travel a longer total distance than ions of lower energy. In addition, time lag focusing (or commonly referred to as delayed extraction) allows the initial energy spread to be partially focused prior to accelerating the ions. The combination of time lag focusing with an ion mirror provides for higher order energy focusing, resulting in significantly enhanced mass resolving power and improved mass accuracy. In many cases, this combination can increase MALDI-TOF mass accuracy to better than 20 ppm for peptides of molecular mass 500–3000 D.

The large number of samples generated by a proteomics approach requires a capability for very high throughput that can be achieved through automation of the entire process. Most commercial MALDI-MS instruments have capabilities for automated data acquisition. However, the amount of interactive control feedback can vary greatly, and this feature should be considered carefully when evaluating this type of analysis. The quality of the data and the speed at which it is obtained can be greatly affected by laser energy and the homogeneity of the analyte spot. To minimize the effects caused by inhomogeneous analyte crystals and searching for "the sweet spot" across a sample spot, an automated MALDI sample preparation robot is used in our laboratory. Currently, there are several automated sample preparation robots available commercially, including ones from Micromass, Bruker, and PerSeptive Biosystems.

The MALDI sample spotter supplied by Genomic Solutions is shown in Figure 4. It is capable of spotting the target configurations of various instrument man-

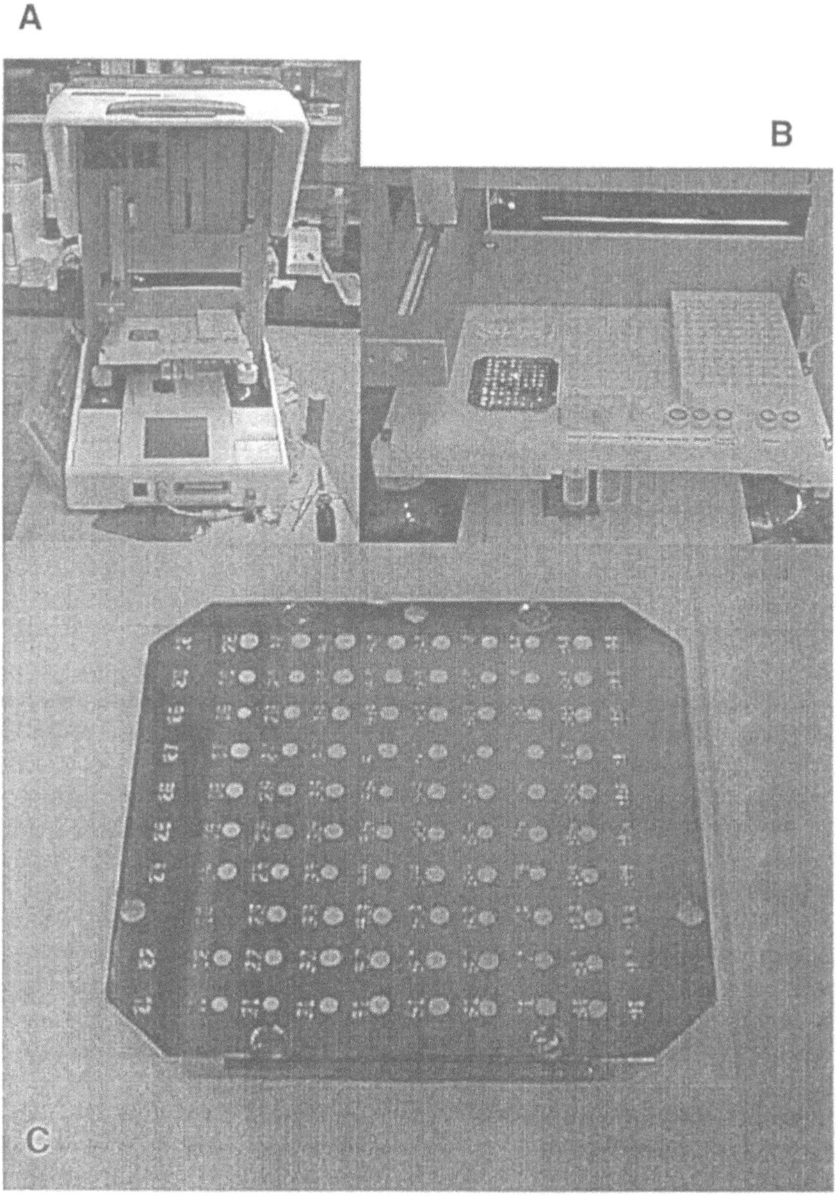

Figure 4 (A) Picture of a Genomic Solutions ProMS automated MALDI sample spotter and (B–C) enlarged views of a MALDI sample target mounted in the unit, showing the result of spotting analyte on the target.

ufacturers' systems. In addition, the system can be programmed with sample preparation protocols to remove gel contaminants (i.e., salts, ammonium bicarbonate, SDS, etc.) that could interfere with or degrade spectral quality. For example, the use of pipette tips packed with reversed-phase media (e.g., C18 "ZipTips" from Millipore) effectively desalts and concentrates peptides for MALDI-MS analysis.

A small aliquot of the digest solution can be directly analyzed by MALDI-MS to obtain a peptide map. The resulting sequence coverage (relative to the entire protein sequence) displayed from the total number of tryptic peptides observed in the MALDI mass spectrum can be quite high, i.e., greater than 80% of the sequence, although it can vary considerably depending on the protein, sample amount, and so forth. The measured molecular weights of the peptide fragments along with the specificity of the enzyme employed can be searched and compared against protein sequence databases using a number of computer searching routines available on the Internet. An example of such an exercise is depicted in Figure 5 and is discussed further in Section III.E.

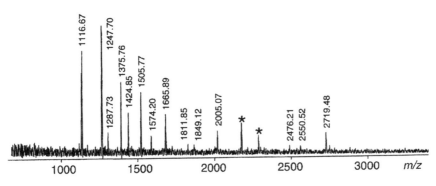

Figure 5 MALDI-MS peptide map of *E. coli* protein, Cell Division Inhibitor MinD (MIND_ECOLI, accession #P18197), separated by 2-DE. The molecular masses labeled on the spectrum were compared with the sequence of the protein for identification ("*" denotes trypsin autolysis peaks). The portions of the protein sequence for the observed tryptic peptides are highlighted on the sequence.

D. HPLC-MS and Tandem Mass Spectrometry

An approach for peptide mapping similar to MALDI-MS involves the use of ESI-MS. ESI is a solution-based ionization method. Analyte solutions flowing in the presence of a high electric field produce submicrometer-size droplets. As the droplets travel toward the mass spectrometer orifice at atmospheric pressure, they evaporate and eject charged analyte ions. These ions are sampled by the mass spectrometer for subsequent mass measurement. A peptide map can be obtained by the direct analysis of the peptide mixture by ESI-MS. A highly applied advantage of ESI is its ease of coupling to separation methodologies such as HPLC. Thus, alternatively, to reduce the complexity of the mixture, the peptides can be separated by reversed-phase HPLC with subsequent mass measurement by on-line ESI-MS (Fig. 2). The measured masses can be similarly compared with sequence databases. An example of an LC-MS application is shown in Figure 6.

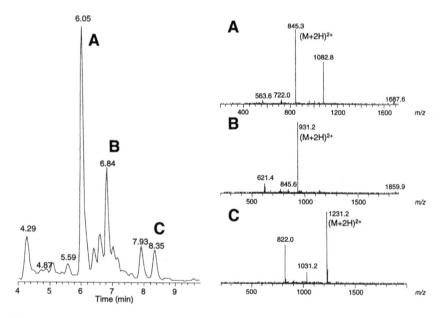

Figure 6 (*left*) HPLC mass chromatogram for the tryptic digest of ovalbumin. (*right*) The resulting mass spectra at the indicated retention times are shown. Approximately 0.25 μg of protein was loaded onto an SDS-PAGE gel, and the protein was stained with zinc imidazole. An electrospray ionization ion trap mass spectrometer (LCQ, Finnigan MAT, San Jose, CA) coupled on-line with a capillary HPLC (MicroPro Syringe Pumping System, Eldex Laboratories, Napa, CA) in junction with a capillary peptide trapping precolumn was used for peptide analysis.

To provide further confirmation of the identification, if a tandem mass spectrometer (or MS/MS) is available, peptide ions can be dissociated in the mass spectrometer to provide direct-sequence information. Peptide fragmentation typically occurs along the polypeptide backbone to produce products termed "y-type" and "b-type" fragment ions (in which the y ions contain the C-terminal portion of the peptide and the b ions contain the N-terminal portion). These product ions from an MS/MS spectrum can be compared to available sequences using powerful software tools as well. In many examples, laboratories may use nanoelectrospray with tandem mass spectrometry to examine the unseparated digest mixtures with a high degree of success [2].

One of the most common tandem mass spectrometers used for proteomics applications is the quadrupole ion trap (QIT) mass spectrometer [1,51–53]. An ion trap is a ion storage device that utilizes radiofrequency (rf) voltage across a ring electrode to contain ions [54]. As the rf amplitude increases, ions of increasing mass become unstable in the trap and are ejected toward a detector. The ion trap mass spectrometer has become a workhorse instrument for proteomics because of its ease of use and because of its high efficiency for generating sequence information. Examples of tandem mass spectra derived from tryptic peptides are shown in Figure 7. For the examples shown, the MS/MS spectra were readily interpreted via computer programs.

For a single sample, LC-MS/MS analysis included two discrete steps: (1) LC-MS peptide mapping to identify peptide ions from the digestion mixture and to deduce their molecular weights, and (2) LC-MS/MS of the previously detected peptides to obtain sequence information for protein identification. An improvement in efficiency and throughput of the overall method can be obtained by performing LC-MS/MS in the data-dependent mode. As full-scan mass spectra are acquired continuously in LC-MS mode, any ion detected with a signal intensity above a predefined threshold will trigger the mass spectrometer to switch to MS/MS mode. Thus, the ion trap mass spectrometer switches back and forth between MS (molecular mass information) and MS/MS mode (sequence information) in a single LC run. This feature was implemented to generate the spectra shown in Figure 7. The data-dependent scanning capability, combined with an autosampler device, can dramatically increase the capacity and throughput for protein identification.

E. Computer-Based Sequence Searching Strategies

The concept of database searching with mass spectral data is not a new one. It has been a routine practice for the interpretation of electron ionization (EI) mass spectra for many years. However, there is a fundamental difference between database searching of EI spectra and proteomic spectra. In the former, an experimentally acquired spectrum is compared with a large collection of spectra acquired from

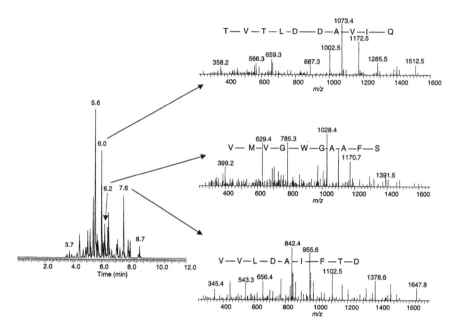

Figure 7 HPLC-MS/MS data–dependent scan results for a tryptic digest of yeast enolase. The ion trap mass spectrometer automatically acquires MS/MS data for peptide peaks
above a defined abundance threshold. The HPLC mass chromatogram is shown on the left,
and representative MS/MS spectra are shown on the right. From top to bottom, the observed
tryptic peptides of enolase are TAGIQIVADDLTVTNPK (residues 312–328), AAQDS-
FAAGWGVMVSHR (residues 358–374), and SGETEDTFIADLVVGLR (residues
375–391).

known, authentic standards. Fundamental features, such as the ions present and
their relative intensities, are compared for establishing a match and a "quality of
fit." This type of computer-based searching is typically referred to as "library
searching." This is in contrast to the strategy employed with proteomic data, where
a list of experimentally determined masses is compared to lists of computer-gen-
erated theoretical masses prepared from a database of protein primary sequences.
With the current exponential growth in the generation of genomic data, these databases are expanding every day.

     There are typically three types of search strategies employed: searching
with peptide fingerprint data, searching with sequence data, and searching with
raw MS/MS data. These strategies will be discussed below. While the strategy
employed often depends on the type of data available, there is also a logical progression, based on the costs of each strategy in terms of time and effort. While
many of the computer-based search engines allow for the purchase of an on-site

Table 1 Web Addresses of Some Representative Internet Resources for Protein
Identification from Mass Spectrometry Data

Program	I. Web address
BLAST	http://www2.ebi.ac.uk/blastall/
Mascot	http://www.matrixscience.com/cgi/index.pl?page=/home.html
MOWSE	http://srs.hgmp.mrc.ac.uk/cgi-bin/mowse
PeptideSearch	http://www.mann.embl-heidelberg.de/Services/ PeptideSearch/ PeptideSearchIntro.html
ProteinProspector	http://prospector.ucsf.edu/
Prowl	http://www.proteometrics.com/

license for use with proprietary data, most are available on the Internet for on-line
access and use with public domain databases (Table 1). One limiting factor that
must be considered for all of the following approaches is that they can only identify proteins that have been identified and reside in an available database or are
highly homologous to one that resides in the database.

1. Searching with Peptide Fingerprints

MALDI peptide fingerprinting is probably the most rapid manner in which to
identify an unknown protein. Computer software is used to theoretically "digest"
the individual protein components of a protein database using the same protease,
generating a list of theoretical peptide masses that would be derived for each entry.
The experimentally determined peptide masses are then compared with the theoretical ones in order to determine the identity of the unknown (as discussed in Sec.
III.C and III.D and depicted in Fig. 8).

The majority of the available search engines allow one to define certain
experimental parameters to optimize a particular search. Among the more typical
are: minimum number of peptides to be matched, allowable mass error, monoisotopic versus average mass data, mass range of starting protein, and type of protease used for digestion. In addition, most permit the inclusion of information
about potential protein modification, such as N- and C-terminal modification, car-
boxymethylation, oxidized methionines, etc. However, most protein databases
contain primary sequence information only, and any shift in mass incorporated
into the primary sequence as a result of posttranslational modification will result
in an experimental mass that is in disagreement with the theoretical mass. In fact,
this is one of the greatest shortcomings of this particular method. Modifications
such as glycation and phosphorylation can result in missed identifications. Furthermore, a single amino acid substitution can shift the mass of a peptide to such
a degree that even a protein with a great deal of homology with another in the data-

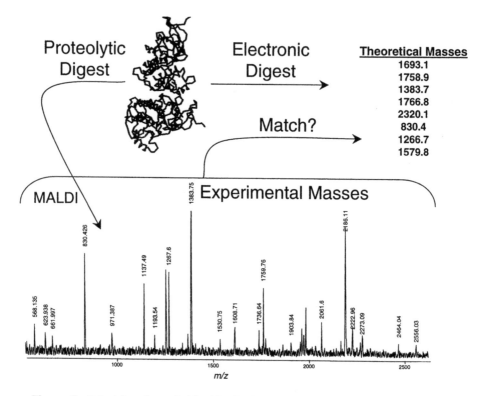

Figure 8 Principles of protein identification by MALDI-MS peptide fingerprinting.

base cannot be identified. Interestingly, one software package, ProteinProspector, has a feature within its MS-Fit subprogram that allows one to search peptide fingerprint data in so-called homology mode. In this mode, the software considers possible mutations of individual amino acid residues in an effort to transform a theoretical peptide mass to match an experimental one. This can be extremely powerful for the identity of a protein that is not in the database yet is significantly homologous to one that is in the database.

A number of factors affect the utility of peptide fingerprinting. The greater the experimental mass accuracy, the narrower you can set your search tolerances, thereby increasing your confidence in the match and decreasing the number of false-positive responses [55]. A common practice used to increase mass accuracy in peptide fingerprinting is to employ an autolysis fragment from the proteolytic enzyme as an internal standard to calibrate a MALDI mass spectrum. Nevertheless, in terms of sample consumption, throughput, and the need for intensive data interpretation, peptide fingerprinting is always a logical first approach for protein identification.

Peptide fingerprinting is also amenable to the identification of proteins in complex mixtures. Peptides generated from the digest of a protein mixture will simply return two or more results that are a good fit. As long as the peptides assigned for multiple proteins do not overlap, then identification is reasonably straightforward. Conversely, peptides that are "left over" in a peptide fingerprint after the identification of one component can be resubmitted for the possible identification of another component.

2. Searching with Sequence Information

Computer-based searching of databases with sequence information is the oldest and probably the most straightforward of the three strategies. Typically, an experimentally determined partial amino acid sequence is compared with the sequences of all of the proteins listed in a database, and a list of those proteins containing the same partial sequence is generated. Virtually all of the web-based search applications are able to search with sequence information. One advantage of this approach is that typical search engines, such as BLAST, allow for increasing levels of ambiguity in the submitted experimental sequence, facilitating the identification of homologous known sequences.

Protein identification via searching with sequence information employs similar strategies irrespective of how the sequence information is obtained. Automated Edman degradation is one of the traditional methods for obtaining sequence information. However, several drawbacks make this approach somewhat less attractive. The collection of data is time consuming, typically requiring 12–24 hr. The subsequent interpretation of the data to extract an amino acid sequence is still largely done by hand, making it a difficult process to automate. And information is limited to the N terminus of the protein; if interior information is desired, the protein must be proteolytically digested and individual peptides separated and collected for off-line analysis.

The ability to rapidly generate amino acid sequence information via MS/MS experiments, whether it is with a triple-quadrupole instrument, an ion trap, or via postsource decay with MALDI-TOF, has revolutionized the practice of generating sequence information. Many software packages can use a combination of sequence information and mass spectral information, such as the molecular weight of the individual peptide under investigation. With an accurate value of the parent ion mass of a peptide, and even partial sequence information, it is possible to get a strong match for an unknown. A disadvantage of this approach is that it requires manual interpretation by the operator, making it more difficult to automate, and can require two separate experiments to get both pieces of information.

Some software packages employ a combination of predictive MS/MS data and sequence information. An example is the so-called error-tolerant software that is part of the PeptideSearch package at the EMBL's web site. This strategy is employed when a certain amount of sequence information is available from an MS/MS spectrum, but not the complete sequence. The starting mass of the partial sequence, followed by the sequence itself and then the ending mass, are submitted for database searching. The partial sequence must be manually derived from the experimental MS/MS data, which requires operator input and is not amenable to automation. However, a weak spectrum in which only 4–5 amino acid residues can be deduced typically does not yield enough information to unequivocally identify a protein or may return a deluge of poor matches. By incorporating the ion mass at which the partial sequence starts and stops, as well as the mass of the peptide itself, PeptideSearch is often able to generate a strong match from marginal data. Potential candidate proteins in the database must contain the partial sequence, must generate a theoretical proteolytic peptide of the correct mass, and must contain the partial sequence positioned appropriately within that theoretical peptide, based on the starting and ending masses of the partial sequence. If a candidate protein meets all of these requirements, then a strong match can be argued for even a very short experimentally derived sequence.

3. Searching with Raw MS/MS Data

Current mass spectral technology permits the generation of MS/MS data at an unprecedented rate. Prior to the generation of powerful computer-based database searching strategies, the largest bottleneck in protein identification was the manual interpretation of this MS/MS data to extract the sequence information. Today many computer-based search strategies that employ MS/MS data require no operator interpretation at all. Analogous to the approach described for peptide fingerprinting, these programs take the individual protein entries in a database and electronically "digest" them to generate a list of theoretical peptides for each protein. However, in the use of MS/MS data, these theoretical peptides are further manipulated to generate a second level of lists that contain theoretical fragment ion masses that would be generated in the MS/MS experiment for each theoretical peptide (Fig. 9). Therefore, these programs simply compare the list of experimentally determined fragment ion masses from the MS/MS experiment of the peptide of interest with the theoretical fragment ion masses generated by the computer program. Again, as with the peptide fingerprint strategy, the operator inputs a list of masses and typically has a choice of a number of experimental parameters that can be used to tailor the search as appropriate. This is a very processor-intensive function and, due to the size of current databases, is only possible on a routine basis due to the explosive increase in desktop computing power.

The recent advent of data-dependent scanning functions on an increasing number of mass spectrometers has permitted the unattended acquisition of MS/MS data. Another example of a raw MS/MS data searching program that takes

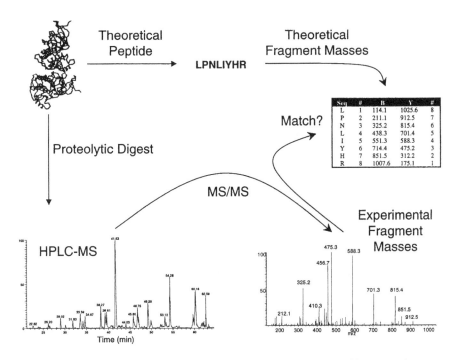

Figure 9   Principles of protein identification by HPLC-MS/MS peptide sequencing.

particular advantage of this ability is the SEQUEST program. The SEQUEST software program inputs data from a data-dependent LC/MS chromatogram, automatically strips out all of the MS/MS information for each individual peak, and submits it for database searching using the strategy discussed above. The appeal of this approach is that each peak is treated as a separate data file, making it especially useful for the on-line separation and identification of individual components in a protein mixture. No user interpretation of MS/MS spectra is involved.

Several different strategies are applicable in the computer-based searching of sequence databases for the identification of unknown proteins. The choice of strategy employed is often dictated by the format of the data available. However, one must always use caution and examine the results with a critical eye. It is the responsibility of the investigator to examine the list of resultant matches with respect to quality of fit. Often this is aided by examining the individual MS/MS spectra and ensuring that most of the abundant ions are being used for identification, not simply those that are in the "grass."

The capacity to perform these searches using web-based programs provides direct access to the rapidly expanding collection of public domain protein databases that are also on the internet. Furthermore, most of the programs take great advantage of HTML's ability to weave various sources of information together through hyperlinks, so that when a strong candidate for a protein identification is found, a wealth of additional information is only a mouse click away.

F. Other Methods Used for Proteomics Research

Seeking to avoid the difficulties associated with extracting proteins embedded in gel matrices, other approaches to proteome analysis dispense with polyacrylamide gel separations and rely on multidimensional chromatography. One such approach has paired size exclusion chromatography with HPLC for intact protein analysis, offering convenient preparative capabilities by directing column effluent to a fraction collector [56]. For identification purposes, ESI-MS mass analysis offers an intact molecular weight accurate to about ±0.1%, and fractions can also be analyzed at significantly lower throughput by Edman degradation for NH_2 terminal sequence determination, enzymatic digestion followed by successive stages of MS and MS/MS for higher confidence identification and/or characterization, or by other assays. While promising, the comprehensive chromatographic method is currently limited by dynamic range (ability to see low-level proteins present at only a few copies per cell in the presence of abundant proteins present at tens of thousands or more copies per cell). Moreover, identification on the basis of molecular weight alone is risky, particularly in complex systems presenting many post-translational modifications; availability of chromatographic retention times does not enhance the confidence of proposed identifications significantly. Finally, membrane proteins and other hard-to-solubilize proteins may not be recovered by this methodology, and tend to be harder to handle as intact proteins versus tryptic peptides.

Capillary electrophoresis (CE) is a very high-resolution technique similar to gel electrophoresis, except that the separations take place in a capillary filled with an electrolyte. The term capillary electrophoresis encompasses all of the electrophoretic separation modes that can take place in a capillary. A schematic of a CE system is shown in Figure 10. In simplest terms, separations are achieved in CE based on differences in the electrophoretic mobilities of charged species placed in an electric field. However, one other phenomenon present in CE also contributes to the movement of analytes in an applied potential field, that being the electro-osmotic flow. Electro-osmotic flow describes the movement of fluid in a capillary under the influence of an applied electric field and is brought about by the ionization of silanol groups on the inner surface of the capillary when in contact with the electrolyte. An electrical double layer is formed when hydrated cations from the electrolyte associate with the negatively charged ionized silanol groups. When a potential is applied, the hydrated cations migrate to the cathode, creating a net flow in the same direction. The velocity of the electro-osmotic flow

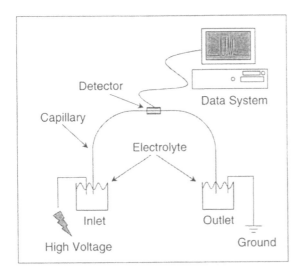

Figure 10   Schematic of a capillary electrophoresis system.

can be directly affected by changes in the field strength, electrolyte pH, and viscosity of the electrolyte solvent system used. The contribution of electro-osmotic flow to the movement of charged species in a capillary can most easily be determined experimentally by observing the migration time to the detector of a neutral marker species. The flow characteristics of electro-osmotic flow are plug-like, in comparison to the laminar flow achieved in LC. As a result, far more theoretical plates can be generated in CE as compared to comparable column lengths in LC. There are any number of excellent texts available that cover in-depth the theories associated with CE [57,58].

As described for high-performance liquid chromatography (HPLC), by far the most widely applied ionization method used in interfacing CE to mass spectrometry for the analysis of biomolecules is electrospray ionization. An uninterrupted electrical contact is essential for both the continued operation of the CE and for the generation of the electrospray when interfacing CE with ESI-MS. Several interfaces have been developed to achieve this electrical contact. The three most widely applicable interfaces are liquid junction, sheath liquid, and sheathless interfaces.

Although detection limits down to attomole (10^{-18} mol) ranges have been reported, CE is generally recognized as having a very low concentration limit of detection (CLOD). To achieve the best resolution and peak shape, it is necessary to inject only very small volumes (low nanoliters) of sample, which forces the use of highly concentrated samples initially. Several groups have developed various preconcentration techniques to attempt to overcome this CLOD [59]. All of these techniques involve trapping or preconcentrating the samples on some type of C18 stationary phase or hydrophobic membrane in the case of tryptic digest mixtures.

Capillary isoelectric focusing (CIEF) has been combined with on-line electrospray ionization Fourier transform ion cyclotron resonance (ESI-FTICR) mass spectrometry to examine desalted, intact *Escherichia coli* proteins [60]. The methodology's promises of simultaneous ppm mass measurement accuracy, high sensitivity, and ultrahigh MS resolution would be particularly attractive for intact protein analyses from proteomics samples. Protein pIs in combination with molecular weight can provide a useful means for proposing protein identifications. However, the CIEF conditions employed for on-line MS have so far employed native or near-native separation conditions, yielding pIs that are not predictable from sequence alone and that do not necessarily correlate with the denatured pIs. MS/MS dissociation techniques compatible with FTICR mass spectrometry, such as infrared multiphoton dissociation (IRMPD) or sustained off-resonance irradiation (SORI), may provide structural information to yield higher confidence protein identifications.

The most developed, automated non-gel methodology for proteome analyses was demonstrated by analysis of *E. coli* periplasmic proteins, partially fractionated by using strong anion exchange chromatography [61]. Each fraction was digested with trypsin and then analyzed by using microcolumn LC/ESI/MS. The tandem mass spectra were used to search the *E. coli* sequence database, from which a total of 80 proteins were identified. The procedure limits the amount of sample handling, and by manipulating the proteins as mixtures, the higher abundance proteins act as carriers for lower abundance proteins, further reducing losses. However, the presence of a single highly abundant protein can potentially suppress the acquisition of tandem mass spectra for lower abundance peptides present in the mixture (dynamic range limitation). Also, because the procedure is a superficial sampling of the peptides present, there is the possibility that a protein may be present but no MS/MS data for peptides from that protein are acquired. For relatively simple mixtures this approach greatly increases the speed and efficiency of analysis.

Relative quantitation can be difficult to achieve with all of the above methods. One trend, designed to deliver quantitative information, has been to isotopically label samples reflecting different conditions [62]. Based on the isotope ratios of tryptic peptides (or appropriately sized intact proteins when FTMS is employed [63]), one can attempt to determine whether a protein is up-regulated or down-regulated. Clearly this methodology can only be employed when it is possible to isotopically label cells, e.g., bacterial cell cultures.

A newer approach to deliverery of quantitative information in all types of samples relies on alkylating cysteines with unique tags (e.g., isotopically encoded) that incorporate biotin functionalities [64]. Cysteine-containing tryptic peptides can be withdrawn selectively from mixtures for subsequent LC/MS/MS analysis, yielding both identification and quantitation. The approach should also reduce limitations on dynamic range because only cysteine-containing proteins would be loaded onto the LC column, albeit at the cost of losing all information about non-cysteine-containing proteins.

IV. CONCLUSIONS

Much of the technological advances to support proteomics research was developed during the past decade. However, it is obvious to those active in the field that many more developments will be unveiled in the near horizon. With improvements in sensitivity, throughput, and ease of use, proteomics will continue to flourish as a promising biomedical research endeavor. The tools used to generate the data will be better crafted, and the way in which the data generated from a proteomics approach are used to further the goals of drug discovery will become more sophisticated.

REFERENCES

1. Arnott D, O'Connell KL, King KL, Stults JT. An integrated approach to proteome analysis: identification of proteins associated with cardiac hypertrophy. Anal Biochem 1998;258:1–18.
2. Shevchenko A, Jensen ON, Podtelejnikov AV, Sagliocco F, Wilm M, Vorm O, Mortensen P, Shevchenko A, Boucherie H, Mann M. Linking genome and proteome by mass spectrometry: large-scale identification of yeast proteins from two dimensional gels. Proc Natl Acad Sci USA 1996;93:14440–14445.
3. Roepstorff P. Mass spectrometry in protein studies from genome to function. Curr Opin Biotechnol 1997;8:6–13.
4. Wilkins MR, Williams KL, Appel RD, Hochstrasser DF. Proteome Research: New Frontiers in Functional Genomics. Berlin: Springer-Verlag, 1997.
5. Celis JE, Oestergaard M, Rasmussen HH, Gromov P, Gromova I, Varmark H, Palsdottir H, Magnusson N, Andersen I, Basse B, Lauridsen JB, Ratz G, Wolf H, Oerntoft TF, Celis P, Celis A. A. comprehensive protein resource for the study of bladder cancer. http://biobase.dk/cgi-bin/celis. Electrophoresis 1999;20:300–309.
6. Dunn MJ. Quantitative two-dimensional gel electrophoresis: from proteins to proteomes. Biochem Soc Trans 1997;25:248–254.
7. Humphery-Smith I, Cordwell SJ, Blackstock WP. Proteome research. Complementarity and limitations with respect to the RNA and DNA worlds. Electrophoresis 1997;18:1217–1242.

8. Wasinger VC, Cordwell SJ, Cerpa-Poljak A, Yan JX, Gooley AA, Wilkins MR, Duncan MW, Harris R, Williams KL, Humphery-Smith I. Progress with gene-product mapping of the mollicutes: *Mycoplasma genitalium.* Electrophoresis 1995;16:1090–1094.

9. O'Farrell PH. High resolution two-dimensional electrophoresis of proteins. J Biol Chem 1975;250:4007–4021.

10. Ingram L, Tombs MP, Hurst A. Mobility-molecular weight relations of small proteins and peptides in acrylamide-gel electrophoresis. Anal Biochem 1967;20:24–29.

11. Weber K, Osborn M. Reliability of molecular weight determinations by dodecyl sulfate–polyacrylamide-gel electrophoresis. J Biol Chem 1969;244:4406–4412.

12. Klose J, Kobalz U. Two-dimensional electrophoresis of proteins: an updated protocol and implications for a functional analysis of the genome. Electrophoresis 1995;16:1034–1059.

13. Lopez MF, Patton WF. Reproducibility of polypeptide spot positions in two-dimensional gels run using carrier ampholytes in the isoelectric focusing dimension. Electrophoresis 1997;18:338–343.

14. Yamada Y. Isoelectric focusing with reduced cathodic drift and migration into the anode chamber. J Biochem Biophys Meth 1983;8:175–181.

15. Bjellqvist B, Ek K, Righetti PG, Gianazza E, Goerg A, Westermeier R, Postel W. Isoelectric focusing in immobilized pH gradients: principle, methodology and some applications. J Biochem Biophys Meth 1982;6:317–339.

16. Bjellqvist B, Sanchez JC, Pasquali C, Ravier F, Paquet N, Frutiger S, Hughes GJ, Hochstrasser D. Micropreparative two-dimensional electrophoresis allowing the separation of samples containing milligram amounts of proteins. Electrophoresis 1993;14:1375–1378.

17. Gorg A. IPG-Dalt of very alkaline proteins. In: Link AJ, ed. Methods Mol. Biol.: 2-D Proteome Analysis Protocols. Vol. 112. Totowa, NJ: Humana Press, 1999;197–209.

18. Rabilloud T. Solubilization of proteins for electrophoretic analyses. Electrophoresis 1996;17:813–829.

19. Link AJ. 2-D Proteome Analysis Protocols. Methods in Molecular Biology, Vol. 112. Totowa, NJ: Humana Press, 1998.

20. Laemmli UK. Cleavage of structural proteins during the assembly of the head of bacteriophage T4. Nature 1970;227:680–685.

21. Wirth PJ, Romano A. Staining methods in gel electrophoresis, including the use of multiple detection methods. J Chromatogr A 1995;698:123–143.

22. Meyer TS, Lamberts BL. Biochim Biophys Acta 1965;107:144–145.

23. Goerg A, Postel W, Guenther S. The current state of two-dimensional electrophoresis with immobilized pH gradients. Electrophoresis 1988;9:531–546.

24. Switzer RC, III, Merril CR, Shifrin S. A highly sensitive silver stain for detecting proteins and peptides in polyacrylamide gels. Anal Biochem 1979;98:231–237.

25. Rabilloud T. Silver staining of 2-D electrophoresis gels. In: Link AJ, ed. Methods in Molecular Biology: 2-D Proteome Analysis Protocols, Vol. 112. Totowa, NJ: Humana Press, 1999;297–305.

26. Rabilloud T. A comparison between low background silver diammine and silver nitrate protein stains. Electrophoresis 1992;13:429–439.

27. Patras G, Qiao GG, Solomon DH. On the mechanism of background silver staining during sodium dodecyl sulfate-polyacrylamide gel electrophoresis. Electrophoresis 1999;20:2039–2045.

28. Hochstrasser DF, Patchornik A, Merril CR. Development of polyacrylamide gels that improve the separation of proteins and their detection by silver staining. Anal Biochem 1988;173:412–423.

29. Giometti CS, Gemmell MA, Tollaksen SL, Taylor J. Quantitation of human leukocyte proteins after silver staining: a study with two-dimensional electrophoresis. Electrophoresis 1991;12:536–543.

30. Gharahdaghi F, Weinberg CR, Meagher DA, Imai BS, Mische SM. Mass spectrometric identification of proteins from silver-stained polyacrylamide gel. A method for the removal of silver ions to enhance sensitivity. Electrophoresis 1999;20:601–605.

31. Steinberg TH, Haugland RP, Singer VL. Application of SYPRO orange and SYPRO red protein gel stains. Anal Biochem 1996;239:238–245.

32. Unlu M, Morgan ME, Minden JS. Difference gel electrophoresis. A single gel method for detecting changes in protein extracts. Electrophoresis 1997;18:2071–2077.

33. Johnston RF, Pickett SC, Barker DL. Autoradiography using storage phosphor technology. Electrophoresis 1990;11:355–360.

34. Towbin H, Staehelin T, Gordon J. Electrophoretic transfer of proteins from polyacrylamide gels to nitrocellulose sheets: procedure and some applications. Proc Natl Acad Sci USA 1979;76:4350–4354.

35. Durrant I, Fowler S. Chemiluminescent detection systems for protein blotting. In: Dunbar BS, ed. Protein Blotting: A Practical Approach. Oxford, UK: IRL Press, 1994: 141–152.

36. Watkins C, Sadun A, Marenka S. Modern Image Processing: Warping, Morphing and Classical Techniques. San Diego: Academic Press, 1993.

37. Sutherland JC. Electronic imaging of electrophoretic gels and blots. Adv Electrophor 1993;6:1–42.

38. Garrels JI, Farrar JT, Burwell CB, IV. The QUEST system for computer-analyzed two-dimensional electrophoresis of proteins. In: Celis JE, Bravo R, eds. Two-Dimensional Gel Electrophoresis of Proteins: Methods and Applications. San Diego: Academic Press, 1984:37–91.

39. Kraemer ET, Ferrin TE. Molecules to maps: tools for visualization and interaction in support of computational biology. Bioinformatics 1998;14:764–771.

40. Tufte ER. The Visual Display of Quantitative Information. Cheshire, CN: Graphic Press, 1983.

41. Gooley AA, Ou K, Russell J, Wilkins MR, Sanchez JC, Hochstrasser DF, Williams KL. A role for Edman degradation in proteome studies. Electrophoresis 1997;18: 1068–1072.

42. Wilkins MR, Ou K, Appel RD, Sanchez J-C, Yan JX, Golaz O, Farnsworth V, Cartier P, Hochstrasser DF, Williams KL, Gooley AA. Rapid protein identification using N-terminal "sequence tag" and amino acid analysis. Biochem Biophys Res Commun 1996;221:609–613.

43. Shevchenko A, Wilm M, Vorm O, Mann M. Mass spectrometric sequencing of proteins from silver-stained polyacrylamide gels. Anal Chem 1996;68:850–858.

44. Houthaeve T, Gausepohl H, Ashman K, Nillson T, Mann M. Automated protein preparation techniques using a digest robot. J Protein Chem 1997;16:343–348.

45. Ashman K, Houthaeve T, Clayton J, Wilm M, Podtelejnikov A, Jensen ON, Mann M. The application of robotics and mass spectrometry to the characterization of the *Drosophila melanogaster* indirect flight muscle proteome. Lett Pept Sci 1997;4: 57–65.

46. Ashman K. Automated in-gel proteolysis for proteomics. Am Biotechnol Lab 1999;17:92–93.

47. Karas M, Bahr U, Ingendoh A, Nordhoff E, Stahl B, Strupat K, Hillenkamp F. Principles and applications of matrix-assisted UV-laser desorption/ionization mass spectrometry. Anal Chim Acta 1990;241:175–185.

48. Fenn JB, Mann M, Meng CK, Wong SF, Whitehouse CM. Electrospray ionization for mass spectrometry of large biomolecules. Science 1989;246:64–71.

49. Cotter RJ. The new time-of-flight mass spectrometry. Anal Chem 1999;71:445A–451A.

50. James P. Of genomes and proteomes. Biochem Biophys Res. Commun 1997;231: 1–6.

51. Yates JR, III. Mass spectrometry and the age of the proteome. J Mass Spectrom 1998;33:1–19.

52. Jonscher KR, Yates JR, III. The quadrupole ion trap mass spectrometer-a small solution to a big challenge. Anal Biochem 1997;244:1–15.

53. Dongre AR, Eng JK, Yates JR, III. Emerging tandem mass spectrometry techniques for the rapid identification of proteins. Trends Biotechnol 1997;15:418–425.

54. McLuckey SA, Van Berkel GJ, Goeringer DE, Glish GL. Ion trap mass spectrometry using high-pressure ionization. Anal Chem 1994;66:737A–743A.

55. Clauser KR, Baker P, Burlingame AL. Role of accurate mass measurement (± 10 ppm) in protein identification strategies employing MS or MS/MS and database searching. Anal Chem 1999;71:2871–2882.

56. Opiteck GJ, Ramirez SM, Jorgenson JW, Moseley MA, III. Comprehensive two-dimensional high-performance liquid chromatography for the isolation of overexpressed proteins and proteome mapping. Anal Biochem 1998;258:349–361.

57. Camilleri P. Capillary Electrophoresis: Theory and Practice, 2nd ed. Boca Raton, FL: CRC Press, 1998.

58. Ding J, Vouros P. Advances in CE/MS. Anal Chem 1999;71:378A–385A.

59. Yang Q, Tomlinson AJ, Naylor S. Membrane preconcentration CE. Anal Chem 1999;71:183A–189A.

60. Yang L, Lee CS, Hofstadler SA, Pasa- Tolic L, Smith RD. Capillary isoelectric focusing-electrospray ionization Fourier transform ion cyclotron resonance mass spectrometry for protein characterization. Anal Chem 1998;70:3235–3241.

61. Link AJ, Carmack E, Yates JR, III. A strategy for the identification of proteins localized to subcellular spaces: application to E. coli periplasmic proteins. Int J Mass Spectrom Ion Proc 1997;160:303–316.

62. Oda Y, Huang K, Cross FR, Cowburn D, Chait BT. Accurate quantitation of protein expression and site-specific phosphorylation. Proc Natl Acad Sci USA 1999;96: 6591–6596.

63. Pasa-Tolic L, Jensen PK, Anderson GA, Lipton MS, Peden KK, Martinovic S, Tolic N, Bruce JE, Smith RD. High throughput proteome-wide precision measurements of protein expression using mass spectrometry. J Am Chem Soc 1999;121:7949–7950.

64. Gygi SP, Rist B, Gerber SA, Turecek F, Gelb MH, Aebersold R. Quantitative analysis of complex protein mixtures using isotope-coded affinity tags. Nat Biotechnol 1999;17:994–999.

5

Where Science Meets Silicon: Microfabrication Techniques and Their Scientific Applications

Tony J. Beugelsdijk
Los Alamos National Laboratory
Los Alamos, New Mexico

I. INTRODUCTION

The historical trend in chemical and biological instrumentation and the development of analysis protocols over several decades has been to work with increasingly smaller sample volumes and quantities of analytes and reagents. This trend has been greatly facilitated by the development of very sensitive measurement technologies, such as mass spectrometry and laser-induced fluorescence. Additional benefits have included reduced reagent costs as well as lower environmental impact.

Microtechnologies merely continue this historical trend, but with a new twist—the jump to an entirely new technology platform. Moreover, new scientific problems can now be studied that take advantage of phenomena unique to micrometer scale domains, such as greatly increased surface to volume ratios. As an example, chemical reactions that are too energetic at a macro scale and that require synthetic detours through less reactive intermediates can often be conducted directly on a micro scale where heat and mass transfer can be controlled much more efficiently. New intermediate products, never seen before, may also result.

The construction of microdevices is based on many of the fabrication technologies employed in the semiconductor industry. However, only recently has its use in microfluidic applications become a reality. A seminal paper that anticipated the use of silicon as a structural material for micromechanical systems is the one written by K. E. Petersen [1]. He suggested and illustrated that microstructures with mechanical functionality were indeed possible with silicon as the construction material. This led gradually to the construction of active microfluidic components, such as valves, pumps, motors, separators, etc., on chips.

Much early research focused on the use of different micromechanical systems and devices, such as pumps and chemical functionalities, for reaction, separation, and detection. As these became more robust and more routine, increased complexity resulted in packaging of entire chemical protocols on a microdevice. On-board detection or interfaces to detection systems are also appearing in research labs and the marketplace [2].

Microdevices are highly suited to field or portable use. We will see increased usage of these devices in medical care and environmental monitoring. Coupled to network systems, these devices can serve as a distributed laboratory. The economies of scale realized in the production of these systems will result in single-use or disposable systems.

This chapter will cover some of the traditional fabrication methods and discuss trends in new materials and techniques. Some discussion will focus on systems packaging and integration techniques and issues. This will be followed by descriptions of a selection of commercial systems that are emerging. It is difficult to predict where these technologies will lead. However, it is safe to assume that they will have a widespread and fundamental impact on many areas of scientific endeavor. These areas include materials research, environmental monitoring, health care, drug discovery, and national security.

The microtechnology field literature is rich [3–5]. It is not the purpose of this chapter to restate this material but rather to provide a quick overview from the perspective of the use of these technologies in the chemical and biological laboratory.

Microtechnologies in the semiconductor industry cover a size regime of roughly 0.1–100 µm. For example, microprocessors are currently being fabricated with 0.18 µm feature sizes that make possible not only faster performance but the packaging of greatly increased functionality on the same size chip. This is the same scale that we will use to describe microtechnologies for chemical and biological applications.

Another new emerging field—nanotechnology—covers the atomic and molecular domains from a few nanometers to about 100 nm. Nanotechnology is defined as the creation of useful materials, devices, and systems through the control of matter on the nanometer length scale and the exploitation of novel properties and phenomena developed at that scale. As such, nano- and microregimes overlap and, indeed, there will be synergies between the two. For example, we will see nanoscale sensors as detection components in microscale laboratory devices. A brief discussion of nanotechnology and its applications will also be mentioned.

II.   TRADITIONAL METHODS OF MICROFABRICATION

The term *microfabrication* broadly refers to all techniques for fabricating devices and systems on the micrometer scale. As such, it borrows heavily from the processes and techniques pioneered in the semiconductor industry. To fabricate such small devices, processes that add, subtract, modify, and pattern materials are heavily used. The term *micromachining* can also be used to describe technologies to make devices other than electronic and semiconductor circuits. Similarly, these technologies can be characterized as additive (i.e., deposition of materials, metals, etc.) or subtractive (i.e., removal of materials through mechanical means, etching, laser processes, etc.). Micromachining processes can further be described as either surface or bulk. Surface techniques act on layers of materials above a base or substrate whereas bulk techniques also involve removal or modification of the substrate.

A.   Lithography and Photolithography

Lithography is the most basic method for the construction of microscale devices and is an old technique first developed in the early 19th century. Used originally and still widely in use today in the printing industry, lithography is also the mainstay of modern semiconductor manufacturing.

Lithography is basically a technique or suite of techniques for transferring copies of a master pattern onto the surface of a solid material. The most widely used form of lithography in the construction of microdevices is photolithography where the master pattern (i.e., a mask) is transferred onto a photosensitive solid material using an illuminated mask. Transfer of the mask pattern can be accomplished through either shadow printing whereby the mask is held close to (10–20 µm) or in contact with the surface of the photosensitive resist layer or by projection printing whereby the pattern is projected through an optical lens system onto the target layer. The latter can take advantage of magnifying or reducing optics to make very small features such as those seen in very large scale integrated (VLSI) devices.

1.   Bulk Micromachining

The exposed resist material is then removed or developed through various etching processes. The exposed portions of the resist layer are removed if positive resist materials are used and, conversely, unexposed portions of the resist are removed if negative resist materials are used. The basic positive resist process is illustrated in Figure 1.

In bulk micromachining, the substrate is removed wherever it is not protected by the resist material during the etching process. Etching can be either

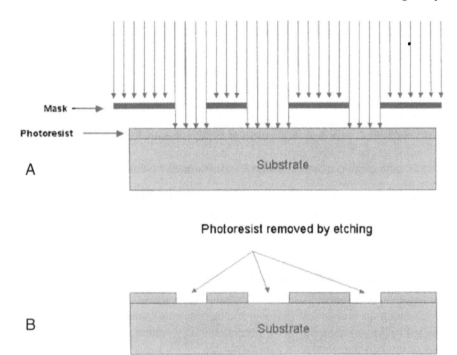

Figure 1 (A) The basic photolithographic process is illustrated wherein a photosensitive resist material on a substrate is exposed through a patterned mask. (B) After exposure the resist material is removed through a developing step. Positive photoresist material is shown in this example.

isotropic or anisotropic. In isotropic etching, removal of material occurs in all directions at the same or approximately the same rate. Isotropic etching tends to produce structures with rounded features. Anisotropic etching, on the other hand, tends to proceed along a preferred direction and results in more sharply defined features. While these terms describe the extremes of potential etching behavior, it is rare that either process operates to the exclusion of the other, and resulting structures are generally along a continuum somewhere between the two extremes.

    a. Isotropic Etching.   Isotropic etching removes material in all directions at the same or nearly the same rates. Deviations from true isotropic behavior are generally attributed to differences in chemical mass transport of etchants to target surfaces. Agitation of the material during etching greatly improves true isotropic performance. Figure 2 shows the individual steps involved in chemical etching, namely, diffusion from the bulk etchant solution and adsorption to the surface of the substrate where chemical reaction occurs. This is followed by desorption of the

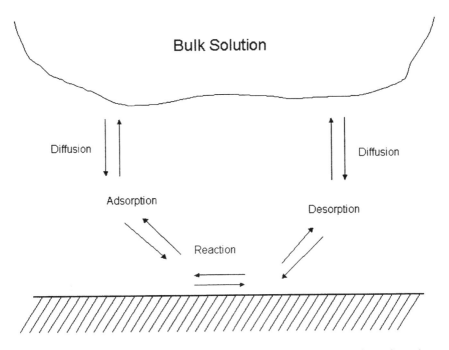

Figure 2 Chemical etching involves five steps: diffusion of reactants to the surface where they are adsorbed, reaction with the surface, and desorption and diffusion of reaction products into the bulk solution.

reaction products and, finally, diffusion of the reaction products back into the bulk solution.

Material removal is often accomplished through etching in acidic media. HNA, a mixture of HF/HNO$_3$/water and acetic acid, is commonly used.

The overall reaction [6] is given by:

$$Si + HNO_3 + 6HF = H_2SiF_6 + HNO_2 + H_2 + H_2O$$

Mechanistically, this reaction can be broken down into several sequential half reactions. Local oxidation of silicon takes place in nitric acid. The anodic reactions are also described as the injection of "holes" into the silicon and are given by:

$$Si = Si^{2+} + 2e^-$$

$$Si + 2H^+ = Si^{2+} + H_2$$

The corresponding cathodic reaction is the attachment of 2OH$^-$ groups to the Si^{2+} to form Si(OH)$_2$ and is given by:

$$2H_2O + 2e^- + 2OH^- + H_2$$

followed by:

$$Si^{2+} + 2OH^- = Si(OH)_2$$

and, finally:

$$Si(OH)_2 = SiO_2 + H_2$$

This is followed by the dissolution of the SiO_2 by HF:

$$SiO_2 + 6HF = H_2SiF_6 + 2H_2O$$

At high HF and low HNO_3 concentrations, the etch rate is controlled by HNO_3 concentration and the rate of oxidation of silicon. Conversely, at low HF and high HNO_3 concentrations, the etch rate is controlled by the ability of HF to remove SiO_2. Addition of acetic acid extends the useful range of oxidizing power of nitric acid over a wider range of dilution. The dielectric constant of acetic acid of approximately 6, compared to water of 81, results in less dissociation of the nitric acid. The etching reaction is diffusion controlled and the concentration determines the etch rate, so that mixing is important for uniform etching behavior. Table 1 summarizes some typical isotropic etching solution concentrations and their effects.

Although isotropic etching agents are simple to use, there are several drawbacks. It is difficult to mask with high precision with a masking agent such as SiO_2 because the masking agent is also etched to a measurable degree. Moreover, the etch rate is sensitive to temperature-stirring conditions. For this reason, anisotropic etching agents were developed.

b. Anisotropic Etching. The discovery of anisotropic etchants in the 1960s addressed the lack of geometrical control presented by isotropic bulk etching agents. These agents preferentially etch along a particular crystalline direction

Table 1   Isotropic HNA-Based Silicon Etching Solutions

Nitric acid	HF	Acetic acid	Comments
100	1	99	Removes shallow implants
91	9		Polishing etch at 5 μm/min with stirring
75	25		Polishing etch at 20 μm/min with stirring
66	34		Polishing etch at 50 μm/min with stirring
15	2	5	Planar etch
6	1	1	Slow polishing etch
5	3	3	Nonselective polishing
3	1	1	Selective etch of n+ or p+ with added $NaNO_2$ or H_2O_2

with a discrimination or anisotropy ratio (AR) that can exceed 500:1. The anisotropy ratio is defined as

$$AR = (hkl)_1 \text{ etch rate}/(hkl)_2 \text{ etch rate}$$

AR is defined as approximately 1 for isotropic etchants and can be as high as 400/1 for the <110>/<111> crystal orientations using potassium hydroxide (KOH).

A wide variety of etching solutions are available for anisotropic etching. Two popular ones are KOH and tetramethylammonium hydroxide (TMAH). Table 2 gives some of the properties of these popular anisotropic etchants. Others include the hydroxides of other alkali metals, such as NaOH, CsOH, and RbOH, ammonium hydroxide, ethylenediamine pyrocatechol (EDP), hydrazine, and amine gallates. For each, a key feature is the fact that the <111> crystal directions are attacked at rates at least 10 times, and typically 20–100 times, lower than other crystalline directions. Anisotropic etching can also be further controlled by the introduction of dopants or by electrochemical modulation.

c. Etch Stopping. It is often desirable to stop the etching process at precisely defined places. Highly doped p^+ regions, generally obtained with gaseous or solid boron diffusion into the silicon substrate, greatly attenuate the etching rate. It is believed that doping leads to a more readily oxidizable surface. These oxides are not readily soluble in KOH or EDP etchants,

Other attenuation methods include electrochemical modulation. This involves holding the silicon positive to a platinum counterelectrode. A very smooth silicon surface can result (referred to as electropolishing). Photon-pumped electrochemical etching is also a popular modulation technique especially for high-aspect-ratio features.

2. Surface Micromachining

Surface micromachining refers to those processes that act on layers above a substrate. Figure 3 illustrates the principle. As in bulk micromachining, both additive

Table 2 Typical Etch Rates and Conditions for Anisotropic Etchants

Formulation	Temp (°C)	Etch rate (μm/min)	<100>/<111> Etch ratio	Mask film
KOH, water, isopropanol	85	1.4	400:1	SiO_2 (1.4 nm/min) Si_3N_4 (negligible)
KOH, water	65	0.25–1.0		SiO_2 (0.7 nm/min) Si_3N_4 (negligible)
TMAH, water	90	3.0	10	SiO_2 (0.2 nm/min)

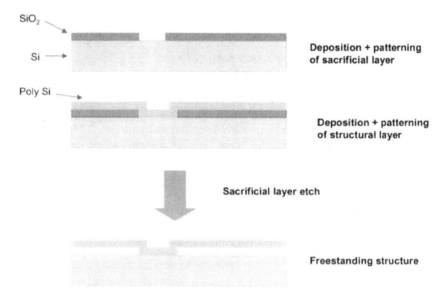

Figure 3   Surface micromachining operates on layers deposited on the surface of a substrate.

and subtractive processes can occur with surface micromachining. A problem unique to surface techniques is sticking whereby supposedly freestanding surface micromachined structures adhere to the substrate after the last rinse.

The primary cause of sticking is the capillary force of water that pulls the structure against the wafer. Ethanol can be added to the rinse water to reduce surface tension. Ethanol and *t*-butyl alcohol followed by freeze drying can also be used as can the addition of antisticking surfaces such as fluorocarbon film.

Many structures have been made with surface techniques. These include digital micromirror devices (DMDs) or arrays (DMMAs), which are used in digital light projectors and now also have seen application in the construction of oligonucleotide hybridization arrays. A picture of nine elements of a DMMA is shown in Figure 4. Other common surface micromachined devices include valves [7] and nozzles [8].

3. Metal Electrodeposition

Electroplating is a very useful process for producing additive metal structures above a substrate. A large number of metals can be electroplated, including copper, gold, silver, nickel, and platinum. These are generally reduced from a salt solution, typically a sulfate or cyanide. Either DC or AC current can be used, with the latter generally resulting in much finer grain growth.

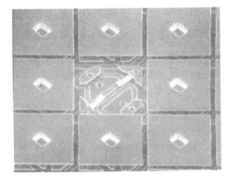 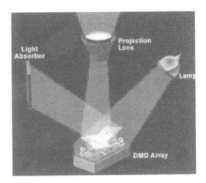

Figure 4 This view of nine digital micromirror device (DMD) array elements shows the mirrors with the central mirror removed to expose the underlying, hidden-hinge structure. These mirror elements are either in an on or off state. In the on state they reflect light onto a screen, while in the off state the light is directed to a beam absorber. The on mirror reflects light into the lens and the off mirror reflects light into a light absorber. Each mirror in the array is individually controlled and is totally independent of all other mirrors. The amount of a particular color in a particular pixel is used to determine the amount of time the corresponding mirror will be in the on state for that movie frame. The mirrors may turn on and off as many as 50,000 times a second, which enables a large number of color possibilities and the elimination of flicker. (Courtesy of Texas Instruments, USA.)

As an alternate to electricity, some metals can be deposited using chemical reducing agents. These are the so-called electroless processes and can be used for gold and nickel. Chemical reducing agents include potassium borohydride (KBH_4) and dimethylamine borane (DMAB) for gold and NaH_2PO_2 for nickel. Aspect ratios for structures generated by electroless plating can reach 10:1.

B.   Newer Techniques and Materials

Many techniques have evolved and been developed during the past 30 years. A few of these are profiled below. This list is far from complete, and there are also many variations on the ones described below. However, these techniques are commonly used, and therefore some familiarity will be useful.

1.   Plasma and Deep Reactive Ion Etching

There are several dry-etching processes that include the use of reactive gas plasmas and ions. External energy in the form of radiofrequency (RF) power drives the chemical reactions. In a plasma etcher, the wafer is one of two electrodes and is grounded. The powered electrode is the same size as the wafer. Plasmas are generally low temperature and operate in the 150–250°C range; however, some operate down to room temperature. In deep reactive ion etching (DRIE), the powered electrode is the wafer with the other electrode being much larger.

Very-high-AR devices (40:1) can be obtained with these techniques. Reactant gases generating ions in the RF field generally have unusually high incident energies normal to the substrate. Some common etch gases and mixtures are $CClF_3 + Cl_2$, $CHCl_3 + CL_2$, SF_6, NF_3, CCl_4, $CF_4 + H_2$, and C_2ClF_5.

2. X-ray LIGA

LIGA is an acronym for the German "Lithographie, Galvanoformung, Abformung," a succession of lithographic, electroplating, and molding processes. LIGA can generate high-aspect-ratio devices in excess of 100:1. Developed by W. Ehrfeld [9], LIGA is a template-guided microfabrication process that uses an extremely well-collimated synchrotron x-ray radiation source to transfer a pattern onto a substrate.

Figure 5 shows the basic steps of the LIGA process. A primary substrate is coated with a conductive top layer. Polymethyl methacrylate (PMMA) is then

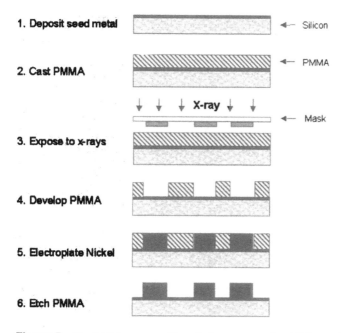

Figure 5 The LIGA process. Steps 1–5 are conventional lithography. Nickel is electroplated in step 6 after which the wafer is lapped to the desired thickness. Step 6 shows the remaining PMMA removed. The structures can then be freed from the seed metal base layer.

applied typically through a series of multiple spin casts or as a commercially pre-pared thin sheet solvent-bonded to the substrate. The PMMA is then exposed through a mask opaque to x-rays and then developed resulting in high-aspect structures. Metal is then electroplated into the PMMA mold, and the resulting assembly is diamond lapped and polished to the desired height. The remaining PMMA is then developed away and a chemical etch removes the conducting top layer, thus freeing the part.

One drawback to LIGA is the need for a synchrotron radiation source that restricts access to the technique dramatically, even though there are many such light sources available worldwide,

Many devices have been constructed using the LIGA process. These include microvalves [10], micropumps [11], fluidic amplifiers [12], and membrane filters [13]. Some of these devices, while manufactured by the LIGA technique, have subsequently proven inferior to or more expensive than those made by other tech-nologies.

3. UV LIGA

To overcome the limitation of synchrotron light source requirement, thick UV-sensitive resists, such as polyimides, AZ-4000, and SU-8, have been developed as alternatives to the x-ray-sensitive PMMA. Epon SU-8 is an epoxy-based, trans-parent negative photoresist material that can be built up into 200-μm-thick layers. Hoechst AZ-4000 is a positive resist material that can be built up into layers 15–80 μm thick with multiple spin coats. These materials and the technique certainly are more accessible than LIGA. Aspect ratios of 5:1 to 15:1 can be achieved with these materials.

4. Polymer Replication

The fabrication of microdevices with conventional plastic molding technologies; such as reaction injection and thermoplastic molding and hot embossing, should not be overlooked. These continue to be by far the cheapest alternatives to making microstructures in materials. The entire CD industry is dependent on these tech-nologies, so that micrometer-size features in plastic are readily achievable. Many of the microfluidic devices currently appearing on the market are made by this technique and are designed to be inexpensive and disposable.

5. Laser Ablation

Powerful laser beams have sufficient energy to ablate silicon through thermal evaporation. The 1.06 μm Nd:YAG and carbon dioxide laser systems are used rou-tinely for drilling silicon. Lasers can be used for subtractive as well as additive processes and have been used for annealing, deposition, and welding. In laser beam cutting, coherent light replaces electrons as the cutting tool. Removal rates tend to be slow. Lasers have also been used to assist in chemical etching to photo-disassociate the reactive etchant.

6. Ion Beam Milling

Ion beam milling is a thermomechanical drilling technique wherein the drill bit is a stream of ions. Typically a liquid metal, such as gallium, is focused to a submicrometer diameter. Like laser ablation, ion beam milling is a slow serial technique. Atomic force microscope tools are made by ion beam milling, but the technique is generally too expensive to use in a mass production mode.

7. Ultraprecision Machining

Single-crystal diamond tools have made ultrahigh-precision mechanical machining possible. A machining accuracy in the low-submicrometer range is possible. Throughput is extremely slow and there are stringent environmental requirements on the machine. This technique will thus find limited use in the mass fabrication of microscale laboratory devices.

8. Porous Silicon as a Sensor Material

Porous silicon was first discovered [14] during electropolishing of silicon in 1956. At low current densities, partial dissolution of Si results during etching with HF with the formation of hydrogen gas:

$$Si + 2F^- + 2H^+ = SiF_2$$

$$SiF_2 + 2HF = Si4_2 + H_2$$

A very porous silicon structure results that can have aspect ratios up to 250. Silicon can be made either microporous or macroporous. The pores follow crystallographic orientation and vary in size from 20 Å to 10 μm. Porous silicon oxidizes readily and etches at a very high rate. A prepattern is generally defined by a photolithographic transfer. The etch pits formed at exposed area of the mask serve as nucleation centers for macropores.

Porous silicon has been used in a number of applications, including electrochemical reference electrodes, high-surface-area gas sensors, humidity sensors, and sacrificial layers in micromachining. Recent research has focused on using porous silicon as a substrate for chemical sensors [15]. The silicon pillars can be derivatized using well-known chemistries and linked to chemical recognition molecules (i.e., antibodies or oligonucleotides). When immersed in a solution of target molecules and exposed to light, an interference pattern results that is extremely sensitive to concentration. These porous silicon sensors can serve either as standalone instruments or as the sensing element in an integrated fluidic chip.

III. SYSTEM INTEGRATION ISSUES

Integration covers a whole spectrum of issues from the semiconductor and fluidic level to the control, to information display and treatment, and to user interface levels. Integration must address electronic interfaces, mechanical and optical interfaces, materials and packaging issues, as well as the chemical compatibility and functionality.

Many single components, such as valves, pumps, separation columns, and optical and electrochemical detectors, have been made in the past 30 years and have been proven to work individually. The focus of much current work is to show how these components can be assembled into a multiple-function device. Activities such as sample preparation, detection, and data presentation are increasingly being collocated.

The choices of materials is wide. Materials must be chosen not only for ease and expense of fabrication but for chemical and biochemical compatibility. Table 3 lists some common choices, along with their advantages and disadvantages.

A. Interfaces

Fluid interconnects do not exist for microfluidic devices and those that have been used vary widely from pipet tips and glue to gas chromatographic fittings and microfabricated fittings [16,17]. In general, the "macro-to-micro" interface issues have not been well resolved. Various technologies including electrokinetic samples made by Caliper allow for the sampling of multiwell microtiter plates.

Table 3 Microchip Systems Material Selection Guide

Material	Advantages	Disadvantages
Silicon	IC compatible, large technology base, bulk etching, surface micromachining, and dry or wet processing; can include electronics	Chemically reactive surface
Glass	Insulating, transparent, good chemical compatibility, bulk etching (like silicon), large lab experience	Little commercial technology base
Plastics	Low cost—used widely in commercial diagnostics systems, replication using hot embossing on a nm scale	Untried commercially on fine resolution, hydrophobic chemicals absorbed

Source: S. Verpoorte and J. Harrison, Short Course on Microfluidics taught at LabAutomation2000, Palm, Springs, CA, January 22–23, 2000.

B. Fluidics and Electronic Integration

Monolithic integration places all components on the same device. Typically, actuators and sensing elements are made in the same process. Little or no assembly is required; monolithic systems are highly reliable and low in cost. The limitations include incompatibilities with process steps, low overall yield due to many points of failure, and high costs for small quantities. Several layers, all with their own processing requirements, can be sandwiched together to make a final assembly in a collective system. The benefits of collective integration include being able to segregate chemical and processing step incompatibilities. Higher individual step yields are countered by the final assembly requirements and are often highly variable. As in collective integration, hybrid integration results in a sandwich construction. The layers of silicon, glass, or plastic can either fluidic, control, or electronic, and are assembled and bonded together.

C. Integral Detection Systems

Sample measurement in chips presents new challenges to detection systems. The most popular modalities are fluorescence, absorbance, luminescence, and chemiluminescence. Other methods include use of mass sensors such as mass spectrometry and acoustic wave devices; electrochemical sensors such as potentiometric, amperometric, and conductivity; and, finally, thermal sensors such as bolometers and thermopiles. All are handicapped to an extent by the small sample sizes encountered on chips and therefore must be very sensitive or coupled to chemistries that exhibit amplification.

IV. APPLICATIONS OF MICROTECHNOLOGIES

A. Bead-based Fiberoptic Arrays

The ability to etch silicon materials predictably has given rise to an interesting technology based on fiberoptics [18–20]. Optical fibers are made from two kinds of glass or plastic: a core and a cladding. The core has a slightly higher refractive index than the cladding, permitting the fiber to transmit light over long distances through total internal reflection. Today's high-bandwidth telecommunications technology is based on optical fibers.

The fibers can be made with 3–7 μm in outside diameters. One thousand of these fibers can be bundled together into a 1-mm-diameter bundle. The ends are then etched with hydrofluoric acid to produce micrometer-size or femtoliter-size pits. Figure 6 shows an image of these wells taken with an atomic force microscope.

It is possible to insert individual microspheres into these wells. The beads are sized so that they self-assemble, one to a well, when the fiber bundles are

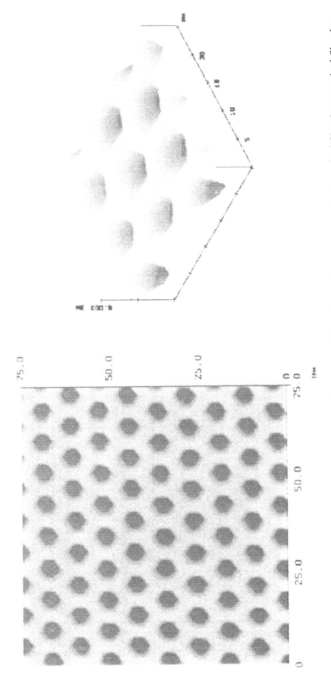

Figure 6 An atomic force microscope image of the wells generated by etching the inner core of each optical fiber in an optical fiber bundle. The capacity of each well is on the order of a few femtoliters. (Courtesy of David R. Walt Group, Tufts University.)

dipped into a 20% solids slurry. One milliliter of such a slurry can contain 100 million beads. Each individual bead can be optically encoded with fluorescent dyes [21] so that it reports a unique optical "bar code" when interrogated with a laser. Figure 7 illustrates the sequence of steps. Moreover, it is possible to construct an array of 384 of these fiber bundles on a 4.5-mm pitch to fit into a standard 384-well microtiter plate. This increases the amount of information gathered in a single experiment to more than 2 million data points. This technology is currently being commercialized by Illumina, Inc. [22].

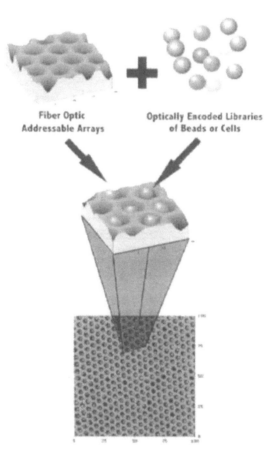

Figure 7 A self-assembled array of optically encoded microbeads into femtoliter-size wells on the ends of individual optical fibers. The identity of the bead is first determined followed by a measurement of the concentration of analyte attached to the bead by selective chemistries. (Courtesy of Illumina Inc.)

Illumina's proprietary Oligator technology complements its BeadArray technology. The Oligator synthesizes in parallel many different short segments of DNA to meet the requirements of large-scale genomics applications. With unique segments of DNA attached to each bead, the BeadArray technology can be used for SNP genotyping.

B. DNA Arrays

Much has been written about oligonucleotide, DNA or cDNA, and RNA microarrays. This technology was first commercialized by Affymetrix, Incyte, and Hyseq. It relies on surface micromachining techniques wherein the "layers" are successively photolithographically masked in light-directed oligonucleotide synthesis steps. For example, the Affymetrix technique works by shining light through a photolithographic mask onto a light-sensitive surface. The surface reactions are controlled so as to carry out the standard phosphoramidite oliognucleotide chemistry. Various cycles of protection and deprotection are required to build up a typical 20-mer oligo at specific sites.

Some of the limitations of this approach to making arrays are that masks are not cheap or quick to make and are specific to the pattern of oligonucleotides that make up the array. A new approach, based on surface micromachining semiconductor technology from Texas Instruments [24], uses a digital micromirror device (DMD). Figure 4 illustrates the DMD device. A DMD consists of individually addressable mirrors on a dense 600×800 array in a 10×14 mm area. There are nearly half a million addressable locations available for light-directed synthesis of oligonucleotides. DMD technology is in common use today in digital light projectors. Recently, a research group at Wisconsin [25] has demonstrated the use of DMD in the construction of oligoarrays. Light from an arc lamp directed by digitally controlled micromirrors cleaves photolabile protecting groups off the ends of DNA molecules. The illuminated areas then couple to the next base to be added while the dark areas remain unreactive.

The ability to spatially control selective chemistries is the basis of much array-based technology. Even higher densities can be obtained with arrays of femtoliter microwells made with standard polymer embossing techniques. Whitesides et al. [26] have described soft lithographic techniques to construct planar arrays of approximately 3-fl wells with 10^7 wells/cm^2. Basically, an array of posts formed in a photoresist on a silicon wafer is used as a "master" to form the arrays of microwells. The master is generated by rapid prototyping or standard photolithography with a chrome mask. The arrays of wells were fabricated by molding an elastomeric polymer against the master. The wells have aspect ratios ranging from 1:1 to 1.5:1. The authors describe a technique for filling the wells that takes advantage of the difference in the interfacial free energies of the substrate and the liquid of interest and controlling the topology of the surface. Liquid is allowed to drain off an array of microwells either by gravity or by pulling the array from a bulk solution.

One application of DNA array technology is that of Hyseq. The HyChip system uses arrays of a complete set of DNA probes in conjunction with a target-specific cocktail of labeled probes to identify differences between a reference and test samples. Since the chip contains all possible probes, the HyChip system has the distinct advantage of being able to sequence DNA from any source. Other available DNA chip technologies require prior knowledge of the gene sequence and mutations prior to chip design, and require no less than one chip for each gene being tested. The HyChip system is therefore universal and requires only a single chip for a wide variety of targets.

The arrays produced by the companies above tend to be very high density with thousands if not millions of uniquely addressable locations. There is also a very large market for lower density arrays produced on coated surfaces by mechanical systems such as robots and cartesian spotting devices. Table 4 lists some of the leading manufacturers of microarray spotting systems, slide suppliers, scanners image processing software, and data analysis software.

C. Electronically Enhanced Hybridization

DNA sequencing by hybridization (SBH) [27,28] and other oligonucleotide hybridization protocols rely on a rather time-consuming hybridization step. Although there are many variables to control for a successful hybdridization, migration of the DNA to the fixed complementary probe tends to be slow. Often this step requires hours to overnight reaction times. Recently, Nanogen has commercialized a chip that electronically drives the target DNA to the probes, greatly speeding up this process [29]. After hybridization, the chip is washed and detection occurs reducing a typical several hour experiment to less than 30 min.

Nanogen's technology allows small sequences of DNA capture probes to be electronically placed at, or "addressed" to, specific sites on the microchip. A test sample can then be analyzed for the presence of target DNA molecules by determining which of the DNA capture probes on the array bind, or hybridize, with complementary DNA in the test sample. In contrast to nonelectronic or passive hybridization with conventional arrays on paper or glass "chips," the use of electronically mediated active hybridization to move and concentrate target DNA molecules accelerates hybridization so that hybridization may occur in minutes rather than the hours required for passive hybridization techniques. In addition to DNA applications, this technology can be applied to a number of other analyses, including antigen–antibody, enzyme–substrate, cell–receptor, isolation of cancer cells from peripheral blood cells, [30], and cell separation techniques.

Table 4 Selected Companies Providing Microarray Technologies, Surfaces, Scanners, Imaging Software, and Data Analysis Tools

Company/institution	Web site
Beecher Instruments	http://www.beecherinstruments.com
BioRobotics	http://www.biorobotics.com
Cartesian Technologies	http://www.cartesiantech.com
Engineering Services	http://www.esit.com/
Genetic Microsystems	http://www.geneticmicro.com
Genetix	http://www.genetix.co.uk
Gene Machines	http://www.genemachines.com
Intelligent Automation Systems	http://www.ias.com
Packard	http://www.packardinst.com
Amersham Pharmacia Biotech	http://www.apbiotech.com
Corning CoStar	http://www.cmt.corning.com
Surmodics	http://www.surmodics.com
Telechem	http://www.arrayit.com
Axon	http://www.axon.com
GSI Luminomoics	http://www.gsilminomics.com
Genomic Solution	http://www.genomicsolutions.com
Molecular Dynamics	http://www.mdyn.com
Virtek	http://www.virtek.com
BioDiscovery	http://www.biodiscovery.com/
Imaging Research	http://imaging.brocku.ca/arrayvision.html
National Human Genome Research Institute	http://www.nhgri.nih.gov/DIR/LCG/15K/img _analysis.html
Stanford University	http://rana.stanford.edu/software/
The Institute for Genomic Research	http://www.tigr.org/softlab/
Silicon Gentics	http://www.signetics.com
Spotfire	http://www.spotfire.com

1.   Electronic Addressing

Electronic addressing is the placement of charged molecules at specific test sites. Since DNA has a strong negative charge, it can be electronically moved to an area of positive charge. A test site or a row of test sites on the microchip is electronically activated with a positive charge. A solution of DNA probes is introduced onto the microchip. The negatively charged probes rapidly move to the positively charged sites, where they concentrate and are chemically bound to that site. The microchip is then washed and another solution of distinct DNA probes can be added. Site by site, row by row, an array of specifically bound DNA probes can be assembled or addressed on the microchip. In the electronic addressing illustration

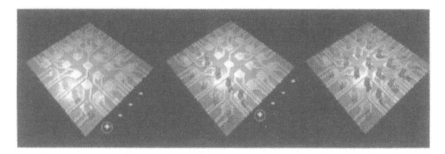

Figure 8   A test site or a row of test sites on the microchip is electronically activated with a positive charge. A solution of DNA probes is introduced onto the microchip. The negatively charged probes rapidly move to the positively charged sites, where they concentrate and are chemically bound to that site. The microchip is then washed and another solution of distinct DNA probes can be added. Site by site, row by row, an array of specifically bound DNA probes can be assembled or addressed on the microchip. (Courtesy of Nanogen, Inc.)

shown in Figure 8, a total of five sets of different capture probes have been electronically addressed to the microchip. With the ability to electronically address capture probes to specific sites, the system allows end-users to build custom arrays through the placement of specific capture probes on a microchip. In contrast to current technologies, these microchip arrays can be addressed in a matter of minutes at a minimal cost, providing research professionals with a powerful and versatile tool to process and analyze molecular information.

2.   Electronic Concentration and Hybridization

Following electronic addressing, electronics are used to move and concentrate target molecules to one or more test sites on the microchip, as shown in Figure 9. The electronic concentration of sample DNA at each test site promotes rapid hybridization of sample DNA with complementary capture probes. In contrast to the passive hybridization process, the electronic concentration process has the distinct advantage of significantly accelerating the rate of hybridization. To remove any unbound or nonspecifically bound DNA from each site, the polarity or charge of the site is reversed to negative, thereby forcing any unbound or nonspecifically bound DNA back into solution away from the capture probes. In addition, since the test molecules are electronically concentrated over the test site, a lower concentration of target DNA molecules is required, thus reducing the time and labor otherwise required for pretest sample preparation.

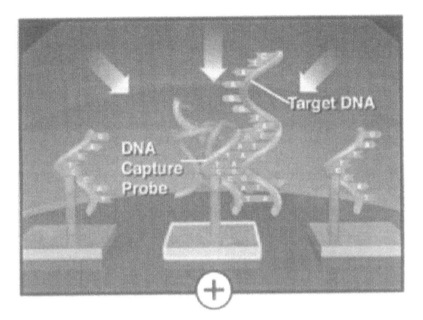

Figure 9 The electronic concentration of sample DNA at each test site promotes rapid hybridization of sample DNA with complementary capture probes. The electronic concentration process has the distinct advantage of significantly accelerating the rate of hybridization. The polarity or charge of the site is subsequently reversed to negative, thereby forcing any unbound or nonspecifically bound DNA back into solution. (Courtesy of Nanogen, Inc.)

3. Electronic Stringency Control

Electronic stringency control is the reversal of electrical potential to quickly and easily remove unbound and nonspecifically bound DNA as part of the hybridization process. Electronic stringency provides quality control for the hybridization process and ensures that any bound pairs of DNA are truly complementary. The precision, control, and accuracy through the use of the controlled delivery of current in the electronic stringency process, as shown in Figure 10, permits the detection of single-point mutations, single-base-pair mismatches, or other genetic mutations, which may have significant implications in a number of diagnostic and research areas. Electronic stringency is achieved without the cumbersome processing and handling otherwise required to achieve the same results through conventional methods. In contrast to passive arrays, Nanogen's technology can accommodate both short and long single-stranded fragments of DNA. The use of longer probes increases the certainty that the DNA that hybridizes with the capture probe is the correct target. Nanogen's electronic stringency control reduces

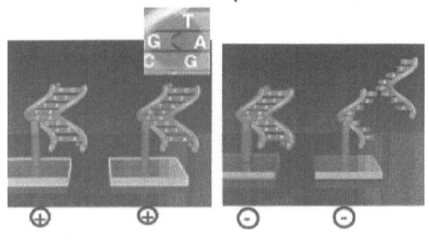

Figure 10   The precision, control, and accuracy through the use of the controlled delivery of current in the electronic stringency process permits the detection of single-point mutations, single-base-pair mismatches, or other genetic mutations. (Courtesy of Nanogen, Inc.)

the required number of probes and therefore test sites on the microchip, relative to conventional DNA arrays. In contrast, traditional passive hybridization processes are difficult to control and require more replicants of every possible base pair match so that correct matches can be positively identified.

D.   Microfluidic Devices

There are many university research laboratories and institutes across the world working in the area of microfluidic devices of all kinds. Much early work was done by such groups as Ramsey's at Oak Ridge National Laboratory [31–33] who, in addition to the groups of de Rooij [34], Manz [35], and Harrison [36,37], for example, continue to be very active.

Microfluidic technologies have over the past decade matured sufficiently so that it has become the basis for many companies. Many of these companies also perform fundamental research while providing their technologies to customers either as products or in early technology access partnerships. Still other companies use microfluidics technology in a specialized application and market the value added in a specialized field of endeavor, such as environmental monitoring, patient diagnostics, genetic testing, or drug discovery. For example, complete instrument systems based on microfluidic separations are emerging, many integrated with detection.

1. Microfluidic Separations

Caliper Technologies was founded on the technologies originating in many of these research labs. During 1999, Caliper introduced its first two LabChip systems—a personal laboratory system for the life sciences market and a high-throughput screening system to aid pharmaceutical companies in discovering new drugs. Codeveloped with Agilent, the first laboratory system consists of the Agilent 2100 bioanalyzer, a desktop instrument designed to perform a wide range of scientific experiments using a menu of different LabChip kits. Each kit contains chips and reagents designed for specific applications. The LabChip system brings the benefits of miniaturized, integrated, and automated experimentation to the researcher's desktop. Agilent launched this product in September 1999. Current applications include DNA and RNA analysis. Figure 11 shows the Agilent 2100 bioanalyzer. The analyzer works with a series of chips optimized for DNA and RNA analysis, e.g., the DNA 7500 LabChip assay kit provides size and concentration information for DNA fragments ranging in size from 100 to 7500 base pairs.

Caliper's LabChip high-throughput screening system utilizes chips that draw nanoliter volumes of reagents from microplates for analysis. The system performs a wide range of experiments using a menu of different chips. Caliper cur-

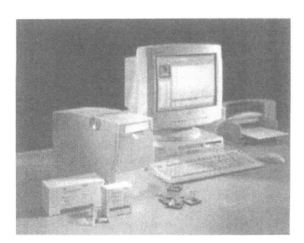

Figure 11   Agilent 2100 bioanalyzer based on the Caliper Lab on a Chip technology. The system operates with several chip kits specific to the analysis of DNA and RNA. Other kits are in development. (Courtesy of Caliper Technologies.)

rently offers chips to perform drug screening for several classes of targets and anticipates offering more chips, currently in development, to increase both capability and throughput.

Using a similar approach, ACLARA Biosciences has demonstrated rapid, high-resolution electrophoretic separations in plastic chips [38–40]. DNA fragment sizing is required in numerous applications and represents an attractive target market wherein ACLARA provides ready-to-use disposable plastic chips, prefilled with a proprietary gel. ACLARA produces plastic chips in polymers thereby enabling the mass production of low-cost disposable chips. They use two main steps in the production of plastic chips: (1) formation of microstructures in a base layer and (2) sealing of the base layer with a cover layer. To form the base layer, microstructure patterns are replicated from a micromachined master (or submaster) onto a polymeric substrate. ACLARA has developed several different replication technologies that span a range of capabilities and economies of scale, enabling the company to select the most appropriate technology for any application under development.

2. Microfluidic Synthesis

Traditional means of transferring fluids with pipets are severely challenged much above 384 wells in a microtiter plate. The microfluidic technology developed by Orchid Biocomputer [41] provides a viable route to achieve much higher levels of densification, unachievable by traditional systems. Orchid is developing modular chip-based systems with 96, 384, 1536, and 12,288 (8×1536) reactor arrays that accommodate 100- to 80-nl sample volumes.

The unique features of the Orchid chips include the ability to process hundreds of reactions in parallel through the use of precise fluidic delivery methods. These chips use hydrostatic pressure pulses with nonmechanical microvalves fabricated in the multilayer collective device to transfer fluids vertically and horizontally into 700-nl microreaction wells. The highly complex three-dimensional architecture of these chips enables the broadest range of capabilities of any chip in the industry. With this enclosed system there is no risk of evaporation or reagent degradation. One important application of Orchid's microfluidic technology is in parallel chemical processing as embodied in the Chemtel chip shown in Figure 12.

3. Chip-Based Flow Cytometry for Medical Diagnostics

A multidisciplinary team at was formed at the University of Washington School of Medicine's departments of bioengineering, mechanical engineering, electrical engineering, and laboratory medicine. The developments resulting from this multidisciplinary research have been licensed from the University of Washington to Micronics, Inc. [42].

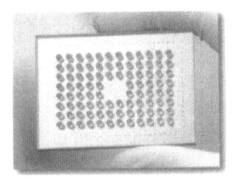

Figure 12 The Orchid biocomputer microfluidic chip. (Courtesy of Orchid Biocomputer.)

Micronics is further developing microfluidics-based systems for application to clinical laboratory diagnostics and analytical and process control chemical determinations. In both instances, the small size and autocalibrating characteristics of the microfluidics technology lends itself to application at the point of the sample. This avoids the transportation of sample to centralized laboratories—a step that results in both delays and degradation of the sample—and it provides answers at the point were decisions can be made immediately.

A major area of Micronics' technology is in microfluidic-based cell cytometry. In operation, biological cells from a sample, such as blood, pass in single file through a channel on which is focused a laser beam. Light scattering measurements are taken at multiple angles, and these multiparameter scatter measurements provide a "fingerprint" for the various types of cells. This technology, known as flow cytometry, is not new. However, Micronics is implementing the technology on a microfluidic scale using new miniaturized optical technology developed recently for CD readers. Micronics microcytometer technology has demonstrated the capacity to count and classify platelets, red blood cells, and various white cell populations by means of laminate-based microfluidic flow channels and light scattering optics. Additional light scattering and data analysis channels will be used to extend the capabilities of the microcytometer toward a complete blood cell assay including a five-part white cell differential.

4. Microfluidics in a Rotating CD

Gyros Microlabs AB has integrated a microfluidics system based on a simple modular design, consisting of a spinner unit, a flow-through noncontact liquid microdispenser, CD with proprietary applications and chemistries, detector(s), and software.

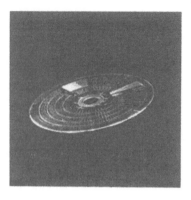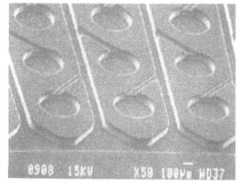

Figure 13 A lab on a CD design and a close-up of individual microchannels. Fluid transport is achieved through the action of centripetal force as the CD spins. (Courtesy of Gyros Microlab AB.)

Many complex steps, such as sample preparation, fluid handling, sample processing, and analysis, can be carried out seamlessly within the confines of a single CD. The CD, shown in Figure 13, is made up of intricate, molded microchannels in plastic, creating interconnected networks of fluid reservoirs and pathways. No pumps are required because spinning the CD moves the liquids around. What makes the technology versatile is the ability to rapidly and easily create application-specific CDs, where the applications are embedded in the intricate microstructures on the CD.

One application explored is high-throughout SNP scoring on a CD in combination with solid-phase pyrosequencing [43]. The centripetal force in the CD device allows for parallel processing without complex tubing connections. One of their current designs integrates the whole process for single-nucleotide polymorphism (SNP) analysis, including sample preparation, achieving more than 100,000 SNPs per day [44].

Gyros has also developed flow-through, noncontact, piezoelectric dispenser allowing them to deposit a precise amount of liquid into each microstructure while the CD is spinning at 3000 rpm, thus managing many operations simultaneously without any evaporation problems. The flow-through principle facilitates the use of thousands of different samples or reagents. Gyros is developing a full range of dispenser variants including arrays, which will revolutionize the way small volumes of liquids can be handled.

As can be seen from the selected examples, many products and services are being developed based on microarray and microfluidic components. Table 5 lists some of the companies along with their web site to which the readers are referred for additional information.

Table 5 Selected Companies and Institutes and Web Sites

Company/institution	Website	Comments
Oak Ridge National Laboratory	http://www.ornl.gov	Large microfluidic development effort
Caliper Technologies	http://calipertech.com	One of the early companies in microfluidic systems, DNA applications
ACLARA Biosciences	http://www.aclara.com/	Microfluidic systems, DNA applications
Illumina	http://www.illumina.com/	Fiberoptic, self-assembling bead arrays, very high-throughput assay technology
Hyseq	http://www.hyseq.com/	Developer of sequencing by hybridization (SBH)
Nanogen	http://www.nanogen.com	Electronically-driven hybridization
Orchid Biosciences	http://www.orchidbio.com	Early microfluidic company focused on chip-based synthesis and SNP scoring
Micronics	http://www.micronics.net/	Licensor of Univ. of Washington microfluidic technologies, microcytometry
Gyros Microlab AB	http://www.gyrosmicro.com/	Lab on a CD disk

V. NANOTECHNOLOGY

Nanotechnology [45] is a very broad emerging discipline; it describes the utilization and construction of structures with at least one characteristic dimension measured in nanometers. Such materials and systems can be deterministically designed to exhibit novel and significantly improved physical, chemical, and biological properties, phenomena, and processes because of their size. Since they are intermediate between individual atoms and bulk materials, their physical attributes are often also markedly different. These physical properties are not necessarily predictable extrapolations from larger scales. Currently known nanostructures include carbon nanotubes, proteins, and DNA.

In biology, recent insights indicate that DNA sequencing can be made many orders of magnitude more efficient with nanotechnology. It can also provide new formulations and routes for drug discovery, enormously broadening the therapeutic potential of drugs. For example, drugs or genes bound to nanoparticles can be administered into the bloodstream and delivered directly to cells. Furthermore, given the inherent nanoscale of receptors, ion channels, and other functional components of living cells, nanoparticles may offer a new way to study these components.

Nanosensors with selectivities approaching those of antigen–antibody or hybridization reactions will greatly influence chemistry and instrumentation development. These sensors would be naturally complementary to microfluidic systems, and we should expect to see these systems integrated in the future.

Scientists are just now beginning to understand how to create nanostructures by design. A more complete understanding will lead to advances in many industries, including material science, manufacturing, computer technology, medicine and health, aeronautics, environment, and energy, to name a few. The total societal impact of nanotechnology is expected to be greater than the combined influences that the silicon integrated circuit, medical imaging, computer-aided engineering, and manufactured polymers have had in this century. Significant improvements in performance and changes of manufacturing paradigms will lead to several industrial revolutions in the 21st century. Nanotechnology will change the nature of almost every man-made object. The major question now is, how soon will this revolution arrive?

VI. SUMMARY

The above examples are merely illustrative and not intended to be a comprehensive coverage of all available systems of current research. This field is changing very rapidly; new products, services based on microfluidic systems, and even new companies are constantly emerging. Most of the above products were made by combinations of the fabrications technologies described in the first part of this chapter. They also illustrate how fundamental developments made in various research groups are migrating to the private sector and eventually to the marketplace.

These devices are the tip of the iceberg. They are indicative of the state of the technology and also serve as a prelude to products to come.

REFERENCES

1.   Petersen, K. E., Silicon as a Mechanical Material, Proc IEEE, vol. 70, no. 5, May 1982, pp. 420–457.
2.   See, for example: Larry Licklider, Xuan-Qi Wang, Amish Desai, Yu-Chong Tai, Terry D. Lee, A micromachined chip-based electrospray source for mass spectrometry, Anal. Chem, 72, 367–75, 2000.
3.   Marc Madou, Fundamentals of Microfabrication, CRC Press, Boca Raton, 1997.

4. Gregory T. A. Kovacs, Micromachined Transducers Sourcebook, WCB/McGraw-Hill, New York, 1998.
5. S. A. Campbell, The Science and Engineering of Microelectronic Fabrication, Oxford University Press, Oxford, UK, 1996.
6. K. R. Williams, R. S. Muller, Etch rates for micromachining processing, J Microelectromech Systems, vol. 5, no. 4, 1996, pp. 256–269.
7. S. Shoji, B. van der Schoot, N. de Rooij, M. Esahi, Smallest dead volume microvalves for integrated chemical analyzing systems, Proceedings of Transducers '91, the 1991 International Conference on Solid-State Sensors and Actuators, San Francisco, CA, June 24–27, 1991, pp. 1052–1055.
8. A. Desai, Y. C. Tai, M. T. Davis, T. D. Lee, A MEMS electrospray nozzle for mass spectrometry, Proceedings of Transducers '97, the 1997 International Conference on Solid-State Sensors and Actuators, Chicago, IL, June 16–19, 1997, pp. 927–930.
9. E. W. Becker, W. Ehrfeld, D. Muchmeyer, H. Betz, A. Heuberger, S. Pongratz, W. Glashauser, H. J. Michel, V. R. Siemens, Production of separation nozzle systems for uranium enrichment by a combination of x-ray lithography and galvanoplastics, Naturwissenschaften, 69, 520–523, 1982.
10. W. K. Schomburg, J. Fahrenberg, D. Maas, and R. Rapp, Active valves and micropumps for microfluidics, J. Micromech. Microeng., 3, 216–218, 1993.
11. R. Rapp, W. K. Schomburg, D. Maas, J. Schulz, W. Stark, LIGA micropump for gases and liquids, Sensors and Actuators A, A40, 57061, 1994.
12. J. Vollmer, H. Hein, W. Menz, F. Walter, Bistable fluidic elements in LIGA technique for flow control in fluidic microactuators, Sensors and Actuators A, A43, 330–334, 1994.
13. W. Ehrfeld, R. Einhaus, D. Munchmeyer, H. Strathmann, Microfabrication of membranes with extreme porosity and uniform pore size, J. Membr. Sci., 36, 67–77, 1988.
14. A, Uhlir, Electrolytic shaping of germanium and silicon, Bell Syst. Tech. J., 35, 333–347, 1956.
15. See article by Robert Service, Versatile chemical sensors take two steps forward, Science, 278, 806, 1997.
16. N. J. Mourlas, D. Jaeggi, N. I. Maluf, G. T. A. Kovacs, Reusable microfluidic coupler with PDMS gasket, Proceedings 10th International Conference on Solid-State Sensors and Actuators, June 7–10, 1999, 1888–89.
17. Nicolas H. Bings, Can Wang, Cameron D. Skinner, Christa L. Colyer, Pierre Thibault, D. Jed Harrison; Microfluidic devices connected to fused-silica capillaries with minimal dead volume, Anal. Chem. 71, 3292–3296, 1999.
18. David R. Walt, Fiber optic imaging sensors, Ac Chem Res, 31, 267–278, 1998.
19. L. C. Taylor, D. R. Walt, Applications of high-density optical microwell arrays in a live-cell biosensing system, Anal. Biochem. (in press).
20. David R. Walt, Fiber-based fiber-optic arrays, Science, 287, 154–152, 2000.
21. K. L. Michael, L. C. Taylor, S. L. Schultz, D. R. Walt, Fiber optic imaging sensors, Anal. Chem. 70, 1242, 1998.
22. See: http://www.illumina.com.
23. S. Fodor, J. L. Read, M. C. Pirrung, L. Stryer, Lu A. Tsai, D. Solas, Light-directed, spatially addressable parallel chemical synthesis, Science, 251, 767–773, 1991.

24. J. B. Sampsell, Digital micromirror device and its application to projection displays, J. Vac. Sci. Technol., B12, 3242–3246, 1994.

25. Sangeet Singh-Gasson, Roland D. Green, Yongijan Yue, Clark Nelson, Fred Blattner, Michael R. Sussman, France Cerrina, Maskless fabrication of light-directed oligonucleotide microarrays using a digital micromirror array, Nature Biotechnol, 17, 974–978, 1999.

26. Rebecca J. Jackman, David C. Duffy, Emanuele Ostuni, Nikolaos D. Willmore, George M. Whitesides, Fabricating large arrays of microwells with arbitrary dimensions and filling them using discontinuous dewetting, Anal. Chem., 70, 2280–2287.

27. R. Drmanac, S. Drmanac, Z. Strezoska, T. Paunesku, I. Labat, M. Zeremski, J. Snoddy, W. K. Funkhouser, B. Koop, L. Hood, R. Crkvenjakov, DNA sequence determination by hybridization: a strategy for efficient large-scale sequencing, Science, 260, 1649–1652, 1993.

28. R. Drmanac, I. Labat, I. Brukner, R. Crkvenjakov, Sequencing of megabase plus DNA by hybridization: theory of the method, Genomics, 4, 114–128, 1989.

29. Jing Cheng, Edward L. Sheldon, Lei Wu, Adam Uribe, Louis O. Gerrue, John Carrino, Michael J. Heller, and James P. O'Connell, Preparation and hybridization analysis of DNA/RNA from *E. coli* on microfabricated bioelectronic chips, Nature Biotechnol., 16, 541–546, 1998.

30. Jing Cheng, Edward L. Sheldon, Lei Wu, Michael J. Heller, James P. O'Connell, Isolation of cultured cervical carcinoma cells mixed with peripheral blood cells on a bioelectronic chip, Analytical Chemistry, 70, 2321–2326, 1998.

31. Stephen C. Jacobson, J. Michael Ramsey, Electrokinetic focusing in microfabricated channel structures, Anal. Chem., 69, 3212–3217, 1997.

32. Stephen C. Jacobson, Timothy E. McKnight, J. Michael Ramsey, Microfluidic devices for electrokinetically driven parallel and serial mixing, Anal. Chem., 71, 4455–4459, 1999.

33. David P. Schrum, Christopher T. Culbertson, Stephen C. Jacobson, J. Michael Ramsey, Microchip flow cytometry using electrokinetic focusing, Anal. Chem., 71, 4173–4177, 1999.

34. C. Belmont-Hebert, M. L. Tercier, J. Buffle, G. C. Fiaccabrino, N. F. deRooij, M. Koudelka-Hep, Gel-integrated microelectrode arrays for direct voltammetric measurements of heavy metals in natural waters and other complex media, Anal. Chem., 70, 2949–2956, 1998.

35. Franz von Heeren, Elisabeth Verpoorte, Andreas Manz, Wolfgang Thormann, Micellular electrokinetic chromatography separations and analyses of biological samples on a cyclic planar microstructure, Anal. Chem., 68, 2044–2053, 1996.

36. Richard D. Oleschuk, Loranelle L. Schultz-Lockyear, Yuebin Ning, D. Jed Harrison, Trapping of bead-based reagents within microfluidic systems: on-chip solid-phase extraction and electrochromatography," Anal. Chem., 72, 585–590, 2000.

37. Jianjun Li, John F. Kelly. Igor Chernushevich, D. Jed Harrison, Pierre Thibault, Separation and identification of peptides from gel-isolated membrane proteins using a microfabricated device for combined capillary electrophoresis nanoelectrospray mass spectrometry, Anal. Chem., 72, 599–609, 2000.

38. Andreas Manz, D. Jed Harrison, Elisabeth M. J. Verpoorte, James C. Fettinger, Aran Paulus, Hans Lüdi, H. Michael Widmer, Planar chip technology for miniaturisation

and integration of separation techniques into monitoring systems: capillary electrophoresis on a chip, J. Chromatogr., 593, 253–258, 1992.

39. Randy M. McCormick, Robert J. Nelson, M. Goretty Alonso-Amigo, Dominic J. Benvegnu, Herbert H. Hooper, Microchannel electrophoretic separations of DNA in injection-molded plastic substrates, Anal. Chem., 69, 2626–2630, 1997.

40. Carlo S. Effenhauser, Gerard J. M. Bruin, Aran Paulus, and Markus Ehrat, Integrated capillary electrophoresis on flexile silicon microdevices: analysis of DNA restriction fragments and detection of single DNA molecules on microchips, Anal. Chem., 69, 3451–3457, 1997.

41. See also *http://www.orchidbio.com*.

42. See: *http://www.micronics.com*.

43. P. Nyrén, A. Lundin, Enzymatic method for continuous monitoring of inorganic pyrophosphate synthesis, Anal. Biochem., 151, 504–509, 1985.

44. T. Nordström, K. Nourizad, M. Ronaghi, P. Nyren, Method enabling pyrosequencing on double-stranded DNA, Anal. Biochem., 282, 186–193, 2000.

45. See:*http://itri.Loyola.edu/nano/IWGN/Research.Directions/* from which this section is excerpted.

6

SNP Scoring for Drug Discovery Applications

John P. Nolan, P. Scott White, and Hong Cai
Los Alamos National Laboratory
Los Alamos, New Mexico

I. INTRODUCTION

An important byproduct of the Human Genome Project is an appreciation of the nature and degree of individual genetic variation [1]. While small insertion and deletions and variation in the length of repetitive DNA elements are common, by far the most frequently occurring type of genetic variation is the single-nucleotide polymorphism (SNP). A SNP is a nucleotide position in genomic DNA where the nucleotide base varies within a population [2]. In humans, it is estimated that between any two genomes, 1 in 1000 bases will be an SNP. When a large population consisting of many genomes is considered, as many as 1 in 100 bases will be polymorphic. Thus, in the human genome, which contains some 3 billion base pairs, there are expected to be more than 3 million SNPs. Many of these SNPs will have biomedical uses ranging from identification of potential drug targets to diagnosis of disease susceptibilities and targeting of therapies. Analysis of millions of SNPs in millions of patients presents a daunting challenge with new types of considerations and requiring the development of new approaches. In this chapter, we will briefly cover some of the uses of SNPs and describe some of the assay chemistries and analysis platforms that will allow SNPs to be used on a large scale for these emerging pharmaceutical applications.

A. SNP Applications

SNPs have several potential applications relevant to drug discovery and development. First, SNPs located in the protein coding or regulatory regions of genes can affect protein function or expression. In some cases, such alterations can be identified as the cause of a disease, thereby pointing to a potential drug target as well as having diagnostic uses. While in some diseases a single mutation can be identified as the cause of a disease, more often disease is expected to be the result of an interacting combination of differences in a number of genes [3]. Case-control association studies that focus on protein-altering SNPs within a set of candidate genes can reveal the involvement of specific genes in such complex diseases [2]. In a set of related applications, SNPs can be used as mapping markers to identify genes that may be associated with a particular disease. In these scenarios, hundreds of thousands of SNPs are scored in affected and control populations consisting of hundreds to thousands of individuals. While the experimental design and statistical considerations for large-scale association or linkage disequilibrium studies are still the subject of debate (discussed and reviewed in [4]), it is hoped that this approach may help address the difficult problem of diseases with complex genetic susceptibilities.

Similarly, amino acid–altering SNPs can affect a patient's response to a drug. Variation among individuals with respect to drug targets as well as drug metabolism can result in important differences in drug efficacy and toxicity [5,6]. As for complex diseases, drug responses will most often have a polygenic character, and patient responses will be determined by an individual variation in the relevant genes. The understanding of pharmacogenetic variation will not only be important for diagnostic uses but for the design of clinical trials for new drugs as well. Ensuring that known drug target and metabolism genotypes are represented in a clinical trial population should make it possible to more precisely predict drug efficacy and safety in the general population. In the broad vision of pharmacogenomics, disease and susceptibilities as well as highly individualized therapies would be ascribed on the basis of a patient's genotype, thereby ensuring safe and optimal treatment for every patient.

B. SNP Discovery and Scoring

A prerequisite for the applications described above is the identification and mapping of SNPs throughout the genome. Most of this task will be accomplished in the course of various large- and small-scale sequencing efforts [7–10]. There are currently active efforts in both the public and private sectors to discover and map SNPs on a genome-wide scale [11,12]. There have been several reviews on the methods and considerations that are relevant for SNP discovery [1,13]. While large-scale sequencing is the source of the majority of newly discovered SNPs, there are also efforts to develop methods of "scanning" genomic DNA for variation, with sequencing being used to confirm and identify SNPs. Although most SNP discovery methods can be configured for subsequent scoring of a SNP in unknown samples, in general scanning methods do not scale well for high-throughput genotyping applications. Scoring of large numbers of known SNPs is more efficient using one or more methods designed to interrogate an SNP directly [14]. In this chapter, we will consider the methods and analysis platforms available for large-scale SNP scoring in a drug discovery environment.

II. GENERAL CONSIDERATIONS

Before discussing in detail the chemistries and platforms used to score SNPs, it is useful to consider the important characteristics of large-scale SNP analysis for drug discovery applications because the requirements in this setting are very different from those of a smaller scale research setting. As discussed above, though estimates vary for applications related to gene discovery, on the order of 100,000 SNP markers will have to be screened in thousands to tens of thousands of individuals. Thus, any single application will likely require the scoring of millions of SNPs. This scale of analysis involves particular consideration of issues of throughput and cost that will influence the choice of assay chemistry and analysis platform. Two issues that are especially important in this regard are the amenability of methods to automation and the multiplexed analysis of many SNPs in each sample.

A. Sample Preparation

In most cases, the starting material for an SNP scoring project will be purified genomic DNA, which is then subjected to polymerase chain reaction (PCR) to amplify the regions containing the SNPs. PCR amplification is a major cost for most SNP scoring methods, and although there is much interest in developing "PCR-less" assays, as yet the combination of sensitivity and specificity of PCR has not been surpassed. Fortunately, PCR reactions are readily set up and performed in microwell plates with commercially available laboratory automation equipment. Additional cost and time savings can be obtained by multiplexing the PCR step, although the technical challenges to performing many PCR reactions in one tube are still significant enough to keep this approach from being routine on a large scale.

Once the DNA template is prepared, some assay chemistry is performed, generally consisting of a hybridization or binding procedure, often coupled to an enzymatic reaction, that allows identification of the nucleotide base located at the SNP position. Such chemistries usually require incubations ranging from minutes to hours, but these need not be rate limiting if they can be performed in parallel in microplates. Specialized enzymes, fluorescent nucleotides, or other reagents are often required and represent another major cost for SNP scoring assays. Again, multiplexed sample processing of many SNPs in a single tube can dramatically decrease the cost per SNP scored, as well as increase throughput.

B. Sample Analysis

If upstream sample processing steps can be conducted in parallel, sample analysis is often the rate-limiting step in SNP scoring applications. The ideal method would permit analysis of the products of SNP scoring reactions directly, without need for further purification, including highly multiplexed analysis of many SNPs per sample, as well as analysis of many samples simultaneously and/or a high serial sample analysis rate. The method should also be integrated with commercial lab automation instrumentation commonly used in a drug discovery environment. While no single analysis platform meets all of these criteria, a few meet several of them, and continued instrument development will likely improve performance in these respects.

C. Automation and Multiplexing

Especially important features for large-scale applications are multiplex and automation capabilities. Microplate-based assays are particularly well suited to automation, and many commercial robotics systems can perform large-scale sample preparation and analysis using microplates. Automation permits processing of large numbers of samples, and microplate assays can be configured to use small volumes (a few microliters) providing a reduction in assay reagent costs. An even bigger reduction in assay costs can be obtained by performing the multiplexed scoring of many SNPs in a single sample. For some SNP scoring chemistries the expensive reagents (enzymes and/or labeled nucleotides) are in excess, so that additional sites can be scored using the same pool of these reagents. This results in a decrease in the cost per SNP scored that is directly proportional to the level of multiplexing.

While microplates are well suited to the parallel processing of many samples, it is difficult to multiplex solution-based SNP scoring assays beyond a few sites. Electrophoresis-based methods can provide a modest degree of multiplexing combined with parallel sample analysis, and automation capabilities are improving. Microarray-based analysis methods are especially well suited for highly multiplexed assays, enabling the analysis of many more SNPs in a single sample than microplate-based assays. Flat microarrays (DNA chips) facilitate the multiplexed scoring of 1000 or more SNPs from a single sample, while soluble microarrays (DNA microspheres) can supports analysis of dozens to a hundred SNPs simultaneously, and potentially many more. Sample preparation and analysis for DNA chips can be automated using vendor-supplied equipment, while multiplexed microsphere-based assays are compatible with parallel sample preparation in microplates and conventional lab automation equipment.

III. SNP SCORING CHEMISTRIES

The objective of an SNP scoring assay is to determine the nucleotide base at specific sites in the genome. A variety of approaches have been developed to score SNPs, some of which exploit differences in physical properties of the DNA and oligonucleotide probes, while others rely on highly specialized enzymes to analyze DNA sequence. These methods vary in their ease of use, flexibility, scalability, and instrumentation requirements, and these factors will affect the choice of approaches employed in a high-throughput screening environment.

A. Sequencing

Conceptually, the simplest approach to scoring SNPs is probably direct sequencing, since sequencing is used to discover and confirm SNPs initially. However, in practice, direct sequencing is a fairly inefficient way to score SNPs. While the speed and throughput of sequencing instruments continues to improve, with capillary-based sequencers capable of generating 96 sequencing reads of 400–500 bases each in 2–3 hrs in general such read lengths will contain only one to a few SNPs on average. Considering this throughput rate (96 SNPs every 2–3 hr per instrument) and sample preparation costs (PCR amplification or cloning followed by one or more sequencing reactions for each target), direct sequencing is not suitable for most large-scale SNP scoring applications. In some highly variable regions of the genome—certain human leukocyte antigen (HLA) genes, for example—a sequencing read may contain dozens of potential SNP sites. In such cases, sequencing can be quite efficient, providing multiplexed SNP scoring in one reaction. However, such cases are rare exceptions, and for most applications sequencing is not a viable high-throughput SNP scoring method.

B. Hybridization

SNPs can often be detected by measuring the hybridization properties of an oligonucleotide probe to a template of interest. The melting temperature for hybridization of an oligonucleotide of modest length (15–20 mer) can differ by several degrees between a fully complementary template and a template that has a one-base difference (i.e., an SNP). By carefully designing oligonucleotide probes and choosing hybridization conditions that allow the probe to bind to the fully complementary template, but not a template containing an SNP, it is possible to use hybridization to distinguish a single-base variant (Fig. 1A).

In practice, this approach generally requires careful optimization of hybridization conditions because probe melting temperatures are very sensitive to

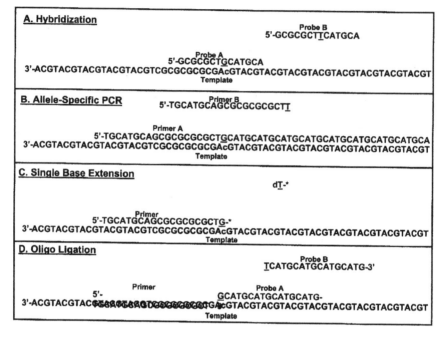

Figure 1 SNP scoring chemistries. **A:** Hybridization-based methods to interrogate a variable site (lowercase) in a DNA template involve the design of probes that, under the appropriate incubations conditions, will anneal only to one specific allele. **B:** Allele-specific chain extension (ASCE) employs primers that anneal at the SNP-containing site such that only the primer annealed perfectly to a specific allele (primer A) is extended, while primer specific for another allele (primer B) is not. **C:** In single-base extension (SBE), a primer is designed to anneal immediately adjacent to the SNP-containing site and a DNA polymerase is allowed to extend the primer one nucleotide using labeled dideoxynucleotides. The identity of the incorporated dideoxynucleotide reveals the base at the SNP site on the template DNA. **D:** The oligonucleotide ligation assay (OLA) uses two types of oligonucleotides. The first (primer) anneals to the template DNA immediately adjacent to the SNP-containing site. The second type (probe) anneals on the other side of the SNP such that that the terminal base will pair with the SNP. If the terminal base is complementary to the base at the SNP site, the first (primer) and second (probe A) oligos will be covalently joined by DNA ligase. If the terminal base of the second oligo (probe B) is not complementary to the SNP base, ligation will not occur.

sequence context as well as to the nature and position of the mismatched base. This difficulty in choosing optimum hybridization conditions (buffer and temperature) can be eliminated by continuous monitoring of probe hybridization as the temperature is increased, allowing the melting temperature for matched and mismatched probes to be determined directly in a process known as dynamic allele-specific hybridization (DASH; Howell, 1999 #46). Alternatively, the use of highly parallel microarrays enables an SNP-containing template to be interrogated by many different hybridization probes for each SNP [15], providing a redundancy of analysis that effectively increases the signal-to-noise ratio. Peptide nucleic acids (PNAs), which are oligonucleotide analogues with a structure that make hybridization very dependent on correct base pairing (and thus very sensitive to mismatches [16,17], can improve hybridization-based assays. Locked nucleic acids (LNAs; Wengel, 1999 #209), another oligonucleotide analogue, are likely to be similarly useful.

C. Allele-Specific Chain Extension

The combination of a hybridization probe with a sequence-sensitive enzymatic step can offer very robust and accurate SNP scoring chemistry. Allele-specific chain extension (ASCE) involves the design of a primer whose 3' terminal base will anneal to the site of the SNP [18,19]. If the base at the SNP site on the template DNA is complementary to the 3' base of the allele-specific primer, then DNA polymerase will efficiently extend the primer (Fig. 1B). If the SNP base is not complementary, polymerase extension of the primer is inefficient and under the appropriate conditions no extension will occur.

Originally implemented as a PCR-based assay, allele-specific PCR (AS-PCR) used gel electrophoresis to detect the PCR product as a positive indicator of the presence of the SNP of interest [18,19]. AS-PCR is widely used in diagnostic assays for several disease-associated mutations [20] as well as for HLA typing [21]. In addition, by using two allele-specific primers, AS-PCR can be used to distinguish whether two SNPs are present on the same chromosome [22]. AS-PCR assays can also be multiplexed to some extent, enabling several SNPs to be assayed in a single sample [23]. More recently, ASCE has been adapted to detection platforms more compatible with large-scale analysis including microarrays [24,25].

D. Single-Base Extension

The ability of DNA polymerase to discriminate correctly paired bases is the principle underlying conventional DNA sequencing as well as ASCE. Another approach employing the sensitive sequence discrimination of DNA polymerases is single-base extension (SBE) of a primer, also known as minisequencing or genetic bit analysis (GBA). In SBE (Fig. 1C), an oligonucleotide probe is designed to anneal immediately adjacent to the site of interest on the template DNA. In the presence of dideoxynucleoside triphosphates, DNA polymerase extends the annealed primer by one base [26,27]. This is essentially the same dye terminator chemistry widely used in conventional sequencing and, as long as the SBE primer is specific, can be very accurate with an excellent signal-to-noise ratio.

Most often, the dideoxynucleotide is labeled. Usually the label is a fluorescent dye, but in some configurations biotinylated dideoxynucleotides can be used and detected with a labeled avidin in a secondary labeling step. If fluorescent dideoxynucleotides are used, all four bases can be scored in a single reaction if each of the four dideoxynucleotides is tagged with a different fluorophore. Thermal cycling of the SBE reaction using a temperature-stable polymerase can provide signal amplification, although at present amplification of the genomic template by PCR is still required.

E. Oligonucleotide Ligation

Another method that takes advantage of enzyme discrimination of correctly paired bases is the oligonucleotide ligation assay (OLA). Two types of oligonucleotide probes are designed: one that anneals immediately adjacent to the SNP site on the template DNA and one that anneals immediately adjacent to the other side of the SNP (Fig. 1D) such that the terminal base will pair with the SNP. If the terminal base of the second primer is complementary to the SNP base, then a DNA ligase enzyme will covalently join the two primers. If the terminal base is not complementary, ligation will be very inefficient. As for SBE, OLA exploits highly specialized enzymes to discriminate correctly matched bases and can be very accurate. In addition, because it uses two primers to interrogate the SNP, OLA can also be configured to detect small insertions or deletion mutations.

Often one primer is immobilized on a solid substrate [28] and the second primer is labeled, either directly with a fluorophore or with a biotin for subsequent detection with labeled avidin. OLA is generally performed on PCR-amplified template DNA, but a variant, the ligase chain reaction (LCR), uses genomic DNA as template for the ligation reaction, the products of which are then amplified [29]. Another variant suitable for use with genomic DNA template is "padlock probe" ligation, which generates a circular oligonucleotide product which can than be amplified many hundred fold using rolling-circle amplification [30,31].

F. Nuclease-Based Assays

Several SNP scoring methods based on nuclease cleavage of oligonucleotide probes have been demonstrated. A relatively straightforward assay targets SNPs that alter the recognition site for a restriction endonuclease, resulting in a change in the electrophoretic migration of the template molecule. More general approaches that can be configured as homogeneous assays are Taq-Man [32] and Invader [33], both based on hybridization combined with an enzymatic 5′-nuclease activity.

In Taq-Man, the 5′-nuclease activity of Taq DNA polymerase cleaves a hybridization probe that specifically anneals to the template DNA during PCR. The Taq-Man hybridization probe is labeled with fluorescent donor and acceptor molecules that exhibit fluorescence resonance energy transfer (FRET) that is released upon cleavage. The Taq-Man probes must be carefully designed to hybridize only to perfectly matched template and not to template with a mismatched base. The Invader assay uses the 5′-nuclease activity of a thermostable flap endonuclease (FEN) enzyme to cleave a 5′ "flap" displaced by an invading probe. Probe cleavage produces a short oligonucleotide bearing a label that can be detected. Alternatively, the short cleavage product can serve as an Invader probe for a second stage of probe cleavage. This results in an amplification of the signal under isothermal conditions, and detection of signals from genomic DNA without PCR has been reported [33]. Both the Taq-Man and Invader assays are gaining popularity for the analysis of single-point mutations. Highly multiplexed analysis of many SNPs simultaneously, such as is desired for large-scale applications, has not yet been demonstrated for these assays.

G. Summary

For large-scale SNP scoring, the SBE chemistry is probably the most robust, flexible, and easily multiplexed chemistry. For SBE, one primer is designed for each SNP, which are then labeled by extension with dideoxynucleotides. The extension of primers with labeled dideoxynucleotides by DNA polymerase is essentially the same chemistry used in conventional sequencing and is generally very accurate. Allele-specific chain extension requires a different primer for each allele, but also benefits from the specificity of DNA polymerase. Ligation assays can be very accurate as well, but they require a primer and a different probe to score each SNP. On the other hand, ligation assays are more readily configured to score small insertions or deletions than SBE. Neither ligation, ASCE, nor SBE assays are well suited to score SNPs in highly variable regions of the genome, as variability in primer binding sites makes primer design more difficult. In these rare instances, conventional sequencing may be the most effective method of assessing genotype.

IV. PLATFORMS

Just as there are a variety of assay chemistries for scoring SNPs, there are several platforms on which samples can be analyzed. Although all chemistries are not compatible with every platform, most can be analyzed by a variety of instruments. Key considerations for large-scale SNP scoring in a drug discovery environment are compatibility with highly parallel and automated sample preparation and the ability to perform multiplexed scoring of many SNPs in each sample.

A. Electrophoresis

Being a standard technique in molecular genetics labs, gel electrophoresis is widely used for SNP scoring. Most often, mobility through the gel or sieving matrix is used to identify a particular DNA fragment by its size. In addition, fluorescence detection of one or more probes can be used to identify primers or incorporated nucleotides. These two features form the basis of automated DNA sequencing but also have applications in SNP scoring. In allele-specific PCR, agarose gel electrophoresis is often used to identify amplified products based on size [23]. For SBE assays, different sized primers, each interrogating a different SNP, can be resolved by electrophoresis, enabling multiplexed analysis of several sites simultaneously [34,35].

The limitations of electrophoresis as a SNP scoring platform stem from fairly low throughput. The current state of the art in electrophoresis for sequencing applications, capillary electrophoresis instruments with 96-sample capacity, can perform an analysis every 2–3 hr. Assuming a size-based primer multiplex to analyze 10 SNPs simultaneously, one could score roughly 4000 SNPs per workday. New generation instruments with 384-capillary capacity could quadruple that throughput.

B. Microplate-Based Assays

Many SNP scoring assays have been adapted to a microwell plate format, enabling highly parallel and automated sample processing and analysis. This platform is compatible with commercial high-throughput sample handling and measurement instruments that are widely used in the pharmaceutical industry. SNP scoring assays in microplates can be configured as heterogeneous (requiring wash steps to remove excess reagents) or homogeneous (no wash steps required), with fluorescence or absorbance detection.

For the heterogeneous approaches, the microwell is often used as a solid support for oligonucleotide probes. For example, OLA and SBE assays have been configured with the SNP primer immobilized on the microplate bottom [28,36]. PCR-amplified template, reporter oligos or nucleotides, and enzyme (ligase or polymerase) are added and the enzymatic reaction causes the immobilized primer to be labeled. Excess reagents are then washed away and the signal remaining in the well is measured.

For homogeneous assays, the microwell serves as a cuvette in which fluorescence is monitored. The key to the most homogeneous assays is the use of

FRET, which results in a change in the fluorescence spectra of a sample when two fluorescent dyes are brought into proximity. In addition to the example of the Taq-Man assay described earlier, FRET-based approaches have been configured for hybridization using molecular beacons [37], OLA [38], and SBE [39].

Fluorescence detection provides sensitive detection for the microwell format, and the use of FRET provides essentially real-time scoring of the SNP. An entire microwell plate can be measured in less than a minute, enabling high sample throughput, and, in the case of 384 or higher densities, the reaction volumes can be quite small (on the order of 10 µl). A disadvantage of microplate-based detection is the limited capacity for the multiplexed detection of many SNPs per sample. The use of differently colored probes can enable simultaneous detection of multiple signals, but because currently available fluorophores have relatively broad emission spectra, it will be very difficult to configure homogeneous solution assays with a multiplex capacity of more than three or four SNPs per sample.

C. Mass Spectrometry

There is a significant effort aimed at adapting mass spectrometry to genomic applications, including SNP scoring. The advantages of mass spectrometry as an analytical tool stem from its capacity to produce very rapid and precise mass measurements. This allows many assays to be configured without the use of exogenous labels. For instance, SBE reactions can be analyzed by measuring the mass of a dideoxynucleotide added to a primer. Because each of the four dideoxynucleotides has a distinct mass, it is possible to identify which nucleotide(s) was added to the primer [40]. In addition, by using several primers of different masses (lengths) to interrogate several SNPs, it is possible to perform a multiplexed analysis on each sample [41].

Current limitations of the mass spectrometry–based SNP scoring include a marked dependence on the size of DNA molecule being analyzed. Single-base resolution decreases for larger oligonucleotides, especially between nucleotides of similar mass such as A and T. The use of mass tagged nucleotides (i.e., isotopically labeled nucleotides) can increase this resolution [41–43] at added expense. Another limitation is the requirement for highly processed and purified samples. Current mass spectrometry–based genotyping protocols call for purification of samples before analysis. This requirement increases the cost and time of the procedure, although these steps can be automated and performed in parallel. It is very likely that some of these limitations will be overcome, given the current high level of interest in adapting mass spectrometry to genomic applications.

D. Flat Microarrays

Perhaps one of the best publicized biological technologies of the last decade is the use of microarrays to perform large-scale genomic analysis [44,45]. These microarrays, typically constructed on glass using photolithographic or robotic printing or spotting processes, can contain hundreds to hundreds of thousands of different DNA molecules on a surface of just a few square centimeters or less. Assays are generally configured using fluorescent reporter molecules, and arrays are read using scanning methods such as confocal microscopy.

For SNP scoring applications, DNA microarrays have generally been used in conjunction with hybridization assays [15]. In these assays, the sensitivity of hybridization to local sequence context of a SNP is overcome by interrogating each SNP with multiple hybridization probes, providing a redundancy to the analysis that reduces ambiguous SNP scoring. Chips designed to interrogate hundreds of SNPs simultaneously have been developed [15], and it should be possible to make chips with even higher SNP scoring capacity. In addition to hybridization-based SNP scoring, the SBE chemistry has been adapted to flat microarrays [27]. Currently, flat DNA microarray technology is expensive and not very flexible. To acquire proprietary or specialized array manufacturing technology and dedicated array analysis instrumentation requires a large initial investment. However, for large-scale SNP scoring applications, the investment may be justified.

E. Soluble Arrays

An approach that has not yet generated the publicity of the DNA chip but will probably have a major impact in a variety of areas is the use of soluble arrays and flow cytometry. Soluble arrays are composed of microspheres that are dyed with different amounts of one or more fluorophores such that many distinct subpopulations of microspheres can be identified on the basis of their fluorescence intensity using flow cytometry. Conceptually, the soluble array approach is similar to that of flat microarrays, with different levels of fluorescence intensity replacing x-y positions on a surface. Currently, soluble microsphere arrays of 100 elements are commercially available ([46]; Luminex Corp., Austin, TX), but this number could in principle be expanded to thousands with the use of additional dyes to create multidimensional arrays.

The analysis of soluble arrays by flow cytometry has a number of advantages over flat surface microarrays. First, oligonucleotides are readily immobilized on microspheres using well-known benchtop chemistry. Second, because each array element is a distinct population of microspheres, array preparation consists of the combining of individual microspheres into a mixture using a pipette. Reconfiguration of the array requires only the modification of individual microsphere populations, followed by the preparation of a new mixture. The use of universal oligonucleotide address tags [47,48] to capture tagged primers after a solution-phase SNP scoring reaction further increases the flexibility of the array by allowing assays to be redesigned. Third, because the array is in a liquid phase, conventional liquid-handling hardware can be used for highly parallel sample preparation in microplates. In addition, improved sample handling capabilities for flow cytometry [49] should boost throughput by more than a factor of 10 from a current 1–2 samples per minute. Fourth, because flow cytometry can discriminate between free and particle-bound probe, under most conditions no wash or purification step is required. Finally, because flow cytometry is capable of measuring tens of thousands of particles per second, soluble arrays can be analyzed in just a few seconds.

A variety of SNP scoring chemistries are compatible with the use of microspheres as solid supports and fluorescence detection by flow cytometry. Hybridization-based assays have been used detect PCR products [50] as well as to interrogate SNPs by multiplexed competitive hybridization [51]. In addition, the OLA and SBE chemistries have been adapted to microspheres [48,52,53]. While the soluble array technology does not yet have the parallel analysis capacity of the flat microarrays, advantages in serial sample throughput, ease of automation, and flexibility will make it attractive for many applications.

F. Summary

Key features of a large-scale SNP scoring platform are the abilities to analyze highly multiplexed assays with high serial sample thoughput in an automated manner (Table 1). Microplates are an excellent platform for automated parallel sample processing but cannot offer a high level of multiplexed analysis. Flat DNA

Table 1 Characteristics of SNP Scoring Platforms

	Hardware costs	Throughput	Automation compatibility	Multiplex capacity
Gels	Low-high	Low-moderate	Low-moderate	Moderate
Microplates	Moderate-high	High	High	Low
Mass spectrometry	High	Moderate-high	Moderate-high	Moderate
Flat arrays/scanner	High	Low	Moderate	High
Microspheres/flow cytometry	Moderate-high	Moderate-high	Moderate-high	Moderate-high
Low	<20K	<1 sample min	Custom HTS	<5 SNPs/sample
Moderate	20–100K	1–10 samples/min	Custom-commercial hybrid	5–50 SNPs/sample
High	>100K	>10 samples/min	Commercial HTS	>50 SNPs/sample

microarrays offer very highly multiplexed analysis (thousands of SNPs) but a low sample analysis throughput. Soluble arrays have a high multiplex capacity (dozens to a hundred SNPs), with a fairly high serial sample throughput. Microplate-based sample processing combined with a highly multiplexed array-based measurement probably represents the most efficient combination of current technologies.

V. CONCLUSIONS AND PROSPECTS

Many strategies are being employed to score SNPs. Large-scale SNP scoring such as is required for drug discovery applications requires special consideration of the issues of throughput and cost. Especially important for optimizing throughput and cost are the ability to automate sample preparation and analysis and the ability to perform multiplexed scoring of many SNPs in a single sample. In this chapter, we have focused on those methods currently available that could be configured for large-scale applications. However, with the intense interest this area of research is generating, improvements in all aspects of sample preparation and analysis are to be expected. In closing, we would like to point to a few areas of likely progress.

Most SNP scoring assays involve PCR amplification of the DNA template. PCR not only improves assay sensitivity but provides added specificity for resolution of specific SNP sites against similar sites in gene homologues or pseudogenes. For the efficient highly parallel analysis of multiple SNPs such as is possible with microarrays, the PCR amplification step must be highly multiplexed. Multiplexed PCR is a challenging problem, requiring the design and pooling of PCR primers that will specifically amplify many sequences under the same conditions yet will not interact with each other to produce primer artifacts. Because this is a generally important problem, with applications beyond SNP scoring, it is hoped that automated informatics and computational tools will be developed to supplement the largely empirical approach to multiplex PCR currently employed.

Applications of DNA microarray technologies will continue to be developed, providing highly parallel multiplexed analysis. Flat surface microarrays should prove to be much more useful for SNP scoring when combined with single-base extension and universal capture tags. The parallel analysis capabilities of soluble microsphere arrays are expected to increase as improved dye chemistry enables the production of multidimensional arrays, providing the parallel analysis throughput of flat microarrays with conventional liquid handling automation. Newer formats, such as microarrays configured on the ends of optical fibers (Chapter 7), may also prove to have unique advantages as detection platforms for SNP scoring applications. Finally, the push of micro- and nanofabrication toward integrated lab-on-a chip approaches will likely have an impact in reducing costs, especially if these can provide a highly multiplexed analysis.

An understanding of human genetic variation, especially in the form of SNPs, offers enormous potential for enhancing and improving the process of drug discovery and development. The realization of this potential depends on the ability to score rapidly and efficiently large numbers of SNPs in large numbers of samples. Technologies that combine automated sample preparation with highly multiplexed analysis will play a central role in meeting these needs.

REFERENCES

1. Schaffer, A. J., Hawkins, J. R. DNA variation and the future of human genetics. Nat Biotechnol 1998;16:33–39.
2. Brookes, A. J. 1999. The essence of SNPs. Gene 1999;234:177–186.
3. Ghosh, S., Collins, F. S. The geneticist's approach to complex disease. Annu Rev Med 1996;47:333–353.
4. Terwilliger, J. D., Weiss, K. M. Linkage disequilibrium mapping of complex disease: fantasy or reality. Curr Opin Biotechnol 1998;9:578–594.
5. Weinshilboum, R. M., Otterness, D. M., Szumlanski, C. L. Methylation pharmacogenetics: catechol O-methyltransferase, thiopurine methyltransferase, and histamine N-methyltransferase. Annu Rev Pharmacol Toxicol 1999;39:19–52.
6. Evans, W. E., Relling, M. V. Pharmacogenomics: translating functional genomics into rational therapeutics. Science 1999;286:487–491.
7. PicoultNewberg, L., Ideker, T. E., Pohl, M. G., Taylor, S. L., Donaldson, M. A., et al. Milling SNPs from EST databases. Genome Res 1999;9:167–174.
8. Gu, Z. J., Hillier, L., Kwok, P. Y. Single nucleotide polymorphism hunting in cyberspace. Hum Mutat 1998;12:221–225.
9. Rieder, M. J., Taylor, S. L., Tobe, V. O., Nickerson, D. A. Automating the identification of DNA variations using quality-based fluorescence re-sequencing: analysis of the human mitochondrial genome. Nucleic Acids Res 1998;26:967–973.
10. Kwok, P. Y., Deng, Q., Zakeri, H., Taylor, S. L., Nickerson, D. A. Increasing the information content of STS-based genome maps: identifying polymorphisms in mapped STSs. Genomics 1996;31:123–126.
11. Collins, F. S., Patrinos, A., Jordan, E., Chakravarti, A., Gesteland, R., et al. New goals for the U.S. Human Genome Project: 1998–2003. Science 1998;282:682–689.
12. Collins, F. S., Brooks, L. D., Chakravarti, A. A DNA polymorphism discovery resource for research on human genetic variation. Genome Res 1998;8:1229–1231.
13. Cotton, R. Slowly but surely towards better scanning for mutations. Trends Geneti. 1997;13:43–46.
14. Landegren, U., Nilsson, M., Kwok, P. Y. Reading bits of genetic information: Methods for single nucleotide polymorphism analysis. Genome Res 1998;8:769–776.
15. Wang, D. G., Fan, J. B., Siao, C. J., Berno, A., Young, P., et al. Large-scale identification, mapping, and genotyping of single nucleotide polymorphisms in the human genome. Science 1998;280:1077–1082.

16. Nielsen, P. E. Applications of peptide nucleic acids. Curr Opin Biotechnol 1999;10: 71–75.

17. Uhlmann, E., Peyman, A., Breipohl, G., Will, D. W. PNA: Synthetic polyamide nucleic acids with unusual binding properties. Angewandte Chem Int Ed 1998;37:2797–2823.

18. Newton, C. R., Graham, A., Heptinstall, L. E., Powell, S. J., Summers, C., et al. Analysis of any point mutation in DNA: the amplification refractory mutation system (ARMS). Nucleic Acids Res 1989;17:2503–2516.

19. Sarkar, G., Cassady, J., Bottema, C. D. K., Sommer, S. S. Characterization of poly-merase chain reaction amplification of specific alleles. Anal Biochem 1990;186: 64–68.

20. Patrushev, L. I., Zykova, E. S., Kayushin, A. L., Korosteleva, M. D., Miroshnikov A. I., et al. New DNA diagnostic system for detection of Factor-V-Leiden. Thrombo-sis Res 1998;92:251–259.

21. Bunce, M., Fanning, G. C., Welsh, K. I. Comprehensive, serologically equivalent DNA typing for HLA-B using sequence-specific primers (PCR-SSP). Tissue Anti-gens 1995;45:81–90.

22. Clark, A. G., Weiss, K. M., Nickerson, D. A., Taylor, S. L., Buchanan, A., et al. Hap-lotype structure and population genetic inferences from nucleotide-sequence varia-tion in human lipoprotein lipase. Am J Hum Genet 63:595–612.

23. Pearson, S. L., Hessner, M. J. A(1,2)BO(1,2) genotyping by multiplexed allele-spe-cific PCR. Br J Haematol 1998;100:229–234.

24. Pastinen, T., Raitio, M., Lindroos, K., Tainola, P., Peltonen, L., et al. A system for spe-cific high-throughput genotyping by allele-specific primer extension on microarrays. Genome Res 2000;10:1031–1042.

25. Tonisson, N., Kurg, A., Kaasik, K., Lohmussaar, E., Metspalu, A. Unravelling genetic data by arrayed primer extension. Clin Chem Lab Med 2000;38:165–170.

26. Syvanen, A. C., Aaltosetala, K., Harju, L., Kontula, K., Soderlund, H. A primer-guided nucleotide incorporation assay in the genotyping of apolipoprotein-E. Genomics 1990;8:684–692.

27. Syvanen, A. C. From gels to chips: "Minisequencing" primer extension for analysis of point mutations and single nucleotide polymorphisms. Hum Mutat 1999;13:1–10.

28. Tobe, V. O., Taylor, S. L., Nickerson, D. A. Single-well genotyping of diallelic sequence variations by a 2-color Elisa-based oligonucleotide ligation assay. Nucleic Acids Rese 1996;24:3728–3732.

29. Barany, F. Genetic disease detection and DNA amplification using cloned ther-mostable ligase. Proc Nat Acad Sci USA 1991;88:189–193.

30. Lizardi, P. M., Huang, X. H., Zhu, Z. R., Brayward, P., Thomas, D. C., et al. Muta-tion detection and single molecule counting using isothermal rolling circle amplifi-cation. Nat Genet 19:225–232.

31. Baner, J., Nilsson, M., Mendelhartvig, M., Landegren, U. Signal amplification of padlock probes by rolling circle replication. Nucleic Acids Res 1998;26:5073–5078.

32. Livak, K., Marmaro, J., Todd, J. A. Towards fully automated genome-wide polymor-phism screening. Nat Gen 1995;9:341–342.

33. Lyamichev, V., Mast, A. L., Hall, J. G., Prudent, J. R., Kaiser, M. W., et al. Polymor-phism identification and quantitative detection of genomic DNA by invasive cleavage of oligonucleotide probes. Nat Biotechnol 1999;17:292–296.

34. Pastinen, T., Partanen, J., Syvanen, A. C. Multiplex, fluorescent; solid-phase minisequencing for efficient screening of DNA sequence variation. Clin Chem 1996;42: 1391–1397.

35. Tully, G., Sullivan, K. M., Nixon, P., Stones, R. E., Gill, P. Rapid detection of mitochondrial sequence polymorphisms using multiplex solid-phase fluorescent minisequencing. Genomics 1996;34:107–113.

36. Livak, K. J., Hainer, J. W. A microtiter plate assay or determining apolipoprotein-E genotype and discovery of a rare allele. Hum Mutat 1994;3:379–385.

37. Tyagi, S., Bratu, D. P., Kramer, F. R. Multicolor molecular beacons for allele discrimination. Nat Biotechnol 1998;16:49–53.

38. Chen, X. N., Livak, K. J., Kwok, P. Y. A homogeneous, ligase-mediated DNA diagnostic test. Genome Res 1998;8:549–556.

39. Chen, X. N., Kwok, P. Y. Homogeneous genotyping assays for single nucleotide polymorphisms with fluorescence resonance energy transfer detection. Genetic Analysis-Biomol Eng 1999;14:157–163.

40. Laken, S. J., Jackson, P. E., Kinzler, K. W., Vogelstein, B., Strickland, P. T., et al. Genotyping by mass spectrometric analysis of short DNA fragments. Nat Biotechnol 1998;16:1352–1356.

41. Haff, L. A., Smirnov, I. P. Multiplex genotyping of PCR products with masstag-labeled primers. Nucleic Acids Res 1997;25:3749–3750.

42. Fei, Z. D., Ono, T., Smith, L. M. Maldi-TOF mass-spectrometric typing of single nucleotide polymorphisms with mass-tagged ddNTPs. Nucleic Acids Res 26:2827–2828.

43. Chen, X., Fei, Z. D., Smith, L. M., Bradbury, E. M., Majidi, V. Stable-isotope-assisted MALDI-TOF mass spectrometry for accurate determination of nucleotide compositions of PCR products. Anal Chem 1999;71:3118–3125.

44. McKenzie, S. E., Mansfield, E., Rappaport, E., Surrey, S., Fortina, P. Parallel molecular genetic analysis. Eur J Hum Genet 1998;6:417–429.

45. Hacia, J. G., Brody, L. C., Collins, F. S. Applications of DNA chips for genomic analysis. Mol Psychiatry 1998;3:483–492.

46. Kettman, J. R., Davies, T., Chandler, D., Oliver, K. G., Fulton, R. J. Classification and properties of 64 multiplexed microsphere sets. Cytometry 1998;33:234–243.

47. Gerry, N. P., Witkowski, N. E., Day, J., Hammer, R. P., Barany, G., et al. Universal DNA microarray method for multiplex detection of low abundance point mutations. J Mol Biol 1999;292:251–262.

48. Cai, H., White, P. S., Torney, D. C., Deshpande, A., Wang, Z., et al. Flow cytometry based minisequencing: a new platform for high throughput single nucleotide polymorphism analysis. Genomics 2000;68:135–143.

49. Edwards, B. S., Kuckuck, F., Sklar, L. A. Plug flow cytometry: an automated coupling device for rapid sequential flow cytometric sample analysis. Cytometry 1999;37: 156–159.

50. Yang, G., Olson, J. C., Pu, R., Vyas, G. N. Flow cytometric detection of human immunodeficiency virus type 1 proviral DNA by the polymerase chain reaction incorporating digoxigenin- or fluorescein labeled dUTP. Cytometry 1995;21:197–202.

51. Fulton, R. J., McDade, R. L., Smith, P. L., Kienker, L. J., Kettman, J. R. Advanced multiplexed analysis with the Flowmetrix(Tm) system. Clin Chem 1997;43:1749–1756.

52. Iannone, M. A., Taylor, J. D., Chen, J., Li, M., Rivers, P., et al. Multiplexed single nucleotide polymorphism genotyping by oligonucleotide ligation and flow cytometry. Cytometry 2000;39:131–140.

53. Chen, J., Iannone, M. A., Li, M., Taylor, J. D., Rivers, P., et al. A microsphere-based assay for multiplexed single nucleotide polymorphism analysis using single base extension. Genome Res 2000;10:549–557.

7
Protein Display Chips

Tina S. Morris
Human Genome Sciences Inc.
Rockville, Maryland

I. INTRODUCTION TO PROTEIN CHIP TECHNOLOGIES

The genome sequencing revolution has presented protein biochemists with blessings and challenges. At the DNA level, high-throughput technologies enabled the rapid discovery progress that the gene discovery community has enjoyed. Innovative, chip-based technologies have provided molecular biologists with a completely new set of tools. At the same time, the incredible amount of information from the various genomic analysis efforts has added additional layers of complexity to the way a lot of biological and medical questions are addressed. The simultaneous genetic analysis of many species and tissue types has broadened our view and quickened our understanding of key physiological processes on a genetic level. As will be discussed in this chapter, technology platforms originally introduced for nucleic acid analysis would eventually also have a significant impact on protein biochemistry in the hands of drug discovery researchers.

The rapid developments in the DNA and RNA analysis field have led the way to smaller sample volumes and rapidly increasing sample throughput. Arraying technologies, as well as microfluidic and robotic systems, have revolutionized industrial molecular biology. However, the fast and furious pace in that area has widened the gap in the understanding of proteins and protein–protein interactions, which has not progressed at the same speed. The reasons for this are both of a philosophical and a practical nature. In the minds of the molecular biology community, proteins for a long time have been not proteins but gene expression products. The umbrella of this term very conveniently shields the molecular complexity and diversity with which proteins present us. This molecular diversity is the main practical reason why the study of proteins is much harder to press into a multiplexed high-throughput format. The beauty of nucleic acid biochemistry lies in the simple variation of a known theme, the repetitiveness of a very limited number of building blocks, with triplet-based sequence as the brilliant key to the language of life. This key encodes the bountiful variety of the protein world, where things become much less predictable. Already the 20 amino acids as components with very different chemical characteristics presents a considerable analytical challenge when one considers the combinatorial possibilities. In addition to that, proteins can undergo posttranslational modifications with other classes of molecules, such as lipids or carbohydrates, which can alter the behavior and characteristics of the entire molecule. Yet from the earliest studies in protein biochemistry, especially in the area of enzymology, the need for efficient as well as meaningful protein analysis has been clear, especially in two aspects: proteins as antagonist targets and lately also as therapeutics themselves in the fight against disease. The increasing pace of discovery in cell biology and molecular biology discovery research has made that need all the more pressing. Protein development efforts drive large programs in the pharmaceutical industry. The focus of these programs has undergone many changes over the years. Enzymology clearly made its mark on drug discovery research early on. The advent of recombinant bacterial and eukaryotic protein expression systems now allows the production of large amounts of functional proteins for small-molecule antagonist screening, structural characterization, and functional studies. Tagging recombinant proteins further facilitated upstream optimization as well as downstream processing and analytical work. Tagging systems represented the first step toward an integrated assay platform for proteins that went beyond polyacrylamide gels. At the same time, advances in the fields of immunology and signal transduction presented new challenges. Functionality of a protein in these areas could not be measured through a catalytic reaction that was monitored as a color change or fluorescence enhancement. Instead, the function of a protein was based on its proper interaction with another protein or other class of effector molecule. This called for the development of new types of assays that allowed real-time monitoring of binding kinetics and the determination of binding specificity in a physiological setting. Also, the genome sequencing efforts led to the discovery of whole families of novel genes with unknown functions. This presented an additional need for interaction studies that would allow identification of binding or reaction partners. High-throughput screening groups started to expand into the areas of rapid biological assays for proteins with unknown activities. Aside from these exploratory and discovery applications, functional assays have become increasingly important at downstream junctures of the drug development process. To catch up with the speed of gene discovery, protein development was in need of sensitive, multiplexed assays that still would have the flexibility to accommodate the diverse needs of the protein world. As it turned out, the technology toolbox that revolutionized the nucleic acid world also changed the way we look at proteins. This chapter will attempt to cover the advances in the area of chip-based protein analysis technologies over the past decade and highlight the most important implications of these technologies for the drug discovery process.

II. SURFACE PLASMON RESONANCE BASED TECHNOLOGY: HOW OPTICAL BIOSENSORS REVOLUTIONIZED PROTEIN–PROTEIN INTERACTION STUDIES

A. Optical Biosensor Technology: Technical Background and Development

Development in the field of optical biosensors received significant impetus from the need of improvement in the area of laboratory-based immunodiagnostics. Optical techniques seemed an obvious choice for this area, since refractive index is one of the few physical parameters that vary upon the formation of an immune complex [1]. While interest in diffraction phenomena and the curious absorption anomalies of metallized optical diffraction gratings in particular dates back to the turn of the century, more systematic theoretical work in the field did not start until the 1950s, with the major advances published again much later [2–5].

Optical biosensor technology relies on a quantum mechanical detection phenomenon called the evanescent field. It is used to measure changes in the refractive index that occur within a few hundred nanometers of a sensor surface. These refractive index changes are caused either by the binding of a molecule to a second molecule that has been immobilized on the surface or by the subsequent dissociation of this complex [6]. There are several ways to create an evanescent field [7–9]. Surface plasmon resonance (SPR), which is the technology platform of the BIACORE instrument, has established itself as the most commonly used over the past 10 years. In SPR, polarized light is shone onto a glass prism that is in contact with a thin gold–glass surface. Light is reflected at all angles off the gold–glass interface, but only at the critical angle the light excites the metal surface electrons (plasmons) at the metal–solution interface. This creates the evanescent field and causes a dip in the intensity of the reflected light. The position of this response is sensitive to changes in the refractive index as well as the thickness of the layer in the vicinity of the metal surface [10]. Resonance is described in an arbitrary scale of resonance units (RU). A response is defined as the RU difference compared with a baseline that is normally established at the beginning of an experimental cycle with the immobilization of the capture protein or molecule. Figure 1 shows the setup of a typical SPR detection system, consisting of a detector, the sensor chip, and an integrated microfluidics system, which allows for the continuous flow of buffer, sample, and reagents.

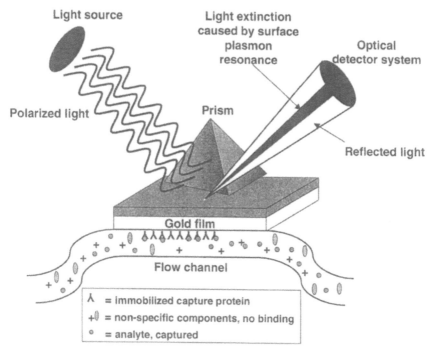

Light source

Light extinction
caused by surface
plasmon
resonance

Optical
detector system

Polarized light

Prism

Reflected light

Gold film

Flow channel

λ = Immobilized capture protein

$+$ = non-specific components, no binding

$\circ$ = analyte, captured

Figure 1 Schematic representation of an SPR detection system.

In a typical experiment, a capture molecule is first immobilized covalently on the sensor surface. Subsequently, the residual binding sites are blocked. After a wash with a buffer of low ionic strength, the interaction sample is passed over the sensor, followed again by buffer. Figure 2 illustrates a typical SPR sensogram. Response is measured with time and is proportional to the mass of the adsorbed molecule [6,11]. As ligand adsorption on the immobilized capture molecule occurs, the adsorption profile allows the determination of the association rate constant, k_{on}. After passing of the sample plug, dissociation of the complex follows as buffer passes over the sensor. The logarithmic decay of the dissociation reaction then allows the calculation of the dissociation rate constant k_{off}. Earlier studies exploring the potential of SPR in the field of biomolecular interactions employed simple adsorption to the metal surface for the immobilization of the capture component. This strategy comes with certain limitations. Some proteins may denature when absorbed directly to the metal; hapten-type ligands are very difficult to immobilize on metal. Furthermore, the performance of the sensor depends on the even and reproducible distribution as well as correct orientation of the adsorbed molecules. With a directly immobilized ligand there can be undesired interaction

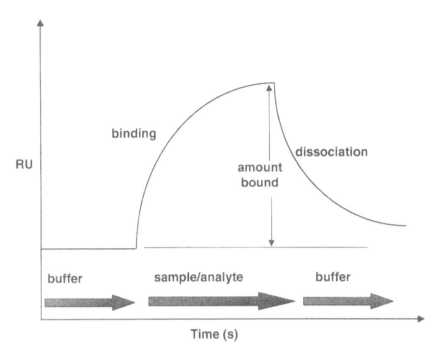

Figure 2 Typical SPR sensogram.

of solutes with the metal as well as exchange processes between ligand and solute. To overcome these limitations, a carboxylated dextran surface coupled to the gold film was developed, which evolved into the standard surface medium for covalent immobilization of capture molecules in the BIACORE system, the CM5 sensor chip. The concept of this surface technology was first described by Johnsson et al. [10]. Their hydrogel-modified surface was designed to minimize nonspecific adsorption of ligands at physiological ionic strength and at the same time facilitate accessibility of the ligand in the subsequent interaction study. Since the BIACORE system has grown into a generally accepted and commercially available analysis platform, the associated surface chemistry has been refined and diversified to accommodate the constantly growing number of applications. Today's gold–dextran surfaces basically have five different layers: the glass basis layer, the gold film, a linker layer, the dextran layer, and a specific layer. In the original surface design the covalent coupling of the biological capture molecules occurred directly by nucleophilic displacement of N-hydroxysuccinimide (NHS) esters on the carboxymethyldextran chains [12]. Modern CM5 surfaces come pre-activated for four different covalent coupling strategies: amine, ligand thiol, surface thiol, or aldehyde. In addition to the covalent binding, hydrophobic surfaces are now available for the capture of membrane complexes, and nickel-chelate surfaces allow the selective binding of His-tagged proteins.

The popularity of biotinylation as an efficient tag for the capture of both proteins and nucleic acids via streptavidin has prompted the development of streptavidin precoated surfaces.

On the instrumentation end, development has yielded a higher degree of sophistication and sensitivity, addressing some of the earlier problems associated with reproducibility and difficulty in detecting low-affinity interactions. At the same time, a greater level of automation has standardized and facilitated the use of the technology, opening it to the nonspecialized user. High-end systems allow the most elaborate kinetic analyses of biological interactions, whereas more simply designed yet fully automated systems allow rapid and reliable screening of a large number of samples.

B. Types of SPR Applications and Experimental Considerations

Since its original development in the area of immunodiagnostics, optical sensor technology has expanded into a wide variety of biological and medical areas of interest. An obvious choice for signal transduction research, SPR has become a standard tool for the analysis of receptor–ligand interactions [13,14]. The field of chaperonins also discovered the technology early on [15–17]. Beyond mere protein–protein interactions, SPR has found applications in small-molecule screening [18] as well as protein–carbohydrate [19] and protein–nucleic acid interactions [20–22]. Even viral particle binding to cell surface receptors has been analyzed by SPR [23]. At downstream junctures of the drug development process, specialized optical biosensors are used for bioprocess monitoring and product analysis [24]. In spite of the great diversity of molecules analyzed, SPR studies mainly fall into two categories as far as experimental goal and design are concerned. Screening applications look for the relatively simple answer of an approximate kinetic ranking, basically to see if an analyte is specifically binding to a given ligand or not. Functional studies look at the mechanism of a certain biological interaction by determining quantitative rate constants. Clearly a functional study with the aim of retrieving key mechanistic data requires a different level of insight and experimental premeditation than a simple "quick and dirty" screen. Yet it is crucial to realize that the mimicking of a biological interaction event on a two-dimensional platform is not a trivial endeavor per se. Failure to understand the key biochemical parameters, caveats, and limitations of the system will inevitably lead to the failure of even the simplest of studies.

The continuously advancing simplification and automation of commercially available SPR systems has made life easier for the inexperienced user, and it has become more and more tempting to forget about the cumbersome underlying theory. Increasing simplicity and user friendliness have allowed an explosion in SPR-related references in the scientific literature. Reviewed over time, the literature reveals a typical trend for an evolving technology platform. Most of the earlier papers in the field were more devoted to the experimental designs, technological details, and most of all the analysis of kinetic data [25–27]. More recent papers are overwhelmingly application driven and for the most part have moved the more dreaded theoretical aspects into the background [28,29]. This development clearly comes at a price, for it appears that less and less effort is spent on both careful experimental design and critical evaluation of the answers provided, leading to a situation where more data actually provide less value but increased confusion instead. Therefore, it seems worthwhile to revisit the key factors that control both the experimental as well as the data analysis parts of SPR experiments.

Clearly, when a reaction that usually occurs in solution is forced into a two-dimensional setup, limitations of mass transfer will have to be considered. At the same time the immobilization of one binding partner on the surface can actually help mimic a biological situation where the capture molecule is immobilized in a molecular superstructure like a membrane. While no systematic efforts have gone into the comparative analysis of SPR and solution binding, several researchers have revisited their SPR-derived affinities using other techniques, such as isothermal titration calorimetry, for confirmation. They have generally found good agreement, provided that the experimental design was chosen wisely [31–33]. Obviously, background understanding of the biological system to be analyzed will help in the design of the study. If the ligand or the analyte is a novel protein of unknown function, the data obtained in the experiment will have to be qualified with the possibility in mind that the binding partners may not have been presented in the correct orientation or configuration for an interaction to take place. When coupling the ligand to the surface in a covalent fashion, e.g., via the primary amines, this basically constitutes a random binding event that may hamper the formation of the correct capture configuration to receive the analyte. Tumor necrosis factor and similar ligands, for example, bind their receptors in a trimeric fashion: three receptor molecules have to form a homologous trimer to receive an analyte trimer. The addition of tags can help to overcome this problem: use of Fc fusions, for example, allows capture on the surface via a protein A bridge that orients all capture molecules in the same way. Also, Fc tags even without the help of protein A force their fusion partner into homologous dimers with other molecules. While this can help to increase the percentage of correctly oriented capture ligands on the sensor surface, it also has to be considered as an additional source of artifacts. Some tags, like Fc's, are quite bulky and can lead to considerable structural changes in the proteins they are attached to. They may destabilize them to the point of breakdown or simply lead them into an inactive configuration. If the fusion breaks down, the empty Fc will still bind to other molecules and produce inactive multimers. Molecule size does matter for another reason in this context: it should be considered in the decision which partner of the binding experiment to immobilize covalently: the bulkier antibody, receptor, fusion protein for example, or the small peptide analyte. In many situations, this decision is made out of necessity rather than choice, as, for example, when one binding partner is available in a purified form but the other needs to be fished out of conditioned cell culture supernatant. Purity and homogeneity of ligand and analyte play a key role in the kinetics of the experiment. If contaminants are present that interfere with binding or act as competitors, this will undoubtedly at least complicate the situation, at most render kinetic data useless. Contaminants can also obstruct the formation of specific multimers necessary for capture. Especially if the stoichiometry of the reaction is unknown, it is important to analyze a wide concentration range of both ligand and analyte. Problems of mass transfer have been extensively studied from a theoretical point of view and the reader is referred to the literature for a comprehensive treatise on the phenomenon [34–36]. In a high-density binding situation the crowding of molecules in the association state will push the balance from desired multimerization to unwanted aggregation. It has been observed that in general valid kinetic measurements are best obtained with low levels of ligand immobilization [37]. If the analyte concentration chosen is too high, the mass transfer limitations hamper its access to and from the surface. The valency of the interaction also needs consideration, since multivalency leads to avidity effects, even in a low-density association. This has been extensively studied using the example of whole antibodies that are at least bivalent [38].

Since SPR analysis represents the in situ monitoring of an interaction with one binding partner in flow, the time component of the setup naturally plays an important role and the optimization of flow rates deserves some consideration. As a general rule, a higher flow rate helps to minimize mass transfer limitations [39]. In a typical BIACORE experiment, the flow rate is kept constant and the sample is delivered to the surface in a small sample plug (typically in a volume between 50 and 200 µl) at a low analyte concentration, preceded and followed by low ionic strength buffer. In this way a discreet amount of analyte is delivered to the chip while the continuous flow necessary for kinetic analysis is maintained. This configuration is useful for first-order or pseudo-first-order kinetics and the determination of affinity constants. However, because of the finite volume of the sample plug and the limited data collection time associated with it, some binding reactions cannot be measured to equilibrium. To do this, the sample has to be recirculated over the surface or delivered in the buffer at a constant concentration [40,41].

The scope of this chapter precludes in-depth discussion if kinetics and data analysis methods that apply to SPR applications, and the reader is referred to the more specialized literature for that area. However, it seems appropriate to at least touch on the most important parameters involved in deriving reliable kinetics and a sound statistical analysis of experimental data. In a very insightful 1994 review Daniel O'Shanessey critiqued SPR studies described in the literature thus far [42].

His article shows that inappropriate interpretation of raw experimental data and incorrect mechanistic assumptions for the kinetics of a reaction are as much a source of error and failure as are faulty experimental design and execution. The single biggest error observed in documented SPR studies to this day is the application of simplistic kinetics and statistical models to reactions that in reality are very complex. This has in part been driven by the goal to create user-friendly software analysis platforms for commercial automated SPR systems. In a lot of cases, to keep things simple, data are attempted to fit the simplest 1:1 interaction model. This works out if the data actually fit this situation, but, as described earlier, the reality is often a lot more complex. Then the derived numbers become apparent rate constants that bear no resemblance to the reality of the molecular interaction. At the same time, use of the wrong statistical fits can be equally detrimental, and the user should invest some effort in the evaluation of linear, nonlinear, and global fitting methods.

C. SPR in the Drug Development Process: Conclusion and Outlook

The usefulness of SPR as a label-free monitoring technique for biological interactions at the many junctures of drug discovery and development is obvious, and the annual number of publications in the field bears substantial testimony to this. With commercially successful and widely used platforms like the BIACORE, the innovative technology has now crossed into the field of established methodology, attracting more and more nonspecialized users. Both increase in sample throughput and advanced automation permit the efficient handling of large numbers of samples. Currently, the more automated systems at the same time apply simpler analysis methods and are designed for "quick and dirty" answers. For these answers to be of any value downstream, SPR systems need to be integrated with complementary analysis tools for the independent confirmation of positives. Eventually hits from screens also have to be revisited with a more sophisticated SPR tool for more meaningful mechanistic studies. As the body of experience with the technology continues to grow and systems at the same time become more and more sophisticated electronically, eventually even high-throughput systems will allow more elaborate answers—that is, provided the right questions are asked.

III. TIME-OF-FLIGHT MASS SPECTROMETRY–BASED TECHNOLOGIES: FROM MALDI TO SELDI AND BIA/MS

A. Matrix-Assisted Desorption Techniques: Technical Background and Development History

Before we attempt to discuss the two currently available true protein chip technologies for mass spectrometry, SELDI and BIA/MS, we need to take a step back.

The development of mass spectrometry from an analytical chemistry technique into a more user-friendly biochemistry and biology tool deserves some attention. The technology was established mainly for purity analysis and molecular weight confirmation of organic chemicals and peptides with molecular weights under 1000 dalton. Fragmentation-related mass limitations initially prevented the analysis of larger molecules. Several desorption techniques like field desorption (FD-MS), secondary ion mass spectrometry (SIMS), fast atom bombardment (FAB-MS), plasma desorption (PDMS), and finally laser desorption/ionization (LDI-MS), extended the molecular weight range of analytes above 100,000 dalton [43]. This obviously made a big difference for the usefulness of mass spectrometry in the area of protein biochemistry. The technique of matrix-assisted laser desorption/ionization (MALDI) was simultaneously and independently discovered in two laboratories in 1987 and reported at international conferences that same year. Results from both groups were first published in 1988 [44,45]. The technology has since then evolved into a standard technique in the area of protein characterization by mass spectrometry. With MALDI it became possible to very accurately and sensitively analyze large, intact biomolecules, even derive information about their quaternary and tertiary structure. Commercially available MALDI platforms have become user friendly as well as much more powerful over the years. Mass accuracy in the 50–100 ppm peptide range is the expected norm. Eventually the field of mass spectrometry started to open to nonexpert users, though real biology applications remained limited. To put this into perspective, it is important to understand the key factors that make a MALDI time-of-flight (TOF) experiment work. Very simply speaking, in a TOF mass spectrometry experiment the protein of interest is turned into a molecular ion. Subsequently the travel time or TOF of this molecular ion through a vacuum tube toward a charged detector is measured. For singly charged ions, the TOF is proportional to the square root of the molecular weight of the analyte. There are different strategies to turn an uncharged molecule into a molecular ion. In the case of MALDI an organic compound, the so-called matrix, in combination with an energy source, usually UV laser, is used. A better term for matrix actually would be "energy-absorbing molecules" (EAM), since that is exactly the purpose of these compounds. After the protein of interest has been mixed with an EAM solution and applied to the instrument probe in a tiny drop, EAM and protein cocrystallize in a dry film. When the laser hits this film, the EAM absorbs the energy, expands into the gas phase, and carries the analyte molecules with it. At the same time a charge transfer between EAM and analyte leads to the creation of intact molecular ions. Usually the EAM is present in vast excess over the analyte. The high matrix/sample ratio reduces association of sample molecules and at the same time provides protonated and free-radical products for the ionization of the molecules of interest. As the sample molecules acquire one or multiple charges they are propelled down the vacuum tube toward a charged detector. Matrices used in MALDI are mostly organic acids. They are prepared as saturated solutions in a solvent system typically consisting of an organic and a strongly acidic inorganic component. Choice of matrix and solvent system very much depends on the nature of the molecule analyzed and are crucial determinants for success or failure of a MALDI experiment. Sinapinic acid (SA) and α-cyano-4-hydroxycinnaminic acid (CHCA) are among the most popular matrix compounds for general protein and peptide analysis. The preparation in 0.5% trifluoroacetic acid and 50% acetonitrile is a good starting point for a first experiment. Purity of the matrix component as well as of the solvent chemicals can critically influence the outcome of the experiment. Accordingly, the choice of highest grade material is well advised. Figure 3 shows a spectrum derived in a typical MALDI experiment. The x axis represents mass/charge (m/z), the y axis percent signal intensity. The two peaks visible represent the singly and doubly charged entities of the same molecule. The singly charged entity is detected at the molecular mass plus 1 (H+), the so-called monoisotopic mass, the doubly charged entity shows at apparently half the molecular mass. In addition to the analyte, matrix molecules are ionized as well and show up at the very low end of the mass spectrum. This has to be kept in mind when attempting to detect very small molecules with molecular masses between 0 and 300 D. When analyzing larger molecules that have hydrophobic qualities, matrix molecules can adhere to the analyte and create artifactual shoulders in the detected peaks. Fortunately, the generally high accuracy of mass detection allows distinction between the different molecular species and substraction of matrix-related peaks. Outside of finding the best matrix and solvent composition for a successful experiment with a particular protein, the purity of the protein and the buffer system used have a crucial influence on the outcome

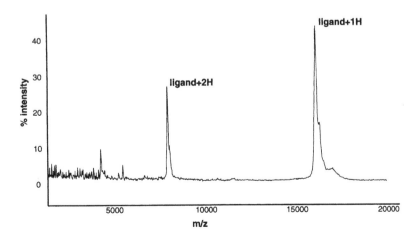

Figure 3   Typical MALDI spectrum of a purified protein.

of the MALDI analysis. Certain ions, such as Na^+, cause a phenomenon called ion suppression that usually results in tremendous chemical noise and inhibited ionization of the protein of interest. Due to this, tris-based buffers as well as other buffers with a high content of sodium ions are unsuitable. Detergents can be very problematic, too. Very few can be considered compatible with the technique. Even under ideal conditions, the protein forms a three-dimensional crystal with the large excess of matrix on the instrument probe. To obtain optimal signal, it is often necessary to search wider areas of the probe surface. This limits the quantitative value of the data. The overall biggest limitations of the MALDI technique are the restrictions it poses on the quality and nature of the sample that can be analyzed. Unless the protein sample is relatively pure and soluble in ionization-compatible buffers, analysis is difficult and requires great skill and understanding in the area of sample preparation. This clearly limits the usefulness of the technique in the area of biological screening and has driven the development of matrix-assisted technologies that address these limitations.

The development has mainly gone in three directions: use of micropipette tip clean-up methods for standard MALDI applications, the direct modification of mass spectrometry probes for specific analyte capture and clean-up (SELDI), and the use of BIACORE chips as MALDI platform (BIA/MS) [46].

B. Surface-Enhanced Laser Desorption/Ionization (SELDI): Protein Display Chips for Mass Spectrometry

The SELDI technique was developed by T. W. Hutchens and T.-T. Yip at Baylor College of Medicine, first experiments were published in 1993 [47]. With a background of protein purification and characterization from very dilute biological samples like tear fluid and urine, Hutchens and Yip had found the available MALDI techniques unsatisfactory and limited for the sensitive characterization of biological samples. They began experimenting with surface modifications of MALDI probes that would selectively tether biomolecules, allow for *in situ* clean-up and concentration, and then release the molecules again in the laser desorption analysis [48,49]. Soon they moved on to chemistries that would allow covalent molecule linkage, similar to the BIACORE chips: immobilize one binding partner covalently, capture a ligand from biological samples, wash away contaminants, and desorb the ligand [50]. As Hutchens' group changed from an academic setting into industry, their new partner Ciphergen Biosystems Inc. obtained comprehensive patent coverage for the chemical modification of mass spectrometry surfaces. SELDI and ProteinChip Arrays have become registered trademarks. Since then, the technique has been refined and, again similar to the BIACORE, been turned into an integrated analysis platform that consists of a chip reader (a linear delayed-extraction TOF device), the arrays, and an analysis software package. Still, being a lot younger than SPR technology, SELDI today is where the BIACORE was probably in 1994. The technology is a few years past its commercial introduction, the first publications are starting to appear outside of the development community [51,52], and users are starting to explore the potential and limitations of this new analysis strategy. Similar to the SPR situation, SELDI has brought a new analysis strategy into the hands of medical and biological researchers, for the most part users with no background knowledge in mass spectrometry. This has somewhat slowed the general acceptance of the technology, since initially a lot of inexperienced users had to discover the laws and limitations of MALDI by trial and error. Core laboratories and established mass spectrometry facilities initially avoided the technology widely, mostly due to the low accuracy of the first-generation mass reader. Ciphergen Biosystems has so far refused to license the surface technology to other instrument manufacturers with the vision in mind to keep hardware, chemware, and software under one roof. This has most certainly slowed the spread and development of the technology. Ciphergen targeted biotech and pharmaceutical industry as initial customers and project collaborators rather than academia. This has led to a large body of unpublished proprietary research, very different from SPR, which stimulated a large interest in the academic community right away that proliferated into a greater number of publications from the start.

C. SELDI Applications: General Principles and Experimental Considerations

Unlike SPR, SELDI quickly came along with a variety of different surfaces, mainly of two categories: preactivated surfaces for the covalent binding of biomolecules via primary amines, and chromatographic surfaces for the selective capture of proteins via charge, hydrophobicity, or metal–chelate interaction.

Preactivated surfaces support applications quite familiar to SPR users: the study of biomolecular interaction. While SPR looks at the affinity as expressed in on and off rates, SELDI takes a snap shot of everything the capture molecule has pulled from a biological sample. Retention can be influenced by the chosen conditions for binding and washing. Molecules bound via the covalently attached capture protein are desorbed in the ionization process. Figure 4 shows a SELDI experiment where a ligand of interest is captured via a receptor from a background of 100% serum. As expected for this medium, a significant amount of nonspecific binding by serum proteins is detected. The experiment shows how the addition of stringency in binding reduces this background but does not completely eliminate it. However, complete background elimination in SELDI is not necessary. If the molecular weight of the ligand is known, competition binders are easily distinguished as the mass spectrometer has a resolution superior to other molecular weight detection methods, generally much better than 0.1%. In an important difference from SPR, SELDI identifies the interacting molecules by molecular weight. This is important in a situation where the ligand of interest is captured from

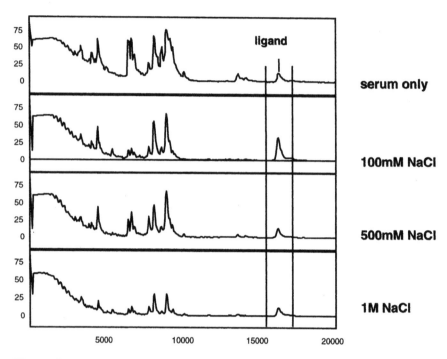

Figure 4 SELDI affinity study of a ligand captured via a receptor from human serum. Effect of different stringency modulators on nonspecific background binding

a complex biological background. In this situation competition binding can lead to confusing results in SPR analysis. SPR and SELDI are very much complementary techniques in this application area: SPR allows the determination of affinities and SELDI contributes protein identification capabilities. SELDI is limited by similar constraints as SPR; in both approaches a biological interaction is forced onto a two-dimensional platform. Different from SPR, though, the binding does not occur in a flow situation but rather in a tiny, stationary drop on the chip. With the limitations of sensitivity in a very small surface area, high density of capture molecules is key. Since kinetic considerations do not apply to the same extent in this analysis strategy, the main concern with high molecule density has to be steric hindrance. From a preparation point of view, SELDI experiments with preactivated chips share some similarity with ELISA techniques. Figure 5 shows a schematic outline of the process. The capture molecule is usually applied to each spot in a volume of less than 2 µl. For a protein, the concentration of the applied solution should be between 0.5 and 1 mg/ml. Because of the primary amine coupling, tris and azide-containing buffers are incompatible. After binding of the capture molecule, residual sites

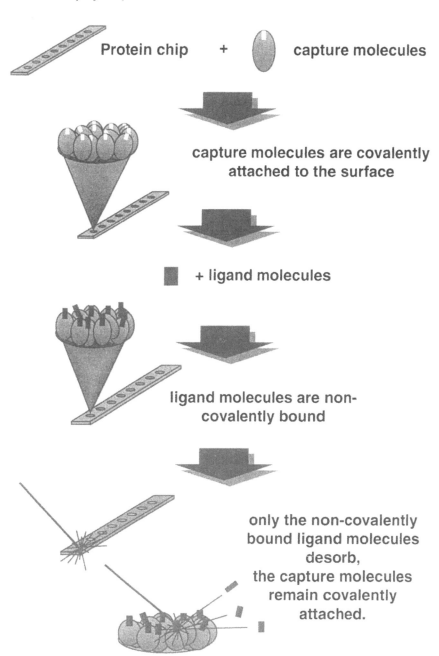

Figure 5 Flow chart of a typical SELDI experiment using preactivated arrays.

are blocked with ethanolamine. To remove noncovalently attached capture molecules remaining on the surface, pH-cycle washes in phosphate and sodium acetate buffers with high salt are recommended. Right before ligand application the chip is washed with PBS. The ligand is applied in a volume between 1 and 10 µl, depending on the concentration. After the ligand binding, the spots on the chip are washed with physiological buffers of appropriate stringency. The latter can be adjusted with salt or detergent. Due to the incompatibility of detergents and sodium salts with the desorption technique, a final wash in carbonate buffer or HEPES is necessary for good detection results. A conventional MALDI matrix mix is finally applied to the semidry sample for cocrystallization. Once dry, the chip is read in the instrument. The even spread of molecules on the surface, forced by the specific capturing, and the layering of matrix on top of the biomolecules dramatically enhance the quality of analysis compared to a conventional MALDI probe. More importantly, the opportunity to wash the surface without removing the protein of interest allows the use of previously MALDI-incompatible buffers and detergents in all steps of the process prior to ionization. This is a significant breakthrough that opened the door to the successful analysis of complex biological samples. On-chip sample clean-up is probably the biggest benefit that the world of mass spectrometry sample preparation has seen in a long time, especially when considering that at the same time a biological affinity interaction is kept intact on a mass spectrometry probe. A carefully designed SELDI binding experiment explores a wide range of ligand concentrations and applies the same data collection parameters across the different spots of the same chip. In this case, quantitative correlation between signal intensity and actual concentration of ligand can be quite impressive. The study of a good range of ligand concentrations as well as the challenge of specificity in a competition binding experiment are as important as in SPR technique to assure quality data. The application type just described finds use at many junctions of the drug development process. In the discovery area, the method is a tool to obtain information about unknown ligands to known capture molecules. With known molecules such as purified antibodies, it is useful to confirm binding activity. In the area of pharmacokinetics it allows the monitoring of molecules in patient serum: if the molecule of interest is a peptide with molecular weight under 10,000, the mass accuracy will even allow reading of the degradation sequence from the molecule, providing it desorbs with decent resolution. In the current absence of post-or in-source decay capabilities for the mass reader, degradation sequence has to be generated by on-probe carboxypeptidase digestions. In direct comparison with ELISA methods, SELDI cannot quite compete with the levels of sensitivity, but the protein identification capability eliminates false positives by revealing cross-reactivity if present. This can be as important as mere sensitivity, especially when dealing will molecule families that have a high level of conservation in structure and sequence leading to immunological cross-reactivity. In one aspect SELDI is more limited than SPR: not all biomolecules are easily ionized and detected. In SPR the mode of detection is more or less independent of the molecular characteristics of the analyte; hence, the broad applicability to proteins, nucleic acids, even carbohydrates. The latter two classes of molecules present special problems for matrix-assisted desorption techniques. They trap a lot of salt in their molecular backbone that causes ion suppression. This also affects the detection of proteins with carbohydrate modifications. Glycoproteins ionize very poorly, which affects the mass accuracy of detection as well as the sensitivity of the assay. SELDI has greatly enhanced the number of ionizable proteins by the simple fact that on-chip washes are very powerful in removing incompatible chemicals and ions even from very difficult molecules. However, some molecules just will not fly, as the mass spectrometrists say. Still, use of DNA or carbohydrates as capture molecules is possible in SELDI, as long as the ligand is easily detected. In SELDI as in SPR the choice of binding partner to immobilize is very important but is often driven by necessity as discussed earlier. If the capture molecule is small, a higher density can be achieved on the chip, and hindrance does not become a problem as quickly as with larger molecules. If the captured target ligand is very large, it is more difficult to ionize and the assay loses sensitivity in the detection step. The random binding to the chip also presents the familiar problem of not having all the capture molecules correctly oriented to receive the ligand. In the case of antibodies and Fc-fusion proteins, protein A coupling is helpful despite the fact that it increases the level of chemical and biological noise in detection. In a protein A sandwich assay both the capture protein and the ligand will get ionized; only the protein A stays attached to the chip. The quality of the protein A used for capture can critically influence sensitivity and noise levels in this type of experiment. In a protein–protein binding experiment, the goal generally is detection of a single binding entity, sometimes multimers of it, or at the most a heteromeric complex. A completely different set of data is obtained when protein chips are used for profiling applications. These applications look at the protein inventory of a biological sample in a given molecular weight range. Protein profiling applications are very interesting in the area of disease research. Comparison of lysates from normal versus diseased cells can reveal the expression of important marker proteins. For cancer research this approach has found a faithful following. Crude cell lysates are spotted on protein chips with different chromatographic surfaces, allowing a multidimensional binding picture based on different types of interaction. Control lysates are read against lysates of interest under the same data collection conditions, and subsequent peak substraction allows the identification of differences. Once a peak of interest has been detected, this protein can be singled out for further analysis. This is made possible by the application of more stringent conditions to the surface. Depending on the type of interaction, this can be achieved in gradient washes of pH, salt, or organic solvent, followed by an ionization-compatible wash. Once a peak is singled out sufficiently, the possibility of on-chip digestion with proteolytic enzymes and subsequent analysis of the peptide patterns can yield important identification information. At the current stage of the technology, protein identification applications are still somewhat limited by the mass accuracy of the protein chip reader, and it is very important to use careful calibration techniques with known peptides of comparable molecular weight to obtain reliable peptide maps. Even with a mass accuracy in the millidalton range, the proteomic researcher is cautioned that the protein chest of nature contains enough redundancy and sequence conservation to make wrong identification calls based on peptide masses. It is therefore necessary to have powerful fragmentation and sequencing capabilities combined with a front end of protein chips to obtain high-resolution data and novel protein information directly from biological samples. Developments in this area are ongoing and already provide exciting glimpses into a very bright future for proteomics by SELDI mass spectrometry.

Aside from the described discovery profiling, chromatographic protein chips are very useful tools in the day-to-day routines of the industrial protein chemistry laboratory. They can be used for expression monitoring and purification screening, as well as a simple identification tool at the end of a high-throughput purification process based on the same type of affinity chromatography.

D. SELDI in the Drug Development Process: A Bright Future

In general, protein chips for mass spectrometry have a very bright future in the drug discovery laboratory. The versatility of SELDI and the speed of the analysis will eventually lead to very elaborate multiplexed systems that provide an incredible amount of information in a very short time. In discovery as well as process development, production, and quality control, the mass accuracy of mass spectrometry joined with a platform for chemical or biological affinity for very small sample volumes will prove to be a very powerful combination. The technology still needs time to mature. As learned from the BIACORE example, a crucial step will be taken when the technology acquires a user base large enough to speed up the elimination of problems with experimental as well as instrument and platform design. It is safe to say that the future of protein biochemistry will be revolutionized by label-free chip technologies, and a few years from now protein gels may have become a thing of the past.

E. BIA/MS: Connecting a Popular SPR Platform to MALDI-TOF

We have already discussed some of the striking similarities that SPR and SELDI share in terms of surface activation and specific capturing of biological molecules on analysis chips. Hence, it is not surprising that researchers have looked at the possibilities of directly connecting a BIACORE platform with a MALDI TOF system.

Two facts have driven the development in this area: the wide acceptance of the BIACORE platform in industrial and academic laboratories, and the comprehensive patent coverage in the hands of Ciphergen Biosystems for the chemical modification of MS probes. BIA/MS circumvents the issue of surface modification specifically for MS and allows users to retrieve additional information from an SPR experiment. Two experimental strategies are mainly used in BIA/MS. In the first technique, the captured molecule of interest is eluted from the BIACORE chip with MALDI-friendly solution (typically a small volume of formic or trifluoroacetic acid) and subsequently applied to the MALDI probe. This has been successful for elution from metal-chelate chips [53]. In an alternative strategy, the BIACORE chip is directly used as a MALDI probe by application of matrix after conclusion of the SPR cycle [54]. Compared to SELDI, the BIA/MS strategy has several disadvantages. As has been discussed earlier, to obtain good results in SPR, it is important to maintain a low molecule density on the chip as well as a low analyte concentration. This challenges the detection capabilities of the best MALDI systems, especially when molecules with poor ionization qualities are analyzed. Furthermore, the BIACORE chip was not designed as a mass spectrometry probe in the first place and thus has several intrinsic problems when used as a probe. Overall, BIA/MS is not a straightforward and easily adapted experimental system. So far, literature in this area has mainly come from two groups [55,56]. BIA/MS advocates stress MALDI sensitivity as well as the technique's tolerance for difficult buffer systems, but the examples demonstrated in the literature so far mainly focus on examples from *E. coli* lysate, where protein abundance and available sample prep options are generally not limiting factors [54]. It remains to be seen how well the technique will fare with difficult biological backgrounds like membrane systems. In those areas the opportunity for higher molecule density and sample clean-up on the SELDI chip will most like prove more advantageous.

IV. CONCLUSION: PROTEIN DISPLAY CHIPS IN DRUG DISCOVERY—THE FUTURE IS HERE

This chapter shows that protein display chips are still very much a developing field, and there are far fewer players than in the respective technology for nucleic acids. Nevertheless, as the genomics field has come of age, development in the protein area has picked up, profiting from the great leaps that have been made in nanoscale analysis for DNA and RNA. Still, for proteins the most exciting discoveries are probably yet to come. Accommodating the incredible diversity of proteins in discovery, development, analysis, and validation is an enormous task, requiring not one or two but at least a handful of technology platforms. These in turn must be integrated to render a multidimensional analysis picture. The overlap between techniques like SPR and SELDI as well as the limitations of both already point us in this direction. The techniques and platforms discussed give us a glimpse of the future that has finally arrived in protein biochemistry.

REFERENCES

1. Cullen DC, Brown RGW, Rowe CR. Detection of immuno-complex formation via surface plasmon resonance on gold-coated diffraction gratings. Biosensors 1987/88;3: 211–225.
2. Wood RW. On the remarkable case of uneven distribution of light in a diffraction grating spectrum. Phil Mag 1902;4:396–402.
3. Ritchie RH. Plasma losses by fast electrons in thin films. Phys Rev 1957;106:874–881.
4. Neviere M. The homogeneous problem. In: Petit R, ed. Electromagnetic Theory of Gratings. Berlin: Springer-Verlag, 1980:123–157.
5. Maystre D. General study of grating anomalies from electromagnetic surface modes. In: Boardman AD, ed. Electromagnetic Surface Modes. Chichester: John Wiley & Sons, 1982:661–724.
6. Leatherbarrow RJ, Edwards PR. Analysis of molecular recognition using optical biosensors. Curr Opin Biotechnol 1999;3:544–547.
7. Malmquist M. BIACORE: an affinity biosensor system for characterization of biomolecular interactions. Biochem Soc Trans 1999;27:335–340.
8. Lowe P, Clark T, Davies R, Edwards, P, Kinning T, Yang D. New approaches for the analysis of molecular recognition using Iasys evanescent wave biosensor. J Mol Recognit 1998;11:194–199.
9. Kurrat R, Prenosil J, Ramsden J. Kinetics of human and bovine serum albumin adsorption at silica–titania surfaces. J Colloid Interf Sci 1997;185:1–8.
10. Johnsson B, Löfås S, Lindquist G. Immobilization of proteins to a carboxy-methyldextran-modified gold surface for biospecific interaction analysis in surface plasmon resonance sensors. Anal Biochem 1991;198:268–277.
11. Martin J, Langer T, Boteva R, Schramel A, Horwich AL, Hartle FU. Chaperonin-mediated protein folding at the surface of GroEL through a "molten globule"-like intermediate. Nature 1991;352:36–42.
12. Cuatrecasas P, Praikh I. Adsorbents for affinity chromatography. Use of N-hydroxy-succinimide esters of agarose. Biochemistry 1972;12:2291–2299.
13. Raghavan M, Chen MY, Gastinel LN, Bjorkman PJ. Investigation of the interaction between the class I MHC-related Fc receptor and its immunoglobulin G ligand. Immunity 1994;1:303–315.
14. Corr M, Slanetz AE, Boyd LF, Jelonek MT, Khilko S, Al-Ramadi BK, Kim YS, Maher SE, Bothwell ALM, Margulies DH. T cell receptor-MHC class 1 peptide interactions: affinity, kinetics, and specificity. Science 1994;265:946–949.
15. Laminet AA, Ziegelhoffer T, Georgopoulos C, Plückthun A. The *Escherichia coli* heat shock proteins GroEL and GroES modulate the folding of the beta-lactamase precursor. EMBO J 1990;9:2315–2319.

16. Zahn R, Axmann SE, Rycknagel K-P, Jaeger E, Laminet AA, Plückthun A. Thermo-dynamic partitioning model for hydrophobic binding of polypeptides by GroEL. J Mol Biol 1994;242:150–164.

17. Lin Z, Eisenstein E. Nucleotide binding-promoted conformational changes release a nonnative polypeptide from the *Escherichia coli* chaperonin GroEL. Proc Natl Acad Sci USA 1996;93:1977–1981.

18. Kragten E, Lalande I, Zimmermann K, Roggo S, Schindler P, Müller P, van Ostrum J, Waldmeier P, Fürst P. Glyceraldehyde-3-phosphate dehydrogenase, the putative target of the antiapoptotic compounds CGP 3466 and R-(-)-Deprenyl. J Biol Chem 1998;273:5821–5828.

19. MaKenzie CR, Hirama T, Deng S-J, Bundle DR, Narang SA, Young NM. Analysis by surface plasmon resonance of the influence of valence on the ligand binding affinity and kinetics of an anti-carbohydrate antibody. J Biol Chem 1996;271:1527–1533.

20. Fisher RJ, Fivash M, Casas-Finet J, Erickson JW, Kondoh A, Bladen SV, Fisher C, Watson DK, Papas T. Real-time DNA binding measurements of the ETS1 recombi-nant oncoproteins reveal significant kinetic differences between the p42 and p51 iso-forms. Protein Sci 1994;3:257–266.

21. Spanopoulou E, Zaitseva F, Wang F-H, Santagata S, Baltimore D, Panayotou G. The Homeodomain region of Rag-1 reveals the parallel mechanisms of bacterial and V(D)J recombination. Cell 1996;87:263–276.

22. Haruki M, Noguchi E, Kanaya S, Crouch RJ. Kinetic and stoichiometric analysis for the binding of *Escherichia coli* ribonuclease HI to RNA-DNA hybrids using surface plasmon resonance. J Biol Chem 1997;272:22015–22022.

23. Lea SM, Poewll RM, McKee T, Evans DJ, Brown D, Stuart DI, van der Merve PA. Determination of the affinity and kinetic constants for the interaction between the human virus echovirus 11 and its cellular receptor CD55. J Biol Chem 1998;273: 30443–30447.

24. Gill A, Bracewell DG, Maule CH, Lowe PA, Hoare M. Bioprocess monitoring: an optical biosensor for rapid bioproduct analysis. J Biotechnol 1998;65:69–80.

25. Borrebaeck CAK, Malmborg A-C, Furebring C, Michaelsson A, Ward S, Danielsson L, Ohlin M. Kinetic analysis of recombinant antibody-antigen interactions: relation between structural domains and antigen binding. Biotechnology 1992;10:697–698.

26. Altschuh D, Dubs M-C, Weiss E, Zeder-Lutz G, Van Regenmortel MHV. Determina-tion of kinetic constants for the interaction between a monoclonal antiboy and pep-tides using surface plasmon resonance. Biochemistry 1992;31:6298–6304.

27. O'Shannessy DJ, Brigham BM, Soneson KK, Hensley P, Brooks I. Determination of rate and equilibrium binding constants for macromolecular interactions using surface plasmon resonance: use of nonlinear least squares analysis methods. Anal Biochem 1993;212:457–468.

28. Cardone MH, Roy N, Stennicke HR, Salveson GS, Franke TF, Stanbridge E, Frisch S, Reed JC. Regulation of cell death protease caspase-9 by phosphorylation. Science 1998;282:1318–1321.

29. Sadir RS, Forest E, Lortat-Jacob H. The heparan sulfate binding sequence of inter-feron γ increased the on rate of the interferon-γ-interferon-γ receptor complex forma-tion. J Biol Chem 1998;273:10919–10925.

30. Ladbury JE, Lemmon MA, Zhou M, Green J, Botfield MC, Schlessinger J. Measurement of the binding of tyrosyl phosphopeptides to SH2 domains: a reappraisal. Proc Natl Acad Sci USA 1995;3199–3203.
31. Thomas C, Surolia A. Kinetics of interaction of endotoxin with polymyxin B and its analogs: a surface plasmon resonance analysis. FEBS Lett 1999;445:420–424.
32. Stuart J, Myszka D, Joss L, Mitchell R, McDonald S, Xie A, Takayama S, Reed J, Ely K. Characterization of interactions between the antiapoptotic protein BAG-1 and Hsc 70 molecular chaperones. J Biol Chem 1998;273:22506–22514.
33. Asensio J, Dosanjh H, Jenkins T, Lane A. Thermodynamic, kinetic and conformational properties of a parallel intermolecular DNA triplex containing 3' and 5' junctions. Biochemistry 1998;37:15188–15198.
34. Glaser RW. Antigen-antibody binding and mass transport by convection and diffusion to a surface: a two-dimensional computer model of binding and dissciation kinetics. Anal Biochem 1993;213:152–161.
35. Schuck P, Minton AP. Analysis of mass transport-limited binding kinetics in evanescent wave biosensors. Anal Biochem 1996;240:262–272.
36. Schuck P. Kinetics of ligand binding to receptor immobilized in a polymer matrix, as detected with an evanescent wave biosensor 1: a computer simulation of the influence of mass transport. Biophys J 1996;70:1230–1249.
37. Edwards P, Lowe P, Leatherbarrow R. Ligand loading at the surface of an optical biosensor and its effect upon the kinetics of protein-protein interactions. J Mol Recognit 1997;10:128–134.
38. Müller KM, Arndt KM, Plückthun A. Model and simulation of multivalent binding to fixed ligands. Anal Biochem 1998;261:149–158.
39. Yu Y-Y, Van Wie BJ, Koch AR, Moffett DF, Davies WC. Real-time analysis of immunogen complex reaction kinetics using surface plasmon resonance. Anal Biochem 1998;263:158–168.
40. Myszka DG, Jonsen MD, Graves BJ. Equilibrium analysis of high affinity interactions using BIACORE. Anal Biochem 1998;265:326–330.
41. Schuck P, Millar DB, Kortt AA. Determination of binding constants by equilibrium titration with circulating sample in a surface plasmon resonance biosensor. Anal Biochem 1998;265:79–91.
42. O'Shanessey DJ. Determination of kinetic rate and equilibrium binding constants for macromolecular interactions: a critique of the surface plasmon resonance literature. Curr Opin Biotechnol 1994;5:65–71.
43. Cotter RJ. Time-of-flight mass spectrometry. Instrumentation and Applications in Biological Research. Washington, DC: American Chemical Society, 1997.
44. Tanaka K, Waki H, Ido Y, Akita S, Yoshida Y, Yoshida T. Protein and polymer analyses up to m/z 100 000 by laser ionization time-of-flight mass spectrometry. Rapid Commun Mass Spectrom 1988;2:151–153.
45. Karas M, Hillenkamp F. Laser desorption ionization of proteins with molecular masses exceeding 10,000 daltons. Anal Chem 1988;60:2299–2301.
46. Papac DI, Hoyes J, Tomer KB. Direct analysis of affinity-bound analytes by MALDI/TOF MS. Anal Chem 1994;66:2609–2613.
47. Hutchens TW, Yip TT. New desorption strategies for the mass spectrometric analysis of macromolecules. Rapid Commun Mass Spectrom 1993;576–580.

48. Ching J, Viovodov KI, Hutchens TW. Surface chemistries enabling photoinduced uncoupling/desorption of covalently tethered biomolecules. J Org Chem 1996;67:3582–3583.

49. Ching, J, Viovodov KI, Hutchens TW. Polymers as surface-based tethers with photolytic triggers for laser-induced release/desorption of covalently bound molecules. Bioconj Chem 1996;7:525–528.

50. Viovodov KI, Ching J, Hutchens TW. Surface arrays of energy absorbing polymers enabling covalent attachment of biomolecules for subsequent laser-induced release/desorption. Tetrahedron Lett 1996;37:5669–5672.

51. Stennicke HR, Salveson GS, Franke TF, Stanbridge E, Frisch S, Reed JC. Regulation of cell death protease caspase-9 by phsophorylation. Science 1998;282:1318–1321.

52. Austen B, Davies H, Stephens DJ, Frears ER, Walters CE. The role of cholesterol in the biosynthesis of beta-amyloid. Neuroreport 1999;10:1699–1705.

53. Thiede B, Wittmann-Liebold B, Bienert M, Krause E. MALDI-MS for C-terminal sequence determination of peptides and proteins degraded by carboxypeptidase Y and P. FEBS Lett 1995;357:65–69.

54. Nelson RW, Jarvik JW, Taillon BE, Kemmons AT. BIA/MS of epitope-tagged peptides directly from *E. coli* lysate: multiplex detection and protein identification at low-femtomole to subfemtomole levels. Anal Chem 1999;71:2858–2865.

55. Sonksen CP, Nordhoff E, Jasson O, Malmquist M, Roepstorff P. Combining MALDI mass spectrometry and biomolecular interaction analysis using a biomolecular interaction analysis instrument. Anal Chem 1998;70:2731–2736.

56. Nelson RW, Krone JR. Advances in surface plasmon resonance biomolecular interaction analysis mass spectrometry (BIA/MS). J Mol Recognit 1999;12:77–93.

8
Integrated Proteomics Technologies and In Vivo Validation of Molecular Targets

Christian Rohlff
Oxford GlycoSciences
Abingdon, United Kingdom

I. PROTEOMICS IN MOLECULAR MEDICINE

The identification and selection of a therapeutic target can determine the success or failure of a drug discovery program. This decision is influenced by the underlying biases of the drug discovery research strategy, which can be a reflection of the applied technologies. Since the vast majority of drug targets are proteins, identification and characterization of a novel molecular target will be greatly facilitated by carrying out the analysis at the protein level, thus focusing "on the actual biological effector molecules" [1] of the gene. This chapter will examine the role of proteomics in drug discovery with a particular focus on preclinical target evaluation. Until we can truly rely on experimental medicine for drug development, disease models will play a pivotal role in molecular medicine for the safety and efficacy evaluation of a new therapeutic. To succeed with this strategy, the relevance of these models must be considered. Proteomics may facilitate this assessment through a comparison of the human disease phenotype to the one obtained in an animal model through a comprehensive analysis of protein expression maps (PEMs) of the relevant body compartments such as bodily fluids and the affected organ tissues.

A. Proteome Terminology

The term proteomics is twinned with another new term, the proteome, which originated in 1995 [2] to describe the complete protein expression profile in a given tissue, cell, or biological system at a given time. Proteomics represents an extension of the earlier established concepts of the genome and genomics. The human genome delineates the entire human genetic information contained in two copies within the nucleus of each cell of the human body with the exception of mature platelets. "Functional genomics is the attachment of information about function to knowledge of DNA sequence," [3] giving an indication of whether a gene is transcribed but not necessarily translated in a disease- or tissue-specific manner. More specifically, functional proteomics describes the biochemical and biological characterization of proteins. These efforts are aimed at identifying structurally and functionally significant sequence motifs in the primary protein sequence with respect to the subcellular location of their activities and to relate these to disease- or tissue-specific changes. Pharmacogenomics is aimed at identifying genetic polymorphic variations in the human population that are relevant to the disease state or the ability to metabolize a drug. Recently, a lot of emphasis in the area of pharmacogenomics has been directed to the identification of the majority of single-nucleotide polymorphisms (SNPs) involved in human disease and drug response. SNPs are single-nucleotide variations between the DNA sequence of individuals that can be substitutions, insertions, or deletions. Information on these variations may allow the clinician of the future to stratify a patient population in clinical trials based on their predicted drug sensitivity-response profile [4]. First applications are emerging, such as chip-based mutational analysis of blood, urine, stool, and breast effusions [5]. However, it remains to be determined what impact the presence of genetic polymorphisms will have on the application of animal models in preclinical development.

Although pharmacoproteomics aims at patient stratification, it is based on protein expression polymorphisms in body fluids and tissues, which could be indicative of susceptibility to disease and responsiveness to drugs in pharmacoproteomic pharmacology or toxicology studies. Longitudinal serum samples from drug-treated animals should identify individual protein markers or clusters thereof that are dose related and correlate with the emergence and severity of toxicity. Structural genomics could be considered an extension of functional genomics using structural information obtained by x-ray crystallography to infer the folding and three-dimensional structure of related protein family members. It can be envisioned that the discipline of structural proteomics could apply the information available on the tertiary structure of a protein or motif to establish its biological significance by systematically mapping out all its interacting protein partners. This information could suggest their role in the pathogenesis of a particular disease and assess its dependence on posttranslational modifications (PTMs). We will illustrate

Table 1 Definition of Terms used in Genomic and Proteomic Research

Term	Definition
Genome	Total genetic information possessed by an individual
Genomics	Characterization and sequencing of the genome
Functional genomics	Systematic analysis of gene activity in healthy and diseased tissues
Structural genomics	Systematic analysis of the three-dimensional structure of a protein of a protein based on homology to a protein with a known structure
Pharmacogenomics	Stratification of patients by their genetic susceptibility to disease and responsiveness to drugs
Phenotype	Observable properties of an organism produced by the genotype (in conjunction with the environment)[a]
	Genetically inherited appearance or behavior of organism[b]
Proteome	Total protein profile of a cell or tissue at a given time
Proteomics	Systematic analysis of a protein expression map in a particular tissue or body fluid
Functional Proteomics	Systematic analysis of protein expression and posttranslational modification of proteins in various cellular compartments of healthy and diseased tissues
Structural proteomics	A proteomics approach for structure determination using native protein array technology
Pharmacoproteomics	Patient stratification based on protein expression polymorphisms in body fluids indicative of susceptibility to disease and responsiveness to drugs

[a]From Ref. 101.
[b]From Ref. 102.

some applications for structural proteomics in Section I.H on the proteomic analysis of protein complexes. Definitions of these terms are given in Table 1.

B. Genome vs. Proteome

Until recently, biological and biochemical analyses were carried out on single molecules. The dramatic advances in genomic sequencing and mRNA-based analyses of gene expression have generated important descriptive information. The field is now quickly evolving from its primary objectives of information collection, organization, and mining to functional and structural genomics, whereby one uses DNA-based technologies to make inferences about an organism's structure and behavior mainly through large-scale analysis of gene expression. Advances in the Human Genome Project together with the availability of an increasing number of methods for gene expression have lead pharmaceutical companies to review their strategies to discover new drugs. However, it is becoming apparent that purely gene-based expression analysis is not sufficient for the target discovery and validation process. There may not necessarily be a tight temporal correlation between gene and actual protein expression [6]. Differences can arise from different stability and turnover of mRNA and protein, posttranscriptional mRNA splicing yielding various protein products, and posttranslational modifications. Proteomics can take these variables into consideration and contribute additional information through expression analysis of subcellular fraction and protein complexes (Fig. 1).

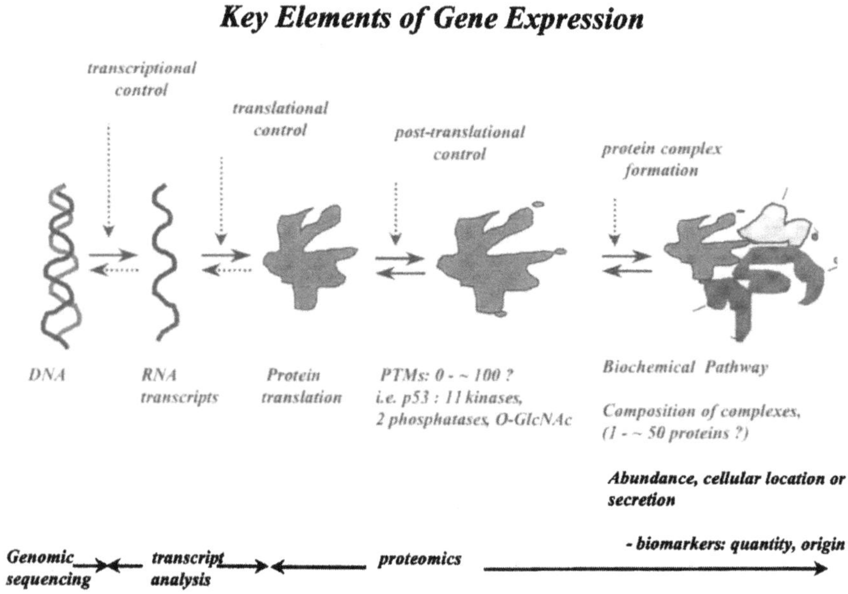

Key Elements of Gene Expression

Figure 1   Genome to proteome. Gene expression can be regulated by the rate of transcription, translation, and further posttranslational regulation of protein expression and activity are known [8]. Each protein may undergo various levels of posttranslational modification (PTM). In some instances, more than 10 serine-, threonine-, and tyrosine-phosphorylated and serine- or threonine O-linked-glycosylated amino acids can be detected on a single protein. Additional PTMs include asparagine-linked glycosylation, farnesylation, and palmitoylation, all of which can affect the activity, stability, and location of a particular protein (see Section I.C). There are an increasing number of examples where enzymes carrying out these PTMs become targets for therapeutic intervention (see Section I.D.) (From Ref.7.)

C. Changes in PTMs Associated with Pathogenesis

An understanding of the control of cellular processes and of the molecular basis of inter- and intracellular signaling can only emerge when the protein and the protein complexes involved in these processes can be elucidated together with the dynamics of their PTMs and associated activities. It is largely through an understanding of such protein-based mechanisms that real insight into molecular bases of complex phenotypic diseases will emerge, leading to more relevant molecular targets for drug discovery. Ample evidence has distinctly validated numerous novel enzymes modulating protein PTMs as targets in many diseases including cancer, diabetes, sepsis as well as certain cardiovascular and neuronal abnormalities [9–15]. Rational design of modulators of these new molecular targets has yielded multiple drug candidates promising more selective therapies. In cancer research, for example, several pharmacological approaches have focused on the enzymatic activity of enzyme-linked cell surface receptor signaling cascades such as the epidermal growth factor (EGF) receptor family signaling pathway illustrated in Figure 2.

D. New Drug Candidates Directed Against Molecular Targets Modulating Protein PTM

As illustrated in Figure 2, tumorigenesis via the erbB receptor signaling cascade has a proven biological significance in experimental tumor metastasis systems [16]. This provides ample opportunities for novel therapeutic modalities at multiple sites within the pathway such as the EGF receptor kinase antagonists [17] and trastuzumab (herceptin), an anti-HER2 monoclonal antibody blocking the activity of HER2 (erbB-2), the second member of the EGF receptor family [18]. The importance of membrane anchoring via acetylation of certain signal proteins, such as Ras, is exemplified by the farnesyltransferase inhibitors, a putative cancer therapy with a better therapeutic index than standard chemotherapy. Originally designed to target tumors with mutant *ras* genes, farnesyltransferase inhibitors also affect growth of tumours with no known *ras* mutations [19]. Several protein kinases, including the immediate downstream effector of ras, raf kinase, and protein kinase C, are targeted clinically via the antisense approach [20,21]. Inhibition of the tumor growth–promoting protein kinase MEK1 (MAPK kinase) leads to arrest at the G_1 phase of the cell cycle. In addition to blocking cancer cell growth, MEK1 inhibitors reverse some of the transformation phenotype, such as resumed flattened morphology and loss of the ability to grow in the absence of a substrate [22]. A detailed understanding of such a pathway in the context of the disease may enable us to select the right drug directed to a particular step the pathway or a combination thereof for each subcategory of the disease.

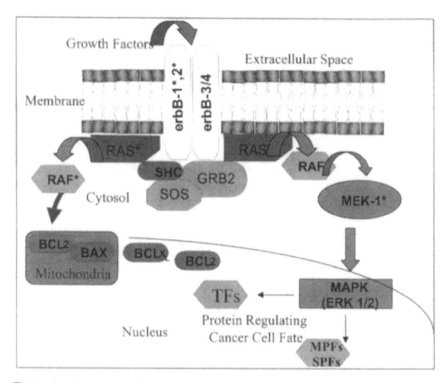

Figure 2   New drug candidates are directed against molecular targets modulating protein PTMs. Extracellular growth factors trigger cell proliferation through their transmembrane receptor tyrosine kinase (RTK) to intracellular signaling pathways such as the mitogen-activated protein kinase (MAPK) cascade. Growth factor binding will change the RTK conformation and activate its intrinsic protein kinase activity resulting in transphosphorylation of a receptor homo- (erb-B1/erb-B1) or heterodimer (erb-B2/erb-B3/4). The activated receptor uses special SH adaptor domains (SH termed for their homology to the oncogene kinase src) to form a sequential complex with several downstream effectors, including Grb2, SHC, and SOS, leading to activation of Ras. Ras will recruit Raf kinase to the membrane, which in turn will activate MEK1 (MAPK kinase) through phosphorylastion on two distinct serine residues. Phosphorylation of ERK1 and ERK2 on threonine and tyrosine residues by MEK1 is critical for cellular transformation and has become a main focus of therapeutic intervention [22,23]. ERK1 and ERK2 phosphorylate a variety of substrates involved in a many cellular aspects of transformation from cytoskeletal changes to cell cycle–dependent gene transcription. Timely expression of heteroprotein complexes is critical for a mammalian cell, such as S-phase and M-phase cell cycle promoting factors composed of cyclin-dependent kinases (CDKs) and regulatory cyclins. They initiate M- and S-phase progression by phosphorylating transcription factors, which in turn drive the expression of cell cycle machinery. Pertubations in the expression in some aspect of these regulatory heteroprotein complexes are the hallmark of almost every form of cancer. *, PTMs of a signaling protein that have become a focus of novel therapeutic modalities.

Initial emphasis in the development of small-molecule protein kinase inhibitors focused on modulating catalytic activity directly. However, homology among the catalytic ATP binding site of hundreds of protein kinases active in a mammalian cell at any given time severely limits the degree of selectivity attainable. A strategy to overcome this has been illustrated by recently developed MEK1 kinase inhibitors that appear to act through an allosteric mechanism of inhibition. This novel class of MEK1 inhibitors display very good toxicity profiles, suggestive of a high degree of selectivity [22]. However, the MAPK signal pathway plays an important role in normal cell signaling for the immune response and neuronal functions, mandating thorough validation in vitro and in vivo [23]. Such validation studies increase the knowledge about the behavior of the small-molecule inhibitor in a complex biological system and may lead to label extension for completely different indications. For example, the MEK1 kinase inhibitors are now being evaluated for their ability to reduce postischemic brain injury [24].

A similar approach of allosteric inhibition of intraprotein binding led to the development of small-molecule inhibitors that block the interactions between the tumor suppressor protein p53 and its inhibitor MDM2. Initial studies on the regulation of p53 focused largely on phosphorylation, the complexity of which is emphasized by at least nine kinases, two phosphatases [25], and cytosolic O-linked glycosylation modulating p53 location, stability, and activity [26]. p53 activity is further regulated by the proto-oncoprotein MDM2, which impedes its transcriptional function and targets p53 oligomers only for ubiqutin-dependent degradation [27]. Small-molecule inhibitors blocking this protein–protein interaction lead to the release of active p53 to activate programmed cell death (Fig. 3). These two examples emphasis the importance of studying protein complexes, as will be discussed in Section I.H, since they may yield an immediate new target for therapeutic intervention.

These small-molecule MDM2 inhibitor mimics the activity of the endogenous cell cycle regulatory protein p19ARF, which also binds MDM2 and stabilizes p53. The diverse expression of the p19ARF/p16INK4a gene exemplifies the complexity of gene expression at another level of regulation. The second p19ARF/p16INK4a gene product originates from an alternative splicing product, which is translated into p16INK4a. p16INK4a has a peptide sequence different from p19ARF because the use of an alternative start exon causes a frameshift and the mRNA is translated in a different reading frame. The alternative splicing occurs in a tissue-specific manner (Fig. 3). Recently, a third splice form, p12 INK4a, was discovered to be of functional significance in pancreatic cancer [30]. Originally studied as a tumor suppressor in cancer, p16INK4a is now being evaluated as a novel therapeutic agent for the management of rheumatoid arthritis [31]. The physiological and therapeutic importance of distinct splice variant isoforms of a protein has already been recognized for seven transmembrane G-protein-coupled receptors [32]. These splice variants arising from exon skipping, intron retention, alternative

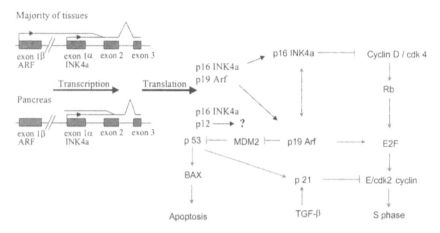

Figure 3 Gene sequence does not predict protein functions; tissue-specific transcription and translation of the p16^{INK4a}/p19ARF gene. The tumor suppressor p16^{INK4a}/ARF gene locus on human chromosome 9p21 is a site of frequent deletion in many cancers including leukemias, gliomas, and non-small cell lung cancers [104]. Three splicing forms of the p16^{INK4a}/ARF gene yield three distinct proteins: p16INK4a, p19ARF, and p12.p16INK4a blocks the cyclinD/cyclin-dependent kinase 4 complex, preventing phosphorylation and inactivation of Rb. Active Rb will inhibit the transcription factor E2F and prevent gene expression of cell cycle machinery protein for S-phase progression causing arrest in G$_1$ phase of the cell cycle. The second splice form p19ARF uses a different start exon and yields a different peptide sequence due to a resulting frameshift. p19ARF prevents MDM2 from binding p53. The third protein product of the p16^{INK4a}/ARF gene p12 composed of the INK4a exon 1a and a novel intron-derived C terminus also inhibits the cell cycle without interacting with the Rb pathway [28]. MDM2 blocks p53 tumor suppressor function by blocking its transcriptional activity and targeting it for ubiquitin-dependent degradation. MDM2 also binds a close homologue of p53, p73α. inhibiting its transcriptional activity without inducing its degradation [29].

start exons, or splicing will also affect ligand binding profiles, G-protein coupling, and receptor desensitization in a tissue-specific manner [32].

In conclusion, discovery and characterization of molecular targets resulting from abnormal cellular function through abnormalities in protein expression and their PTMs cannot be achieved through descriptive genetic analysis. Exploring how the protein products of individual genes interact dynamically to control cellular processes, as well as how these protein interactions and activities are controlled by PTMs, will lead to greater insight into the control of the complex and dynamic processes of protein PTM that are central to cellular behavior and cellular responses. Understanding the control of subcellular protein expression and PTMs will lead to our understanding with greater precision the molecular basis of abnormalities in cellular control processes and protein networks, leading ultimately to more specific and more relevant molecular targets for disease control [33]. This implies a central role for the proteomic analysis of molecular targets in the evaluation process in vitro and in vivo. Although proteins reflect the physiology of normal and diseased tissue more closely than transcript analysis, the technology requirements for reproducibility, sensitivity, and throughput of two-dimensional (2-DE). Gel electrophoresis hampered the fast and direct access to this information. Significant advances in the technology combined with new approaches to disease models and access to clinically relevant tissues may provide us with a molecular fingerprint of disease at the protein level and identify further targets for therapeutic intervention.

E. Protein Expression Mapping

Protein expression mapping aims to define global protein expression profiles in tissues, cells or body fluids. A protein expression profile may be representative of a given time point in an experiment or a disease state and become the basis for a comparative analysis. The most common implementation of proteomics is based on 2-DE of proteins in a complex mixture and their subsequent individual isolation, identification, and analysis from within the gel by mass spectrometry (MS). If multiple isoforms of a protein exist within the sample due to PTMs and splice variants as described above, they may be identified because PTMs affect the charge and molecular weight of protein isoforms altering their mobility in the 2D gel.

In the proteomic process, proteins are initially extracted from tissues, whole cells, or cell organelles using extraction procedures well documented in the literature [34]. The proteins are solubilized in 2D sample buffers and run on 2D polyacrylamide gels by separating them according to their charge (pI) in the first dimension using isoelectric focusing. They are then separated by size, using sodium dodecyl sulfate–polyacrylamide gel electrophoresis (SDS-PAGE), in the second dimension. Most commonly proteins within the gel are visualized by Coommassie blue or silver staining. The proteins referred to as features in the raw primary image represent the proteome. At Oxford GlycoSciences (OGS), the image is scanned through fluorescent detection and digital imaging to yield a PEM. An electronic database containing all PEM (now in digitized form) can be constructed. Each protein feature in each PEM is assigned a molecular cluster index (MCI). Each MCI has attributes of pI, relative molecular mass, quantity in each sample, frequency in each sample set, and a linkage to the feature ID in each gel for subsequent analysis of any proteins in any archived gel. By this process all protein features in a sample are linked to MCIs and are then available for quantitative analysis. A comparison of the proteomes generated from normal and disease samples is summarized in the

Proteograph. The PC-Rosetta software is capable of rapidly identifing those proteins that are unique in PEMs of control and diseased samples, or those that show increased or decreased expression. It provides information on its pI and molecular weight and in large sample sets statistical data on differentially expressed proteins are computed (Fig. 4). Several other commercial companies also provide basic image analysis tools, such as Melanie (BioRad; http://www.bio-rad.com) and Phoretix 2D (Phoretix International; http://www.phoretix.com).

Many modifications have been made at OGS to improve handling, throughput, sensitivity, and reproducibility of 2-DE. For example, proprietary attachment chemistry causes covalent attachment of the gel to the back plate. This greatly enhances reproducibility by avoiding warping and other distortions of the gel. Fluorescent dyes that bind noncovalently to SDS-coated proteins facilitates detection of protein spots in the gel over a greater linear range than densitometric methods while not interfering during the MS analysis [35].

Zoom gels can be used to further expand the resolution of a gel or to analyze a particular area of the gel containing a protein of interest with greater accuracy. For this purpose, proteins separated in the first dimension on three IEFs pH 4–6, pH 5–7, and pH 6–8 rather than on a standard IEF (pH 3–10). Through this process the number of features resolved can be increased considerably. For example, the number of features resolved from a cell extract of Huh7 human hepatoma cells can be increased from approximately 2000 feature to more than 5000 features (Fig. 5).

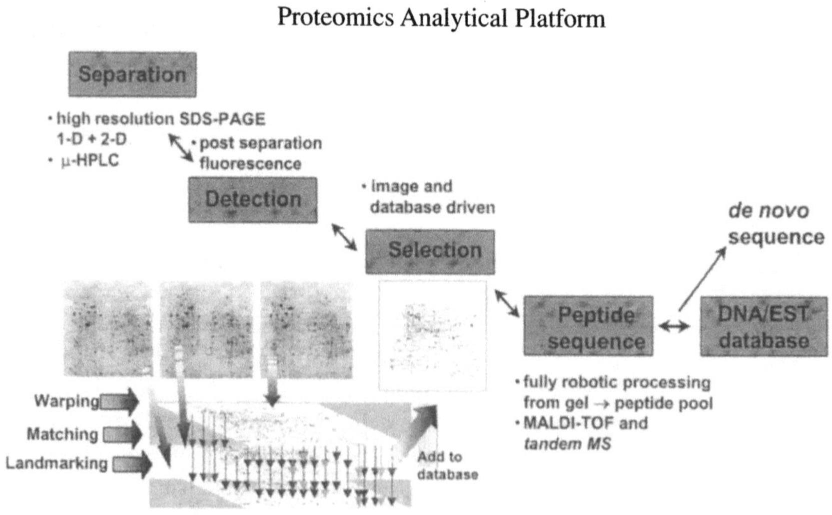

Proteomics Analytical Platform

Figure 4 Components of the proteomic process.

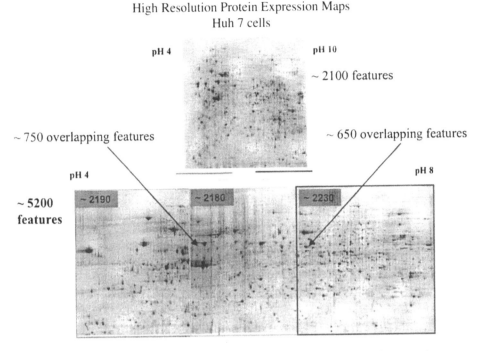

Figure 5 Zoom gels can be used to further expand the resolution of a gel or to analyze a particular area of the gel containing a protein of interest with greater accuracy. This example shows cell extracts from Huh7 human hepatoma cells separated in the first dimension on a standard IEF (pH 3–10) or on three IEF pH 4–6, pH 5–7, and pH 6–8. Through this process the number of features resolved can be increased significantly.

Selected features are isolated from the gels and chemically or enzymatically fragmented in the gel slice [36,37] or after electrotransfer onto a suitable membrane for MS analysis [38–41]. The resulting peptides can be separated by on-line capillary HPLC for subsequent MS analysis through matrix-assisted laser desorption ionization (MALDI) MS [42,43], tandem mass spectrometry (MS/MS), or electrospray ionization (ESI) MS/MS or as described by others [44,45]. Protein identification is based on searching the resulting peptide fragmentation spectra against genomic and expressed sequence tag (EST) databases using either the automated SEQUEST program or proprietary algorithms. Thus protein identification has moved from the traditional laboratory N-terminal sequencing method to a highly dynamic fast MS–based method that correlates MS data of peptides with the information contained in sequence databases [46].

As pointed out by Haynes et al. [46], "there are a number of alternative approaches to proteome analysis currently under development. There is a considerable interest in developing a proteome analysis strategy, which bypasses 2-DE altogether, because it is a relative slow and tedious process, and because of perceived difficulties in extracting proteins from the gel matrix for analysis. However, 2-DE as a starting point for proteome analysis has many advantages compared to other techniques available today. The most significant strengths of the 2-DE-MS approach include the relatively uniform behavior of proteins in gels, the ability to quantify spots and the high resolution and simultaneous display of hundreds to thousands of proteins within a reasonable time frame." In addition, a comparative analysis carried out with digitized PEMs, described above, enables us to compare hundreds of samples/PEMs obtained from "normal" and "disease" samples each containing thousands of proteins. In concurrence with a statistical analysis of the fold changes for each protein, a disease specific protein marker can be selected out of several hundred thousand proteins queried.

One recently described alternative 2-DE independent approach for a comparative global proteome analysis [47] is based on a new isotope-coded affinity tags (ICAT) method combined with direct MS/MS analysis. The approach relies on an isotopically coded linker coupled to an affinity tag specific for sulfhydryl groups in the side chains of cysteinyl residues in the reduced protein sample. Two versions of ICAT, an isotopically light and a heavy form, are used to label protein mixtures from state A and state B of the sample. The samples are mixed and digested for direct MS analysis as described above. Relative signal intensities for identical peptide sequences can be quantified by being traced back to the original sample based on the respective ICAT. This allows for simultaneous identification and quantification of components of protein mixtures in a single, automated operation from a fairly limited amount of sample such as LCM (see below).

F. Cellular Proteomics

To understand the molecular basis of a disease as the difference between normal and diseased tissues and organs, it is necessary to interpret the complex interactions between many different cell types at the protein level. In addition, it may be necessary to isolate and characterize abnormal cells within or adjacent to unaffected areas of the diseased tissue or organ. A recently developed technology called laser capture microdissection (LCM) [48] has made this difficult task achievable with a minimal effect on the gene and protein expression profile present in vivo. LCM allows for a precise identification and isolation of specific cells and their application to RT-PCR [48], cDNA microarray [49], enzyme activity [48], and proteomic analysis [50]. Cells in frozen tissue slices are first identified through a conventional staining method of choice, before they are selected through a microscope. A solid-state near-infrared laser beam is then focused on the target cells, causing their selective adhesion to a transfer film. The film is lifted away from the surrounding tissue and placed directly into DNA, RNA, enzyme assay, or protein lysis buffer. Since Emmert-Buck et al. published their original findings in 1996, LCM has become routine for the identification of tumor-specific mRNA/gene expression analysis in a variety of cancers. The technology progressed in the meantime from applications in conjunction with cDNA microarrays to profile gene expression of adjacent neuronal subtypes [49]. At the same time, Banks et al. [50] described the first proteomic analysis of LCM-purified normal and malignant human cervix and renal cortical tissues. These technological advances provide us with an opportunity to map out complex interaction of many cell types throughout human anatomy in both the normal and diseased states at an unprecedented level of complexity and detail. In oncology research, such valuable information can give an understanding of the alterations taking place in the cells surrounding the diseased tissue, such as stromal and endothelial cells, as well as the cancer cell itself. These additional insights provide us with an opportunity to broaden our therapeutic approaches as illustrated by novel cancer therapeutics targeted against tumors and/or surrounding activated vascular endothelial cells [51,52]. But more importantly for the purpose of this review, we can now assess how closely our chosen animal models mimic the in vivo situation in the patient. For example, in tumor angiogenesis and metastases, researchers are faced with the dilemma that xenograft tumors (human tumors implanted underneath the skin of mice with faulty immune systems) don't behave like naturally occurring tumors in humans [51,53], as will be discussed further in Section II.C. In such a case, a proteomic comparison of LCM-purified stromal and endothelial cells from a human biopsy and the mouse model may be revealing and identify critical differences in the two protein expression profiles that may be linked to the deficiencies of the animal model.

G. Proteomic Analysis of Body Fluids

Body fluids represent a central link between various body compartments to exchange metabolic "fuels" and dispose of metabolic waste products and toxins. The complex mixtures of proteins present in systemic fluids such as serum or plasma are secreted from many organs, such as liver, pancreas, lung, and kidney, and are central to energetic drug metabolism and catabolism and homeostasis. For example, many steroids and peptide growth factor–binding proteins constantly present in the serum are responsible for a tight regulation of these potent circulating cell regulatory molecules. Many alterations in the physiological or disease states of an animal or human change the levels of the proteins in body fluids. Information about the magnitude of the change of identified proteins and clusters thereof may be of diagnostic, prognostic, or therapeutic significance. Proteomics body fluid analyses have been carried out for plasma, serum, cerebrospinal fluid

(CSF), urine [54], joint fluid [55], tears [56], pancreatic fluid [57,58], amniotic fluid [59], ascitic fluid [60], pleural fluid [61], cyst fluid [62], sweat [63], milk [64], and seminal fluid [65].

The objectives of these studies were to discover and characterize disease-specific proteins in body fluids by building databases of high-resolution PEMs from the relevant body fluids obtained from individuals. Interrogation of these databases may reveal proteins whose expression is significantly increased in a disease-related manner for subsequent molecular characterization. Routine application of this approach for a rapid and reliable identification of disease-specific protein markers had been severely limited by the interference by high-abundance proteins such as albumin, haptoglobin, IgG, and transferrin. For example, without removal of these high-abundance proteins, no more than 300–500 individual features can be separated in CSF (see Figs. 6A and 6B). OGS has refined the use of proteomics for these type of analyses through immunoaffinity-based depletion methods in which these four highly abundant proteins are removed from the sample to be analyzed. After such an enrichment, many additional features previously masked by the high-abundance proteins become visible (see Figs. 6C and 6D). Now up to approximately 1500 features of a CSF sample can be separated through 2-DE. As with analysis of cell extracts (Fig. 5), zoom gels may used to further enhance the resolution and sensitivity of the separation. This approach can be extended to all known body fluids and the removal of any known interfering high-abundance proteins prior to a proteomic analysis. PEMs obtained from human biofluids may serve as a reference point for the selection of the appropriate animal model. A comparison of body fluid PEMs between randomly mutagenized mice and human disease samples may establish a link between the disease and a single genetic abnormality.

H. Analyses of Protein Complexes

Once a putative therapeutic target protein has been identified, the need to assign a biological function and establish the relevant pathway for such a protein drives our attempts for cataloging binding partners. As discussed in Section I.C, changes in cellular location and protein binding partners in response to stimuli-driven PTMs may suggest protein function. For example, proteomic mapping of purified protein complexes has lead to the discovery of novel signal proteins such as FLICE [66], IKK [67], and components of the spliceosome complex [68]. For this purpose, the cell lysate is enriched for protein partners of the protein complex either with a tagged version of the protein such as FLAG [69] or GST [70] or through well-established immunoaffinity-based technologies. Again it is 2-DE that will assist a reliable and quick identification of those proteins or isoforms thereof that are changed within the complex in the disease only, guiding the investigator toward the disturbances in a given pathway pertinent to the disease. In the case of the Ras

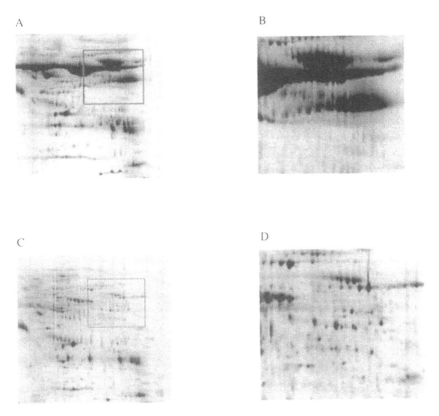

Figure 6   (A) PEM of human CSF without removal of high-abundance proteins. (B) Expanded region of the PEM highlighted in the box in the PEM in Figure A. (C) PEM of human CSF with removal of high-abundance proteins. (D) Expanded region of the PEM highlighted in the box in the PEM in Figure A. (From Ref. 105.)

pathway, multiple alterations cause uncontrolled proliferation and the loss of the ability to carry out programmed cell death (apoptosis), thereby promoting carcinogenesis (Fig. 2). The proto-oncogene Raf kinase prevents apoptosis by phosphorylation-dependent activation of the Bcl-2 protein (Fig. 2), a mechanism down-regulated by the anticancer agent taxol in ovarian cancer [71]. The exact mechanism by which Bcl-2 and $BclX_L$ (a related protein) prevent cell death is not known. However, it has been suggested recently that alterations in the mitochondrial membrane permeability through a Bcl-2/$Bclx_L$ Bnip3L (Bcl-2-interacting protein3-like) protein heterocomplex may be a prerequisite for apoptotic cell death [72]. In a classic proteomic mapping exercise summarized in Figure 7, Gygi

Discovery & Identification of
Bcl-x$_L$ - associated proteins

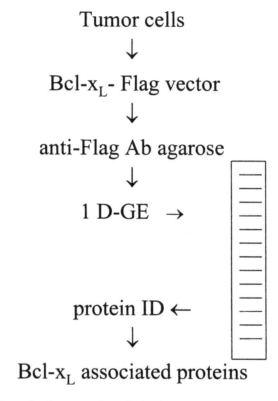

Tumor cells
↓
Bcl-x$_L$- Flag vector
↓
anti-Flag Ab agarose
↓
1 D-GE →

protein ID ←
↓
Bcl-x$_L$ associated proteins

Figure 7 Example of a proteomic analysis of protein complexes as described previously [1].

et al. [1] were able to identify 23 BclX$_L$ associated proteins, many of which have already a proven association with apoptosis (see figure 7).

One can imagine how this process can be continued iteratively until an end point for a particular pathway has been reached or sufficient novel putative targets have been selected. The throughput of this technique may be further accelerated in some instances by applying technologies such as ICAT-MS/MS analysis decribed above and further improvements in MS now facilitate characterization of even complex mixtures of proteins [47].

I. Combined mRNA/Protein Expression Analysis for Pathway Mapping and Candidate Target Selection

Although mRNA expression analysis may have no direct utility in the analysis of protein complexes, combined with proteomics it may yield useful information for additional target validation experiments. Effective integration of nucleic acid- and protein-based technologies may accelerate the selection of the best candidate target. Whereas the target discovery process described above is largely protein driven, knockout technologies and overexpression strategies rely on molecular biology. In a case where a protein is down-regulated in the disease, one can envision the use of inducible gene expression vectors as a quick means to restore protein expression and normal cell function, i.e., reintroduction of a tumor suppressor such as p53. More commonly, an overexpressed disease-specific protein becomes the target for a therapeutic inhibitor strategy. If access to preexisting small-molecule inhibitors are not available or cannot be generated easily, the gene can be readily ablated through antisense strategy. An antisense oligonucleotide can be synthesized or an antisense cDNA can be expressed in the cell in an inducible gene expression vector. In some cases, ribozyme constructs (small DNA fragments with intrinsic endonuclease activity that binds the target mRNA through a small DNA sequence complementary to a coding region in the target mRNA) are more useful. However, the effectiveness of these strategies is again monitored most accurately at the protein level. In particular, for the antisense strategy it is important to determine that the antisense selective blocks the expression of the target protein only and doesn't result in nonspecific effects on protein expression. In the case of cell surface protein targets, quickly advancing phage display technologies now promise functional inhibitory antibodies within months. With these tools one can now establish if interfering at different levels in the pathway will affect the protein expression profile differently and which resembles the protein expression profile of the normal state most closely. This approach is facilitated by the fact that in most cases whole clusters of proteins rather than a single protein will be changed. By using new bioinformatics tools, clusters of proteins can be used in a specific protein expression map to describe a phenotype, thus increasing the predictive value of the analysis.

II. IN VIVO VALIDATION OF MOLECULAR TARGETS

As we enter a new millennium, rapid advances in molecular medicine may provide us with a molecular fingerprint of the patient and disease phenotype that could represent the molecular and genetic bases for a preclinical animal model to evaluate novel candidate therapeutic targets. Preclinical evaluation of candidate targets requires complex animal models that will represent as many of the aspects of the drug discovery process as possible in order to identify the successful therapy. At the stage where small-molecule inhibitor leads have been identified, the relevance of the disease model becomes even more important to investigate mode of action, efficacy, and safety of these leads. To illustrate this, we will continue to use examples of oncology and central nervous system (CNS) research with particular emphasis on Alzheimer's disease.

A. Disease Model Relevance

The assessment of lead compounds in the most suitable animal model is of great importance because many agents that looked highly promising in vitro or in animal models fail because of insurmountable toxicity problems or lack of efficacy in humans. Knockout and transgenic technologies have made the creation of mouse models of genetic disorders almost routine. As we will discuss below, specific gene mutations and conditional knockouts are now achievable in a tissue- and/or time-dependent manner. An analysis of the complexity of most human disease necessitates a global comparison of the protein phenotype, well suited to a gene-related proteomic analysis (see Section II.E).

B. Animal Models of Alzheimer's Disease

Alzheimer's disease (AD) is a progressive neurodegenerative disorder that first presents clinically with memory impairment followed by continuous deterioration of cognitive function. The pathology is characterized by the presence of neurofibrillary tangles (NFTs) within critical neurons and neuritic plaques causing synaptic and neuronal death. NFTs are largely composed of hyperphosphorylated tau, a structural microtubule-associated protein. The plaques contain deposits of the amyloid-β protein (Aβ), a cleavage product of the β-amyloid precursor protein (APP). Of the two isoforms of Aβ present in brain tissue and CSF, Aβ_{42} aggregates more readily into plaques than Aβ_{40} [73,74]. In fact, the APP gene was the first gene identified causing familial Alzheimer's disease (FAD). Mutations in APP affect its cleavage and the generation of Aβ (for review, see [75]). In addition, mutations in the presenilin genes *PS1* and *PS2* are also observed in FAD and patients with *PS1* mutations display increased Aβ_{42} deposition as well [76,77]. The formation of amyloid plaques has been recognized as an early, necessary step in the pathogenesis of Alzheimer's disease [75]. Many transgenic mice have been used to model the biochemical and neuropathological effects of the known genes implicated in FAD. Animals overproducing human FAD APP in neurons produce AD-like amyloid deposition [78,79] with a morphology and regional distribution similar to that of humans [80]. While some of these transgenic mice strains show increased Aβ levels, amyloid, and correlative memory deficits [81], NFTs or severe neuronal death were not observed in any of these models [80]. In addition, in some models cognitive impairments appear prior to plaque formation [82]. Synaptic alterations in these mice have not yet been identified. It appears likely that sporadic forms of AD as well as FAD, as modeled by FAD mutants, originate from multiple causes. As a result, the complex phentotypic changes in many interacting cell types in critical areas of the brain must be evaluated comprehensively. This analysis should be carried out through a global analysis of the biological effector molecules, i.e., the protein expression of normal and diseased CSF and CNS tissue. This may be achieved through a systematic correlation of each gene mutation to complex changes in protein expression pattern through applications such as gene-related functional proteomics (Section II.E) supported by pharmacoproteomics (Section II.F) in transgenic animal models and human tissue with clinical aspects of the phenotype.

C. Animal Models of Cancer

An increasing number of studies in the analysis of signal transduction pathway of human cancers reveal that many regulatory proteins generate stimulatory and inhibitory signals at the same time. For example, in early stages of cancer, transforming growth factor β (TGF-β) can inhibit cancer growth via induction p21 (Fig. 3). However, in cancer cells where the Ras signal cascade is activated (Fig. 2), TGF-β promotes invasiveness and tumor metastases [52]. Attempts to study cancer in an in vivo model such as the human xenograft are further complicated by the fact human tumor–derived factors may interact differently with mouse host than human host machinery. For example, cancer-associated fibroblasts (CAFs) now have a recognized role in tumorigenesis of transformed epithelial cells [52,83]. While this opens exciting new avenues for therapeutic intervention, it also points to further difficulties for the reliable use of human xenograft models in rodents. This might explain why some metastatic human tumors do not spread to other tissues in mice [51]. In fact, the National Cancer Institute (NCI) has encountered serious challenges in their efforts to establish a meaningful screening system for candidate anticancer drugs. For example, the human xenograft models employed for the NCI in vivo screen show very limited predictive information for the clinical setting. When the NCI tested 12 anticancer agents used in patients against xenograft models, more than 60% of the tumors did not show a response [53]. In other cases, tumors showed opposite behaviors in vitro and in vivo. Tumors with a deletion in the p21 gene (Fig. 3) respond to radiation therapy in vivo, whereas the same tumor is equally resistant to radiation in an in vitro clonogenic assay [84]. In addition to similar findings in other models, this suggests that efficacy of currently available chemotherapy may be linked to genetic mutations such as those associated with checkpoint or cell cycle–related genes [85]. This has lead many investigators to a molecular characterization of new targets and away from classical drug screening efforts in models with poor predictability. A comprehensive summary of animal models of cancer was recently reviewed [86].

D. Knockout and Mutagenesis Models, and Tissue-Specific Inducible Gene In Vivo Models

The examples discussed in Section II.A and II.B signify the importance of gene targeting technologies in mouse models of human disease (for review, see [87–90]). Recent advances in creating conditional and tissue-specific knockouts enable us to study the disease in a more relevant temporal and organ-specific context. For example, until recently it was not possible to study the *BRAC1* gene responsible for about 50% of heredity breast cancer in animal models, since homozygous Brca 1 null mice would die early in embryogenesis. Conditional knockouts were generated with the Cre-loxP approach (for review, see [91,92]) in mice expressing Cre recombinase with a mammary epithelial cell–specific promoter allowed for an analysis of a selective inactivation of the *BRCA1* gene in mammary glands [93]. These mice develop mammary tumours and have abnormally developed mammary glands that would form the basis of a better understanding of *BRCA1* in tumorigenesis. Similar advances have been made for CNS models using the tetracyline-regulated system. Vectors have been reengineered for CNS-specific gene expression and led to the development of an inducible gene expression system specific to several brain regions including the CA1 region of the hippocampus, cerebellum, and striatum [94]. It is now conceivable that in the near future tedious gene knockout technology may be replaced by new tissue-specific gene-targeting systems that use rapid retroviral vectors in genetically engineered mice expressing the receptor for the retrovirus in a particular organ or tissue [95]. These approaches or a combination thereof may be particular useful in conjunction with proteomics. For example, the viral receptor responsible for organ-selective infection by the retrovirus could also provide the molecular basis for immunobased cell purification procedure or a fluorescent tag to be recognized during LCM/proteomics. Such systems allow for a rapid and reproducible expression of many single genes or a combination thereof as well as selective purification of those cells only for a detailed molecular characterization of the disease at the protein level.

E. Gene-Related Functional Proteomics

The definition of the phenotype of an organism was recently given as "the integral of fulfilled gene functions and environmental effects" wherein "the protein of a gene offers all the molecular structures and properties needed to fulfill the functions of a gene" [96]. Considering that any phenotype may be the result of more than one gene, it is important to determine the extent by which each gene contributes to the phenotype in order to determine the function of a particular gene. New approaches in gene-related functional proteomics (reviewed in [96]) may allow us to gain new insights into the relationship between the genotype of an organism and the phenotype of its proteins. A disease such as AD defined by its clinical symptoms may be described by the phenotype at the morphological, physiological, biochemical, and molecular level and enable us to subdivide a disease into mechanistic subclasses of individual steps in the pathogenesis according to the proteins affected. This could facilitate the evaluation of many putative therapeutic targets specific to different aspects/pathways/stages of the disease.

In order to evaluate the role of a single gene product/protein in a disease, we need to consider existing protein polymorphisms, such as PTM-specific isoforms. Some of the origins of these protein polymorphisms may be revealed by mouse genetics. Tracing the origin of PTM variant protein through genetic techniques in animal models can lead to the definition of a protein's origins at the genetic level as discussed above for body fluid analysis. Furthermore, a 2-DE comparison of 10,000 protein features obtained from the brains of various genetically distant mouse strains revealed variations in more than 1000 protein features. Identification of the subset of protein isoforms unique to a particular mouse strain correlated with genetic linkage studies and gene mapping may reveal some of the responsible relevant genes [96]. For example, the tau polymorphism results in more than 100 protein spots in a 2-DE gel of human brain proteins caused by various levels of phosphorylation and multiple splice variants [97].

In addition, 2-DE may identify PTM variants originating from gene mutations causing amino acid substitutions in flavin adenine dinucleotide from various mutations in APP, PS1, or PS2, all causing increased cerebral production and deposition of Aβ peptide in amyloid plaques (reviewed in [98]). A protein polymorphism characterized at the molecular and genetic level will reveal more detailed information about its origins and significance in the diseased tissue. Studies of its relevance in normal tissues and other organs not affected by the disease or its occurrence at a particular age of the animal can be compared between the animal model and that observed in the patient. Contrary to the above example, where multiple proteins result in the same phenotype (e.g., increased amyloid deposition), a single protein affects the phenotype of several other proteins simultaneously and a similar analysis can be applied.

In conclusion, it is important to define the origins of a detected protein polymorphism at the molecular and genetic level in particular for any multifactorial disease. A phenotypic analysis originating at the protein level rather than the gene level seems more likely to identify the primary defective protein linked to the disease as well as other proteins affected by the defective proteins. At this stage it is appropriate to identify the gene linked directly to the defective proteins.

F. Pharmacoproteomics

The application of preclinical drug development may be summarized as one aspect of pharmacoproteomics. Within preclinical development, proteomics can be used beyond the evaluation of a model and confirm modes of action of candidate drugs, once the appropriate model has been selected. For the majority of cancers, diagnostic, prognostic, or therapeutic proteins identified in serum may have great potential, since blood samples are readily available for proteomic analysis. In the CNS, the CSF bathes the brain almost completely. Therefore, it seems likely to contain many important secreted proteins and neuropeptides mediating interaction of different cell populations and reveal insights in disease-related changes when CSF from patients with neurodegenerative disease is compared with that of normal patients. Protein expression changes within these body fluids underlying specific disease states can be compared with the animal model counterparts. The degree of similarity may guide the investigator to the most relevant model available for the in vivo evaluation of candidate drugs.

At this stage in development, proteomics can be applied to identify serum protein markers associated with overt toxicity and efficacy or lack thereof. Such markers may be predictive of toxicity in a particular organ or indicative of efficacious therapy. This approach offers greater sensitivity than conventional toxicology and enables candidate drugs to be screened for toxicity at the earliest possible stage of development. Thus, pharmacoproteomics may allow us to refine a multifactorial disease into subcategories more suitable for a particular therapy or less likely to bring about undesirable side effects. These findings maybe applied during clinical development to enhance the successful selection of lead candidates for clinical trials (Fig. 8).

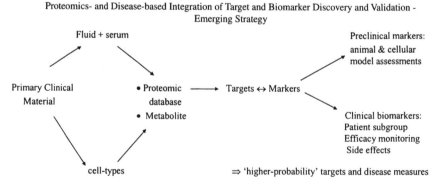

Figure 8 Emerging strategy for proteomic applications drug discovery.

III. PROTEOMIC TECHNOLOGY IN THE MOLECULAR CHARACTERIZATION OF NOVEL THERAPEUTIC TARGETS: FUTURE PERSPECTIVES

Most human disease, as defined in clinical pathology, should be regarded as multifactorial, and its complexity must be understood at the molecular level. It has been recognized that all complex diseases, such as cancer, must be characterized in terms of the host organism [99]. Disease models will continue to play a significant role in modern drug discovery. Rapid genomic and proteomic discovery technologies reveal great insight into the disease phenotype at the gene and protein level. This increasing knowledge can be applied to a more mechanistically based and target-driven discovery process. In preclinical development, more emphasis will be based on a refined molecular characterization of the target rather than classical efficacy assessments in animal models. Proteins represent the main biological effector molecules of any given cell and appear most suitable for the target evaluation process. Classical proteomic approaches offer the unique opportunity to identify disease-specific changes in protein expression profile in a complex system comprising up to 10,000 proteins. This strategy will generate an increasing number of disease-specific protein markers that can be utilized for the evaluation of preclinical models.

The following important questions can now be addressed:

1. Does cluster analysis of multiple protein changes reveal similar changes between normal and disease in humans and in the selected model?
2. Are these changes reversed in the validation studies with candidate target protein inhibitors?
3. Are these changes unique to a particular step in the pathway in a cell type–specific manner indicative of selectivity/specificity?
4. Do small-molecule inhibitors modulate protein expression profiles of human disease and correlate with those observed in the validation studies?
5. Do clinical lead compounds affect the same cluster of proteins in the animal model as in samples obtained in clinical studies from humans?

Interfaces with other technologies, such as protein chip arrays [100], will quickly expand to a more versatile platform with the ability to evaluate biological systems of great complexity at great speed. An integrated proteomics tool can assign up to several hundred disease-specific proteins in body fluids and purified authentic tissues with statistical confidence. This information becomes valuable in a comparative analysis between the preclinical model and the clinical situation, which can feed back into a refined experimental design (see Fig. 8). Rapid advances in genetically engineered animal models should enable researchers to tailor design models in such a way that complex gene–protein interactions can be studied in a temporal and spatial context reflective of the clinical situation and with easy access to proteomic analysis.

ACKNOWLEDGMENTS

I thank Jim Bruce and Robin Philp for the images of human CSF and Huh7 zoom gels and Dr. Robert Burns and Dr. Raj Parekh for their helpful comments on the manuscript.

REFERENCES

1. Gygi SP, Han DKM, Gingras AC, Sonnenberg N, Aebersold R. Protein analysis by mass spectrometry and sequence database searching: tools for cancer research in the post-genomic era. Electrophoresis 1999;20:310–319.
2. Wasinger VC Cordwell SJ, Cerpa-Poljak A, Yan JX, Gooley AA, Wilkins MR, Duncan MW, Harris R, Williams KL, Humphery-Smith I. Progress with gene-product mapping of the Mollicutes: *Mycoplasma genitalium.* Electrophoresis 1995;16: 1090–1099.
3. Goodfellow P. A celebration and a farewell. Nature Genet 1997;16:209–210.
4. Dawson, E. New collaborations make pharmacogenomics a SNP. Molecular Medicine 1999;5:280.
5. Sidransky D. Nucleic acid-based methods for the detection of cancer. Science 1997;278:1054–1058.
6. Gygi SP, Rochon Y, Franza BR, Aebersold R. Correlation between protein and mRNA abundance in yeast. 1999; Mol Cell Biol 3:1720–1730.
7. Parekh RP, Lyall A. Proteomic as an emerging technology in pharmaceutical R&D. J Commercial Biotechnol (in press).
8. Zong Q, Schummer M, Hood L, Morris DR. Messenger RNA translation state: the second dimension of high-throughput expression screening. Proc Natl Acad Sci USA 1999;96:10632–10636.
9. Hunter, T.: Oncoprotein networks. Cell 1997;88:333–346.
10. Hakomori S. Tumor malignancy defined by aberrant glycosylation and sphingo-(glyco)lipid metabolism. Cancer Res 1996;56:5309–5318.
11. Sayed-Ahmed N, Besbas N, Mundy J, Muchaneta-Kubara E, Cope G, Pearson C, el Nahas M. Upregulation of epidermal growth factor and its receptor in the kidneys of rats with streptozotocin-induced diabetes. Exp Nephrol 1996;4:330–339.
12. Hasselgreen PO, Fischer JE. The ubiquitin-proteasome pathway: review of a novel intracellular mechanism of muscle protein breakdown during sepsis and other catabolic conditions. Ann Surg 1997;225:307–316.
13. Beaulieu M, Brakier-Gingras L, Bouvier M. Upregulation of alpha1A- and alpha1B-adrenergic receptor mRNAs in the heart of cardiomyopathic hamsters. J Mol Cell Cardiol 1997;29:111–119.
14. Makino I, Shibata K, Ohgami Y, Fujiwara M, Furukawa T. Transient upregulation of

the AT2 receptor mRNA level after global ischemia in the rat brain. Neuropeptides 1996;30:596–601.

15. Yao GL, Kato H, Khalil M, Kiryu S, Kiyama H. Selective upregulation of cytokine receptor subchain and their intracellular signalling molecules after peripheral nerve injury. Eur J Neurosci 1997;9:1047–1054.

16. Mansour SJ, Matten WT, Hermann AS, Candia JM, Rong S, Fukasawa K, Vande Woude GF, Ahn NG. Transformation of mammalian cells by constitutively active MAP kinase kinase. Science 1994;265:966–970.

17. Woodburn JR, Barker AJ, Gibson KH, Ashton SE, Wakeling AE, Curry BJ, Scarlett L, Henthorn LR. ZD1839, an epidermal growth factor tyrosine kinase inhibitor selected for clinical development (abstr). Proceedings of the American Association for Cancer Research 1997;38:633.

18. Shak S. Overview of the trastuzumab (Herceptin) anti-HER2 monoclonal antibody clinical program in HER2-overexpressing metastatic breast cancer. Herceptin Multinational Investigator Study Group. Semin Oncol Aug 26, 1999; 4 Suppl 12:71–77.

19. Gibbs JB, Oliff A. The potential of farnesyltransferase inhibitors as cancer chemotherapeutics. Annu Rev Pharmacol Toxicol 1997;37:143–66.

20. Monia BP, Johnston JF, Geiger T, Muller M, Fabbro D. Antitumor activity of a phosphorothioate antisense oligodeoxynucleotide targeted against C-raf kinase. Nature Med 1996;2:668–675.

21. Glazer RI. Protein Kinase C as a target for cancer therapy. Antisense Nucl Acid Drug Dev 1997;7:235–238.

22. Sebolt-Leopold JS, Dudley DT, Herrera R, Van Becelaere K, Wiland A, Gowan RC, Tecle H, Barret S.D, Bridges A, Przybranowski S, Leopold WR, Saltiel AR. Blockade of the MAP kinase pathway suppresses growth of colon tumors in vivo. Nature Med 1999;7:810–816.

23. Duesberry NS, Webb CP, Vande Woude GF. MEK wars, a new front in the battle against cancer. Nature Med 1999;7:736–737.

24. Alessandrini A, Namura S, Moskowitz MA, Bonventre JV. MEK1 protein kinase inhibition protects against damage resulting from focal cerebral ischemia. Proc Natl Acad Sci USA 1999;96:12866–12869.

25. Milczarek GJ, Martinez J, Bowden GT. p53 Phosphorylation: biochemical and functional consequences. Life Sci 1997;60:1–11.

26. Shaw P, Freeman J, Bovey R, Iggo R. Regulation of specific DNA binding by p53: evidence for a role for O-glycosylation and charged residues at the carboxy-terminus. Oncogene 1996;12:921–930.

27. Maki CG. Oligomerization is required for p53 to be efficiently ubiquinated by MDM2. Biol Chem 1999;275:16531–16535.

28. Lukas J, Sørensen CS, Lukas C, Santoni-Rugiu E, Bartek J. p16INK4a, but not constitutively active pRb, can impose a sustained G1 arrest: molecular mechanisms and implications for oncogenesis. Oncogene 1999;18:3930–3935.

29. Balint E, Bates S, Vousden KH. MDM2 binds p73α without targeting degradation. Oncogene 1999;18:3923–3930.

30. Robertson KD, Jones PA. Tissue specific alternative splicing in the human INK4a/ARF cell cycle regulatory locus. Oncogene 18:3810–3820.

31. Taniguchi K, Kohsaka H, Inoue N, Terada Y, Ito H, Hirokawa K, Miyasaka N. Induc-

tion of the p16INK4a senescence gene as a new therapeutic strategy for the treatment of rheumatoid arthritis. Nature Med 1999;7:760–767.

32. Kilpatrick GJ, Dautzenberg FM, Martin GR, Eglen RM. 7TM receptors: the splicing on the cake. Trends Pharmacol 1999;20:294–301.

33. Parekh R. Rohlff C. Post-translational modification of proteins and the discovery of new medicine. Curr Opin Biotechnol 1997;8:718–723.

34. Link A. 2-D Proteome Analysis Protocolls. Methods in Molecular Biology. Vol. 112. Totowa, NJ: Humana Press, 1999.

35. Page MP, Amess B, Townsend RR, Parekh R, Herath A, Brusten L, Zvelebil MJ, Stein RC, Waterfield MD, Davies SC, O'Hare MJ. Proc Natl Acad Sci USA 96:12589–12594.

36. Rosenfeld J, Capdevielle J, Guillemot JC, Ferrara P. In-gel digestion of proteins for internal sequence analysis after one- or two-dimensional gel electrophoresis. Anal Biochem 1992;203:173–179.

37. Shevchenko A, Wilm M, Vorm O, Mann M. Mass spectrometric sequencing of proteins silver-stained polyacrylamide gels. Anal Chem. 1996;68:850–858.

38. Aebersold RH, Leavitt J, Saavedra RA, Hood LE, Kent SBH. Internal amino acid sequence analysis of proteins separated by one- or two-dimensional gel electrophoresis after in situ protease digestion on nitrocellulose. Proc Natl Acad Sci USA 1987;84:6970–6974.

39. Hess D, Covey TC, Winz R, Brownsey RW, Aebersold R. Analytical and micropreparative peptide mapping by high performance liquid chromatography/electrospray mass spectrometry of proteins purified by gel electrophoresis. Protein Sci 1993;2:1342–1351.

40. Van Oostveen L, Ducret A, Aebersold R. Colloidal silver staining of electroblotted proteins for high sensitivity peptide mapping by liquid chromatography–electrospray ionization tandem mass spectrometry. Anal Biochem 1997;247:310–318.

41. Lui M, Tempst P, Erdjument-Bromage H. Methodical analysis of protein–nitrocellulose interactions to design a refined digestion protocol. Anal Biochem 1996;241:156–166.

42. Mann M, Wilm M. Error-tolerant identification of peptides in sequence databases by peptide sequence tags. Anal Chem 1994;66:4390–4399.

43. Courchesne PL, Patterson SD. Identification of proteins by matrix-assisted laser desorption/ionization mass spectrometry using peptide and fragment ion masses. Meth Mol Biol 1999;112:487–511.

44. Haynes P, Miller I, Aebersold R, Gemeiner M, Eberini I, Lovati RM, Manzoni C, Vignati M, Gianaza E. Proteins of rat serum: I. Establishing a reference two-dimensional electrophoresis map by immunodetection and microbore high performance liquid chromatography–electrospray mass spectrometry. Electrophoresis 1998;19:1484–1492.

45. Ducret A, Gu M, Haynes PA, Yates JRIII, Aebersold R. Simple design for a capillary liquid chromatography-microelectrospray-tandem mass spectrometric system for peptide mapping at the low femtomole sensitivity range (abstr). Proceedings of the ABRF'97 international symposium: Technique at the genome/proteome interface 1997;69.

46. Haynes PA, Gygi SP, Figeys D, Aebersold R. Proteome analysis: biological assay or data archive? Electrophoresis 1998;19:1862–1871.

47. Gyigi SP, Rist B, Gerber SA, Turecek F, Gelb MH, Aebersold R. Quantitative analysis of complex protein mixtures using isotope coded affinity tags. Nature Biotechnol 1999;10:994–999.

48. Emmert-Buck MR, Bonner RF. Smith PD, Chuaqui RF, Zhuang Z, Goldstein SR, Weiss RA, Liotta L. Laser capture microdissection. Science 1996;274:998–1001.

49. Luo L, Salunga RC, Guo H, Bittner A, Joy KC, Galindo JE, Xiao H, Rogers KE, Wan JS, Jackson MR, Erlander MG. Gene expression profiles of laser-captured adjacent neuronal subtypes. Nature Med 1999;5:117–122.

50. Banks RE, Dunn MJ, Forbes MA, Stanley A, Pappin D, Naven T, Gough M, Harnden P, Selby PJ. The potential use of laser capture microdissection to selectively obtain distinct population of cells for proteome analysis—preliminary findings. Electrophoresis 1999;20, 689–700.

51. Bibby MC. Making the most of rodent tumour systems in cancer drug discovery. B J Cancer 1999;79:1633–1640.

52. Elkeles A. Oren M. Cancer: molecular players and unifying principles. Mol Med 1999;5:334–335.

53. Gura, T. System for identifying new drugs are often faulty. Science 1997;278:1041–1042.

54. Sanchez JC, Hochstrasser, D. Preparation and solubilization of body fluids for 2-D. Meth Mol Biol 1999;112:87–93.

55. Argiles A. Amyloid deposit in hemodialysis patients: immunochemical analysis. Nephrologie 1987;8:51–54.

56. Janssen PT, Van Bijsterveld QP. Comparison of electrophoretic techniques for the analysis of human tear fluid pattern. Clin Chim Acta 1981;114:207.

57. Scheele GA. Two-dimensional gel analysis of soluble proteins. J Biol Chem 1975;250:5375–5385.

58. Cassara G, Gianazza E, Righetti PG, Poma S, Vicentini L, and Scortecci V. Isoelectric focusing studies on human pancreatic secretion. J Chromatogr 1980;221:279.

59. Jones MI., Spragg SP., and Webb T. Detection of proteins in human amniotic fluid using two-dimensional gel electrophoresis. Biol Neonate 1981;39:171–177.

60. Toussi A, Paquet N, Huber O, Frutiger S, Tissot JD, Hughes GJ, et al. Polypeptide marker and disease patterns found while mapping proteins in ascitis. J Chromatogr 1992;582:87–92.

61. Dermer GB. Enhancement techniques for detecting trace and fluid-specific components in two-dimensional electrophoresis patterns. Clin Chem 1982;28:881–887.

62. Brunet JF, Berger F, Gustin T, Laine M, Benabid HL. Characterisation of normal brain-reactive antibodies in glioma cyst fluids. J Neuroimmunol 1993;47:63–72.

63. Marshall T, Williams KM. Analysis of human sweat proteins by two-dimensional electrophoresis and ultrasensitive silver staining. Anal Biochem 1984;139:506–509.

64. Anderson NG, Powers MT, Tollaksen SL. Proteins of human Milk. Identification of major components. Clin Chem 1982;28:1045–1050.

65. Edwards JJ, Tollaksen SL, Anderson NG. Proteins of human semen. Two-dimensional mapping of human seminal fluid. Clin Chem 1981;27:1335–1340.

66. Muzio M, Chinnaiyan AM, Kischkel FC, O'Rourke K, Shevchenko A, Ni J, Scaffidi C, Bretz JD, Zhang M, Gentz R, Mann M, Krammer PH, Peter ME, Dixit VM. FLICE, a novel FADD-homologous ICE/CED-3-like protease, is recruited to the CD95 (Fas/APO-1) death–inducing signaling complex. Cell 1996;85(6):817–827.

67. Mercurio F, Zhu H, Murray BW, Shevchenko A, Bennett BL, Li J, Young DB, Barbosa M, Mann M, Manning A, Rao A. IKK-1 and IKK-2: cytokine-activated IkappaB kinases essential for NF-kappaB activation. Science 1997;278:860–866.

68. Neubauer G, Gottschalk A, Fabrizio P, Séraphin B, Lührmann R, Mann M. Identification of the proteins of the yeast U1 small nuclear ribonucleoprotein complex by mass spectrometry. Proc Natl Acad Sci USA 1997;94:385–390.

69. Chubet RG, Brizzard BL. Vectors for expression and secretion of FLAG epitope-tagged proteins in mammalian cells. Biotechniques 1996;1:136–141.

70. Hunter T, Hunter GJ. GST fusion protein expression vector for in-frame cloning and site-directed mutagenesis. Biotechniques 1998;2:194–196.

71. Blagosklonny M, Giannakakou P, El-Deiry WS, Kingston DGI, Higgs PI, Neckers L, Fojo T. Raf-1/Bcl-2 phosphorylation: a step from microtubule damage to cell death. Cancer Res 1997;57:130–155.

72. Imazu T, Shimizu S, Tagami S, Matsushima M, Nakamura Y, Miki T, Okuyama A, Tsujimoto Y. Bcl-2/E1B 19 kDa-interacting protein 3-like protein (Bnip3L) interacts with Bcl-2/Bcl-x_L and induces apoptosis by altering mitochondrial membrane permeability. Oncogene 1999;18:4523–4529.

73. Harper JD, Wong SS, Lieber CM Lansbury PT Jr. Observation of metastable ab amyloid protofibrils by atomic force microscopy. Chem Biol 1997;4:119–125.

74. Walsh DM, Lomakin A, Benedek GB, Condron MM, Teplow DB. Amyloid beta-protein fibrillogenesis. Detection of a protofibrillar intermediate. J Biol Chem 1997;272:22364–22374.

75. Selkoe, D.J. Translating cell biology into therapeutic advances in Alzheimer's disease. Nature 1999;399 (Suppl):A23–A31.

76. Lemere CA, Lopera F, Kosik KS, Lendon CL, Ossa J, Saido TC, Yamaguchi H, Ruiz A, Martinez A, Madrigal L, Hincapie L, Arango JC, Anthony DC, Koo EH, Goate AM, Selkoe DJ, Arango JC. The E280A presenilin 1 Alzheimer mutation profuces increased $A\beta_{42}$ deposition and severe cerebellar pathology. Nature Med 1996;2:1146–1148.

77. Mann DM, Iwatsubo T, Cairns NJ, Lantos PL, Nochlin D, Sumi SM, Bird TD, Poorkaj P, Hardy J, Hutton M, Prihar G, Crook, R, Rossor MN, Haltia M. Amyloid beta protein (A-beta) deposition in chromosome 14-linked Alzheimer's disease: predominance of A-beta (42(43)). Ann Neurol 1996;40:149–156.

78. Higgins LS, Cordell B. Genetically engineered animal models of Alzheimer's disease. Meth Enzymol 1996;10:384–391.

79. Duff K. Recent work on Alzheimer's disease transgenics. Curr Opin Biotechnol 1998;9:561–564.

80. Higgins LS. Animal models of Alzheimer's disease. Mol Med 1999;5:274–276.

81. Hsiao K, Chapman P, Nilsen S, Eckman C, Harigay Y, Younkin S, Yang F, Cole G. Correlative memory deficits, A elevation, and amyloid plaques in transgenic mice. Nature 1996;274:99–102.

82. Moran PM, Higgins LS, Cordell B, Moser PC. Age-related learning deficits in transgenic mice expressing the 751-amino acid isoform of human b-amyloid precursor protein. Proc Natl Acad Sci USA 1995;92:5341–5345.

83. Olumi AF, Dazin P, Tlsty TD. A novel coculture technique demonstrates that normal human prostatic fibroblasts contribute to tumor formation of LNCaP cells by retarding cell death. Cancer Res 1998;58:4525–30.

84. Wouters BG, Giaccia AJ, Denko NC, Brown JM. Loss of p21Waf1/Cip1 sensitizes tumors to radiation by an apoptosis-independent mechanism. Cancer Res 1997;57:4703–4706.

85. Waldman T, Zhang Y, Dillehay L, Yu J, Kinzler K, Vogelstein B, Williams J. Cell-cycle arrest versus cell death in cancer therapy. Nature Med 1997;9:1034–1036.

86. DePinho R, Jacks T (eds). Mouse models of cancer. Oncogene 1999, 18:Review Issue.

87. Yamamura K. Overview of transgenic and gene knockout mice. Prog Exp Tumor Res 1999;35:13–24.

88. Aguzzi A, Raeber AJ. Transgenic models of neurodegeneration. Neurodegeneration of (transgenic) mice and men. Brain Pathol 1998;8:695–697.

89. Sturchler-Pierrat C, Sommer B. Transgenic animals in Alzheimer's disease research. Rev Neurosci 1999;10:15–24.

90. Macleod KF, Jacks T. Insights into cancer from transgenic mouse models. J Pathol 1999;187:43–60.

91. Plück A. Conditional mutagenesis in mice: the Cre/loxP recombination system. Int J Exp Pathol 1996;77:269–278.

92. Stricklett PK, Nelson RD, Kohan DE The Cre/loxP system and gene targeting in the kidney. Am J Physiol May 27, 1999;276(Suppl):F651–657.

93. Xu X, Wagner KU, Larson D, Weaver Z, Li C, Ried T, Hennighausen L, Wynshaw-Boris A, Deng CX. Conditional mutation of Brca1 in mammary epithelial cells results in blunted ductal morphogenesis and tumor formation. Nature Genet 1999;22:37–43.

94. Chen J, Kelz MB, Zeng G, Sakai N, Steffen C, Shockett PE, Picciotto MR, Duman RS, Nestler EJ. Transgenic animals with inducible, targeted gene expression in brain. Mol Pharmacol 1998;54:495–503.

95. Federspiel MJ, Bates P, Young JAT, Varmus HE, Hughes SH. A system for tissue-specific gene targeting: transgenic mice susceptible to subgroup A avian leulosis virus-based retroviral vectors. Proc Natl Acad Sci USA 1994;91:11241–11245.

96. Klose J. Genotype to phenotype. Electrophoresis 1999;20:643–652.

97. Janke C, Holzer M, Goedert M, Arendt T. Distribution of isoforms of the microtubule-associated protein tau in grey and white matter areas of human brain: a two-dimensional gel electrophoretic analysis. FEBS Lett 1996;379:222–226.

98. Selkoe DJ. Alzheimer's disease: genotypes, phenotypes and treatments. Science 1996;275:630–631.

99. Lane D. The promise of molecular oncology. Lancet 1998;351(Suppl 2):17–20.

100. Senior K. Fingerprinting disease with protein chip arrays. Mol Med 1999;5: 326–327.

101. King RC, Stansfield WD. A Dictionary of Genetics. New York: Oxford University Press, 1990, p. 239.

102. Varmus H Weinberg RA. Genes and the biology of cancer. 1992 Scientific American Library, New York.

103. Rohlff C. Proteomics in molecular medicine: applications in central nervous system disorders. Electrophoresis 2000;21:1227–1234.

104. Nobori T, Miura K, Wu DJ, Lois A, Takabayashi K, Carson DA. Deletions of the cyclin-dependent kinase-4 inhibitor gene in multiple human cancers. Nature 1994; 368:753–756.

105. Rohlff C. Proteomics in neuropsychiatric disorders. Int J of Neuropsychopharmacology 2001;4:93–102.

9
High-Throughput Screening as a Discovery Resource

John P. Devlin
MicroSource Discovery Systems, Inc.
Gaylordsville, Connecticut

I. BACKGROUND

Over the past decade we have witnessed the most dramatic change in drug discovery since the launch of antibiotic research in the 1940s. High-throughput screening (HTS) evolved from a part-time, low-priority activity in the late 1980s to become the core of discovery operations in most pharmaceutical companies before the turn of the century. That development not only created unprecedented opportunities in the identification of new bioactive molecules; it also established a unique working relationship and dependence among different scientific and support disciplines that had never been achieved. Discovery became an integrated multidisciplinary activity.

Prior to 1990, new drug discovery was largely a departmental effort based on the contributions of innovative chemists and biologists. Biotechnology had made its entry but the impact on "small-molecule" discovery was, at best, vague. In most major companies, considerable emphasis was still based on analogue synthesis, with breakthroughs dependent on the serendipitous finding of novel activities in new structural classes devised by chemists or on the skilled observations of biologists in the recognition of unusual activities in conventional bioassays. The standard therapeutic targets, which encompassed the commercial gamut of therapeutic significance, were believed to be well represented in clearly defined pharmacological models and presumably supported by comprehensive structure–activity relationships (SAR) bases in medicinal chemistry. The situation was stagnant and breakthroughs became less common. The number of new-development compounds in a company's pipelines were dwindling and costs increasing. "Me-too" chemistry was also losing its appeal as markets became saturated and shares in those markets shrank to single digits. Management became concerned and reached out for new opportunities.

Concurrent with the above were the dramatic developments in genetic engineering and molecular biology, along with the emergence of economical access to biological reagents not previously imagined. The ability to explore specific macromolecular interaction in rapid biochemical and cellular screens became an economic reality. Targets and protein ligands were soon identified (e.g., the interleukins) that promised new forms of therapy and the hope of useful intervention with small molecules. Whole-animal or tissue models, which had been the mainstay of primary screening for decades, slowly disappeared from the discovery armamentarium and were replaced by biochemical and cellular assays that reflected mechanistic responses rather than whole-organism behavior. Screening became specific and economical.

With new biomolecular assays available and the ability to screen larger numbers of test compounds than the conventional pharmacological models, management turned to the chemist with the anticipation of satisfying the need for the compounds required as screening candidates. Here lay the first problem. Designing a synthesis program that would ultimately yield a new molecule that interferes at a biological target is an impossible task when there is no chemical precedence to guide the initial probes. "Rational" drug design had been touted as the answer, but despite two notable successes (e.g., cimetidine and captopril) it was clearly limited in application by strict demands of support data at the molecular and biological levels. The real answer was to resort to the almost "unscientific" task of screening all possible structural types in the new assay with the hope that some chemical lead (a "hit") would surface. It was the only solution, but corporate infrastructure was not prepared.

This "random screening" approach was not well received by industrial scientists who were accustomed to more aesthetic research activities. Nevertheless, it was reluctantly accepted as a part-time activity of a few biochemistry and pharmacology laboratories. With the absence of a central focus, budgets were small and progress was slow. Available instrumentation was based on a variety of liquid handlers redesigned from diagnostic applications. HTS robotics was in its infancy. Information systems were primarily developed in-house with the exception of established core software for data (e.g., Oracle) and chemical structure management (e.g., MDL's Chembase); again the market was not fully developed and incentives were few.

In 1990, assay throughput was at best 100 compounds per week, but that level was sufficient to handle the limited compound collections available. Compound archives most companies were large but highly focused and low in diversity. The organic chemist reluctantly took on a new responsibility in the discovery process: manual selection of a few thousand representatives from the corporate compound archives that would reflect the structural scope available. The many gaps in diversity in these small collections were filled by purchase of compounds from conventional chemical suppliers, occasionally by direct purchase from academic chemists worldwide and from the new breed of "compound brokers" that had emerged.

Reluctance to share experiences in early HTS development was also a problem. In 1992, The first conference dedicated to HTS technologies was held at SRI International (Menlo Park, CA) [1]. The purpose of that meeting was to bring together scientists involved or interested in HTS with the intention of stimulating dialogue in the implementation of this new technology and discussing common problems in organization, technical integration, data management, and personnel issues. Finding the audience for this event was difficult at that time because screening had no internal management focus and the individuals involved were distributed throughout the departmental structure of most companies. Nevertheless, 140 participants gathered to discuss screening challenges and solutions. Open discussion periods provided enough catalysis to stimulate dialogue and to make the conference a grand success. A byproduct of the conference was the launch of the first publication on screening technologies, *Screening Forum,* which provided information and technology reports on HTS topics [2].

So it began. HTS, now synonymous with "grunt work," was a part of the weekly schedule of R&D and accepted as such. Enthusiasm was initially low but, fortunately, a new breed of scientist emerged who recognized the challenge and the potential rewards of screening and was able to convince management of the immense potential if the technology were provided sufficient opportunity and resources. Such scientists were quick to take up the challenge of penetrating interdepartmental barriers and blending complex technologies, current instrumentation, and the available data management tools into functional and productive discovery machines. While instrumentation designed for HTS had yet to be developed, innovative adaptation of available instrumentation (e.g., from Beckman, Tecan, Packard, and Wallac) initially proved satisfactory. Notable was Tomtec's 96-well plate duplicator (Quadra) as an important asset at this early stage. The drive and foresight of these pioneers was the catalyst necessary to demonstrate the productivity of HTS and its importance as a discovery process.

As with any new technology, the standardization of tools became a critical matter. Fortunately, the 96-well microplate had already been proven in diagnostic applications and quickly became the standard screening vessel. Its origin can be traced to 1960 [3]; however, it wasn't until the mid-1970s when Ken Walls at the U.S. Centers for Disease Control and Prevention (CDC) started using it for enzyme-linked immunosorbent assay (ELISA) testing that it's benefit in automated assays became apparent. Robotic systems were developed to accommodate the microplate and integrated test systems established. It was a natural transition to apply these systems to the demands of the new and now lucrative market of screening.

Targets and assays were primarily developed in house since they represented the company's proprietary interests and technologies; however, novel and more sensitive detection systems evolved externally that provided useful tools in optimal protocol development. New microplate designs [4] were similarly created in the support industries that saved time and reagents in assay development and operation. Packaged data management systems evolved from companies such as Molecular Design (now MDL Information Systems) and Tripos, which formed the core of chemical structure management. The SD file became the standard file format for structure display and storage. Compound libraries could be created by purchase of small samples from a growing list of brokers who gleaned their collections from academic laboratories and "chemical factories" throughout the world. However, the cost of establishing the all-important structurally diverse, compound library was formidable and a serious bottleneck for startup companies.

In 1993, MicroSource Discovery Systems [5] pioneered the provision of test compounds in microplate format. This approach provided efficiency, economy, and diversity in a single product with full data support. It was based on the realization that even with a modest level of assay miniaturization, a few milligrams of a test compound were sufficient to support years of screening. Purchases of the standard 50 mg sample were unnecessary, and the cost of acquisition of large libraries was cut by as much 90%. Diversity was drawn from world leaders in chemical synthesis, and samples were provided in a format that avoided handling, documentation, and storage. Today MDSI has evolved into a leading provider of natural products and drug standards in microplate formats.

By 1994, HTS had become an integral part of the drug discovery process. Large companies reorganized their internal structure to accommodate the multidisciplinary character of this new technology. The hierarchical distinction between HTS and conventional "research" was resolved by the recognition of the distinct differences in the tools and goals of these activities and their equivalent and complementary contributions to the development of new drugs. Screening operations became centralized and new positions created. Topics such as assay miniaturization, integrated automation, compound acquisition, and data management became key activities in discovery operations. New companies sprang up that were based solely on new assay targets and the ability to screen efficiently. A myriad of support industries were also created to provide tools and resources that facilitated screening and improved return. Test compounds, automation systems, and even cloned target receptors [6] became available from outsource groups.

In 1994 the second forum on HTS technologies was held in Princeton, New Jersey. It was a sellout in attendance with almost 400 participants squeezed into a small conference space. The meeting was a tremendous success and launched HTS as a formidable tool in discovery. That conference also provided the seed for the beginning of the Society for Biomolecular Screening, which today is the foremost source of information on HTS technologies [7].

II. WHERE WE ARE

HTS, as applied in the pharmaceutical industry today, refers to the integrated technologies that permit the rapid evaluation of millions of compounds annually in scores of bioassays in search for new therapeutic agents. There are three objectives: *de novo* discovery, hit development, and the preliminary assessment of the metabolism and toxicity of lead candidates. The first two are widely applied and complementary; the last is new to HTS but is rapidly becoming an important facet of drug development.

De novo discovery addresses the search for compounds that interact with a new biochemical or cellular target for which there is no precedence in chemical structure. The identification of both ligands and antagonists for most orphan receptors is an excellent example of such applications. The discovery of drugs against diseases that cannot be satisfactorily treated with existing therapies or for which no treatment is available is another. *De novo* HTS requires the use of large compound collections with as broad a structural diversity as possible and bioassays that accentuate the specific character of each target. The goal is to find one or more "hits" that can provide a chemical focus for further screening. Such hits need not be at the activity level anticipated for a development candidate; structural information about a weak inhibitor is much better than no information at all. *De novo* HTS generally addresses a broad spectrum of targets.

Unlike *de novo* HTS, hit development begins with some level of chemical intuition. Such information may have been gleaned from *de novo* programs (see above), from historical data on the character of ligands or antagonists, or from computational analysis of the structure of the target receptor. This is the area where the use of high-throughput organic synthesis (HTOS) has provided the greatest benefit and has resulted in important advances in optimization of a lead and dramatic reduction in the time required for lead development. These benefits are discussed in greater detail below. Bioassays employed in developmental HTS focus on the overall activity profile anticipated for the test substance.

Preliminary assessment of the metabolism and toxicity of new drug candidates is a critical part of drug development. The requirements for such assessments are heavily regulated and, with the companion characteristics of absorption and distribution, constitute key elements in the success of any new drug application and its subsequent introduction. These processes are critically dependent on in vivo studies that are costly and time consuming. Failure of a compound in any of these aspects usually results in its removal from development; the investment made to that point is essentially lost. Recent developments in the miniaturization of metabolic and toxicological assessment procedures permit high-throughput assessment of lead candidates at a preselection stage. Such in vitro information has yet to be accepted by regulatory bodies; however, it does provide an important preview of the performance of a lead. The use of such data in the selection of candidates for development can significantly improve compound survival rates and shorten development time.

The primary components of any HTS program can be roughly divided into three areas: test substance supply, bioassay development and implementation, and informatics (data management). How these are organized is another dimension that segregates low from high, high from ultrahigh, and so on. The result is the same: discovery. Instrumentation and systems integration have become integral parts of all aspects of HTS and need not be addressed separately.

III. TEST SUBSTANCE SUPPLY

A structurally diverse test substance supply is the key to discovery. It is *the* critical resource i.e., the sole factor that determines the success level for every assay. Careful attention to the quality of the test substance resource is an essential aspect of HTS management. Essentially, a well-managed, structurally diverse test substance supply holds a company's equity in new drug discovery. This is true for any screening program, low and high capacity, in both small and large corporations.

A large variety of sources for test substances are available for HTS programs. Accessing any of these in a naïve "numbers-only" approach can be disastrous. Heavy dependence on commercially available combinatorial libraries is not advisable. Structural diversity alone dictates the number of test substances required. A small but carefully selected collection of 10,000 compounds may be a much better resource for discovery than a mass produced library with millions of components. Design and maintenance of an appropriate test substance resource is an important facet of corporate survival.

A. Compound Library Development

The demand for large and complex chemical libraries as test resources in HTS programs continues to grow to meet the dramatic increase in throughput potential of today's HTS systems. However, it is noteworthy that a small low-capacity screen can still yield important advances. This principle is manifested by the early screening successes in the potent PAF inhibitor WEB-2086 and the human immunodeficiency virus (HIV) reverse transcriptase inhibitor nevirapine. Both of these were discovered in libraries of less than 10,000 compounds without any indication of structural guides, certainly not "pharmacophores."

Despite the above comments, numbers are important if the compounds selected for inclusion in the corporate HTS pool have reasonable structural diversity; essentially, the higher the number of diverse test compounds, the better the chance of success. Today's million-compound libraries have simply improved the odds.

Compound collections that are truly diverse in skeletal and functional array are especially important in achieving a meaningful probe into the unknown three-dimensional space of a new receptor or enzyme. The classical approach in *de novo* discovery has been to draw on the structural riches of a well-designed and stocked compound collection that represents not only the scope of in-house synthesis but also the diversity available from external suppliers: direct chemical sources, brokers, and microplated compound libraries. The structural richness of the numerous pure natural products and their derivatives that are commercially available [5,11] must also be included since these displays cannot be mimicked by current HTOS.

Claims that high-throughput solid-phase and solution-phase chemical synthesis is a reliable source for the generation of limitless diversity are unfounded. This position is softened when such libraries are multitemplate based and constitute millions of representatives. Companies such as ArQule and Pharmacopeia offer such access but cost again becomes significant. The unquestioned strengths of these sources are in the rapid development of series with some chemical insight. This aspect is addressed below.

Compound management and acquisition has become an important facet of HTS structure and function. It requires a continuous awareness of what is in hand, what has been depleted, and what is necessary to enhance the chemical and topological character of the corporate collection. The responsibility lies not only in filling gaps in the functional parameters and their display within the collection but also in avoiding those substances that are inherently reactive with biological systems. Certain groups that are chemically reactive can give meaningless false positives that waste time and money and interrupt the discovery process. Acid chlorides, anhydrides, active esters, and the like are among these. Many halogenated compounds also fit into the category of nonspecific alkylating agents—α-haloketones, halomethyl aromatics, 2-halopyridines, and other reactive heterocycles—are common constituents in commercial collections. There are other groups that are cytotoxic and unwelcomed components; most organometallics, nitroso, and alkyl nitro and nitroso groups are among these. Hydrazines, hydrazides, and similar structures should not be removed entirely since these structural features have found their way into several important drugs; however, their ease of preparation makes them a more than necessary component in available collections. The same applies to aryl nitro representatives. Instability is another concern: *tert*-butyl esters, acetals, aminals, and enol ethers are some examples. Other groups that have been the subject of extensive analogue development (e.g., adamantane and perhaloalkanes) should also be carefully filtered. Redundancy is another problem. Analogue representation is necessary to efficiently represent a new compound class; however, excessive representation can become an unnecessary expense and distraction.

It is nevertheless important to be sensitive to the rigors of implementing some of these rules. Some published guidelines recommend the removal of compounds that are potential substrates for Michael addition, for example, α,β-unsaturated ketones. Such restriction is important if the group is especially activated, but that is frequently not the case—progesterone and a myriad of similar molecules are potential Michael addition candidates. Other restrictions, such as molecular size, number of rotatable bonds, and chemical functional density, are fine on paper but destructive if applied generically in library design. The end product can lead to a library that is pretty in presentations but sterile in discovery! These matters become serious concerns when the tailoring of the corporate compound collection is assigned to individuals insensitive to the potential of discovery in complex systems that violate one or more of the above guidelines. There is no substitute (yet) for the practiced eye of a medicinal chemist.

Software packages are available [8] that claim to provide assessments of diversity and recommendations for its enhancement. Very large libraries must depend on these or other computational techniques in such assessments, but caution must be exercised to the extent that such packages are used. The utility of many of these programs is strained when the assessment attempts to include complex molecular arrangements. Diversity assessment is especially important in small collections (about 10,000 compounds); however, it is best in these instances to resort to manual review.

B. HTOS Applications

HTOS (also termed combinatorial chemistry) has had a dramatic impact on both the organization and productivity of industrial medicinal chemistry. It was first applied in new drug discovery in the late 1980s in the form of combinatorial peptide coupling. Solid-phase synthesis of peptides, which had been developed by Bruce Merrifield (Rockefeller University) 20 years earlier, was used to create large polypeptides by affixing one end to a solid support (e.g., a resin bead) and adding the individual units sequentially by standard peptide coupling techniques. Subsequent chemical cleavage from the resin yielded the target polypeptide. The application of these techniques to the simultaneous synthesis of families of related peptides was pioneered by Mario Geysen (Glaxo) in the mid-1980s. The concept was further applied to new drug discovery in the synthesis of large libraries (20,000 to more than 1 million) of peptides fixed to beads or silicon chips and the assessment of the binding of these fixed libraries to labeled soluble targets (e.g., Selectide, Affymax, and others). Research managers were attracted to these systems by the remarkable numbers of test substances and the simplicity of the detection systems. Unfortunately, the impact of fixed supports in the binding of biomolecules and the limitations of peptides as structural leads in development were underrated. Soluble peptide libraries (e.g., Houghton Pharmaceuticals) were similarly offered as discovery tools, but again applications were limited and interest and corporate support waned.

Despite the shortcomings of large peptide libraries discussed above in *de novo* drug discovery, the use of peptide HTOS technologies in the identification of their direct roles in receptor responses *per se* or as surrogates for ligand definition in orphan receptor research brings forth a new and important role for these HTS approaches (see below).

The slump in the popularity of peptide-based HTOS in the early 1990s quickly turned around as the concept was applied to the synthesis of nonpeptide libraries using diverse synthetic techniques. Mike Pavia (then at Sphinx) was an important pioneer in the development of these technologies and their implementation in microplate format. His innovation and that of his associates facilitated the introduction and adaptation of HTOS into HTS applications and encouraged the automation/robotics industries to develop instrumentation that would meet the needs of industrial chemistry. It revived HTOS as a discovery technology with little apparent interruption, but once more the enthusiasm was unchecked and promises of satisfying the needs of discovery programs in structural diversity became unrealistic (see Fig. 2).

Early HTOS also launched support industries that could take a chemical lead or hunch and expand it into large libraries that encompass relevant structural diversity. Companies such as ArQule and Pharmacopeia offered efficient application of HTOS in the exploitation of solution- and solid-phase syntheses in the development of libraries that addressed specific client targets. These two successful corporations have, in their years of operation, amassed libraries including millions of components. Notwithstanding the above-mentioned limitations of HTOS in the generation of structural diversity, these massive libraries can offer a first-pass opportunity in discovery simply on the basis of the huge library populations and the diversity of the templates.

Reactions performed on solid supports have a number of process advantages over classical solution methods. The ability to drive reactions to completion with large excesses of reagents is one such advantage; the ease with which the product is cleaned at each step is another. The reaction kinetics is often found to be different between solid-phase and solution syntheses and is often favorable to the solid-phase approach. But there are shortcomings. Many reactions are impossible or at least exceedingly difficult to perform on solid phase due to the sensitivity of the linker or the resin itself. The inherent need to base such syntheses on common platforms also produces redundancy in the library generated. The common linkage site on each molecule further dampens structural diversity. Multiple platforms and nonfunctional linkage residues offer partial solutions to these problems. Nevertheless, today's HTOS compound libraries sorely need to be supplemented by selected products of classical synthesis and pure natural products to attain a meaningful three-dimensional, functional display for a *de novo* discovery program. This aspect is best illustrated by assessing how a hypothetical HTOS program would be designed if the goal were to *rediscover* (from scratch) representative nonplanar drugs, e.g., glucocorticoids, lipid-lowering agents (e.g., mevalonin), taxol, etc. Would today's solid-phase or even solution-phase synthesis collections achieve such a goal?

There are new directives in process that will provide some solutions to these problems. For example, the introduction of naturally derived, three-dimensional platforms can dramatically broaden the scope of HTOS. Variables will increase dramatically and thereby create another dimension in numbers as libraries of millions of compounds become commonplace. MicroBotanica [5] has identified proprietary natural templates as the cores of unique libraries and cheminformatics tools. These templates offer three-dimensional access not available to conventional laboratory-based synthons. ArQule, a leader in the progressive development of diverse and directed HTOS libraries, has made significant advances in improving the efficiency of HTOS in both solid- and solution-phase modes. Their home page [9] is worthy of a visit.

Simultaneously, HTOS was applied to bringing an HTS hit or otherwise identified bioactive entity to lead status and its rapid development into a clinical candidate. In most cases, HTOS has replaced the drudgery of "one-at-a-time" analogue synthesis in the generation of SAR data and dramatically reduced development time. Essentially, all possible analogues are prepared rather than a small population selected by medicinal chemistry on the basis of immediate relevance and economics. HTOS libraries provide the full SAR analysis with little reference to what would formerly be perceived as redundant. Such a "bulk" approach leads to a more definitive analysis of SAR and a better selection of candidates. This application is clearly the most important contributions that high-throughput technologies have made to medicinal chemistry and perhaps to drug discovery in general. Its impact is best appreciated in consideration of development time and on-market patent life (Fig. 1). Today an annual market return of $1 billion is not unusual for a new therapeutic entity. That translates into $83 million for every month that the new drug is on the market and under patent protection. The development time for a new drug can easily consume half of its patent life. HTOS can reduce development time and dramatically increase market returns.

Figure 1 illustrates the time line of drug development from discovery to introduction. It does not reflect the additional savings that HTOS provides in hit-to-lead generation. That aspect can provide an additional year of benefit in earlier recognition of the lead. While that generally does not impact patent life (a subsequent event), it does give the advantage of "first on the market" in a highly competitive

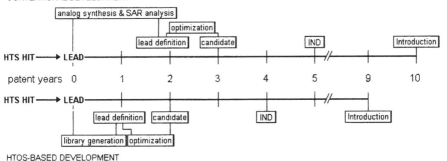

CONVENTIONAL DEVELOPMENT

HTOS-BASED DEVELOPMENT

Figure 1 Impact of HTOS on new drug development.

field. The illustration (Fig. 1) also does not take into consideration the emerging benefits of high-throughput ADME and toxicity profiling discussed below.

C. Natural Products as a Discovery Resource

The unique structural diversity inherent in natural products continues to be an important HTS resource. As with HTOS and other technologies, trends have had a disturbing influence on the adoption of natural products as a primary discovery resource (Fig. 2). Notable is the stability of microbials as a discovery resource, but

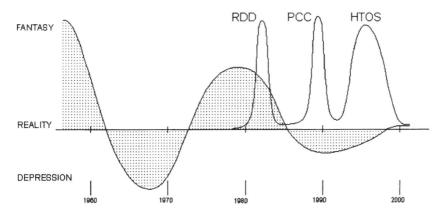

Figure 2 The rise and fall of technological hype in the use of plant natural products and sequential influence of early attempts in rational drug design (RDD), peptide combinatorial chemistry (PCC), and HTOS in HTS programs.

plants have had a sine-wave history and continue to be susceptible to technological pressures and prejudices.

Microbials are by far the most widely used natural resource in industrial screening programs. They have been mainstay in HTS applications in several major companies, with little fluctuation in their use over time. The reason is threefold: economics, reproducibility, and a continued history of new biomolecular discovery. Once a company has established and staffed a microbiological facility on site, costs are manageable and predictable.

The use of microorganisms over the past 60 years in antimicrobial research and development has established a sound technological basis for the culture, preservation, and manipulation of bacteria and fungi. Clear projections of scope and cost can be made for their use at the semi-microscale in discovery and the macroscale in commercial processes. Microbials are accountable for most of the antibiotics in therapeutic use today and, in addition, have served as biochemical factories for chemical modifications that cannot be reasonably achieved otherwise. In the past two decades, we have seen the successful use of microbials in broader pharmacological screening with remarkable success—ivermectin, FK-506, rapamycin, mevalonin, to name only a few. They can also provide unique chemical substrates for further manipulation in the chemist's laboratory and in this application constitute the basis for important semisynthetic variations in antibiotics and other products. The shortcomings of microbials are (1) the limited biochemical scope compared to plant resources and (2) the critical need for dereplication at an early stage in screening. Novelty in new structural types is less common in microbial screening.

Marine organisms offer a remarkable variety of chemical variation. Many such natural products are not available from other natural sources and certainly not through laboratory synthesis. Unfortunately, access to this resource is very expensive, limited to initial structural leads, and rarely amenable to commercial development. Even recollection for research purposes is limited by cost and environmental concerns.

Plants, although entrenched in the early history of drug development, have not been used as a discovery resource to the extent that microbials have in recent times. In the 1950s and early 1960s there was a flurry of tissue- and animal-based screening based on plant extracts (Fig. 2). Important discoveries in the alkaloid classes (e.g., reserpine) created an inordinate level of optimism and many companies established extensive plant-based screening programs in *in vivo* systems. Unfortunately, the narrow focus on alkaloids in both collection (selected plant families) and chemistry (nitrogen-containing constituents) led to a great deal of redundancy, so that by the mid-1960s many of these expensive industrial research programs were closed as discovery attended to the more lucrative area of analogue synthesis.

The revival in plant natural products research in the 1970s, on the heels of the then-fashionable, marine-based research, was cut short by the introduction of rational drug design through computational modeling. The high level of hype associated with this area was short lived (Fig. 2) but soon replaced by a similar optimism with peptide-based combinatorial chemistry (see above). Plant natural products as a classical (and expensive) program again lost favor.

This persistent quick-change attitude in research management reflected its frustration with conventional discovery resources, its determination to be at the cutting edge of new technologies and among the first to harvest the benefits. Happily, stability is returning as HTOS finds its place in drug development and the significance of assuring structural diversity in test substance supply is addressed in practical terms. Plant-derived natural products begin to resurface and to take their rational place as a source of immense structural diversity.

The lack of adoption of plant sources as a test resource is somewhat paradoxical. The plant genome is much larger than other natural sources (bacteria, 1000 genes; fungi, 10,000 genes; plants, more than 100,000 genes) and therein offers a broader biochemical network for the generation of unique chemical structures. Unfortunately, until recently, the technologies and protocols of collection, processing, recollection, and scale-up had changed little in 50 years. Each sample collected individually demanded shipping, storage, and handling expenses; the attention of a chemist and considerable laboratory-based preparation time prior to assay were also required. Few attempts had been made to adapt these classical collection and preparative techniques to modern screening programs and budgets. As a result, plant-based research commanded a much higher cost per test sample than microbials, and it is this cost, and the requirement for a dedicated research team, that turned program directors away from the use of plants as a significant HTS resource.

Companies that have continued to use plants over the past two decades have done so at low throughput with the evaluation of only a few hundred species per year. In 1993, MicroBotanica addressed the economics and efficiency of plant collection with the goal of making this unique source available to screening programs at a throughput level that permits broad evaluation in modern HTS systems and a cost that is compatible with HTS budgets. It established a joint program with three groups in Peru: Perubotanica srl, Universidad Nacional de la Amazonia Peruana, and Conservacion de la Naturaleza Amazonica del Peru. The goal was biodiscovery and the collection, classification, documentation, and development of the plant resources in the Amazon Basin with strict compliance with the terms of the Convention on Biological Diversity [10].*

The technical approach is based on the position that the initial collection of test materials for HTS should be only what is required for the first pass and the initial confirmation of a hit, i.e., about 1 mg of a crude extract. Larger scale collec-

---

*We are pleased to find chemical companies such as Gaia Chemical Corporation that specialize in the provision of pure natural products as a discovery resource [11].

tion and extraction must be implemented only on the identification of hits. Such a "microcollection" program dramatically reduced costs and increased the number of plants sampled. It also permitted extraction in the field and thereby eliminated on-site specimen processing as well as lab handling time and expenses. This consortium can also respond immediately to a hit with sufficient material for confirmation and secondary profiling, and simultaneously to be able to assure recollection and the receipt of larger scale extract preparation in a timely manner—usually 2–3 weeks.

Another issue of special concern in the implementation of a plant-based natural product program is the sensitivity of many HTS assays to interference by polyphenols and tannins through nonspecific binding. Such substances are common constituents in plants and their removal prior to bioassay is frequently required. This issue has also been addressed by MicroBotanica through the development and application of proprietary liquid-liquid partitioning amenable to automation or the more conventional use of polyamide binding. Today MicroBotanica boasts ready access to samples of more than 30,000 extracts from approximately 13,000 plant specimens and the ability to follow through from recollection to isolation on any hit. MicroBotanica's participation in the Amazon consortium also makes it a unique source for collection and research on any plant endogenous to the Amazon Basin [5].

D. Structure-Based Design

The use of the structure of the target as a basis for computational design is not a new concept. Twenty years ago it ran rampant through the pharmaceutical industry (Fig. 2). Research management, heady with the developments in molecular modeling software and x-ray crystallography that were current, was impressed with the purported ability to design new drugs on the basis of target structure alone. Misinformation, misinterpretation, and bad timing took its toll. Structural analyses were weak and presumptive; computational power was overestimated and projections totally unrealistic. Fortunately, only a few companies made major commitments in this area, but those that did lost a great deal in program deletions, time, and credibility. Today the *de novo* design of an active molecule for a new biomolecular target is still fanciful. Finding structural precedence in small-molecule interaction is the key. Enter HTS and the revival of structure-based drug design.

Today structure-based drug design (SBDD) encompasses the integrated use of computational design software, HTOS, and HTS. In principle, SBDD is based on the sequence illustrated in Figure 3.

Information based on x-ray crystallographic data, nuclear magnetic resonance, and other analytical techniques facilitates the definition of the molecular dimensions and functionality of the target and its active site (Fig. 3A). Computational techniques are applied to the identification of the optimal small-molecule

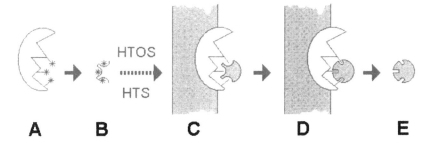

Figure 3 Structure-based drug design (**A**). Definition of target dimensions (**B**). Computational analysis of structural features for small-molecule interaction (**B–C**). HTOS generation of relevant compound libraries and identification of first hit through HTS (**C–D**). Optimization of the hit to one or more leads (**E**).

characteristics for interaction at the target site. This information is then used to screen real or virtual libraries for compounds suitable as first probes. A test library is then generated, acquired, or synthesized through HTOS and screened in the relevant assay(s). If hits are not realized, the process is repeated by retooling the target definition or anticipated small-molecule characteristics. Once significant data are obtained (Fig. 3C), larger libraries are prepared and the molecule is optimized to lead status. Conventional medicinal chemistry usually takes over at this point to provide the optimum candidate(s) for development. The system works. Of course, it still has both the requirement of a considerable knowledge base for the target and the risk associated with projections of biomolecular interaction to therapeutic significance. Nevertheless, it is reassuring to know that such a simple but elegant approach can be successfully implemented, provided all the tools are present and realistically evaluated.

SBDD is also applied to assessing the significance of the myriad of therapeutic targets anticipated from comparative analyses in functional genomics (see Section IV.B). While estimates of new and therapeutically relevant receptors are in the hundreds, finding those in the sea of information is a herculean task. The relevance of these targets, the identification of natural and artificial ligands, and the discovery of small molecules that can modulate their effects are goals in the practical application of this immense information base. Information gleaned from these studies will find application in drug discovery, diagnostics, toxicology, and other areas yet to be fathomed.

A recent and dramatic example of efficient application of SBDD was in the identification of inhibitors of nuclear factor of activated T cells (NFAT) in the search for new modulators of the immune response that do not have the limitations of cyclosporine or FK-506. Patrick Hogan and collaborators [12] applied HTOS in the form of peptide libraries of more than a billion units to identify optimal amino acid composition at seven sites of a hexadecapeptide sequence associated with calcineurin binding. This is an area that is by definition peptide in content and well suited to peptide HTOS. Transfer of the information gleaned into a useful immune-suppressive drug is yet to be achieved, but the ground is laid and open to innovation.

IV. BIOASSAY DEVELOPMENT AND IMPLEMENTATION

The identification of a cellular or molecular target for drug discovery and the development and validation of a relevant bioassay are critical early milestones in an HTS program. There must be a persuasive reason to believe that the cellular or molecular (enzyme, receptor, protein–protein, or protein–DNA interaction) target is involved in a pivotal step in the targeted disease process. That link—the molecular target to the disease process—requires exhaustive analysis. Today with the cost of screening at \$3–5 per well (compound and reagents) at the 96-well plate level, the assessment of a 50,000-member library will cost as much as \$250,000 before personnel costs and overhead are considered. Many of us can recount pre-HTS times when certain animal or biochemical assays formed the core of a discovery program only to prove of little or no value in the identification of a clinically active agent. Relevance must be carefully balanced against cost (Fig. 4).

Once a target has been selected, the next step is to develop a bioassay that is appropriate and compliant with the parameters applied in the corporate HTS system. Typically such assays have to be hearty and avoid the use of temperamental or unstable reagents. Each assay must be amenable to miniaturization at least to the 96-well microplate level but preferably beyond. Miniaturization to 384 is

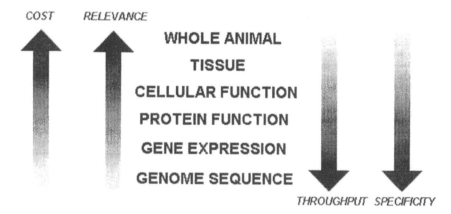

Figure 4   Relationship of bioassay targets to relevance and HTS compatibility.

commonplace, but further reduction is encouraged with the potential of lower cost and simultaneous higher throughput and data analysis. Cost savings are in attention time and the amount of compound and reagents used. By the simple shift from 96 to 384 wells the practical reaction volume and, correspondingly, the required reagents and compound are reduced by 75%. The latter is of special significance since many compounds, especially pure natural products, are in limited supply and conservation of such supply is often critical. Shifts to 1536 plates or high-density formats have corresponding benefits, although sample handling becomes a problem. Moreover, some detection systems are unreliable beyond 384.

Assays and even therapeutic targets have a defined lifetime. Frequently, even the most comprehensive and structurally diverse compound collection will not yield a hit in some assays. Such events generally are attributed to the inability of a small molecule to interfere in a complex biological process. Protein–protein interactions are often difficult to disrupt or block. At some point, usually the exhaustion of the current compound library, the decision is made to remove the assay for reevaluation. Occasionally this may result in a minor variation in reagents or protocol, or may lead to elimination of the assay or even the base target. The number of compounds screened through any bioassay may range from 10,000 to millions depending on the culture of the organization, the extent and diversity of the chemical resources, and a judgment as to the importance of the target.

Assays are generally established to permit a return of 0.05% or less hits. High-density systems with large numbers and low diversity in the test substances used may be a log or two lower. The frequency with which assays are removed from an HTS program on the basis of "no yield" can be reduced by critical analysis of the assay and the dose level prior to introduction into the HTS program. This is especially true in *de novo* applications where there is no drug reference to guide appropriate test concentrations and time. Nevertheless, the effects of a broad group of bioactive compounds on the assay response can be a useful directive. Fortunately, compound collections such as GenPlus (960 bioactive compounds) and NatProd (720 natural products) are available from MicroSource Discovery Systems [5] in microplate format. Such collections can be valuable tools in defining the sensitivity and specificity of any new assay. These are preplated at standard concentrations (mg/ml or 10 mM dimethyl sulfoxide) and can be easily blended into an assay validation protocol.

The living cell is the preferred format in discovery programs, offering a test response at the "organism" level while still allowing automation and high throughput. Cells can be engineered to house complex receptor systems tailored to represent a myriad of therapeutic targets. Detection modes are colorimetric, fluorescent, chemiluminescent, and radioisotopic systems. While regulatory and disposal problems continue to encourage the displacement of radioisotopes by other detection modes, innovations in simple and sensitive homogeneous systems, such as the recent SPA developments by Amersham [13], maintain a stable market.

Validation of a lead prior to further development involves the testing of the lead for efficacy in an animal model. The biological connection of a target to a disease, and the utility of such a target in drug discovery and development, is speculative without whole-animal data. Once a lead has been identified, it is essential to establish a "proof of concept" through in vivo evaluation. The selection of such a model is a process that should be concurrent with the development of the HTS assay. Such models may already be established, but it is likely that, with the emergence of novel genomics-based targets, they will require creative pharmacology and critical validation before confidence is established.

Activity in a whole animal is still not definitive for activity in humans, but the absence of activity draws attention to the need to reconsider the utility of the target. It is best to have such revelations early in a discovery program. The timeline and milestones applied in the recent collaboration of Axys and Merck in the identification and development of a small-molecule inhibitor of cathepsin K as a therapeutic modality in osteoporosis is a good illustration of this approach [14].

All of these technologies are not only complementary but feed back on one another with dramatic amplification of discovery potential. This can be of significant benefit as new activities in new indications are uncovered; however, there is a serious danger of misdirection. Incorrect information derived from a missed false-positive, incorrect analysis of an assay output or poor assay design can expand into unproductive and expensive voids. Any new development in HTS in design, discovery, or data analysis must be carefully assessed before it becomes an integral part of the process.

A. Fluorescence Detection Systems

Fluorescence technologies are dominant in HTS. Numerous well-characterized fluorescence tags suitable for differentially labeling specific cell components and protein probes are now commercially available [15]. Many quantitative techniques have been developed to harness the unique properties of fluorescence; several of these are represented in the following chapters in this book.

An excellent example of such technology is provided by K.A. Giuliano (Cellomics) in Chapter 8 in the development and advantages of functional screening based on high-resolution fluorescence imaging of multiple targets in intact cells. In Chapter 13, Scheel et al. (EVOTEC BioSystems) discuss the application of multiple fluorescence readout methods in the development of single-molecule detection technologies that enable a variety of parameters to be evaluated in a single sample.

Fluorescence resonance energy transfer (FRET) is a new, ultrahigh-throughput technology developed by Aurora Biosciences, one of the most progressive biotech companies in HTS technologies. FRET uses a coumarin-linked phospholipid asymmetrically bound to the plasma membrane as the donor and negatively charged oxonol acceptors which partition across the plasma membrane as a function of the transmembrane electric field. In Chapter 14, Paul England discusses the use of FRET in cell-based and reporter–receptor binding, protein–protein interactions, and other applications. Aurora's platform [16] also includes ultrahigh-throughput screening technologies and discovery modules, which allows for computer-directed delivery and bioassay of more than 100,000 selected compounds per day in 96 or 384 well plates.

Homogeneous time-resolved fluorescence, as well as its chemical basis and application in a broad scope of cellular and biomolecular assays, is described by Upham and Mathis in Chapter 15.

B. Comparative Functional Genomics

The identification of genome-based targets and representative bioassays is a more recent facet that already has spawned opportunities that were unimagined a decade ago. The use of human functional genomic data as a basis for new drug discovery is taking a commanding lead in industrial HTS programs. The technologies used in this area are not new, but the huge amount of data that has become available is, and their comparative analysis in normal and disease states constitutes one of the most rapidly growing and promising areas in the identification of new therapeutic targets.

Comparative functional genomics focuses on the identification of human genes associated with disease response in the whole organism and their role in the proliferation or suppression of the disease state. Such analysis has yielded hundreds of new targets that have no precedence in therapy or medicinal chemistry; many more are anticipated. The definition of the significance of these "orphan" receptors relies on classical strategies of genetic engineering and disease–gene modeling. These orphan receptors require validation before becoming an integral part of a discovery program; the identification of associated ligands is a first step.

Needless to say, these technologies have produced considerable hype in the projection of their impact on health management. Such hype is seen both in the marketplace and in industrial research planning. Fortunately, we are probably at the peak of the hype curve and look forward to tangible contributions in new target modeling and ultimately in therapeutic benefit.

Proteomics, an essential supportive technology in functional genomic applications, addresses characterization of the physicochemical properties of a protein expressed by a newly discovered disease-relevant gene and its production in large amounts through transfected cell cultures. Such probes have also been conducted in the HTS mode. These proteins, if beneficial, may lead to therapeutic agents in their own right, but for our purpose they can serve as tools for *de novo* assay development. Antibodies to such proteins provide insight into their function and location, and may also serve in therapy or assay development as specific antagonists.

C. ADME and Toxicological Profiling

ADME (adsorption, distribution, metabolism, and excretion) and toxicological studies are critical parts of any drug development program and essential for compliance with regulatory guidelines. Historically they were conducted only on drug candidates that had survived the rigors of chemical optimization, process development, and pharmacological profiling. The reason for this segregation was simply that such studies invariably involved whole-animal models and therefore were time consuming and expensive. It was not economically sound to expend such resources on candidates that were not firmly committed to development by other selection criteria. Unfortunately, when an ADME problem finally was detected it was at late investigational new drug (IND) preparation or even in the clinic. Such events created serious disruption of the development process and often resulted in closure of the project and a lost opportunity.

Parallel development of several candidates from the same compound class has been standard procedure to avoid project termination in the event of the emergence of an untoward effect. The considerable cost imparted by this approach was justified as being necessary for project survival.

Today the situation is changing rapidly and dramatically. ADME and toxicology technologies have evolved to permit the use of rapid and less expensive methods that have made the early assessment of drug candidates very attractive to the pharmaceutical industry. Major companies are shifting ADME assessment to become an integral part of the candidate selection process. Costs are still substantial but justified.

The goal is to move the assessment of drug metabolism and toxicity up in the discovery/development process (Fig. 5). Metabolic profiles of a large group of compounds that are considered for development can provide important information at the preselection level, save considerable time, and significantly reduce the cost of new drug development. Structural characteristics of test compounds that

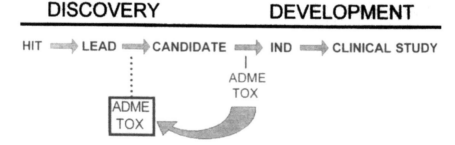

Figure 5 Current shift in emphasis of ADME assessment in the drug development process.

impart resistance to rapid metabolism are often independent of the biotarget pharmacophore and yield a different SAR analysis. Early ADME assessment can uncover such compounds before they are discarded on the basis of activity alone.

The principal source of drug metabolism is the cytochrome P450 enzymes, which constitute a superfamily of monooxygenases (requiring NADPH). They are found primarily in the endoplasmic reticulum of the liver although a prominent member is also found in the gut. In vitro ADME assays can be based on human liver microsomes or hepatocytes, which incorporate the full complement of P450s and other microsomal and cytosolic enzymes, or individual enzymes. Most P450s have been identified and many are available through recombinant techniques; their monoclonal antibodies are also commercially available [17]. Information can be obtained in vitro systems about patterns of metabolism, which P450s are involved, metabolite hepatotoxicity, and drug–drug interactions. Such analyses are amenable to HTS. Metabolite isolation and identification is an HTS challenge that can build on the technology already in place in HTOS and combinatorial technologies.

Albert P. Li (In Vitro Technologies) discusses HTS applications in ADME and toxicology in Chapter 17 of this book. The ease of isolation of human hepatocytes and their importance in metabolic and toxicological studies are underscored. These hepatocytes are stable and can be cryopreserved, thereby providing a regular supply of hepatocytes for screening without dependence on frequent access to fresh human liver.

Gentest [18] has described a microplate-based fluorimetric approach to rapid screening of test compounds for their susceptibility to and effects on P450 enzymes. The technology is efficient (100 compounds in 4 h) but limited in scope.

If a drug has an inhibitory effect on one enzyme and enhances the effect of another, its blood level in diverse ethnic populations can be dramatically different and create risks of ineffective dose or toxicity. It is likely that more stringent assessment requirements will be forthcoming for drugs that demonstrate inhibitory or enhancing activities on metabolic enzymes. HTS again can provide the tools.

V. INFORMATICS

The analysis and efficient use of the massive amount of data generated in HTS and related sciences has created the new discipline of bioinformatics, which has opened doors to new modes of discovery. Bioinformatics combines software, hardware, and database architecture to facilitate the storage, retrieval, and analysis of HTS data and to cross-reference such data to archival information on the basis of structure, physiochemical characteristics, biological profile, and therapeutic application. Such analyses enhance the efficiency of lead detection but also can provide unanticipated "finds" in areas not previously considered; serendipity continues to play an important role.

The complex network of biological and physicochemical interactions of test compounds with receptors, endogenous proteins, metabolites, and other cellular constituents provides a "pedigree" of behavior that constitutes the equity of the corporate screening resource. This pedigree also includes its chemical character, which incorporates chemical functionality and topological display. It is also important to add any data are associated with compound handling characteristics (solubility, instability, etc.), chemical character (reactivity, chelation potential, etc.), as well as the potential for interference in bioassay detection systems (e.g., color, fluorescence, etc.).

It is not enough to record that a compound is active or inactive in one or more assays. Any unusual observation with a test compound must be stored within its pedigree and not lost in a project's archives. It is important to tabulate these findings with assay conditions and activity levels, although the simple "yes/no" record for many of today's high-density assays limits such input. Much of this information is not readily available for large collections but can be accumulated in time as aspects of these and other features surface. ADME information is also an important aspect of such an information base but today, that is especially limited. Storage and handling of these data and their integration into analytical and decision making protocols yields an valuable information pool. This is the basis of HTS informatics.

Variation in the nature of assay protocols and performance must be addressed in the design of the information handling system. Protocol compliance and experimental error—mechanical, biological, or chemical interference—are important factors in defining the integrity of the data retrieved. False positives and negatives and the relationship of their incidence to assay or compound character are other aspects that can improve data quality and future performance.

Today the new term "data mining" brings forth the realization that the data retrieved in an HTS run have value that goes beyond the initial assay intention. Such information can lead to pattern analysis that will impact future inquiries. Negative and positive data hold equal value and constitute valuable equity in a company's HTS operations. This aspect is of special importance as we enter into the realm of unknown receptors and ligands. The acquisition of data and its management, storage, and analysis is addressed in Chapter 21 of this book.

VI. MANAGEMENT AND PERSONNEL ISSUES

Centralization of HTS activities was an early organizational change in R&D. It was essential on the basis of coordination of robotics, assay development and integration, data retrieval and management, and, most importantly, personnel development. I began this chapter by acknowledging the arrival in the early 1990s of a new breed of scientist who recognized the challenge and the potential rewards of screening and the important catalyst that such individuals provided in the rapid growth and success of HTS. That breed has evolved into a new professional elite that forms the core of discovery operations in many companies.

The specific goals of HTS have made it a separate and important corporate entity. This has been a natural process as technologies and information output have become exclusive to the discipline. Personnel have also become highly specialized, with attention and skill directed to aspects not previously part of conventional discovery operations.

Even the equipment employed for HTS in major companies has introduced new dimensions, requiring huge space allocations and large staff commitments. Witness the means employed for the storage, retrieval, and dispensing of dry compounds and solution samples. Such systems significantly improve HTS efficiency and accuracy but can require thousands of square feet for operation. Notable is the Haystack system from Automation Partnership [19], which has become the standard system for most large HTS operations. Haystack can automatically handle millions of samples as well as providing scheduling and tracking support. The more recent addition, the HomeBase system extends that capacity to include microplate management up to densities of 1536 wells with dispensing potential from 0.5 to 250 µl. Such equipment and associated robotics support constitute a "production-level" operation. This physical feature and the corresponding emphasis on massive data management and analysis separates the operation from the mainflow of research activity. While such separation is inevitable, there remains the need to ensure that feedback is given to the HTS team on the development of any hits and leads uncovered.

In small and large corporations, the integration of multidisciplinary technologies and personnel into a productive and innovative HTS team is as important as the anticipated advances in throughput and discovery. The latter follows automatically from a well-integrated, self-supportive team. Excellent reviews and commentaries by others on these all-important "people" aspects have been published elsewhere [20,21].

VII. PROJECTIONS

Throughput has been increased with higher density microplates, free-form systems, chips, and other innovative devices that take advantage of the recent advances in microfluidics and associated micronization of sample transfer, assays, and readouts. These advances also significantly reduce operational costs.

Microfabrication and microfluidic technologies are in a growth phase and creating a significant impact on innovation in screening design. They are a lucrative outsource activity and likely to remain so as the scope of these technologies continues to be explored. Application in miniaturization in drug discovery and genomics are two areas that impact our interests. Aclara BioSciences [22] employs plastic and glass microfluidic array chips in sample processing and analysis at picoliter volumes. Caliper Technologies [23] applies similar microchip technologies in facilitating liquid handling and biochemical processes. Their "Lab-on-a-Chip" technology uses nanoliter volumes of reagents in enzyme, receptor binding, and functional cell-based assays as well as systems that address toxicological and pharmacokinetic parameters.

Aurora Biosciences [16] has developed the NanoWell™ assay plate, which boasts 3456 miniaturized wells suitable for fluorescent assay applications. The assay volume used in these plates is 100 times smaller than the conventional 96-well format. This reduces the cost per test and the amount of compound needed. The required microfluidic technologies have also been developed by Aurora for compound transfer (<1 nl) at rates of up to 10,000 wells per hour; fluorescence detectors capable of handling more than 500,000 assays per day are also in place.

How small can we go? Biosensors based on molecular recognition force measurements between individual molecules using atomic force microscopy (AFM) have been described [24]. These include interactions between individual ligand–receptor, antibody–antigen, and DNA–DNA molecules. Using the similar single-molecule measurements, discrimination between two chiral molecules has also been achieved at the single-molecule level by chemical derivatization of the scanning probe tip in AFM [25]. These assay technologies are far from high throughput but offer considerable promise for such at the monomolecular level.

We have overcome the demands of sample throughput up to the point where meeting the demands of compound supply and diversity is a strain. Robotics, detection systems, sample density, and data management have increased to a level that was not conceivable a few years earlier. Unfortunately, assay systems that provide relevance as well as throughput are few and far between. All too often, relevance is set aside as a matter for secondary evaluation rather than the primary screen. Such an approach is fine providing there is an appropriate second screening stage to bring both numbers and relevance to acceptable levels. The challenge now is in the development of systems that allow significant flexibility for assay enhancement in therapeutic relevance and the increase of information gleaned from each. Increase in the latter is important but not at the expense of the former.

REFERENCES

1. The First Forum on Data Management Technologies in Biological Screening (Chairman, John P. Devlin). SRI International, Menlo Park, CA, April 22–24, 1992.
2. *Screening Forum* stopped hard copy distribution in 1998, but its archives and current articles may still be found on the internet at *www.msdiscovery.com*.
3. *Screening Forum*, 3(2), 1 (1995).

4. See *www.bd.com,* *www.dynextechnologies.com,* *www.greineramerica.com,* *www. polyfiltronics.com,* and *nunc.nalgenunc.com* for additional information.

5. See *www.msdiscovery.com.*

6. See *www.biosignal.com* as an example.

7. See *www.sbsonline.org.*

8. See *www.tripos.com, www.msi.com, www.daylight.com, www.mdli.com, www.oxmol. com,* and *www.synopsis.co.uk* as examples.

9. See *www.arqule.com* and *www.pcop.com* as examples.

10. J.P. Devlin, Chemical diversity and genetic equity: synthetic and naturally derived compounds, in J.P. Devlin (ed.), The Discovery of Bioactive Substances: High Throughput Screening, Marcel Dekker, New York, 1997, pp. 3–48.

11. See *www.gaiachem.com.*

12. J. Aramburu, M.B. Yaffe, C. Lopez-Rodrigez, L.C. Cantley, P.G. Hogan, A. Rao, Science 285:2129 (1999).

13. See *www.amersham.com.*

14. See *www.axyspharm.com* and *www.Merck.com.*

15. See *www.probes.com.*

16. See *www.aurorabio.com.*

17. See *www.panvera.com.* as an example.

18. See *www.gentest.com.*

19. See *www.autoprt.com.*

20. John Babiak, Management and service issues in a centralized robotics HTS core, in J.P. Devlin (ed.), The Discovery of Bioactive Substances: High Throughput Screening, Marcel Dekker, New York, 1997, pp. 461–470.

21. Mark Beggs, John S. Major, Flexible use of people and machines, in J.P. Devlin (ed.), The Discovery of Bioactive Substances: High Throughput Screening, Marcel Dekker, New York, 1997, pp. 3–48.

22. See *www.aclara.com.*

23. See *www.calipertech.com.*

24. Richard Colton (Naval Res Lab, DC), in Proceedings of Cyprus '98: New Technologies and Frontiers in Drug Research, Limassol, Cyprus, May 4–8, 1998. Downloadable at *www.msdiscovery.com.*

25. Rachel McKendry (U Cambridge, UK), in Proceedings of Cyprus '98: New Technologies and Frontiers in Drug Research, Limassol, Cyprus, May 4–8, 1998. Downloadable at *www.msdiscovery.com.*

10
Fluorescence Correlation Spectroscopy (FCS) and FCS-Related Confocal Fluorimetric Methods (FCS+plus): Multiple Read-Out Options for Miniaturized Screening

Cornelia Rufenach, Andreas Scheel, Sylvia Sterrer, and Rodney Turner
Evotec BioSystems AG
Hamburg, Germany

I. INTRODUCTION: A RATIONALE FOR NEW READ-OUT METHODS IN DRUG DISCOVERY

The process of drug discovery has been in a state of rapid change over the past decade. The advent of genomics and combinatorial chemistry has lead to an increased reliance on efficient and effective techniques for screening large numbers of chemical compounds against an increasing number of potential pharmaceutical targets. The discipline of high-throughput screening (HTS) has been at the center of a revolution in drug discovery. Not only has HTS emerged as an important tool in the early stage of drug discovery, it is also the stage for the interaction of profound biological and chemical diversity with new technologies in the area of automation, robotics, and bioinformatics [1,2]. The way in which assays are performed for screening is changing significantly. Whereas once assay volumes of 100–150 µl were common for such screening techniques as enzyme-linked immunosorbent assay (ELISA) and radioligand binding assays, modern miniaturized HTS favors homogeneous "add-and-read" assay formats with volumes as low as 1 µl per well. Miniaturization will become the rule throughout the drug discovery process as compounds will be needed for more assays while being synthesized in smaller quantities. The process of HTS is also seeing increased application of industrial standard automation and robotics technology to improve efficiency. In parallel developments, novel detection technologies and assay strategies are being implemented to improve the effectiveness of the process. Therefore, novel detection technologies will be tested in an environment that requires the maximum determination of biological information in the shortest amount of time with a minimum of reagent and compound, and with maximal precision.

The technology described in this chapter has emerged from physics laboratories and the analysis of rapid chemical reactions to find application in drug discovery. Use of the confocal optical systems described herein facilitates the analysis of biological interactions at the molecular level. Changes in the molecular environment of a fluorescently labeled biological molecule result in the change in signal used by fluorescence correlation spectroscopy (FCS) and related technologies. The changes in molecular environment typically occur as a result of binding or biological processing and therefore provide an ideal basis for screening assays [3].

The challenges with regard to modern assay techniques and the related technologies are large. These include the need to maintain sensitivity as volumes, and therefore quantities of reagents and compounds, decrease as much as 100-fold; to obtain as much information as possible from a single measurement; to help eliminate the disturbances often encountered in compound screening, such as compound autofluorescence and turbidity; and to be compatible with homogeneous assay formats. The following pages describe how FCS+plus meets most of these challenges.

II. SINGLE-MOLECULE CONFOCAL FLUORESCENCE DETECTION TECHNOLOGY

Fluorescence-based confocal detection technologies allow molecular interactions to be studied at the single-molecule level. Combining laser spectroscopy with confocal microscopic optical systems, the laser beam can be highly focused in such a way that only molecules in a volume of 1 fl (a billionth of a millionth of a liter) are hit by the light—a volume that equals roughly the size of a bacterial cell [4]. With the laser illuminating such minute parts of the sample, even volumes of 1 μl or less are sufficient for sample testing. On the basis of this technology, new methods have been developed in recent years that allow molecular properties of fluorescent biomolecules to be studied in 1-μl sample volumes, enabling a wide range of solution-based and cellular assays to be established for HTS.

The ability to make full use of the fluorescent molecule and all of its properties should be the benchmark of any fluorescence-based assay technology. While most assay strategies make use of only a single fluorescent property, the broad applicability of a screening system requires that flexibility of assay design be extended to the read-out technology by including a variety of detection modes. While most scientists may associate the use of fluorescence in biological assay systems solely with the measurement of fluorescence intensity, the measurement of additional fluorescent properties, such as lifetime, polarization, fluorescence energy transfer, and quenching, can yield a wealth of information from a single measurement. This ability to collect multiple data points per measurement not only provides an internal control but also contributes to screening efficiency by enabling rapid multiparameter evaluation of compound–target interactions.

A. FCS⁺plus: Multiparameter Fluorescence Read-out Technology

FCS is used to determine the translational diffusion of fluorescent molecules [5]. Each fluorescent molecule that diffuses through the illuminated confocal focus of the laser gives rise to bursts of fluorescent light quanta. The length of each photon burst corresponds to the time the molecule spends in the confocal focus. The photons emitted in each burst are recorded in a time-resolved manner by a highly sensitive single-photon detection device. The detection of diffusion events makes possible the determination of a diffusion coefficient. Upon binding of a fluorescently labeled ligand to its receptor, the molecular weight and therefore the diffusion coefficient changes. Thus, the diffusion coefficient serves as a parameter to distinguish between free and bound ligand. Hereby, the confocal optics eliminate interference from background signals and allow homogeneous assays to be carried out.

Since translational diffusion relies on significant changes in molecular weight upon molecular interaction, new methods were developed at Evotec that use a variety of fluorescence parameters as read-out. These new methods, collectively called FCS⁺plus, evaluate fluorescence signals from single molecules on the basis of changes in fluorescence brightness, fluorescence polarization, fluorescence lifetime, fluorescence spectral shift, by fluorescence energy transfer or by confocal imaging (Table 1). Brightness analysis is a unique read-out method that allows one to determine concentrations and specific brightness values of individual fluorescent species within a sample [6]. As a measure of fluorescence brightness, the number of photon counts per defined time interval in the confocal volume is detected. Changes of molecular brightness during a binding event can be due to two mechanisms: (1) If one of the two partners is labeled with a fluorescent dye, quenching of fluorescence may occur upon binding. (2) Amplification of the molecular brightness takes place when both partners are labeled or a particle offers multiple binding sites for the fluorescent ligand (e.g., receptor-bearing vesicles or beads/bacteria with one binding partner immobilized on the surface). This technique has wide applications since it can be used to study the interactions of pro-

Table 1 Read-out Modes offered by FCS⁺plus

Method	Principle
Translational diffusion (fluorescence correlation spectroscopy, FCS)	Translational diffusion properties of molecules are dependent on the molecular weight. Diffusion coefficients of fluorescently labeled molecules therefore change upon interaction and enable distinction between free and bound state of the molecule.
Fluorescence brightness	The number of photon counts per defined time interval in the confocal volume serves as a measure of molecular fluorescence brightness. Changes in fluorescence brightness of a fluorescent molecule upon binding are monitored.
Fluorescence polarization	The fluorescence polarization of a molecule is directly proportional to its molecular volume. Changes in the molecular volume due to binding or dissociation of two molecules, conformational changes, or degradation can be detected as changes in polarization values of the fluorescently labeled molecule.
Fluorescence lifetime	Fluorescence lifetime describes the average time that a fluorescent molecule remains in the excited state. The lifetime of the fluorescent signal is dependent on the molecular environment of the fluorescent tag, allowing monitoring of molecular interactions.
Fluorescence energy transfer	The emitted light of a fluorophore serves as the energy source to excite a second fluorophore. Energy transfer between a donor fluorophore on molecule A to acceptor fluorophore on molecule B depends on proximity and can therefore serve as a measure for interaction of A with B.
Spectral shift	The excitation and/or emission wavelength of a fluorescent tag is dependent on the molecular environment. Changes of the spectral properties of a fluorescent molecule induced by molecular binding serve as a read-out for binding.
Confocal imaging	Fluorescence changes on the cell surface or within cells caused by biological reactions are visualized by confocal imaging techniques combined with two-dimensional scanning.

teins with similar molecular weight and binding of ligands to membrane receptors (see below).

Changes in any of the molecular parameters described in Table 1 can be used as a read-out to characterize molecular interactions. In most cases, the same optical and electronic configurations are utilized, merely employing a different algorithm for analysis. This means that all fluorescent parameters noted above can be monitored using the same detection unit. Some of the fluorescence parameters described in Table 1 can even be monitored simultaneously in a single measurement (multiplexing), resulting in exceptional data quality regarding reproducibility and statistics. A comparison of Evotec's detection technology with other commonly used fluorescence methodologies is shown in Table 2.

B. Advantages of Using FCS⁺plus for Miniaturized HTS

The major advantages of FCS⁺plus technologies over other detection technologies are summarized in the following sections.

1. Inherent Miniaturization

All macroscopic fluorescence methods, whether based on intensity, polarization, or lifetime detection, measure by averaging all signals across an optical collection volume, which is usually a significant portion of the sample well. For such ensemble measurements, lowering the assay volume results in a lower number of fluorescence signals contributing to the ensemble measurement. In most cases, this results in reduced assay performance, with the signal decreasing relative to background as the assay volume decreases toward the 1-μl range. With FCS⁺plus, fluorescence parameters are measured from individual molecules in a detection vol-

Table 2 Comparison of Evotec's Technology and Other Fluorescence Methodologies

| Feature | Conventional fluorescence methods | | | | Technologies at Evotec | |
	FI	FP	FRET	HTRF	FCS	FCS⁺plus[a]
Homogenous	o	+	+	+	+	+
Mass independent	+	−	+	+	−	+
Signal independent of assay volume	−	−	−	+	+	+
Single-molecule sensitivity	−	−	−	−	+	+
Insensitive to autofluorescence	−	−	o	+	o	+
No significant inner filter effects	−	−	−	o	+	+
Multiplexing	−	−	−	−	+	+
Components to be labeled	1 or 2	1	2	2	1	1 or 2

FI, fluorescence intensity (total); FP, fluorescence polarization; FRET, fluorescence resonance energy transfer; HTRF, homogeneous time-resolved fluorescence.
+, advantage always featured; o, not always featured; −, disadvantage/not a feature.
[a]FCS⁺plus comprises the detection of fluorescence brightness, polarization (FP), molecular diffusion, and lifetime. In addition, assay systems based on FI and FRET can be applied with FCS⁺plus.

ume of 1 fl regardless of sample volume. The signal-to-background ratio is effectively independent of the sample volume. Using FCS⁺plus as a detection technology, miniaturized screening is possible in assay volumes of 1 µl and lower without loss of signal. Miniaturization applied to large-scale screening has a considerable effect on the costs: to run a screen with 100,000 compounds, the reagent savings of 100-µl versus 1-µl assay volumes can make a difference of US$1 Mio versus US$10,000 assuming average costs for reagents including standard purified proteins. The cost savings will increase all the more if precious reagents are needed.

2.   Homogeneous Assay Format

Since the bound and unbound state of a fluorescent biomolecule can be distinguished by different fluorescent parameters (Table 1), no physical separation of bound and unbound ligand is required. The elimination of washing and separation steps make such "add-and-read" assay formats easily amenable to automation and rapid to perform.

3.   Increased Safety of Reagents

Fluorescence detection technologies avoid the use of hazardous radiochemicals and production of large-scale radioactive waste.

4.   Elimination of Background Effects

Due to the short pathlength of the confocal optical configuration, background effects and signal reduction caused by turbidity and ink-like solutions can be substantially reduced in comparison with other methods. In addition, other disturbing background effects, such as those from light-scattering or autofluorescent compounds, can be eliminated by registering only the signal of the fluorophore used for labeling.

5.   Single-Component Labeling

In most cases, fluorescent labeling of one binding partner with standard dyes is sufficient using FCS⁺plus. FCS⁺plus is therefore more widely applicable than fluorescence resonance energy transfer (FRET) or homogeneous time-resolved fluorescence (HTRF), where both partners have to be labeled.

6.   Multiple Read-out Modes

Since FCS⁺plus encompasses a variety of read-out modes (Table 1), it offers unique flexibility: the most suitable read-out mode can be selected for each assay system. FCS⁺plus is applicable to study protein–nucleic acid, protein–peptide, and protein–protein interactions, enzymatic reactions, interactions of ligands with membrane fractions or live cells, detection of secretory products, and to study intracellular events such as reporter gene activity or translocation events. Some of the read-out modes described in Table I can even be applied in parallel (multiplexing).

7. Multiple Read-out Parameters

FCS+plus provides an intrinsically information-rich output for each measurement: each read-out mode allows the detection of several read-out parameters, such as the total concentration of fluorescent species as well as absolute concentrations of bound and free ligand. These additional parameters provide valuable intrawell controls and help to eliminate false-positives results.

8. Throughput

FCS+plus measurements are fast, typical read-out times are 1–2 sec per well, allowing for high throughput. However, high-performance and high-throughput screening in a miniaturized format can only be carried out when combining the FCS+plus technology in an automated HTS system with microfluidics and robotics technology working with the same level of precision. Using the EVOscreen® system, a fully automated ultra high-performance screening platform, a throughput of up to 100,000 compounds per day can be achieved for most FCS+plus assays.

C. Case Studies I: Using FCS+plus Multiparameter Read-outs

We have chosen a number of different biological systems as case studies that demonstrate the unique potential of the FCS+plus technology in meeting the demands of modern drug discovery described in the introduction.

a. Effect of Assay Miniaturization. Since FCS+plus uses highly focused confocal optics, the volume illuminated by the laser beam is as small as a bacterial cell. The signal-to-background ratio is therefore effectively independent of the sample volume. This is demonstrated in Figure 1, where the DNA binding properties of topoisomerase were studied. Since the molecular weight of fluorescently labeled oligonucleotides increases by approximately a factor of 17 upon binding to topoisomerase, this event can be monitored using FCS. As shown in Figure 1, the performance of the assay in a miniaturized 1-µl format is identical to that in a "large"-scale format of 20 µl with respect to both statistics and the observed protein–DNA affinity.

This demonstrates that in comparison to other methods currently used in industrial HTS, such as ELISA, fluorescence polarization (FP), SPA, and HTRF, assay miniaturization down to a 1-µl assay volume is achieved without compromising assay performance.

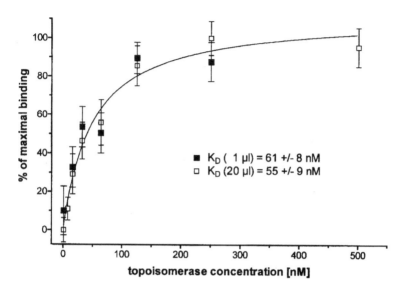

Figure 1 FCS⁺plus allows assay miniaturization to 1-µl formats. The interaction of topoisomerase with a fluorescently labeled oligonucleotide was monitored using FCS in 1-µl and 20-µl assay volumes. Maximal binding was normalized to 100%.

Besides the need for a sensitive detection technology, screening in a miniaturized format requires significant expertise with liquid handling of nanoliter volumes. In addition, evaporation and adsorption effects must be overcome. Typically, target characterization and assay development are initially carried out in volumes of 20 µl. Subsequently, the assay volume is reduced to 1 µl for HTS adaptation and screening.

b. Multiparameter Read-out. The success of HTS strategies in drug discovery depends on the reliable determination of the compound activity, thus distinguishing between promising potential drug candidates and useless false positives (where inactive compounds score active in the assay). Elimination of false positives is a drain on the time and resources because it requires retesting. While the use of fluorescence is usually associated solely with the measurement of fluorescence intensity, FCS⁺plus allows the determination of several fluorescence parameters in a single measurement. Therefore, FCS⁺plus delivers more information on a compound, allowing for efficient elimination of false positives in the primary screen.

To demonstrate FCS⁺plus multiparameter read-outs, a model system based on biotin-streptavidin was used. Binding of fluorescently labeled biotin (molecular weight 1 kD) to streptavidin (molecular weight 60 kD) can easily be monitored by FCS. This allows one to determine the diffusion rates of free and bound biotin, and the distribution of fluorescent biotin between these two species. A test run was carried out in a miniaturized format in an HTS mode (1-μl sample volume, 2-sec read time per well) using unlabeled biotin as a competitor.

A sample of 40 wells from a single row of a high-density plate is shown in Figure 2. Three fluorescence parameters are obtained from a single measurement within each well: (1) fluorescence count rate (average fluorescence intensity in the sample), (2) particle number (a measure of the total number of fluorescent biotin molecules present in the confocal volume) and (3) ratio of bound to total biotin (ratio of streptavidin-bound biotin relative to total biotin).

Other detection systems based on radioactivity or fluorescence typically deliver a single read-out parameter per well, usually the amount of complex formed. In this case, well 6 would score as a hit. The additional read-out parameters obtained by FCS+plus show that both count rate and concentration of biotin (particle number) in this well are increased. This can be attributed to the failure of a dispenser to deliver the appropriate amount of streptavidin to this well. The resulting lower volume yields an increase in count rate and particle number (the

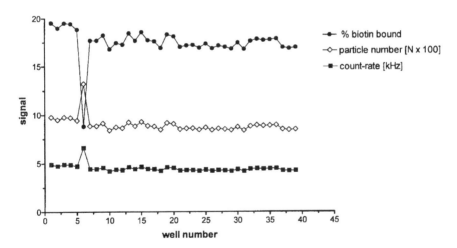

Figure 2 FCS+plus offers multiparameter read-outs. Binding of fluorescently labeled biotin to streptavidin was studied with FCS on EVOscreen. Shown is a segment from a nanocarrier (total assay volume of 1 μl). The data was fit using a two-component fit procedure assuming the presence of a fast-diffusing component (free fluorescent biotin) and a slowly diffusing component (fluorescent biotin–streptavidin complex). The fit prodedure yields the percentage of fluorescent biotin present in the two fluorescent components ("% biotin bound" and "% biotin free"), total fluorescence intensity (count rate) and total concentration of fluorescent biotin (particle number).

final concentration of biotin is higher due to the lower volume), whereas the lower amount of streptavidin results in a decrease in the amount of complex formed. Thus, with the additional information obtained from the FCS$^+$plus read-out parameters, well 6 is discarded as a false positive.

This example shows how the simultaneous analysis of multiple fluorescence parameters helps to significantly improve the precision of primary screening by efficient elimination of false-positive results. Using the EVOscreen platform, the screening database automatically eliminates false positives on-line during the primary screen if control parameters within a well, such as total count rate or particle numbers, deviate from a previously defined range.

D. Case Studies II: Flexibility of Multiple Read-out Modes

Ideally, a detection technology must allow maximal flexibility in assay design since assay types developed and screened in pharmaceutical companies vary enormously. Since FCS$^+$plus encompasses a variety of different read-out modes, for each specific assay system the most suitable read-out mode can be selected. In the following section, we have chosen several important target classes/assay systems in order to demonstrate the degree of flexibility and performance offered by FCS$^+$plus.

1. Enzyme Assays

Kinases are important therapeutic targets in drug discovery programs. We have selected p60c-src as an example of tyrosine kinases that are involved in controlling important cellular functions such as mitogenesis. Kinase activity is usually monitored by quantitating the amount of phosphorylated peptide formed using an anti-phosphotyrosine antibody. Since the molecular weight of a phosphopeptide increases significantly upon antibody binding, enzymatic activity can easily be determined with FCS using a fluorescently labeled peptide as substrate.

Other detection methods, such as FP and HTRF, are also applicable. In comparison with these methods, FCS offers significant advantages. Using FCS, assays can be designed not only to determine the end-point activity of a given kinase, but also in a kinetic mode where enzyme activity is monitored over time.

Thus, during the assay development phase new kinases are characterized by determining kinetic constants such as k_{on} and k_{off}. During assay adaptation to a miniaturized HTS format, suitable assay conditions are investigated as shown in Figure 3. In this experiment, different amounts of enzyme were used and the amount of product formed was monitored over time in a 1-µl format. After successful completion of this stage, the assay was run in an HTS mode on the EVO-screen platform (1 µl per assay, end-point mode) in order to identify compounds that inhibit kinase activity. Thus, FCS$^+$plus can be used for target characterization, assay development, for miniaturized, fully automated HTS and for hit profiling,

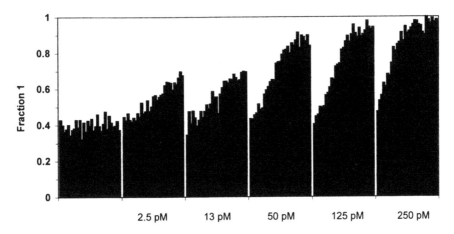

Figure 3 Enzyme kinetics in 1-μl assay volumes. Src kinase activity was determined on a nanocarrier (1-μl assay volume) using FCS. The production of phosphorylated peptide was monitored for 30 min using increasing enzyme concentrations.

yielding a maximum of information using a minimum of assay components and compounds. Using the EVOscreen system, a throughput of up to 100,000 compounds is achieved within 24 hours for this type of assay.

2. GPCR Assays

G-protein-coupled receptors (GPCR) belong to another important target class because they are involved in a variety of diseases such as asthma, AIDS, neurodegenerative and cardiovascular diseases [7]. However, technologies currently used have significant disadvantages as they typically involve the use of radioactively labeled ligands. This means exposure to hazardous radioactivity, limited shelf lifes of labeled components, and the production of radioactive waste on a large scale. Also, radioactive assays are still carried out in the standard 96-well format using volumes of 100–150 μl and are not easily amenable to miniaturization beyond the 384-well format (30–50 μl per well).

These assays involve the use of membrane fractions prepared from receptor-expressing cells; therefore, standard FCS can not be applied because of the very slow diffusion rate of membrane vesicles. To overcome this restriction, a new read-out method was developed based on brightness analysis. This method complements FCS since it measures the brightness of fluorescent species and not diffusion times; as a result, it is entirely mass independent. It allows one to study the interaction of proteins with similar molecular weight but is also applicable to monitor interactions of soluble ligands with receptor-bearing vesicles. The principle of brightness analysis in this case is multiple fluorescently labeled ligands binding to a receptor-bearing membrane vesicle. Bound ligand can be distinguished from unbound because a membrane vesicle with many fluorescent ligand molecules bound is significantly brighter than a single fluorescent ligand molecule.

Figure 4 shows an example of such an assay using the chemokine receptor CXCR2 and its ligand, fluorescently labeled interleukin 8 (IL-8). The results from 500 wells during a screening run using the EVOscreen platform are displayed. The competitor added was easily identified since the assay yields a nice screening window with a signal-to-background ratio of approximately eightfold.

Using radioactive methods, only the amount of bound ligand can be determined. In contrast, with brightness analysis, the concentration of both bound and free ligand is obtained from a single measurement, thus providing a valuable internal control.

3. Cellular Assays

A further challenge to modern HTS is the use of living cells. Cellular assays provide a more physiological approach and put functional data into a biological context. However, the requirements for miniaturized HTS on cellular assays are high:

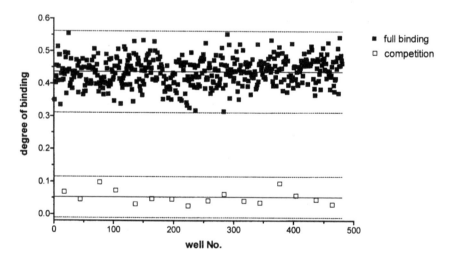

Figure 4   Test screen of the chemokine receptor CXCR2 in a miniaturized format. A sample of 500 wells from a Nanocarrier is shown from a fully automated test screen using EVOscreen. 100 nl of 10% DMSO with (□) or without (■) competitor were added from 96-well plates to nanocarriers. Ligand (100 nl) and membranes (800 nl) were added by dispensers and the assay was analyzed by brightness analysis. The solid line represents the mean of each sample and the dotted line represents the mean ± three standard deviations.

assays must be single step and, homogeneous, which presents a technical challenge.

FCS⁺plus is applicable to a wide variety of cellular assay systems. One example is shown in Figure 5, where binding of a fluorescent ligand to cell surface receptors was monitored with live cells. In this experiment, the activity of a chemical compound was analyzed for competing with IL-8 binding to CXCR2 receptors expressed on the cell surface. In this case, a variation of the brightness analysis read-out described above was used to study the binding event. Here the cells were placed at the bottom of a well and fluorescently labeled ligand was added. Cell-bound fluorescence was quantitated by scanning with the confocal volume through the cells.

In addition to cell surface binding, secretory products from cells into the surrounding medium as well as gene induction using reporter systems can be measured by FCS⁺plus. Due to the small confocal detection volume, subcellular resolution is obtained with FCS⁺plus by using confocal imaging techniques. This makes assay systems accessible to HTS where the distribution of fluorescence across a cell changes while the total fluorescence remains unaltered, e.g., during translocation events.

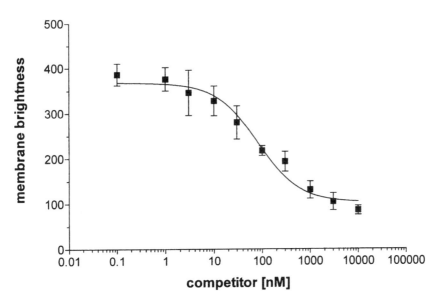

Figure 5 Studying ligand–receptor interactions using live cells. Live cells expressing the chemokine receptor CXCR2 were incubated with fluorescently labeled IL-8 in the presence of increasing concentrations of a low molecular weight compound analyzed by brightness analysis. The membrane brightness was determined by FCS⁺plus.

The combination of sensitivity and miniaturization capabilities of FCS+plus offers a further major advantage: primary cells can be used in HTS because restrictions resulting from the availability of primary tissue are overcome by the very small numbers of cells needed for each assay (1000–2000 cells per well).

III. SUMMARY

FCS and related confocal fluorescence-based detection technologies provide a valuable platform for assay development, high-throughput screening, and subsequent optimization of assays. The technology is applicable to a wide variety of target classes and assay techniques, allowing great flexibility in assay design. Screening applications as varied as the kinetic study of compounds acting on tyrosine kinases, the binding characteristics of compounds acting on G-protein-coupled receptor systems, and the study of binding to and secretion from living cells have been accomplished with this technology.

FCS+plus technologies overcome the use of hazardous radioactive probes, are amenable to miniaturization, can be used in a kinetic or end-point mode, and deliver internal control values for each sample measured. Because of the inherently small detection volume, the techniques are independent of sample size, suffering no loss of sensitivity in low volume assays, and therefore ideally suited for assay miniaturization. The multiple parameters read in a single measurement improve the precision of each measurement taken. The potential to impact all areas of drug discovery has yet to be fully exploited, but FCS+plus is a technology platform that we feel will contribute significantly to improvement of the drug discovery process.

ACKNOWLEDGMENTS

We thank Drs. Martin Klumpp, Dirk Ullmann, and Julian Wölcke for providing data, and Drs. Andy Pope and Ken Murray for providing reagents.

REFERENCES

1. Houston JG, Banks MA. The chemical-biological interface: developments in automated and miniaturised screening technology. Curr Opin Biotechnol 1997;8:734–740.
2. Turner R, Sterrer S, Wiesmüller KH. High throughput screening. In: Ullmann's Encyclopedia of Industrial Chemistry, Weinheim: VCH. In press.
3. Turner R, Ullmann D, Sterrer S. Screening in the nanoworld: single molecule spectroscopy and miniaturized HTS. In: Handbook of Screening, Dr. James Swarbrick's the Drugs and the Pharmaceutical Sciences Series. In press.

4. Auer M, Moore KJ, Meyer-Almes FJ, Guenther R, Pope AJ, Stoeckli KA Fluorescence correlation spectroscopy: lead discovery by miniaturised HTS. DDT 1998;3:457–465.
5. Eigen M, Rigler R. Sorting single molecules: application to diagnostics and evolutionary biotechnology. Proc Natl Acad Sci USA 1994;91:5740–5747.
6. Kask P, Palo K, Ullmann D, Gall K. Fluorescence intensity distribution analysis (FIDA) and its application in biomolecular detection technology. Proc Natl Acad Sci USA 1999;96:13756–13761.
7. Horn F, Vriend G. G protein–coupled receptors in silico. J Mol Med 1998;76:464–468.

11

Homogeneous Time-Resolved Fluorescence

Loraine V. Upham and Betty Howard
Packard BioScience, Downers Grove, Illinois

Jocelyn W. Burke
Packard BioScience, Meridan, Connecticut

Gerard Mathis
CIS Bio International, Bagnols sur Cèze, France

I. INTRODUCTION TO HOMOGENEOUS TIME-RESOLVED FLUORESCENCE

The evolution of high-throughput screening (HTS) has created the need for more sensitive, rapid, and easily automated assays. Combinatorial chemistry, expanding compound libraries, increasing numbers of drug targets, and increasing pressure for discovery of new chemical entities in the pharmaceutical industry have fueled the expansion of HTS methods [1]. The advent of homogeneous, "mix-and-measure" assays lead to a significant leap in the throughput of typical HTS. Homogeneous assays eliminate the need to separate bound from free label, which also reduces waste and error. Furthermore, homogeneous assays are easier to automate since they require only addition steps. Scintillation proximity assay (SPA) (Amersham International, Amersham, UK) was the first mix-and-measure assay developed. With the TopCount scintillation and luminescence microplate counter (Packard Instrument Company, Meriden, CT) and the MicroBeta microplate scintillation counter (EG&G Wallac, Turku, Finland), SPA assays made HTS a reality [2]. However, SPA assays still require a radiolabeled binding partner, long counting times for accurate measurements, and correction for quench and color interference effects of biological compounds. In addition, SPA assays involve a scintillating solid-phase bead, which settles out of solution [3]. The need for a nonradioisotopic, truly homogeneous alternative led to the development of homogeneous time-resolved fluorescence (HTRF), an in-solution, homogeneous, nonradioisotopic method. This chapter describes the theory and application of HTRF—a sensitive, robust, homogeneous, fluorescence method for high-throughput screening.

II. UNIQUE PROPERTIES OF HTRF CHEMISTRY

A. Specific Requirements of Homogeneous Assays

Based on the specific requirements of homogeneous assays, a new class of long-lived fluorescent tracers was utilized to create this novel assay method. The following sections describe the unique challenges of creating a fluorescence-based, homogeneous method in general, and the unique solution provided by HTRF chemistry.

1. Unique Tracers

Assaying a specific effect on biological targets without the luxury of a separation step requires unique tracers. Natural fluorescence of proteins and other compounds in biological samples and media creates limitations for the use of conventional fluorescent labels. Upon laser excitation, conventional fluorophores shift to a longer wavelength and are measured immediately based on the change in wavelength [4]. Most background signals are prompt in nature, and also dissipate within 50 µsec after excitation, making them difficult to separate from specific signal. HTRF utilizes the rare-earth lanthanide ion europium (3+), which exhibits a signal as long-lived as several hundred microseconds, permitting time-resolved measurement and elimination of prompt background fluorescence [5].

2. Signal Modulation

Another requirement of homogeneous assays is a method of modulating signal between the affected and unaffected assay targets. Making the distinction between the bound and unbound target molecules by a method other than separation is necessary. HTRF technology utilizes a carefully selected pair of fluorescent molecules to generate signals specific to the bound and unbound states. The "donor" molecule is europium cryptate, referred to as (Eu)K. When excited, (Eu)K transfers energy to an "acceptor" molecule, a modified (stabilized) allophycocyanin called XL665. A long-lived signal at a specific wavelength is generated only when a binding event between donor and acceptor molecules occurs. For example, when the target molecules are unbound as a result of the presence of an inhibitor, the specific signal is not generated [6]. Such signal modulation is required for a truly homogeneous assay.

3. Resistance to Biological Media

Since no separation step is involved in a homogeneous assay, biological assay components and media remain in the presence of the target molecules of interest during measurement. The signal of a homogeneous assay should be resistant to unrelated, nonspecific effects of biological assay components, such as media and natural products, if involved. HTRF technology is measured by a patented "ratio-metric" method, described later in detail, which eliminates or corrects for non-specific interference from biological assay components [7].

B. Lanthanide Cryptates: A New Type of Fluorescent Label

1. Chelates as Fluorescent Labels

The rare-earth lanthanides, europium, terbium, dysprosium, and samarium, are naturally occurring fluorophores, and their chelates have a number of applications in immunological and biological assays [8]. In lanthanide chelates, the lanthanide is the fluorescent label. It is held by chelation that permits conjugation with biological components. Since lanthanide chelates are not fluorescent when conjugated to biological components, a dissociative enhancement step is required to free the lanthanide ion from the conjugated chelate, to make a new and different ion complex that can generate measurable fluorescence, as in the DELFIA chemistry (EG&G Wallac, Turku, Finland). The exception is the LANCE (EG&G Wallac, Turku, Finland) chemistry, which has demonstrated a measurable signal in homogeneous form, but with a substantially diminished signal-to-noise ratio, relative to the DELFIA heterogeneous method [8]. Lanthanide chelates are subject to potential dissociation of the ion, which can undermine the integrity of the label, increasing background and nonspecific binding contributions. In addition, lanthanide chelates are subject to inactivation by EDTA, and require separation and washing steps for best results [9]. These limitations of chelates are overcome by the use of the novel family of lanthanide cryptates as fluorescent labels, for which Professor Jean Marie Lehn was awarded the 1987 Nobel Prize in Chemistry (shared with J. Pederson and D. Cram).

2. Cryptates as Fluorescent Labels

Lanthanide cryptates are formed by the inclusion of a lanthanide ion in the cavity of a macropolycyclic ligand containing 2,2'-bipyridine groups as light absorbers (Fig. 1). The cryptate can undergo intramolecular energy transfer when the cavitated species is europium (3+). The cage-like structure of the cryptate protects the central ion, making it stable in biological media. Well-known heterobifunctional reagents can be used to conjugate the diamine derivative of the europium tris-

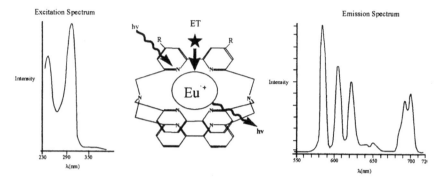

Figure 1 Europium trisbipyridine cryptate has an excitation peak at 337 nm and an emission peak at 620 nm.

bipyridine cryptate, (Eu)K, to biological assay components, such as proteins, peptides, receptors, nucleic acids, and antibodies without loss of reactivity. Even upon conjugation to such components, the photophysical properties of (Eu)K are conserved, making it particularly useful for homogeneous assays as a fluorescent label. No dissociation enhancement step is required, and cryptates are stable and kinetically very inert, as the activation energy required to reach the transition state of dissociation is significantly higher for cryptates than for chelates [10]. For (Eu)K excitation at 337 nm yields an emission spectrum with a strong peak at 620 nm, as shown in Figure 1 [11].

3.   Use of XL665 as Acceptor

The best choice for an acceptor molecule for the (Eu)K donor will complement the cryptate fluorescence energy spectrum, accept the transfer of energy efficiently, be stable in common assay media, and lend itself to appropriate chemistry for conjugation with biological components. For HTRF assays, the best choice for acceptor molecule is one of the main constituents of the phycobilisomes of red algae. These protein–pigment complexes absorb light and channel it to the cell's photosystem. In the phycobilisome, the last component that transfers light is allophycocyanin (APC), a phycobiliprotein of 105 kD with an absorption band ranging from 600 to 660 nm and an emission maximum at 660 nm. APC, when modified by cross-linking, emits at 665 nm and is called XL665 (Fig. 2).

XL665 has a high molar absorptivity at the cryptate emission wavelength, which enables very efficient energy transfer of about 75% for a donor–acceptor distance of 7.5 nm. Spectral emission is high where the cryptate signal is insignificant, making it particularly complementary (Fig. 3). The quantum yield of energy

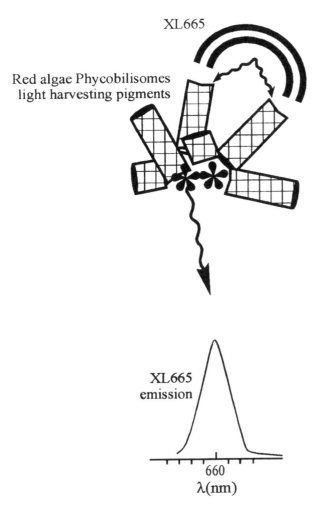

Figure 2 XL665, cross-linked allophycocyanin has a strong emission peak at 665 nm.

is high at about 70%. XL665 is stable and not quenched by the presence of biological media [11].

4. Signal Amplification of the Cryptate Fluorescence

Forster theory (1948) defines the nonradiative energy transfer that occurs between fluorescence resonance energy transfer (FRET) pairs, such as the (Eu)K donor

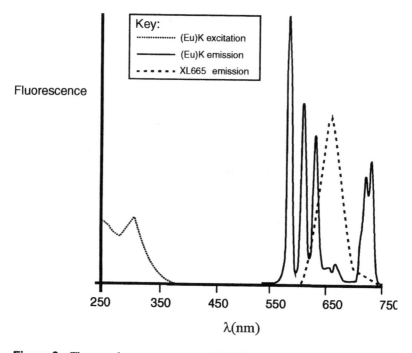

Figure 3   The complementary spectra of (Eu)K and XL665.

molecules and the XL665 acceptor molecules of HTRF. The efficiency of transfer is a function of the distance ($1/d^6$) between the donor and acceptor pairs [12]. Figure 4 illustrates the energy transfer between (Eu)K and XL665 in HTRF. (Eu)K excited separately has a spectrum that allows only about 60% of the signal to be measured. Paired with XL665, the signal is amplified by the transfer of energy to the XL665 spectrum, which provides a spectrum that allows one to measure essentially all emitted energy, at the shifted wavelength. Therefore, by being paired with XL665, the (Eu)K signal is effectively amplified [13].

C.   HTRF Signal and Measurement

The specific FRET pair of (Eu)K and XL665 exhibits both temporal and spectral emission characteristics that provide opportunities for measurement in unique ways. The Discovery HTRF microplate analyzer (Packard Instrument Company, Meriden, CT) was developed and optimized specifically for the detection of HTRF assays for HTS (Fig. 5). Since no separation occurs between bound and free assay

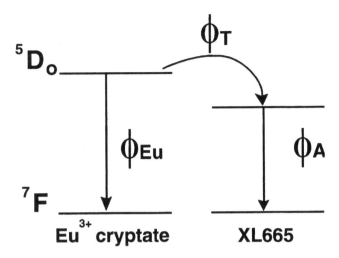

Figure 4 Energy transfer and amplification between (Eu)K and XL665. When the fluorescence is measured at the emission wavelength of the XL665, an amplification is obtained when (ϕ_A) $(\phi_T) > \phi_{EU}$, where ϕ_A, and ϕ_{EU} are the quantum yields of XL665 and europium ion, respectively, and ϕ_T is the transfer efficiency.

components, the signals from each individual fluorophore may be distinguished from the signal of the bound pair based on both time and wavelength. The Discovery takes into consideration the following characteristics of HTRF chemistry to make the most efficient and useful measurement.

1. Time-Resolved Measurement

Background and nonspecific fluorescence from microplates, media, and biological components has a short lifetime of emission. Unbound or isolated XL665 also emits a short-lived signal when excited at 337 nm. Unbound or isolated (Eu)K emits a long-lived signal at 620 nm, easily separated by optical discrimination. Together, the (Eu)K XL665 pair emits a long-lived signal at 665 nm (Fig. 6).

The Discovery excites each sample with a nitrogen laser excitation pulse at 337 nm. Measurements are taken after a 50-μsec delay, allowing any short-lived fluorescence to dissipate before the emission light is collected. Time-resolved fluorescence (TRF) measurement has been incorporated into a number of fluorometers, such as the Victor (EG&G Wallac) and the Analyst (LJL Biosystems), although the excitation sources vary.

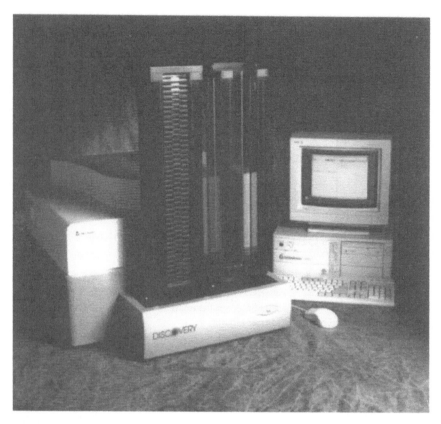

Figure 5 Discovery HTRF Microplate Analyzer. (Courtesy of Packard Instrument Company, Meriden, CT.)

2. Dual-Wavelength Measurement

Although time-resolved measurement is a feature now copied in and common to various vendors' instruments, simultaneous dual-wavelength detection is unique to the sophisticated Discovery instrument. Figure 7 illustrates the optical design of the Discovery used to make measurements of HTRF assays at 620 nm and 665 nm simultaneously. Together, time-resolved measurement and simultaneous dual-wavelength detection distinguishes the bound from free fluorophores. In addition, the extent to which binding has occurred can be measured independent of interference effects from media, biological components, and physical assay complications such as turbidity. Figure 8 shows the detection of an HTRF assay by the Dis-

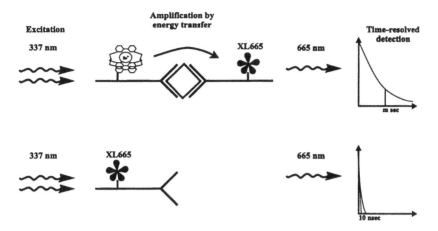

Figure 6 Principle of time-resolved detection of HTRF. The time delay of 50 μsec allows short-lived background fluorescence and the signal from free XL665 to dissipate.

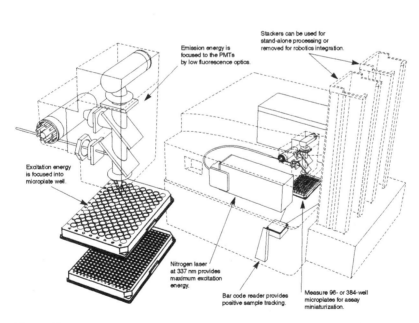

Figure 7 Optical configuration of the Discovery HTRF Microplate Analyzer. A nitrogen laser provides the excitation energy of 337 nm. Simultaneous dual wavelength detection provides measurements at 620 nm and 665 nm after a time delay.

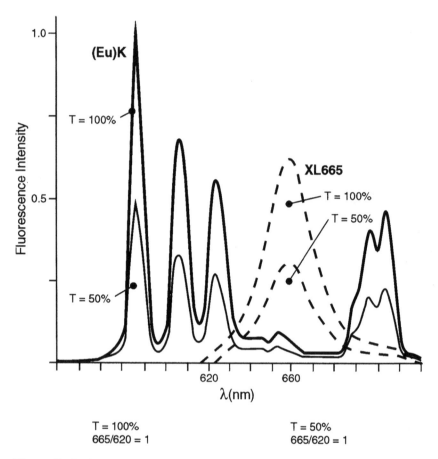

Figure 8 Ratio measurement of 620 nm and 665 nm wavelengths. The long-lived signals, 620 nm emission from free (Eu)K and the 665 nm emission from the bound (Eu)K and
XL665 pair, provide a method for correcting for color or turbity in the reaction.

covery. During the course of 1 sec per well, excitation by the nitrogen laser at 337
nm elicits a long-lived signal at 620 nm from free (Eu) K and long-lived signal at
665 nm from the europium cryptate bound to XL665 by biomolecular interaction
[6]. The ratio of the two simultaneous measurements is a specific measure of the
extent to which the labels are bound in the assay. Inhibitors of binding or enzyme
effects on the binding partners can be measured directly without separation of
individual assay components or biological media.

3.   Data Reduction

Assay data can be presented in terms of the ratio of the 665/620 nm measurements, R, to correct for any interference from media or absorption of excitation or emission wavelengths by the media. ΔR is the change in ratio that occurs with respect to the blank or negative sample. It is used to express the specific signal in the assay. ΔF is an instrument-independent measurement that shows the signal-to-noise ratio of the assay [14]. Both measurements utilize the patented ratio method of detection, which eliminates interference from test compounds, or turbidity of test samples. Discovery can provide raw 665-nm counts, raw 620-nm counts, or ratios. This patented technique is unique to HTRF measurement and is proprietary to this detection technology.

$$\Delta R = (\text{ratio of the sample} - \text{ratio of the negative sample}) \times 10,000 \qquad (1)$$

$$\Delta F = \frac{\Delta R}{\text{ratio of negative sample}} \times 100 \qquad (2)$$

The following sections describe recent and meaningful applications of HTRF chemistry for HTS.

III.   APPLICATIONS OF HTRF FOR HIGH-THROUGHPUT SCREENING

HTRF assays can be constructed using several formats. The direct-assay format requires that the binding partners of interest be directly conjugated to the (Eu)K and the XL665 fluorophores. The advantages of this format are that the assay optimization depends only on the particular interaction of the binding partners, with no consideration of antibody affinities. A disadvantage is that a substantial quantity of the binding partners is required because some material is lost in purification of direct conjugates. In addition, the integrity of the binding interaction may be affected by the direct conjugation. The more commonly used indirect method utilizes a high-affinity pair, like streptavidin/biotin, or antibodies specific to the binding partners to construct the assay. The semidirect method involves one directly labeled binding partner and another indirectly labeled partner [15].

HTRF assays are typically run in a 200-μl volume in a 96-well plate or 70-μl volume in a 384-well plate. The Discovery measures plates in either format. HTRF assay technology is not appropriate for intracellular assays but is particularly suitable for kinetic studies due to the fast read times and ability to measure each sample repeatedly over time. Most widely performed assays include immunoassays, enzyme assays, receptor binding assays with purified receptors or membrane fragments, protein–protein interactions, and nucleic acid hybridizations. The following are examples of HTRF assays and results as measured on the Discovery instrument.

A. Immunoassays

Immunoassays can be created using HTRF as it was first developed for clinical applications and sold under the name of TRACE chemistry by CIS Bio International. These are conducted as sandwich assays in which monoclonal antibodies raised against the target are conjugated directly with (Eu)K and XL665. The following example shows a comparison of the HTRF assay to a commonly used ELISA assay method.

The ELISA version of this cytokine assay requires the first antibody to be bound to the well of a microplate. The second antibody to the same cytokine is linked to the reporter enzyme [15]. This assay requires three separate wash steps, four reagent additions, four incubations, and can be used to screen a maximum of 10,000 assay points per day. The HTRF assay, as shown in Figure 9, requires no separation steps, one reagent addition, one incubation at room temperature, and can be used to screen up to 10,000 assay points in 2 hr. Samples contained red blood cells up to 5% by volume. Figure 10 shows the comparison of the OD of the ELISA assay at 405 nm with the ratio measurement of the HTRF assay. Both methods are capable of detecting picogram quantities of cytokine in complex samples; however, HTRF is considerably easier to perform for HTS purposes. An HTRF prolactin immunoassay has also been described previously [11].

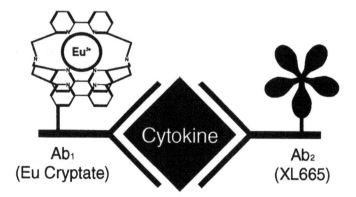

Figure 9 HTRF immunoassay configuration. Polyclonal antibodies are conjugated directly with (Eu)K and XL665. Presence of cytokine is measured by the binding of both antibodies.

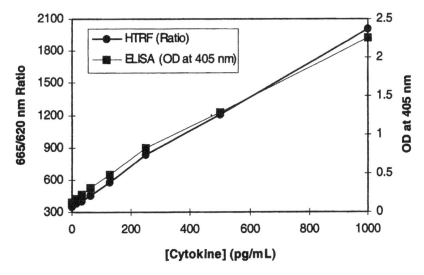

Figure 10 Comparison of ELISA and HTRF methods for detection of cytokines. Both are capable of picogram levels of detection, but the HTRF assay is fewer steps.

B. Enzyme Assays

Enzyme-mediated reactions that cleave, synthesize or modify compounds represent a significant group of targets for HTS. The HTRF assays can be constructed such that enzyme activity can be measured by the absence or presence of high signal. Protein tyrosine kinases play a critical role in the cellular signal transduction pathways, with significant implications for mechanisms of allograft rejection, allergic response, and autoimmune diseases. Hundreds of tyrosine kinases have been identified and many are still to be discovered through genomic research [17,18]. The following is an example of an HTRF tyrosine kinase assay.

Biotinylated polypeptide substrates are incubated with kinase enzymes to catalyze the phosphorylation reaction. Europium cryptate conjugated with PY20 antibody recognizes those peptides that are successfully phosphorylated. Streptavidin conjugated to XL665 binds to the biotinylated substrate, whether or not it is successfully phosphorylated. Those peptides that are phosphorylated effectively bring to together the HTRF pair such that a high signal is achieved upon excitation at 337 nm with the nitrogen laser of the Discovery (Fig. 11).

A number of known inhibitors were titrated against five src-family tyrosine kinases tested using this HTRF format. The IC_{50}s values obtained from the HTRF assay were very similar to those achieved using a comparable radiometric scintillation proximity assay (SPA) (Amersham, UK) [19]. Figure 12 shows the inhibition curves as measured by HTRF.

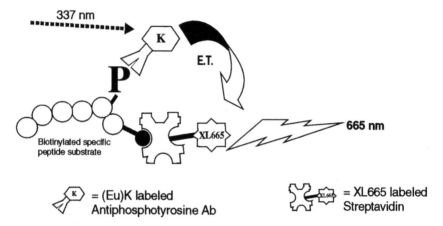

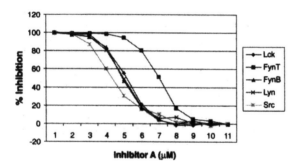

Figure 11 Tyrosine kinase assay using HTRF reagents. Biotinylated substrate binds streptavidin-XL665 and antiphosphotyrosine-(Eu)K recognizes those peptides that are phosphorylated.

Figure 12 Titration of kinase inhibitor for src-1 family of enzymes.

Sensitivity is a critical issue in HTS when the cost of reagents must be considered and the availability of enzyme and sample materials is limited. In order to determine sensitivity of the HTRF chemistry for kinase activity, varying concentrations of lck enzyme was added reactions containing peptide and ATP. At time points up to 80 min reactions were stopped and measured in the Discovery. As little as 20 pM lck enzyme gave significant results with a signal-to-noise background of 10:1 after 40 min (Fig. 13). This result demonstrates that the HTRF assay method provided about two orders of magnitude more sensitivity than the SPA assay method, making it the first nonradioisotopic alternative capable of yielding results that could be achieved previously only with the use of radioisotopes. The

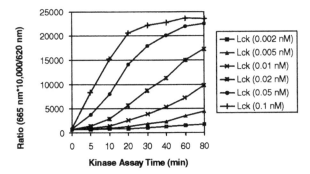

Figure 13   Time course of the lck kinase assay. Concentration of enzyme varies from 0.002 nM to 0.1 nm.

high sensitivity of this HTRF method saves both enzyme and library samples and enables screening of weaker inhibitors not easily measured by less sensitive methods such as SPA.

Additional examples of the application of HTRF specifically to kinase assays have been published [20,21]. Other HTRF enzyme assays that have been published include a viral protease assay [22] and a ubiquitination assay [23].

C. Receptor Binding Assays

Biomolecular interactions between nuclear receptors and their coactivators are associated with transcriptional regulation and are therefore seen also as an important target for HTS in drug discovery. Ligand binding promotes the association of nuclear receptors with nuclear proteins, such as CREB-binding protein (CBP) and steroid receptor coactivator (SRC-1), which are believed to function as coactivators of transcriptional activity [24]. Following is a description of how HTRF methods were used to characterize and screen for potential agonists to these ligand-dependent interactions.

Nuclear receptors contain a well-conserved, 200- to 300-mer amino acid ligand binding domain in which a number of functionalities are encoded, including ligand and coactivator binding and transactivation. The ligand binding domains (LBDs) of peroxisome proliferator–activated receptor (PPARγ) were used as a model in this study. PPARγ-LBD was expressed and purified as a GST fusion protein from *E. coli* strain DH5. Both coactivators CBP $_{1-453}$ (amino acids 1–453) and SRC-1 $_{568-780}$ (amino acids 568–780) were biotinylated [24].

In this assay, (Eu)K is covalently bound to anti-GST antibody to create (Eu)K-∞-GST for labeling the nuclear receptor. The secondary fluorophore, XL665, is covalently bound to streptavidin (SA-XL665) to label the biotinylated coactivators. Both SA-XL665 and (Eu)K-∞-GST are available as "generic" or

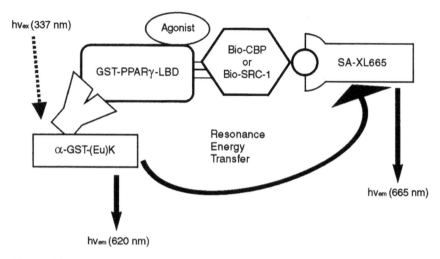

Figure 14 HTRF strategy for detection and quantification of interaction between receptor and coactivator.

"off-the-shelf" reagents from Packard Instrument Company. Figure 14 illustrates the indirect-assay format used to create the HTRF assay of nuclear receptors and coactivators. Agonist-induced interaction between the nuclear receptors and their coactivators brings the two fluorophores in proximity and results in a high signal.

Known agonists have been shown previously to activate ligands for PPARγ in mammalian cell–based assays [24]. Using the HTRF assay approach described above, increasing concentrations of thiazolidinediones (TZDs) were added to reaction mixtures. Figure 15 shows that TZDs induced a dose-dependent, specific interaction between PPARγ-LBD and the nuclear receptor binding domain of CBP with similar EC_{50}s values obtained by transactivation studies. This assay indicates that HTRF assay methods can provide a powerful alternative to cell-based assays for screening large compound libraries for potential agonist drug candidates [25].

D. Protein–Protein Interactions

A number of HTRF protein–protein interactions have been described previously. The JUN:FOS assay was done by directly labeling the FOS protein with (Eu)K and using biotinylated JUN to bind with the streptavidin-XL665 [26]. Now antispecies or antiepitope tag antibodies conjugated with (Eu)K are available and used more often than direct labeling and streptavidin-XL665 [14]. The following example is an HTRF protein–protein assay using the indirect method.

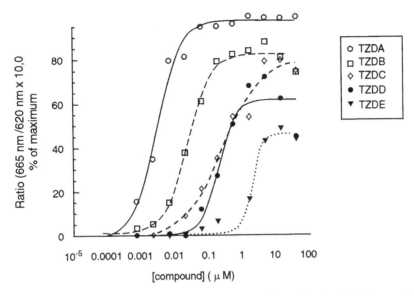

Figure 15   Effects of TDZs on PPARγ-CBP interactions using the HTRF approach.

Ligation of CD28 and CD86 leads to signals that are required for the production of interleukin-2, a process that is implicated in the regulation of T-cell anergy and programmed cell death [27–30]. An HTRF assay was constructed to screen for small-molecule antagonists of this interaction, which could be considered possible drug targets. The acceptor, XL665, was covalently bound to anti-human antibody that recognizes the Fc region. CD28 was expressed as a fusion protein to the human immunoglobulin (Ig) domain. The other binding partner, CD86, was expressed as a fusion protein with a rat Ig domain, recognized by biotinylated sheep anti-rat antibody. Streptavidin-EuK binds to complete the HTRF reaction [31] (Fig. 16).

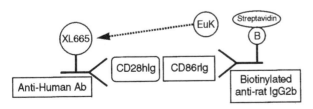

Figure 16   HTRF assay configuration for detection of small molecule inhibitors of CD28/CD86 interaction.

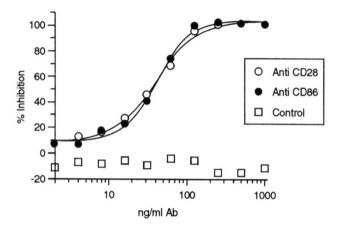

Figure 17 Dose response curves illustrating the inhibition of binding by blocking antibodies.

Dose–response curves were created with blocking antibodies that prove that the binding of CD28/CD86 proteins causes the signal generation (Fig. 17). Since the affinity of interaction between CD28 and CD80 was shown to be relatively low (200 nM–4 µM) by different methods [8,9], ELISA methods resulted in dissociation of the bound complex during washing and SPA methods required high levels of radioactivity. The HTRF method uses readily available generic reagents, was shown to be resistant to color quench effects, and requires few steps, thereby minimizing the errors associated with pipetting. In addition, this modular approach makes development of other related assays for specificity testing easier than direct-labeling approach [31].

Another published HTRF assay for measuring protein–protein interactions is given in "stoichiometry of a ligand-gated ion channel determined by fluorescence energy transfer" by Farrar et al. [32]. HTRF was used to elucidate the stoichiometry of subunits within an oligomeric cell surface receptor in a way that could be applied generally to other multisubunit cell surface proteins.

E. Nucleic Acid Hybridizations

DNA hybridization and related enzyme assays using nucleic acid binding partners can be conducted in solution using HTRF. A simple measure of hybridization was conducted using one oligonucleotide directly labeled with (Eu)K, while the complementary strand was biotinylated and labeled with streptavidin-XL665. The extent to which the complementary strands are bound can be measured by the HTRF signal that results from the proximity of the two fluorophores [11]. The following assays were more recently developed to measure nucleic acid–related enzyme activity.

1. DNA Nuclease Assay

A 21-bp oligonucleotide was directly labeled with (Eu)K on the 3′ end and biotinylated on the 5′ end. Streptavidin-XL665 was added to complete the FRET reaction (Fig. 18). Increasing amounts of DNase enzyme were added to show the specific signal decrease as activity increases. This assay may be used to screen for DNase inhibitors [33] (Fig. 19).

2. Reverse Transcriptase Assay

Inhibitors of reverse transcriptase activity remain a major target for viral research in drug discovery. The following HTRF assay configuration enables one to screen for increases of inhibition of enzyme activity in high throughput. Oligonucleotide primers labeled directly with (Eu)K are added to RNA templates (Fig. 20). Addition of RTase and biotinylated dUTP to nucleotide building blocks creates a biotinylated double-stranded molecule labeled with (Eu)K, to which streptavidin-XL665 is added to complete the reaction. Complete reverse transcriptase activity results in a high HTRF signal. Inhibition would decrease the signal to the extent to which the enzyme is blocked. Increasing amounts of reverse transcriptase enzyme results in higher activity as the HTRF fluorophores are brought into proximity while the double-stranded molecules form [30,34] (Fig. 21).

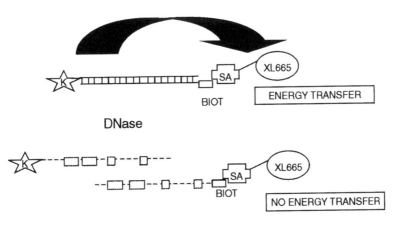

Figure 18   HTRF assay for the detection of nuclease activity.

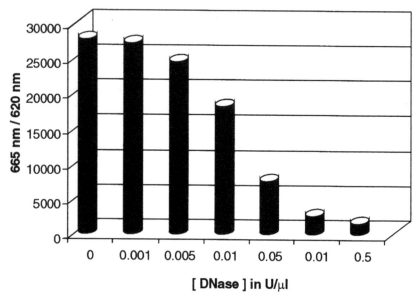

Figure 19   Increasing amounts of DNase enzyme decreases the HTRF signal.

IV.   HTRF ASSAY OPTIMIZATION

The following sections are included to provide insight into how one might best develop and optimize an HTRF assay. HTRF assays are normally performed with only a few steps, mainly additions, so there are a smaller number of considerations when designing an HTRF assay than there may be with a more complicated method. The main considerations for optimizing an HTRF assay are buffer selection, whether label (Eu)K or XL665 should be used for each assay component, and what controls should be run.

A.   Buffer Selection and Stability

Homogeneous assays by nature involve no washing step, so that all buffer and assay components are present during the ultimate measurement of activity or binding. As a result, the following work has been done to help determine how HTRF assays, specifically the (Eu)K component, are likely to perform in various buffers. Europium cryptate was added to 200-μl samples of the most commonly used buffers, with and without 50 mM potassium fluoride (KF). Potassium fluoride provides a Fms ion, which has been shown to form ion pairs with Eu^{3+}. Fluorescence

Reverse Assay Format

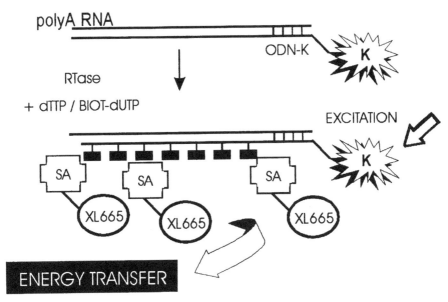

Figure 20   HTRF Reverse transcriptase assay configuration.

lifetime was measured to determine if KF had an affect on the stability of the signal of the (Eu)K component as measured at its emission peak of 620 nm. Figure 22 shows that in all cases lifetime of the signal from the (Eu)K label was stabilized and, in effect, equalized by the presence of fluoride ions, illustrating the protective effect of the F^- ion.

B.   Choice of Label for Each Assay Component

Europium cryptate and XL665 are both available conjugated with streptavidin, biotin, antispecies, and antiepitope antibodies, as well as a number of other biological components. However, the following recommendations apply. Due to the difference in sizes of the fluorophores, it is better to use europium cryptate label on the smaller assay component and the XL665 on the larger assay component. In terms of the smaller component, if it can be biotinylated, it is likely acceptable to label it with europium cryptate. XL665 should be used on the component that is

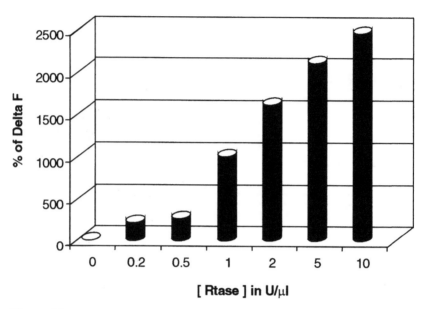

Figure 21   Increasing amounts of reverse transcriptase enzyme increase the HTRF signal.

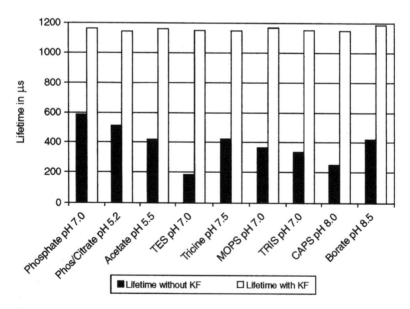

Figure 22   Effects of various buffers and KF on stability of (Eu)K.

in excess in the assay, and europium cryptate should be used on that component that is most sensitive to change.

C. Suggested Assay Controls

For the purposes of assay development and analysis of screening results, the following controls should be run for each assay. A buffer blank should be created that includes buffer only at the volume of the assay. A (Eu)K blank should be included that contains buffer and europium cryptate at the concentration used in the assay. This control enables one to do a (Eu)K background subtract or "K blank" subtract out the small peak that exists at the 665-nm wavelength. Finally, as always, a negative control should be created that includes total assay conditions with something to make it negative, like completely inhibited or inactivated. Using ratio and ΔF calculations and the above controls helps get the most reproducible and precise data from the HTRF assay.

V. CONCLUSION

HTRF chemistry was developed to help overcome some of the obstacles to HTS in general. It is homogeneous, so that separation steps are eliminated. It is fluorescent in nature but has the time-resolved, simultaneous, dual-wavelength detection that enables one to achieve high fluorescent signal with extremely low backgrounds. HTRF is best measured on the Discovery HTRF microplate analyzer because it was designed specifically and optimized for the particular wavelengths of HTRF. However, a number of detection systems are now available for measuring TRF and HTRF applications. The HTRF reagent list is growing; thus, fewer assays require customized conjugation with (Eu)K and XL665. Many of the applications described utilize off-the-shelf reagents that are readily available and require no license fee. As a result, this tool is widely accepted in the literature as one of the few truly homogeneous methods available to meet the HTS demands of drug discovery today.

REFERENCES

1. Fox S. Packard applies HTRF tool to high-throughput screens. Genet Eng News 1996;16(19).
2. Upham L. Conversion of 96-well assays to 384-well homogeneous assays. Biomedical Products (HTS supplement) 1999; Jan. p. 10–11.
3. Park YW, Garyantes T, Cummings RT, Carter-Allen K. Optimization of ^{33}P scintillation proximity assays using cesium chloride bead suspension. TopCount Topics TCA-030. Packard Instrument Company, 1997.

4. Lakowicz JR. Principles of Fluorescence Spectroscopy, 2nd ed. New York: Plenum Publishing, 1999.

5. Mathis G. Rare earth cryptates and homogeneous fluoroimmunoassays with human sera. Clin Chem 1993;39(9):1953.

6. Packard Instrument Company. The principles of time-resolved fluorescence. Application Note HTRF-001, 1997.

7. U.S. Patent 5,527,684.

8. Hemmilä I, Hill S, Elcock C. Development and optimization of robust assays using lanthanide based time-resolved fluorescence detection. Drug Disc Technol '98, London, UK. April 27–30, 1998.

9. Alpha B, Lehn J, Mathis G. Energy transfer luminescence of europium(III) and terbium(III) cryptates of macrocyclic polypyridine ligands. Angew Chem Int Ed Engl 1987;26:266.

10. Mathis G. Counterpoint: HTRF technology. J Biomol Screening 1999;4(6):309–313.

11. Kolb A, Burke J, Mathis G. Homogeneous, time-resolved fluorescence method for drug discovery. In: Assay Technologies and Detection Methods. New York: Marcel Dekker, 1997:345–360.

12. Forster T. Zwischen molekare energiewanderung und fluoreszenz Ann Physik 1948;2:55.

13. Mathis G. Amplification by energy transfer and homogeneous time-resolved immunoassay. Sixth International Symposium on Quantitative Luminescence Spectrometry in BioMedical Sciences, University of Ghent, Belgium, 1993.

14. Upham L. HTRF Epitope tag antibody reagents for assay development and high throughput screening. Application note AN4003-DSC, Packard Instrument Company, July 1999.

15. Wild D. The Immunoassay Handbook. New York: Stockton Press, 1994.

16. Upham LV. Three HTRF methods provide sensitivity for miniaturization in high thoughput screening. Lab Robot Automat 1999;11:324–329.

17. Hanks ST, Quinn AM, Hunter T. Science 1988;241:42–51.

18. Hanks ST, Hunter T. FASEB J 1995;9:576–596.

19. Park YW, Cummings RT, Wu L, Zheng S, Cameron PM, Woods A, Zaller DM, Marcy AI, Hermes JD. Homogeneous proximity tyrosine kinase assays: scintillation proximity assay versus homogeneous time-resolved fluorescence. Anal Biochem 1999;269:94–104.

20. Rogers MV. Light on high-througput screening: fluorescence-based assay technologies. Drug Discovery Today, 1997;2:156–160.

21. Kolb AJ, Kaplita PV, Hayes DJ, Park YW, Pernell C, Major JS, Mathis G. Tyrosine kinase assays adapted to homogeneous time-resolved fluorescence. Drug Disc Today 1998;3:333–342.

22. Cummings RT, McGovern HM, Zheng S, Park YW, Hermes JD. Use of a phosphotyrosine-antibody pair as a general detection method in homogeneous time-resolved fluorescence: application to human immunodeficiencey viral protease. Anal Biochem 1999;269:79–93.

23. Yabuki N, Watanabe SI, Kudoh T. Nihira SI, Miyamoto C. Application of homogeneous time-resolved fluorescence (HTRF) to monitor poly-ubiquitination of wild-type p53. Comb Chem High-Throughput Screening 1999;2:279–287.

24. Lehmann JM, Moore LB, Smith-Oliver TA, Wilkison WO, Wilson TM, Kliewer SA. An antidiabetic thiazolidinedione is a high affinity ligand for peroxisome proliferator-activated receptor γ. J Biol Chem 270:12953–12956.

25. Zhou G, Cummings RT, Li Y, Mitra S, Wilkinson HA, Elbrecht A, Hermes JD, Schaeffer JM, Smith RG, Moller DE. Nuclear receptors have distinct affinities for coactivators: characterization by fluorescence resonance energy transfer. Mol Endocrinol 1998;12:1594–1604.

26. Mathis G, Preaudat M, Trinquet E, Pernelle C, Trouillas M. A new homogeneous method using rare earth cryptate and amplification by energy transfer for the characterization of the FOS and JUN leucine zipper peptides dimerization. Fourth Annual Conference of the Society for Biomolecular Screening. Philadelphia, September 1994.

27. Ellis JH, Burden MN, Vinogradov DV, Linge C, Crowe JS. Interactions of CD80 and CD86 with CD28 and CTLA4. J Immunol 1996;56:2700.

28. June CH, Bluestone JA, Nadler LM, Thompson CB. The B7 and CD28 receptor families. Immunol Today 1994;15:321.

29. Linsley PS. Distinct roles for CD28 and cytotoxic T lymphocyte-assocoiated molecule-4 receptors during T cell activation? J Exp Med 1995;182:289.

30. Lenschow DJ, Walunas TL, Bluestone JA. CD28/B7 system of T cell costimulation. Annu Rev Immunol 1996;14:233.

31. Mellor GW, Burden MN, Preaudat M, Joseph Y, Cooksley SB, Ellis JH, Banks MN. Development of a CD28/CD86 (B7-2) binding assay for high throuput screening by homogeneous time-resolved fluorescence. J Biomol Screening 1998;3:91–99.

32. Farrar SJ, Whiting PJ, Bonnert TP, McKernan R. Stoichiometry of a ligand-gated ion channel determined by fluorescence energy transfer. J Biol Chem 1999;274:15:10100–10104.

33. Alpha-Bazin B, Mathis G. New Homogeneous assay formats for the measurement of nuclease and reverse transcriptase activity. Fourth Annual Conference of the Society for Biomolecular Screening, Baltimore, September 21–24, 1998.

34. Alpha-Bazin B, et al. Europium cryptate tethered nucleoside triphosphate for non-radioactive labeling and HTRF detection of DNA and RNA. Fifth Annual Conference of the Society for Biomolecular Screening, Edinburgh, Scotland, September 13–16, 1999.

12

ADME-Tox Screening in Drug Discovery

Albert P. Li
In Vitro Technologies, Inc.
Baltimore, Maryland

I. INTRODUCTION

With the advances in combinatorial chemistry, genomics, and high-throughput screening assays for therapeutic targets, the discovery of chemical entities with potential therapeutic properties has become extremely efficient. There is no longer a lack of "hits" once a molecular therapeutic target has been identified. The question now is, of the many hits, how does one choose a drug candidate that will be most likely to be successful in the clinic?

A. Why Drugs Fail in the Clinic

Drugs fail in the clinic for two major reasons: inefficacy and toxicity. ADME-tox properties—absorption, distribution, metabolism, elimination, toxicity—are critical factors in both of these major causes of failure. Inefficacy can be due to the inability of a drug candidate to be delivered to the desired target tissue. For instance, an oral drug can fail if it cannot be effectively absorbed into the systemic circulation or if it is rapidly eliminated after absorption and therefore can not reach the therapeutic concentration. A drug often is withdrawn after clinical trials due to unexpected toxicity. There are many cases in which a commercial drug is withdrawn from the market due to toxicological implications.

Withdrawal of a drug candidate at the stage of clinical trial or withdrawal of a drug after commercialization is extremely costly. In fact, I believe that before one chooses a drug candidate for preclinical development, one should have enough information to ensure that the drug will have appropriate ADME-tox properties in both laboratory animals and human beings.

B. Challenges with Accurate Prediction of Human Drug Properties

A major challenge that we face in choosing a drug candidate is the difficulty in predicting human drug properties. Experimentation with laboratory animals obviously is not adequate, as most drug candidates that fail in the clinic are chosen after favorable results have been obtained in laboratory animals during preclinical trials. That laboratory animals and human subjects differ in ADME-tox drug properties is well established. A major reason for the species–species differences in drug properties, besides such physical factors as size, is the differences in drug-metabolizing enzymes. For instance, it is now known that laboratory animals and humans have major differences in the major drug-metabolizing enzymes such as the cytochrome P450 isoforms. The involvement of different enzymes in the metabolism of a drug candidate in a rat and a human will lead to differences in the rate of metabolic clearance and in the profile of the metabolites, resulting in different levels of toxicological effects.

As species differences in drug metabolism is believed to be a major factor responsible for the known species–species differences in drug toxicity, an experimental system containing human drug-metabolizing enzymes should be useful in the prediction of human drug properties.

C. Optimization of Drug Properties

The old paradigm of drug discovery and development is to first find a chemical moiety with the appropriate pharmacological activity and to then subject the moiety through vigorous animal models for the evaluation of ADME-tox properties. One would hope for appropriate bioavailability and low toxicological properties. This "cross your fingers and hope for the best" tactic is highly inefficient in two aspects: (1) the preclinical animal studies are expensive and time-consuming and (2) as described earlier, because of species–species differences, a drug that is found to have acceptable properties in laboratory animals may still be problematic in man.

The emerging paradigm of drug discovery now is to include ADME-tox screening using human-based experimental systems in the selection of lead chemical entities for further development. The lead chemicals chosen for further development after such a screen would have both acceptable pharmacological and ADME-tox properties, and therefore should have a higher probability of success in the clinic than drug candidates that are not "optimized."

II. EXPERIMENTAL SYSTEMS FOR THE OPTIMIZATION OF ADME-TOX PROPERTIES

For the past years, human-based ADME-tox systems have been developed for the evaluation of human-specific drug properties. Recently, these systems have been applied early in the drug discovery phase to aid the selection of lead molecules for further development. In general, the assays are used to optimize for intestinal absorption, metabolic stability, toxicity, and drug–drug interaction potential.

A. Intestinal Absorption

Oral delivery is the most desirable route of drug administration. Therefore, it is important to develop drugs that can be absorbed effectively through the intestinal mucosa. Intestinal mucosa permeability of a chemical depends on its physical properties such as lipophilicity, which can be estimated based on the chemical, partitioning properties from aqueous phase to organic phase. In general, octanol-water partitioning (log P) is used to describe a chemical's lipophilicity and therefore its permeability through the lipid bilayer cell membrane. The knowledge of log P and also pK_a will help one to estimate the permeability of a chemical through the intestinal mucosa with a certain degree of success.

Besides passive diffusion, a chemical may be absorbed via energy-dependent processes such as active transport. Furthermore, after a chemical enters the intestinal mucosa, it can be removed from the cell via a transporter called P-glycoprotein (Pgp). Pgp is responsible for the multiple drug resistance of cancer cells. In intestinal mucosa cells, Pgp is responsible for the low oral availability of drugs that are its substrates, as these drugs are transported back into the intestinal lumen (efflux) after absorption by Pgp.

1. In Vitro Models for the Prediction of Intestinal Permeability

Physicochemical factors such as pK_a, lipophilicity, and solubility are important and can be measured. However, intestinal permeability cannot be predicted from these values alone. For the screening of a large number of chemicals, an in vitro model of the intestinal mucosa is needed. These models include artificial membranes (immobilized artificial membranes) and cell-based permeability models.

As artificial membranes have no biological activities, they simply represent a chemical diffusion model and will not be discussed further here. The application of artificial membranes in drug screening has been previously reviewed (Yang et al., 1997; Lundahl and Beigi, 1997; Kansy et al., 1998).

Here I will concentrate on the well-accepted cell-based model for intestinal permeability: the Caco-2 cell system. Another promising cell-based model is the Madin Darby canine kidney (MDCK) cells. The MDCK model will not be discussed here. Caco-2 cells are in general believed to be more appropriate than MDCK cells because (1) the expression of transporter proteins is much lower than that in Caco-2 cells and (2) the Caco-2 cell is of human origin whereas the MDCK cell is of canine origin. However, extensive research is being carried out on the incorporation of human transporters in MDCK cells (Pastan et al., 1988; Zhang and Benet, 1998; Soldner et al., 1999) to enhance the application of these cells in the prediction of human intestinal drug uptake.

2.   Caco-2 Screening Assay for Intestinal Absorption

A wealth of data have been collected on the barrier characteristics of Caco-2 cells. These cells, although originated from a human colon adenocarcinoma (Fogh et al., 1977), are found to behave like normal, differentiated enterocytes when cultured as confluent cells. The confluent monolayer culture has tight cell junctions and are found to express the active efflux protein Pgp.

The cells are routinely cultured in transwells for drug uptake studies. In a transwell culture, the cells are grown on a semipermeable membrane. After confluency, the drug to be evaluated is added to the medium above the Caco-2 cells (lumen or A compartment). Uptake of the drug is then monitored by quantifying the amount of the drug in the medium on the opposite side of the membrane (basolateral or B compartment). A-to-B transport is then calculated by the ratio of the amount of drugs in the basolateral compartment to that in the lumen compartment. The Caco-2 system can be used to evaluate uptake of drugs across the cytoplasm (transcellular uptake), between cells (paracellular uptake), as well as uptake involving transporters (active uptake). The role of Pgp in the uptake of a particular drug can also be evaluated via the use of a known Pgp inhibitor, such as verapamil. Uptake of a Pgp substrate (e.g., vinblastine) would be enhanced by the inhibition of its efflux from the Caco-2 cells in the presence of the Pgp inhibitor.

The advantages of the Caco-2 system include the abundance of published information concerning the cells, the overall good correlation with drug absorption potential in human in vivo, and the presence of active transporters such as Pgp (Stewart et al., 1995; Gan et al., 1998; Chong et al., 1997). The limitations of the Caco-2 system include the following:

1.   High laboratory-to-laboratory variation in results has been observed. This is believed to be mainly a function of the subpopulations of the cells that each laboratory has, as well as other technical factors such as passage number and culture conditions. A possible solution to this problem is to establish a universal stock of Caco-2 cells as well as a single procedure for the culturing of the cells and the performance of the assay.

2.   The routine procedure for a differentiated confluent cell layer is to culture the cells for 21 days. This "21-day" system is difficult due to pos-

sible contamination of the cultures during this prolonged culture period. Several laboratories, including ours, have developed conditions that would allow the Caco-2 cells to express differentiated properties after a shorter period of time. In our laboratory, a proprietary 3-day culture system has been developed.

3. Permeability, measured either by electrical resistance or the permeability of probe substrates, appears to be significantly higher in Caco-2 cells than in ileum.

The application of Caco-2 cells in drug discovery is the rank ordering of compounds based on permeability. The throughput for this screening is enhanced by several key technological advancements: (1) development of 3-day culture systems; (2) automation of cell culture; and (3) automation of permeability assay.

To minimize day-to-day variations in response, we have painstakingly standardized our procedures in the Caco-2 cell culture (Li et al., 2001). A large number of vials of cells from a single passage have been cryopreserved for experimentation. Cells are passaged using standardized procedures including split ratio, cell density at plating, and feeding frequencies. A 3-day culturing procedure is used for the development of confluent and differentiated monolayers. A comparison of permeability for Caco-2 cells cultured as 3-day cultures and the standard 21-day cultures is shown in Figure 1.

The protocol outline for the screening of intestinal absorption is shown in Table 1. In our laboratory, we routinely use 3-day Caco-2 cells cultured on 24-well transwells for high-throughput permeability studies. Transmembrane resistance, mannitol/propranolol permeability, and Pgp activity (measure by the evaluation of vinblastine permeability in the presence and absence of the Pgp inhibitor, verapamil) are used for the evaluation of cell quality. In general, the chemicals are evaluated at a single concentration of 50 μM. Higher concentrations may also be used, but solubility and cytotoxicity can be complicating factors at higher concentrations. Transport from A to B (apical to basal) is used for the evaluation of permeability, using LC/MS as the standard analytical tool to quantify the amount transported. The reproducibility of the 3-day Caco-2 permeability is illustrated by results from our laboratory with 10 compounds performed in 5 independent experiments. All five experiments show the same rank ordering of the 10 compounds in permeability, thereby supporting the use of this assay for routine screening (Fig. 2).

B. Drug Metabolism

An orally delivered drug will be subjected first to metabolism by the drug-metabolizing enzymes in the intestinal mucosa. The metabolites as well as the unmetabolized parent, once absorbed, are firstly carried by the blood into the liver, where extensive biotransformation occurs. Biotransformation controls several key drug properties, including metabolic stability, toxicity, and drug–drug interaction

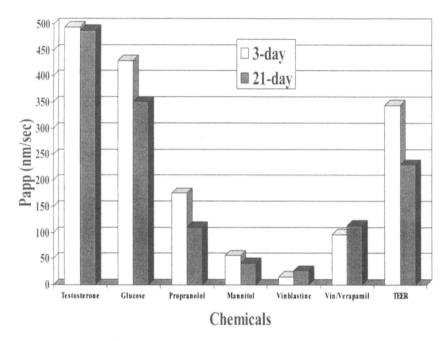

Figure 1 Permeability (Papp) of model chemicals in Caco-2 cells cultured as the conventional 21-day culture and as 3-day culture using a proprietary protocol developed in our laboratory. The chemicals chosen are known to permeate through Caco-2 monolayer cultures transcellularly (testosterone), via active transport (glucose), and paracellularly (propranolol and mannitol). Vinblastine is a Pgp substrate and verapamil is a Pgp inhibitor. The enhanced permeability of vinblastine in the presence of verapamil therefore reflects the presence of Pgp in both the 21-day and 3-day cultures. The transepithelial electrical resistance (TEER) values of the two cultures are also presented.

potential. Approaches to screen for these metabolically related drug properties are presented here.

1. Drug Metabolism Pathways

It is important to describe the major drug-metabolizing enzymes before proceeding to the rationale behind the selection of various screening systems. Drug metabolism in general is divided into two major pathways: phase I oxidation and phase II conjugation.

    1.   Phase I oxidation: During phase I oxidation, the relatively hydrophobic organic molecules are oxidized, mainly by the cytochrome P450s (CYP), a family of heme-containing proteins. In humans, the major CYP isoforms are 1A2, 2C9, 2C19, 2D6, 2E1, and 3A4. CYP3A4 has

Table 1 Screening for Intestinal Absorption in Caco-2 Cells

Experimental model: Caco-2 cells plated in transwells in 24-well tissue culture plates.
Incubation conditions: Caco-2 cells are plated in individual transwells in 24-well tissue culture plates and cultured to establish the cultures. After 3 days, the cells are tested for electrical resistance (ER) as a measure of the formation of tight junctions between cells. Only cells with an ER of $\geq 200\ \Omega \cdot cm^2$ will be used. Test article (at 1 concentration) is applied to the apical side of Caco-2 cells and incubated for 45 min (37°C, 5% CO_2).
Test article concentration: 50 μM
Replicates: $N = 2$
Controls: Mannitol (low permeability), propranolol (high permeability), and vinblastine (Pgp substrate) with and without verapamil (Pgp inhibitor).
Analysis: The medium from the basolateral well is analyzed using LC/MS to quantify the amount of test article transported.

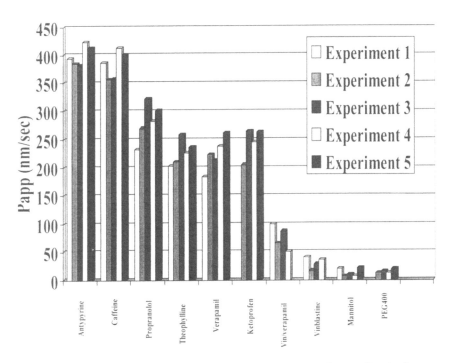

Figure 2. Permeability of 10 compounds in 5 independent experiments. Results demonstrate the high reproducibility of the 3-day Caco-2 culture for the evaluation of permeability. These 10 compounds are chosen from a list of compounds recommended for the validation of Caco-2 permeability assay by the U. S. Food and Drug Administration.

been shown to metabolize more than 50% of existing drugs. All of these CYP isoforms are present in the human liver, with CYP3A4 also present in the intestinal mucosa. It is now realized that other oxidative pathways, such as flavin monooxygenases (FMOs), can also play important roles in phase I oxidation. The FMO family of proteins include a minimum of five members: FMO1, FMO2, FMO3, FMO4, and FMO5, with FMO3 being the major isoform expressed in human livers. Phase I oxidation in some cases would result in the generation of reactive metabolites, which may lead to serious toxicological consequences

2. Phase II conjugation: During phase II conjugation, the parent xenobiotic or its phase I metabolites are conjugated to highly polar small molecules such as glucose (glucuronidation), sulfate (sulfation), and glutathione (GSH conjugation). Glucuronidation is carried out by the microsomal enzyme UDP-glucuronosyltransferase (UGT). Sulfation is carried out by cytosolic sulfotransferases: phenol sulfotransferase (PST) and estrogen sulfotransferase (EST). Phase II enzymes are also abundant in the liver.

Orally delivered drugs are firstly subjected to metabolism in the intestinal mucosa, which is now known to contain a high concentration of the 3A4 isoform of cytochrome P450. The metabolites plus the parent molecules that enter the systemic circulation are then further subjected to metabolism in the liver. The parent drug and its metabolites are then subjected to elimination either into feces via bile excretion in the liver, or into urine via the kidneys. In the kidney, further metabolism may occur. Drug metabolism is critical to three important drug properties: metabolic stability, toxicity, and drug–drug interaction.

a. Metabolic Stability. A successful drug candidate will have an appropriate metabolic stability. Too low a stability would cause difficulties in achieving a steady desirable plasma concentration. An ideal drug is one that is metabolically inert but is readily eliminated from the body at a reasonable rate.

b. Toxicity. Metabolism can both decrease and increase the toxicity of a drug candidate. The metabolic process may be detoxifying, turning a toxic parent drug into a nontoxic metabolite. An example is terfenadine, a nonsedative antihistamine with cardiotoxic potential that is metabolized to the nontoxic and rapidly eliminated acid metabolite. On the other hand, the metabolic process can lead to the formation of toxic metabolites. For instance, acetaminophen is metabolized to the highly toxic quinone metabolites.

c. Drug–drug Interaction. Coadministered drugs may affect each other's metabolism, leading to serious problems (Li and Jurima-Romet, 1997a). For instance, terfenadine, a nondrowsy antihistamine used for the treatment of allergy symptoms, is known to be affected by the antifungal ketoconazole. Ketoconazole, a potent inhibitor of CYP3A4, can inhibit the metabolism of terfenadine, thereby elevating plasma terfenadine to cardiotoxic levels. This type of interaction, where one drug inhibits the metabolism of a coadministered drug, is called an inhibitory drug–drug interaction. Another type of drug–drug interaction is inductive drug–drug interaction. Rifampin, a macrolide antibiotic, is known to be a potent inducer of several drug-metabolizing enzymes, especially CYP3A4. Rifampin is known to reduce plasma level of coadministered drugs that are metabolized by the enzyme pathways that it induces. The affected drugs include ethinylestradiol (EE2) (substrate of CYP3A4, UDP-glucuronyltransferase (UGT), and estrogen sulfotransferase (EST), Li et al., 1999b; Song et al., 1998), cyclosporine (substrate of CYP3A4), and prednisolone (substrate of CYP3A4). While inhibitory drug–drug interactions would lead to toxicity due to the unexpected elevation of the plasma level of the affected drug, inductive drug–drug interactions would lead to nonefficacy due to the reduction of the plasma level of the affected drug to nonefficacious levels. In either case, serious adverse effects can be precipitated that sometimes may lead to death.

2. In Vitro Hepatic Experimental Systems for Drug Metabolism

Screening for metabolic stability can be performed with in vitro systems containing metabolic enzymes. As the liver is the major organ for drug metabolism and often the target of drug toxicity, in the past decade several in vitro hepatic experimental systems have been developed. These include the following:

1. *Liver-S9:* The supernatant of the liver homogenate after centrifugation at $9000g$ is a commonly used source of liver drug metabolizing enzymes. The S-9, also called postmitochondrial supernatant, contains cytosolic enzymes as well as microsomal enzymes (see below). Liver S-9 from rats treated with P450 inducers (e.g., Arolclor 1254) has been used commonly as an exogenous metabolic activating system for in vitro genotoxicity assays. By selecting different cofactors, liver S-9 can be used to study phase I or phase II metabolism. For phase I oxidation, NADPH-regenerating system is used as cofactor. For phase II conjugation, one can use UDPGA as cofactor for glucuronidation, and PAPS as cofactor for sulfate conjugation.

2. *Microsomes:* Microsomes are membrane vesicles of the endoplasmic reticulum that can be prepared by centrifugation of the liver S-9 at $100,000g$. The microsomal pellet consists of both rough and smooth endoplasmic reticulum. As all CYPs are present in the smooth endoplasmic reticulum, microsomes are routinely used to evaluate CYP-mediated phase I oxidation, using NADPH-regenerating system as cofactor. As UDPGT is also an endoplasmic reticulum-bound enzyme, phase II glucuronidation can be studied using UDPGA as cofactor.

3. *Hepatocytes:* Hepatocytes are intact parenchymal cells of the liver that
    can be isolated at high viability. Hepatocyte isolation is accomplished
    using collagenase digestion and can be purified against nonparenchy-
    mal cells by differential centrifugation. Intact hepatocytes probably
    represent the most physiologically relevant model of the liver as the
    cells are self-sufficient in cofactors and contain all of the drug-metabo-
    lizing enzymes in the liver. Also, as hepatocytes are live cells, they can
    be used to evaluate toxic potential. Hepatocytes, especially human
    hepatocytes, represent an attractive experimental system for the evalu-
    ation of drug properties (Fabre et al., 1990; Guillouzo et al., 1997, 1998;
    Li, 1994, 1997). Because of the general difficulty in the availability of
    fresh human livers, research with human hepatocytes had been limited
    until the recent development of successful cryopreservation procedures
    (Li et al., 1999a, 1999c; Hengstler et al., 2000). Cryopreserved human
    hepatocytes can be used routinely as short-term (up to approximately 6
    hr) suspension cultures for the evaluation of drug metabolism,
    inhibitory drug–drug interactions, and cytotoxicity (Li et al., 1999a).
    The similarity between freshly isolated and cryopreserved human hepa-
    tocytes in phase I P450 isoform activities and phase II glucuronidation
    and sulfation activities are shown in Figure 3.
4. *Liver slices:* Precision-cut liver slices are mechanically generated, thin
    (200–300 μm thick) slices of the liver. Liver slices have the same
    advantages of the hepatocytes, consisting of intact liver cells with com-
    plete metabolic pathways and cofactors. A further advantage is the pres-
    ence of nonparenchymal cells, which may be important for certain
    aspects of toxicity (e.g., cytokine-induced apoptosis). The major disad-
    vantage is the artifactual diffusion barrier for cells in the center of the
    slice. In general, liver slices are adequate for qualitative studies in drug
    metabolism but may underestimate the rate of metabolism for chemi-
    cals with diffusion problems.

3. Screening Assays for Metabolic Stability

Screening assays for metabolic stability are routinely performed using either
human liver microsomes or cryopreserved human hepatocytes.

1. *Microsome screen:* As most xenobiotics (approximately 70%) are
    metabolized by microsomal enzymes such as CYP450 isoforms, human
    liver microsomes are used routinely for the evaluation of metabolic sta-
    bility (Carlile et al., 1999; Obach, 1999; Obach et al., 1997; Iwatsubo
    et al., 1996; Kanamitsu et al., 2000). A typical screening assay (Table
    2) is the incubation of a single concentration (e.g., 10 μM) of com-
    pounds for a single time period (e.g., 30 min) in buffer containing

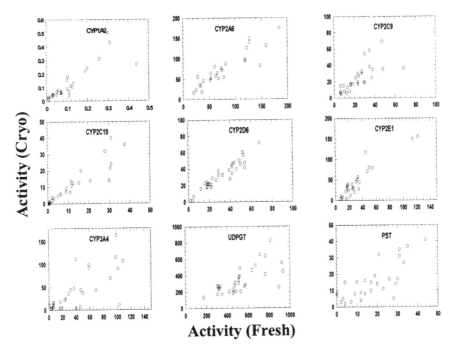

Activity (Fresh)

Figure 3 Effects of cryopreservation on xenobiotic metabolism enzyme activities in human hepatocytes. Activities from human hepatocytes isolated from 30 donors were shown. The activities after cryopreservation were plotted against activities of the same lots of hepatocytes before cryopreservation. The results show that hepatocytes had similar activities before and after cryopreservation. The activities evaluated were phenacetin O-deethylation (CYP1A2), coumarin 7-hydroxylation (CYP2A6), tolbutamide 4-hydroxyla-tion (CYP2C9), S-mephenytoin 6-hydroxylation (CYP2C19), dextromethorphan O-demethylation (CYP2D6), chlorzoxazone 6-hydroxylation (CYP2E1), testosterone 6-hydroxylation (CYP3A4), umbelliferone glucuronidation (UDPGT), and umbelliferone sulfation (PST).

microsomes and cofactors, followed by measurement of disappearance of the parent molecule. LC/MS is the analytical instrument of choice for the quantification of parent disappearance.

2. *Hepatocyte screen:* The success in cryopreservation allows hepato-cytes, especially human hepatocytes, to be used in screening assays. The advantage of hepatocytes is the presence of practically all of the liver metabolism pathways in these cells. While microsomal systems measure mainly phase I oxidation, hepatocytes can perform both phase I and phase II pathways. Some drugs are metabolized mainly by phase

Table 2 Screening for Metabolic Stability in Human Liver Microsomes

---

Experimental model: Pooled human liver microsomes.

Incubation conditions: Microsomes (0.5 mg/ml) are combined with test article and NADPH-regenerating system (NRS) in test tubes in a 37°C water bath, and incubated for 30 min. NRS is added to start the reaction. Reactions are terminated at the appropriate time by the addition of an equal volume of methanol or acetonitrile.

Test article concentration: 10 μM

Replicates: $N = 2$

Controls: Vehicle control (microsomes incubated without test article but with vehicle); metabolic positive control (7-ethoxycoumarin metabolism); negative control (microsomes combined with test article, then methanol added before the NADPH-regenerating system).

Analyses: HPLC or LC/MS (as appropriate) is used to measure the concentration of each parent compound that remains after the incubation period.

II conjugation pathways (e.g., zidovudine) and therefore would be metabolically stable when incubated with microsomes. In hepatocytes, however, the metabolic stability of a drug would be a factor of phase I oxidation, phase II conjugation, or other pathway (e.g., esterase activity). Freshly isolated and cryopreserved human hepatocytes are found to be competent in the metabolism of xenobiotics via P450 pathways, non-P450 oxidative pathways, glucuronidation, sulfation, O-methylation, and N-acetylation (Li et al., 1999a, b; Song et al., 1998). Therefore, metabolic stability values obtained with hepatocytes should be more relevant than those obtained using liver microsomes. The major limitation in the use of hepatocytes is the limited extent of metabolism. The assay is similar to that for microsomes except that cofactors are not required and that the test compound concentration is lower (5 μM) than that used for microsomes to compensate for the lower amount of metabolizing enzyme activity. A typical screening assay for metabolic stability in human hepatocytes is shown in Table 3. For new chemicals with unknown metabolic pathways, hepatocytes represent the most appropriate system for metabolic stability evaluation. The major reason is that in hepatocytes all the drug-metabolizing enzyme pathways are present, whereas in microsomes only the oxidative pathways are present under normal experimental conditions (with NADPH as cofactor). The use of microsomes to screen for metabolic stability toward oxidative metabolism will generate results that may or may not be relevant to humans in vivo. A compound may not be oxidized in vivo but would be oxidized in vitro by microsomes. An example of this is our recent study

Table 3 High-Throughput Screening for Metabolic Stability in Human Hepatocytes

Experimental model: Cryopreserved human hepatocytes pooled from multiple donors.
Incubation conditions: Hepatocytes are added to uncoated 96-well tissue culture plates
(5×10^4 cells in 100-µl culture media per well). Test article will be added at 1 concentration, and the cultures are incubated for 4 hr ($37°C$, 5% CO_2).
Test article concentration: 5 µM
Replicates: $N = 2$ for all experimental and control groups
Controls: Vehicle control (hepatocytes incubated without test article but with vehicle);
metabolic negative control (heat-inactivated hepatocytes incubated with test article);
metabolic positive control (7-ethoxycoumarin metabolism).
Analyses: HPLC or LC/MS (as appropriate) is used to measure the concentration of each
parent compound that remains after the incubation period.

on EE2 metabolism (Li et al., 1999b). EE2 is mainly metabolized via direct conjugation to sulfate and glucuronide in humans in vivo. With intact human hepatocytes, the correct pathways were identified. However, with liver microsomes, we only observed oxidation to 2-OH EE2. Our results illustrate the importance of using the appropriate experimental system for metabolism studies. Several independent laboratories have data demonstrating that results with intact hepatocytes can be used to quantitatively predict hepatic metabolic clearance in vivo (Houston and Carlile, 1997; Lave et al., 1997a, b; Hayes et al., 1995; Lacarelle et al., 1991).

III. TOXICOLOGY

For obvious reasons, a drug must have an acceptable therapeutic index, i.e., a high safety margin between the therapeutic dose and the toxic dose. Prediction of toxicity has been a major challenge for the pharmaceutical industry. As recently as 1999, drugs have been restricted or withdrawn from the market because of unforeseen toxicity, especially idiosyncratic drug toxicity (toxicity that occurs rarely but with grave consequences).

Hepatotoxicity is the most common drug toxicity. Screening for hepatotoxicity therefore is appropriate. The known species differences in drug metabolism probably account for most of the known species differences in drug toxicity. Therefore, screening for human hepatotoxicity should involve a system that encompasses human drug metabolism pathways. Human hepatocytes represent such a system. Because of the difficulty in obtaining fresh human livers for the isolation of hepatocytes, cryopreserved human hepatocytes represent the most pragmatic model.

A. Screening Assays for Human Hepatotoxicity

As parenchymal cells are generally the target for hepatotoxic drugs, human hepatocytes represent a relevant experimental system for the evaluation of human hepatotoxic potential of new chemicals (Li, 1994, 1998; Li et al., 1997). We have recently developed a screening assay for drug toxicity using cryopreserved human hepatocytes (Li et al., 1999a). The assay is shown in Table 4. Hepatocytes pooled from multiple donors are used. The procedure is an addition-only procedure, therefore allowing automation. In general, the procedure involves the addition of human hepatocytes into a 96-well plate, followed by the addition of test chemicals at specified concentrations. After an incubation period (e.g., 4 hr), reagents are added to assay for cell viability. We have been successful in using MTT reagents (a measurement of mitochondrial metabolism) for the quantification of cell viability (Li et al., 1999a). Recently, we have further increased the throughput and decreased the cost via the use of 384-well plates and using cellular ATP content as the measurement of viability. A schematic of the experimental protocol for the assay is shown in Figure 4. Dose-dependent induction of cytotoxicity by known human hepatotoxicants was observed using this assay (Fig. 5).

B. Other Cytotoxicity Screening Assays

The assays described for human hepatocytes can be applied to other cell types. Rodent hepatocytes can be used for the prediction of in vivo rodent hepatotoxicity (Davila et al., 1998; Ulrich et al., 1995; Guillouzo et al., 1997; Li, 1994). The capability to predict rodent toxicity will allow researchers to screen out potentially problematic compounds. Comparing results of human hepatocytes to those obtained from hepatocytes of nonhuman animals will also allow one to choose the

Table 4 Screening for In Vitro Human Hepatocyte Cytotoxicity

Experimental model: Cryopreserved human hepatocytes pooled from multiple donors.
Incubation conditions: Cryopreserved hepatocytes are incubated with test articles in 96-well tissue culture plates (50,000 cells per well in 100-μl volume) for 4 hr (37°C, 5% CO_2). At 4 hr, MTT reagent is added. These cultures are incubated for an additional 3 hr, during which time viable cells will convert the MTT to a colored product. The MTT product is extracted from the cells with acidified isopropanol, then aliquots of the MTT extracts are analyzed spectrophotometrically.
Test article concentrations: 100 μM
Replicates: $N = 2$ for all experimental and control groups
Controls: Positive control (tamoxifen); negative control (incubation media only, no test article).
Analyses: 96-well plate reader.

HTS Hepatotoxicity Protocol
(Quantification of cellular ATP)

• T=0: Add 10 μL of 2X test chemicals and 2,000 hepatocytes in 10 μL to 384-well plate (per well).

• Incubate 2 hr at 37°C, 5% CO_2.

• T=2 hr: Add 10 μL lysis buffer, wait 2 minutes.

• T=2 hr + 2 min: Add 10 μL luciferin/luciferase substrate, wait 10 minutes.

• T=2 hr+ 12 min: Measure luminescence of each well.

Figure 4 Experimental procedures for the high-throughput screening of hepatotoxicity in cryopreserved human hepatocytes using cellular ATP content as an end point. This is an addition-only assay, utilizing an end point that can be measured using a 384-well plate reader. The cost of reagents per well is calculated to be approximately $0.25.

most appropriate animal species for toxicity evaluation or to determine if the toxicity observed in nonhuman animals is relevant to humans (Li, 1994). Continuous cell lines can also be used for the measurement of "intrinsic toxicity," i.e., the capacity of a chemical to kill living cells in the absence of metabolism. End points for toxicity include release of cytoplasmic enzymes such as alanine aminotransferase, aspartate aminotransferase and lactate dehydrogenase, inhibition of macromolecular synthesis (e.g., protein synthesis; RNA synthesis), the induction of apoptosis, and the induction of stress proteins (Li, 1994). Using genomic and proteomic technologies, high-content assays using alterations in gene expression profile and protein profile as end point are now being evaluated in numerous laboratories.

IV. DRUG–DRUG INTERACTIONS

Adverse drug reactions can result from drug–drug interactions. Examples are plentiful: Fatalities have been reported for patients taking the antihistamine terfendadine and the antifungal ketoconazole. We now know that this is due to the inhibition of the major CYP isoform for terfenadine metabolism, CYP3A4, by

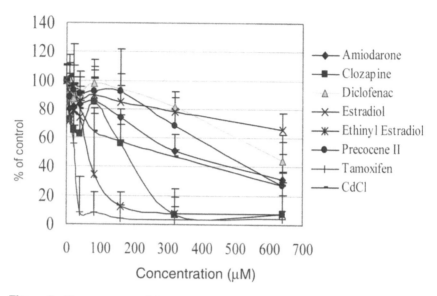

Figure 5 Dose–response of the induction of cytotoxicity, measured as a decrease in cellular ATP, in human hepatocytes. The known hepatotoxic drugs tamoxifen, ethinyl estradiol, and clozapine were found to be have high degrees of cytotoxicity. Cadmium chloride, amiodarone, precocene II, and diclofenac showed cytotoxicity at relatively higher levels. Estradiol had very low, if any, cytotoxicity. The results demonstrate that this assay can be used to routinely screen compounds for potential hepatotoxicity in humans.

ketoconazole. The result is the elevation of plasma terfenadine to a cardiotoxic level. Another example is the decrease in effectiveness of oral contraceptives in women who were also administered rifampin. Rifampin is now known to enhance the metabolism of EE2, the active ingredient of oral contraceptives, thereby lowering the plasma level of EE2 to nontherapeutic levels. Drug–drug interactions therefore can have both toxicological and pharmacological consequences. An optimized drug should have minimum drug–drug interaction potential.

Drug–drug interactions in the past were discovered after the drugs involved were already in the marketplace. This is highly undesirable ethically as well as financially for the pharmaceutical companies involved. Based on the thorough understanding of the mechanisms involved in pharmacokinetic drug–drug interactions, it is now scientifically acceptable to screen for drug–drug interaction potential using in vitro systems. The in vitro assays are developed based on the two major mechanisms of pharmacokinetic drug–drug interactions: inhibition and induction of drug-metabolizing enzymes (Lin and Lu, 1998; Strolin Benedetti and

Bani, 1998; Schmider et al., 1999; Li and Jurima-Romet, 1997a, b; Li and Kedderis, 1997; Li, 1997; Fischer et al., 1997; Ito et al., 1998)

A. Screening for Enzyme Inhibition

CYP isoforms CYP1A2, CYP2A6, CYP2C9, CYP2C19, CYP2D6, CYP2E1, and CYP3A4 are the most important drug-metabolizing enzymes. It is therefore desirable to screen for the ability of a new drug candidate to inhibit these isoforms. Screening can be performed using liver microsomes (e.g., Ito et al., 1998), hepatocytes (Li and Jurima-Romet, 1997; Li et al., 1999a), or cDNA-expressed microsomes (Crespi and Penman, 1997).

Human hepatocytes, human liver microsomes, or cDNA-expressed microsomes are incubated with the drug candidate followed by the addition of CYP substrates. Inhibition is indicated by the decrease in activity compared with that of the solvent control. For liver microsomes and hepatocytes, as all the liver CYP isoforms are present, the substrates used need to be specific to the individual isoforms for one to elucidate the inhibitory potential of each test article toward the specific isoform. The isoform-specific substrates include the following: phenacetin for CYP1A2, coumarin for CYP2A6, tolbutamide for CYP2C9, S-mephenytoin for CYP2C19, dextromethorphan for CYP2D6, chlorzoxazone for CYP2E1, and testosterone for CYP3A4. Examples of screening assays with microsomes or hepatocytes are shown in Table 5.

A high-throughput screening assay for CYP inhibition has been developed with microsomes genetically engineered to express only one specific CYP isoform (Crespi et al., 1997). As only one isoform is present, relatively nonspecific substrates can be used, therefore allowing the use of fluorometric substrates. Measuring activity using fluorometry is extremely high throughput in comparison with the isoform-specific substrates required with HPLC and LC/MS. The fluorometric substrates include the following: 3-cyano-7-ethoxycoumarin (CEC) for CYP1A2, CYP2C9, CYP2C19, CYP2D6 and 4-trifluoromethylcoumarin for CYP3A4 (Table 6).

The choice of system—hepatocytes, liver microsomes, cDNA-expressed microsomes—for CYP inhibition evaluation is contingent on the purpose of the screening. Hepatocytes represent the most ideal system as they can allow one to predict inhibitory effects based on plasma concentration (extracellular concentration). Results with liver microsomes and cDNA-expressed microsomes reflect the effects of the chemicals at the concentrations at the enzyme level, whereas results with hepatocytes reflect the effects outside the cells, therefore equivalent to plasma level. Because of active transport, bioaccumulation, or active excretion, intracellular concentration may not be the same as the extracellular concentration. As in most cases, one would not have information on intracellular drug concentrations in the liver; it is necessary to predict inhibitory effects based on plasma

Table 5 Screening of the Inhibitory Potential on CYP 1A2, 2A6, 2C9, 2C19, 2D6, 2E1, and 3A4 in Human Liver Microsomes or Human Hepatocytes

Experimental model: Human liver microsomes or cryopreserved human hepatocytes.
Incubation conditions:
Microsomes: Microsomes are preincubated with test article at 10 μM for 15 min. CYP isoform-specific substrate are added, and the incubation is continued for an additional 15 min.
Hepatocytes: Hepatocytes are added to uncoated 24-well tissue culture plates (0.5×10^6 cells in 0.5-ml culture media per well). Test article (10 μM) and CYP isoform-specific substrate is added, and the incubation is continued for 1 hr.
Test article concentrations: 10 μM
Replicates: $N = 2$
CYP isoform substrates: Phenacetin (1A2); coumarin (2A6); tolbutamide (2C9); *S*-mephenytoin (2C19); dextromethorphan (2D6); chlorzoxazone (2E1); testosterone (3A4).
CYP isoform inhibitors (positive controls): Furafylline (1A2); tranylcypromine (2A6, microsomes); diethyldithiocarbamate (2A6, hepatocytes); sulfaphenazole (2C9); omeprazole (2C19); quinidine (2D6); 4-methylpyrazole (2E1); ketoconazole (3A4).
Controls: Negative control (microsomes or hepatocytes incubated with substrate only, no test article); positive control (microsomes or hepatocytes incubated with substrate and chemical inhibitor of each isoform-specific substrate); chromatographic interference control for each substrate (microsomes or hepatocytes incubated with the test article in the absence of inhibitors or substrates).
Analyses: HPLC analysis of metabolite formation from each substrate.

Table 6 Screening for CYP Isoform Inhibitory Potential Using Expressed Recombinant Human Enzymes CYP 1A2, 2A6, 2C9, 2C19, 2D6, 2E1, and 3A4

Experimental model: Expressed recombinant human P450 isoforms 1A2, 2A6, 2C9, 2C19, 2D6, and 3A4.
Incubation conditions: Expressed isoforms will be incubated with test articles and NADPH-regenerating system (NRS) for 60 min (37°C water bath).
Test article concentrations: 10 μM
Replicates: $N = 3$ for all experimental and control groups
Controls: Negative control (no test article) and positive controls (known inhibitors for each CYP isoform).
Substrates: 3-Cyano-7-ethoxycoumarin for CYP 1A2, 2C9, 2C19, 2D6, and 4-trifluoromethylcoumarin for CYP3A4.
Analysis: Flourometric measurements.

drug concentration. Recently, it was shown that microsomal incubation with drugs would lead to ubiquitous binding of the drugs to the microsomal membrane at nonenzymatic sites, an artifact of this in vitro system that may explain the under-prediction of in vivo inhibitory effects in microsomal assays (Obach, 1997, 1999; Obach et al., 1997; McLure et al., 2000). Results with intact hepatocytes therefore may be the most physiologically relevant. The specificity of various CYP isoform inhibitors in human hepatocytes is shown in Figure 6 (Li et al., 1999a). We have previously shown that ketoconazole is a more potent inhibitor of terfenadine metabolism in intact human hepatocytes than liver microsomes (Li and Jurima-Romet, 1997). Another example of differences between intact hepatocytes and liver microsomes is the inhibitory effects of α-naphthoflavone, a CYP1A inhibitor. The inhibitory effects of α-naphthoflavone is significantly higher in intact human

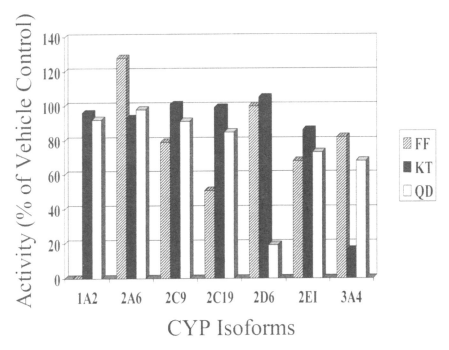

Figure 6 Effects of known P450 inhibitors furafylline (FF), ketoconazole (KT), and quinidine (QD) on the activities of isoform-specific substrate metabolism in human hepatocytes. FF, KT, and QD were found to inhibit CYP isoforms 1A2, 3A4, and 2D6, respectively. The results are consistent with the known inhibitory effects of these model P450 inhibitors. The human hepatocytes used were previously cryopreserved cells, pooled from 10 individual donors. The results demonstrate that cryopreserved human hepatocytes can be used routinely to screen for P450 inhibitory potential.

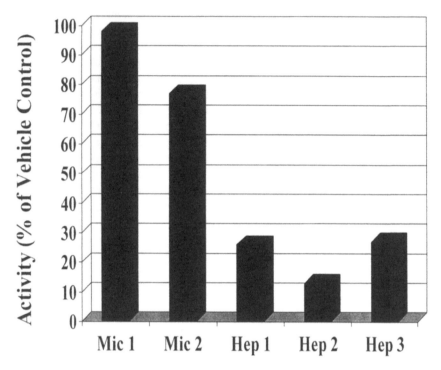

Figure 7   Effects of 25 μM α-naphthoflavone, a known CYP1A inhibitor, on CYP1A activity measured as phenacetin O-deethylation, in liver microsomes (two experiments: Mic 1 and Mic 2), and in human hepatocytes (three experiments: Hep 1, Hep 2, Hep 3). The results show that hepatocytes are more sensitive to the inhibitory effects of α-naphthoflavone than liver microsomes. The mechanism for the difference could be bioaccumulation of the inhibitor into hepatocytes so that the intracellular concentration is higher than the nominal extracellular concentration. Ubiquitous binding of the inhibitor to liver microsomes can also play a role in this difference. The inhibitor may bind to nonenzymatic regions of the microsomal membrane, thereby leading to a lower effective concentration for interaction with CYP1A.

hepatocytes than in liver microsomes (Fig. 7). Another advantage of the use of human hepatocytes is that one can evaluate inhibitory effects on phase II conjugation, as illustrated by the inhibitory effect of salicylamide on sulfation and glucuronidation of 7-OH-coumarin (Fig. 8).

Because of the above-mentioned multiple factors which may affect the final outcome in hepatocytes, liver microsomes, where the enzymes are exposed to the inhibitors directly, are more appropriate for the elucidation of the mechanism of

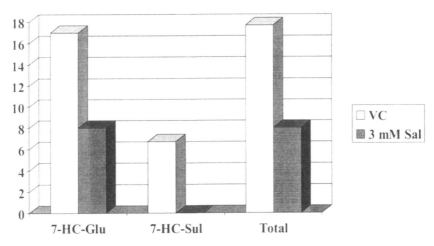

Figure 8 Screening for inhibition of phase II conjugating enzymes in human hepatocytes. The effects of salicylamide on 7-hydroxycoumarin (umbelliferone) conjugation were evaluated, showing almost total elimination of sulfation and approximately 50% inhibition of glucuronidation.

inhibition, especially when enzyme kinetic approaches are used. Of course, the recent findings on binding of drugs to microsomes demonstrate the complexity of modeling enzyme inhibition even using this relatively simple experimental system (Obach, 1997, 1999; Obach et al., 1997; McLure et al., 2000).

One drawback to the use of microsomes and hepatocytes is that results on P450 isoform activities are quantified using HPLC, which is not yet high throughput. Expressed P450 systems have only one isoform and therefore can use substrates that are not isoform-selective but the metabolism of which can be measured based on fluorescence. One drawback of the expressed P450 systems is that contribution of other isoforms (which may metabolize the test chemical to metabolites with higher or lower inhibitory potential) is not accounted for; another drawback is the previously mentioned complication of differential intracellular and extracellular concentrations.

As a summary, for the evaluation of P450 inhibition, screening for inhibitory effects on selected P450 isoforms is usually performed in a high-throughput manner using expressed P450. For selected compounds, the results may be confirmed with liver microsomes or hepatocytes. Liver microsomes can be used to further evaluate the K_i and mechanism of inhibition. Hepatocytes are used to generate data to aid the prediction of in vivo effects at plasma drug concentrations.

B. Screening for Enzyme Induction

Human hepatocytes are routinely used as an experimental system for the evaluation of CYP induction potential (Merrill et al., 1995; Li et al., 1995, 1997a, b; Li, 1997; Li and Kedderis, 1997; Silva et al., 1998; Ramachandran et al., 1999; Sahi et al., 2000; Xu et al., 2000). All the known CYP inducers for humans in vivo, such as rifampin, phenobarbital, omeprazole, phenytoin, and troglitazone, are also inducers in cultured human hepatocytes (Li et al., 1997a; Sahi et al., 2000; Ramachandran et al., 1999). To screen for human CYP induction potential, freshly isolated human hepatocytes are routinely used. The cells are cultured for 2–3 days after isolation followed by a 2- to 3-day treatment period. After treatment, isoform-specific substrates are added onto the cells to evaluate the rate of metabolism. Induction is indicated by an increase in activity above that of the solvent control.

To increase the throughput, this assay can be performed in 24-well plates. Because of the need to use freshly isolated human hepatocytes and the required 4- to 5-day experimental period, the assay therefore is not yet considered to be high throughput. We and others have shown that cryopreserved hepatocytes remain responsive to CYP inducers and therefore may be appropriate for use in this assay (Ruegg et al., 1997; Silva et al., 1999; Hengstler et al., 2000). It is possible that in the near future cryopreserved hepatocytes will be found appropriate for the evaluation of CYP induction.

The CYP induction assay with human hepatocytes has been extensively reviewed (Li, 1997; Li et al., 1997a) and has been applied in our laboratory toward the evaluation of structure–induction potential relationships of rifamycin B antimicrobials—rifampin, rifapentine, and rifabutin (Li et al., 1997b)—and toward various proton pump inhibitors—omeprazole, lanzoprazole, and pantoprazole (Masubuchi et al., 1998). Typical results on the evaluation of enzyme induction potential of a drug candidate are shown in Figure 9. Compound X was found to be a potent inducer of CYP1A2, a weak inducer of CYP3A4, and a noninducer of all other isoforms evaluated. We have also begun studying the induction of phase II conjugation. We recently showed that rifampin induced EE2 sulfation (Li et al., 1999b), therefore providing evidence for a new, and apparently more appropriate, mechanism for rifampin–oral contraceptive interactions. Examples of an induction screening assay is shown in Table 7.

The evaluation of enzyme induction potential is definitely not high throughput. Although cryopreserved human hepatocytes can be used for enzyme induction studies (Ruegg et al., 1997), in general, freshly isolated hepatocytes are the cells of choice. The use of mRNA measurement for induction (Mattes and Li, 1997) may allow higher throughput, taking advantage of the latest advances of rapid gene expression screening. Recently, via the elucidation of the mechanism of CYP3A4 induction, cell lines have been engineered containing the responsive element (PXR) linked to a reporter gene (e.g., luciferase), thereby allowing high-throughput screening of CYP3A inducers. Again, due to the lack of other drug-

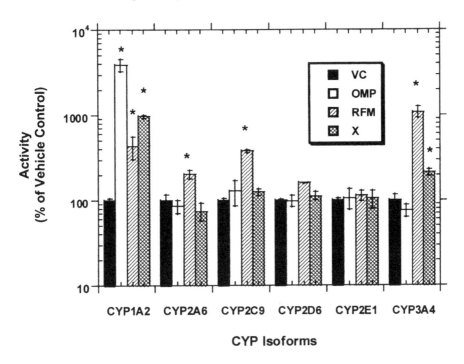

Figure 9   Screening for induction of P450 isoforms. Human hepatocytes from a single donor were cultured for 2 days followed by treatment with omeprazole (OMP, 50 μM), rifampin (RFM, 25 μM), compound X (50 μM) and solvent only [vehicle control, VC (0.1% DMSO)]. The activities relative to that of VC (VC = 100%) are shown. The results show that the experiment was acceptable, as the known inducers OMP and RFM yielded induction of CYP1A2 and CYP3A4, respectively. Compound X was found to be a potent inducer of CYP1A2 and also an inducer of CYP3A4. The results presented here were part of a larger study in which multiple concentrations of compound X were evaluated, and the observation was reproduced in experiments with hepatocytes from three donors.

metabolizing enzyme pathways in these engineered cells, results need to be confirmed with intact human hepatocytes before definitive conclusions can be made on induction potential.

V.   FUTURE APPROACHES

To effectively apply ADME-tox screening in drug discovery and development, one must increase the efficiency of the process as well as improve the quality of the

Table 7   Screening of Induction Potential for CYP 1A2, 2A6, 2C9, 2C19, 2D6, 2E1, and 3A4 in Human Hepatocytes

---

Purpose: To investigate the potential of test articles to induce CYP 1A2, 2A6, 2C9, 2C19, 2D6, 2E1, and 3A4 activity in human hepatocytes.

Experimental model: Hepatocytes isolated from a freshly procured human liver.

Incubation conditions: Hepatocytes are plated in collagen-coated 24-well tissue culture plates (3.5×10^5 cells in 0.5-ml culture media per well). The cells are then incubated for 48 hr to establish the cultures, followed by dosing with test articles at each of 3 concentrations or with known inducer, for a total treatment duration of 48 hr.

Test article concentrations: 1, 10, 100 μM.

Replicates: $N = 3$ for all experimental groups and $N = 6$ for all control groups.

Controls:
- Positive controls: rifampin for CYP3A; omeprazole for 1A; phenobarbital for 2B and 3A
- Vehicle control (hepatocytes incubated without test article but with vehicle).

CYP450 isoform substrates: Ethoxyresorufin (1A2); coumarin (2A6); tolbutamide (2C9); S-mephenytoin (2C19); dextromethorphan (2D6); chlorzoxazone (2E1); testosterone (3A4).

Analyses: HPLC analysis is used to quantify metabolite production.

---

screen. Approaches below are directions which are being developed by practitioners in high-throughput screening and should improve efforts in this important discipline of drug discovery and development.

1. *Miniaturization:* Almost all the assays described here involve the use of 96-well plate format. The use of the next higher density plates, especially 384-well plates, is definitely technically feasible for the cytotoxicity assay and the CYP inhibition assay with cDNA-expressed microsomes.

2. *Automation:* Automation of the procedures described in this chapter is an approach that is already adopted by several industrial laboratories to enhance throughput and accuracy. In the near future, ADME-tox screening can be foreseen to be fully automated both in the performance of the experimental procedures and in data reporting and analysis.

3. *Genomics/proteomics:* Categorization of drug properties, especially toxicological properties based on the spectra of gene expression or protein synthesis, is one of the most active areas of research. Gene chips are available commercially for the evaluation of gene expression of a large number of human or laboratory animal genes. Two-dimensional gels coupled with LC/MS or nuclear magnetic resonance allows better definition of protein spectrum. Informatics software is also available for

data analysis. The key is to develop a reproducible experimental system and the use of an appropriate battery of drugs with known properties to validate the approach. This is an exciting area that may allow us to define drug properties accurately in the future. The areas in which we desperately need help include idiosyncratic drug toxicity and carcinogenicity.

4. *Analytical chemistry:* It is well recognized that the major bottleneck in ADME-tox screening is analytical chemistry. Low-throughput analytical procedures, such as HPLC and LC/MS, are necessary in the evaluation of intestinal absorption, metabolic stability, and drug–drug interaction potential. Improvements in this area can be made via automation, pooling of multiple samples, elimination of solid-phase extractions, and use of surrogate end points that would replace the standard analytical end points. This is an extremely important area, but unfortunately, it is also the most technical challenging in throughput enhancement. Recent developments to enhance throughput include the development of automated systems for LC/MS analysis (Korfmacher et al., 1999; Linget and du Vignaud, 1999).

5. *Virtual screening:* The highest throughput approach is to perform screening without actual experimentation. Drugs can now be designed to interact with specific molecular targets (e.g., HIV protease inhibitors). Data are accumulating for the correlation of chemical structure to ADME-tox properties, with the hope that in the future one will be able to predict human drug properties. Several models for toxicity prediction are now available, but in general they are not yet considered predictive. The ability to design drugs to have the "perfect" combination of pharmacological activities and ADME-tox properties is a worthwhile but extremely challenging goal.

VI. CONCLUSIONS

The major advantage of in vitro human-based experimental systems is that they can be used to study human-specific drug properties, which may not be possible with laboratory animals. The lack of in vivo factors for in vitro systems, however, cannot be ignored. Experimentation with laboratory animals is still extremely important for the evaluation of in vivo factors that cannot be modeled successfully in vitro. These in vivo factors include multiple organ effects, extrahepatic metabolism including intestinal flora metabolism, drug distribution, secondary effects, and long-term exposure effects. Our use of the term "screening" does not imply that data interpretation is unnecessary and that sound scientific principles need not be applied. The most productive approach to the use of in vitro systems is to study drug properties using assays performed under physiologically relevant experimental conditions with mechanistically relevant end points. It is important to know the limitations of each assay so that sound data interpretation can be performed. Where the current assays are limited, one should strive to develop approaches to overcome the limitations. Research should continue to understand the mechanism of drug effects to aid the development of appropriate screening assays. Areas that are important but lacking appropriate testing systems include idiosyncratic drug toxicity, blood–brain barrier models, and models for drug transporters. Using data obtained with a comprehensive battery of well-validated in vitro systems will no doubt enhance one's ability to select drug candidates with the best probability of success in the clinic for drug development.

REFERENCES

Carlile DJ, Hakooz N, Bayliss MK, Houston JB (1999). Microsomal prediction of in vivo clearance of CYP2C9 substrates in humans. Br J Clin Pharmacol 47:625–635.

Crespi CL, Penman BW. (1997). Use of cDNA-expressed human cytochrome P450 enzymes to study potential drug–drug interactions. Adv Pharmacol 43:171–188.

Crespi CL, Miller VP, Penman BW. (1997) Microtiter plate assays for inhibition of human, drug-metabolizing cytochromes P450. Anal Biochem 15;248(1):188–190.

Chong S, Dando SA, Morrison RA (1997). Evaluation of Biocoat intestinal epithelium differentiation environment (3-day cultured Caco-2 cells) as an absorption screening model with improved productivity. Pharm Res 14:1835–1837.

Davila JC, Rodriguez RJ, Melchert RB, Acosta D Jr. (1998). Predictive value of in vitro model systems in toxicology. Annu Rev Pharmacol Toxicol 38:63–96.

Fabre G, Combalbert J, Berger Y, Cano JP (1990). Human hepatocytes as a key in vitro model to improve preclinical drug development. Eur J Drug Metab Pharmacokinet. 15:165–171.

Fischer U, Rohde B, Wacke R, Stange J, Nitschke FP, Adam U, Drewelow B (1997). Prediction of in vivo drug interaction from in vitro systems exemplified by interaction between verapamil and cimetidine using human liver microsomes and primary hepatocytes. J Clin Pharmacol 37:1150–1159.

Fogh J, Fogh JM, Orfeo T (1977). One hundred and twenty-seven cultured human tumor cell lines producing tumors in nude mice. J Natl Cancer Inst 59:221–225.

Gan LS, Yanni S, Thakker DR (1998). Modulation of the tight junctions of the Caco-2 monolayers by H2-antagonists. Pharm Res 15:53–57.

Guillouzo A, Morel F, Langouet S, Maheo K, Rissel M (1997). Use of hepatocyte cultures for the study of hepatotoxic compounds. J Hepatol 26 Suppl 2:73–80.

Guillouzo A. (1998). Liver cell models in in vitro toxicology. Environ Health Persp 106:Suppl 2:511–532.

Hayes KA, Brennan B, Chenery R, Houston JB (1995). In vivo disposition of caffeine predicted from hepatic microsomal and hepatocyte data. Drug Metab Dispos 23:349–353.

Hengstler JG, Utesch D, Steinberg P, Platt KL, Diener B, Ringel M, Swales N, Fischer T, Biefang K, Gerl M, Bottger T, Oesch F (2000). Cryopreserved primary hepatocytes as a constantly available in vitro model for the evaluation of human and animal drug metabolism and enzyme induction. Drug Metab Rev 32:81–118.

Houston JB, Carlile DJ (1997). Prediction of hepatic clearance from microsomes, hepatocytes, and liver slices. Drug Metab Rev. 29:891–922.

Ito K, Iwatsubo T, Kanamitsu S, Nakajima Y, Sugiyama Y (1998). Quantitative prediction of in vivo drug clearance and drug interactions from in vitro data on metabolism, together with binding and transport. Annu Rev Pharmacol Toxicol 38:461–499.

Iwatsubo T, Hirota N, Ooie T, Suzuki H, Sugiyama Y (1996). Prediction of in vivo drug disposition from in vitro data based on physiological pharmacokinetics. Biopharm Drug Dispos 17(4):273–310.

Kanamitsu S, Ito K, Sugiyama Y (2000). Quantitative prediction of in vivo drug–drug interactions from in vitro data based on physiological pharmacokinetics: use of maximum unbound concentration of inhibitor at the inlet to the liver. Pharm Res 17:336–343.

Kansy M, Senner F, Gubernator K. (1998). Physicochemical high throughput screening: parallel artificial membrane permeation assay in the description of passive absorption processes. J Med Chem 41:1007–1010.

Korfmacher WA, Palmer CA, Nardo C, Dunn-Meynell K, Grotz D, Cox K, Lin CC, Elicone C, Liu C, Duchoslav E (1999). Development of an automated mass spectrometry system for the quantitative analysis of liver microsomal incubation samples: a tool for rapid screening of new compounds for metabolic stability. Rapid Commun Mass Spectrom 13:901–907.

Lacarelle B, Marre F, Durand A, Davi H, Rahmani R (1991). Metabolism of minaprine in human and animal hepatocytes and liver microsomes—prediction of metabolism in vivo. Xenobiotica 21:317–329.

Lave T, Dupin S, Schmitt C, Valles B, Ubeaud G, Chou RC, Jaeck D, Coassolo P (1997). The use of human hepatocytes to select compounds based on their expected hepatic extraction ratios in humans. Pharm Res 14:152–155.

Lave T, Dupin S, Schmitt C, Chou RC, Jaeck D, Coassolo P (1997). Integration of in vitro data into allometric scaling to predict hepatic metabolic clearance in man: application to 10 extensively metabolized drugs. J Pharm Sci May; 86:584–590.

Li AP (1994). Primary hepatocyte culture as an in vitro toxicological system. In: Shayne G, ed. In Vitro Toxicology. New York: Raven Press, pp. 195–220.

Li AP, Kaminski DL, Rasmussen A (1995). Substrates of human hepatic cytochrome P450 3A4. Toxicology Dec 15;104(1–3):1–8.

Li AP, Rasmussen A, Xu L, Kaminski DL (1995). Rifampicin induction of lidocaine metabolism in cultured human hepatocytes. J Pharmacol Exp Ther 274:673–677.

Li AP (1997). Primary hepatocyte cultures as an in vitro experimental model for the evaluation of pharmacokinetic drug–drug interactions. Adv Pharmacol. 43:103–130.

Li AP, Jurima-Romet M (1997a). Overview: pharmacokinetic drug-drug interactions. Adv Pharmacol 43:1–6.

Li AP, Jurima-Romet M (1997b). Applications of primary human hepatocytes in the evaluation of pharmacokinetic drug-drug interactions: evaluation of model drugs terfenadine and rifampin. Cell Biol Toxicol 13:365–374.

Li AP, Beck DJ, Loretz LJ, Xu L, Rasmussen A, Merrill JC, Kaminski DL (1997). Primary human hepatocytes as an in vitro toxicology system. In: Sahem H, Katz SA, eds.

Advances in Animal Alternatives for Safety and Efficacy Testing. New York: Taylor and Francis, pp. 359–368.

Li AP, Kedderis GL (1997). Primary hepatocyte culture as an experimental model for the evaluation of interactions between xenobiotics and drug-metabolizing enzymes. Chem Biol Interact. 107:1–3.

Li AP, Maurel P, Gomez-Lechon MJ, Cheng LC, Jurima-Romet M (1997a). Preclinical evaluation of drug–drug interaction potential: present status of the application of primary human hepatocytes in the evaluation of cytochrome P450 induction. Chem Biol Interact 107:5–16.

Li AP, Reith MK, Rasmussen A, Gorski JC, Hall SD, Xu L, Kaminski DL, Cheng LK (1997b). Primary human hepatocytes as a tool for the evaluation of structure–activity relationship in cytochrome P450 induction potential of xenobiotics: evaluation of rifampin, rifapentine and rifabutin. Chem Biol Interact 107:17–30.

Li AP (1998). Applications of primary hepatocytes in drug metabolism and toxicology. Comm Toxicol 6:199–220.

Li AP, Hartman NR, Lu C, Collins JM, Strong JM (1999). Effects of cytochrome P450 inducers on 17alpha-ethinyloestradiol (EE2) conjugation by primary human hepatocytes. Br J Clin Pharmacol 48:733–742.

Li AP, Gorycki PD, Hengstler JG, Kedderis GL, Koebe HG, Rahmani R, de Sousas G, Silva JM, Skett P (1999b). Present status of the application of cryopreserved hepatocytes in the evaluation of xenobiotics: consensus of an international expert panel. Chem Biol Interact 121:117–123.

Li AP, Lu C, Brent JA, Pham C, Fackett A, Ruegg CE, Silber PM (1999a). Cryopreserved human hepatocytes: characterization of drug-metabolizing enzyme activities and applications in higher throughput screening assays for hepatotoxicity, metabolic stability, and drug-drug interaction potential. Chem Biol Interact 121:17–35.

Li AP, Lu C, Silber PM, Dixon K (2001). Caco-2 cells screening assay for intestinal absorption. In: Ernst SC, ed. High Throughput Screening. Morris Plains, NJ: Cahners Press, pp 6–9.

Lin JH, Lu AY (1998). Inhibition and induction of cytochrome P450 and the clinical implications. Clin Pharmacokinet 35:361–390.

Linget JM, du Vignaud P (1999). Automation of metabolic stability studies in microsomes, cytosol and plasma using a 215 Gilson liquid handler. J Pharm Biomed Anal 19: 893–901.

Lundahl P, Beigi F (1997). Immobilized liposome chromatography of drugs for model analysis of drug–membrane interactions. Adv Drug Deliv Res 23:221–227.

Masubuchi N, Li AP, Okazaki O. (1998). An evaluation of the cytochrome P450 induction potential of pantoprazole in primary human hepatocytes. Chem Biol Interact 114:1–13.

Mattes WB, Li AP (1997). Quantitative reverse transcriptase/PCR assay for the measurement of induction in cultured hepatocytes. Chem Biol Interact 107:47–61.

McLure JA, Miners JO, Birkett DJ (2000). Nonspecific binding of drugs to human liver microsomes. Br J Clin Pharmacol 49:453–461.

Merrill JC, Beck DJ, Kaminski DA, Li AP (1995). Polybrominated biphenyl induction of cytochrome P450 mixed function oxidase activity in primary rat and human hepatocytes. Toxicology 99:147–152.

Obach RS (1999). Prediction of human clearance of twenty-nine drugs from hepatic microsomal intrinsic clearance data: an examination of in vitro half-life approach and nonspecific binding to microsomes. Drug Metab Dispos 27:1350–1359.

Obach RS (1997). Nonspecific binding to microsomes: impact on scale-up of in vitro intrinsic clearance to hepatic clearance as assessed through examination of warfarin, imipramine, and propranolol. Drug Metab Dispos 25:1359–1369.

Obach RS, Baxter JG, Liston TE, Silber BM, Jones BC, MacIntyre F, Rance DJ, Wastall P (1997). The prediction of human pharmacokinetic parameters from preclinical and in vitro metabolism data. J Pharmacol Exp Ther 283:46–58.

Pastan I, Gottesman MM, Ueda K, Lovelace E, Rutherford AV, Willingham MC (1988). A retrovirus carrying an MDR1 cDNA confers multidrug resistance and polarized expression of P-glycoprotein in MDCK cells. Proc Natl Acad Sci USA 85: 4486–4490.

Ramachandran V, Kostrubsky VE, Komoroski BJ, Zhang S, Dorko K, Esplen JE, Strom SC, Venkataramanan R (1999). Troglitazone increases cytochrome P-450 3A protein and activity in primary cultures of human hepatocytes. Drug Metab Dispos. 27: 1194–1199.

Sahi J, Hamilton G, Sinz M, Barros S, Huang SM, Lesko LJ, LeCluyse EL (2000). Effect of troglitazone on cytochrome P450 enzymes in primary cultures of human and rat hepatocytes. Xenobiotica 30(3):273–284.

Schmider J, von Moltke LL, Shader RI, Harmatz JS, Greenblatt DJ (1999). Extrapolating in vitro data on drug metabolism to in vivo pharmacokinetics: evaluation of the pharmacokinetic interaction between amitriptyline and fluoxetine. Drug Metab Rev 31:545–560.

Silva JM, Day SH, Nicoll-Griffith DA (1999). Induction of cytochrome-P450 in cryopreserved rat and human hepatocytes. Chem Biol Interact 121:49–63.

Silva JM, Morin PE, Day SH, Kennedy BP, Payette P, Rushmore T, Yergey JA, Nicoll-Griffith DA (1998). Refinement of an in vitro cell model for cytochrome P450 induction. Drug Metab Dispos 26:490–496.

Soldner A, Christians U, Susanto M, Wacher VJ, Silverman JA, Benet LZ (1999). Grapefruit juice activates P-glycoprotein-mediated drug transport. Pharm Res 16:478–485.

Song WC, Qian Y, Li AP (1998). Estrogen sulfotransferase expression in the human liver: marked interindividual variation and lack of gender specificity. J Pharmacol Exp Ther 284:1197–1202.

Stewart BH, Chan OH, Lu RH, Reyner EL, Schmid HL, Hamilton HW, Steinbaugh BA, Taylor MD (1995). Comparison of intestinal permeabilities determined in multiple in vitro and in situ methods: relationship to absorption in humans. Pharm Res 12:693–699.

Strolin Benedetti M, Bani M (1998). Design of in vitro studies to predict in vivo inhibitory drug–drug interactions. Pharmacol Res 38:81–88.

Ulrich RG, Bacon JA, Cramer CT, Peng GW, Petrella DK, Stryd RP, Sun EL (1995). Cultured hepatocytes as investigational models for hepatic toxicity: practical applications in drug discovery and development. Toxicol Lett 82–83:107–115.

Xu L, Li AP, Kaminski DL, Ruh MF (2000). 2,3,7,8-Tetrachlorodibenzo-p-dioxin induction of cytochrome P4501A in cultured rat hepatocytes. Chem Biol Interact 124:173–189.

Yang CY, Cai SJ, Liu H, Pidgeon C (1997). Immobilized artificial membranes-screens for drug–membrane interactions. Adv Drug Deliv Rev 23:229–256.

Zhang Y, Benet LZ (1998). Characterization of P-glycoprotein mediated transport of KO2, a novel vinylsulfone peptidomimetic cysteine protease inhibitor, across MDR1-MDCK and Caco-2 cell monolayers. Pharm Res 15:1520–1524.

13

Screening Lead Compounds in the Postgenomic Era: An Integrated Approach to Knowledge Building from Living Cells

Kenneth A. Giuliano, Ravi Kapur, Keith R. Olson, Chandrasekaran Vasudevan, Jian Wang, and Elizabeth S. Woo
Cellomics, Inc.
Pittsburgh, Pennsylvania

I. INTRODUCTION

The new face of drug discovery is focused on the living cell with its myriad ionic, metabolic, macromolecular, and organellar networks as the ultimate target of drug activity. E. B. Wilson essentially set the stage for a cell-centric approach to drug discovery in his introduction to a textbook that was one of the earliest attempts to combine cytology, physiology, embryology, genetics, biochemistry, and biophysics into the newly coined discipline of cellular biology [1]. Among other insights, he stressed the importance of measurements made on living cells in the presence of "changed conditions in the physical or chemical environment." Since then, there have been countless reports on the characterization of isolated components of living cells. There have also been reports where components from single cells have been characterized. One early approach to single-cell biochemistry, which appeared around the same time that Watson and Crick described the structure of cellular DNA, involved the extraction of nucleic acids from single neurons, their hydrolysis, electrophoresis on copper fibers, and analysis with ultraviolet light [2]. Although knowledge of the components of the chemistry of life has soared during the latter part of the 20th century, resulting in the modern disciplines of genomics and proteomics, there remains the great challenge of discovering the functional integration and regulation of these living components in time and space within the cell. We envision that the integration of genomics and proteomics with a new knowledge base built from temporal and spatial data on the chemical and molecular interrelationships of cellular components will provide an extremely rich platform for drug discovery.

II. GENOMICS AND PROTEOMICS AS THE FOUNDATION FOR CELL-BASED KNOWLEDGE

Whereas other chapters in this book specifically expand on the role of genomics and proteomics in modern drug discovery, we view the genome and proteome as important building blocks for the construction of new cell-based knowledge. The genomics era, begun more than a decade ago, has realized a one-dimensional description of human and other organismal genes, each a potential new drug target. Even those genes coding for molecules other than functional proteins are theoretically new drug targets.

The level of DNA organization in the genome is surprisingly simple. There are an estimated 100,000 genes in the human genome and they are encoded within about 3 billion base pairs of nucleotides. The precise sequence of genes within the context of these billions of units, which are themselves organized into larger structures such as chromosomes, has been the primary goal of the human genome project. The enormous impact of genomics on drug discovery can be attributed first to advances in automated sequencing instrumentation and reagents. A successive and arguably more important phase of genomics is the association of gene expression to normal and disease physiology. This phase has been empowered by technologies and platforms to measure message level changes in response to drug treatment and new informatics strategies to organize DNA sequence information into logical, searchable, and meaningful databases. Proteomic analysis has become the logical extension of genomics and its associated databases. The daunting task of defining the protein complement expressed by a genome within cells, tissues, and organisms can be rationalized with several arguments [3]. These include the much less than perfect correlation between mRNA and protein expression levels; post-translational modifications of proteins that affect intracellular localization, activity, or both; and proteome dynamics that reflect the physiological state of the cell, tissue, or organism. Nevertheless, the proteome of a single native organism has yet to be completely described let alone a mapping of drug activity overlaid onto one. Although proteomic databases are continually growing, both the methodology to measure proteomic changes and the approaches to extract, analyze, and characterize proteomic data have yet to be attacked as systematically as the genomic platform development has been. It remains unclear if current sample preparation methods and two-dimensional protein electrophoresis, the highest resolution approach available for proteome mapping, will be perfected to the point where an entire proteome can be mapped [4], especially as sample sizes diminish toward the single-cell level. Several factors make proteome analysis inherently more complicated than genomic analysis. For example, many genes in the human genome code for multiple proteins depending on mRNA processing; proteins can be posttranslationally modified; and proteins may have several distinct functions. Overlaid on the complexity of individual protein molecules are the temporal and spatial interactions between proteins and other molecules. At any one time, there is on the order of tens of thousands of different proteins arranged within a cell. Each protein may have up to hundreds of thousands of copies. Thus, out of the relative simplicity of the genome comes an astronomical number of molecular and biochemical reactions, nearly all of which are mediated by proteins, occurring in time and space within a living cell. As we move into the postgenomic era, the complementarity between genomics and proteomics will become apparent and the connections between them will undoubtedly be exploited. However, neither genomics, proteomics, nor their simple combination will provide the data necessary to interconnect molecular events in living cells in time and space, especially the network of events that targeted drugs inevitably interrupt or modulate.

III. CREATION OF NEW BIOLOGICAL KNOWLEDGE

A new perspective on drug discovery is cell centric rather than focused on isolated genes or proteins. Because the cell is the smallest unit of life that can live independently, it must be highly organized to perform life functions. This organization begins at the one-dimensional level encoded by its DNA. The intrinsic information of cellular structure and function is encoded by the simple language of the genome. The translation of genomic language into the proteins and other macromolecules that participate in every chemical reaction occurring within a living cell represents an even higher level of organization than the blueprint held within the DNA. However, cells are not composed of a random collection of these macromolecules, which includes the entire proteome. Additional orchestration of the highly organized interactions of ions, metabolites, and organelles makes cells living entities. The knowledge base of the living cell is built by connecting layers of these interactions into the pathways and networks that govern all aspects of cellular life. We have extended cell-based knowledge to include cellular responses to drugs, including pharmacokinetic effects as well as pharmacodynamic effects on multiple cellular targets, pathways, and networks under the heading of "PharmacoCellomics™." All deep biological information will be captured, defined, organized, and searchable in the Cellomics Knowledgebase of cellular knowledge. Just as automated genome analysis and bioinformatics tools are pushing the genomics era to a conclusion, automated cell analysis systems and cellular knowledge will be key to the era of the cell. Coupling of cellular knowledge to the drug discovery process will be essential for faster and more effective drug discovery. Such a process, composed of automated whole-cell-based detection systems, fluorescent reagents, and informatics and bioinformatics, is referred to as high-content screening (HCS).

IV. HCS OF TARGET ACTIVITY IN LIVING CELLS

The wealth of information obtainable from genomic and proteomic databases has led to at least one bottleneck in the early drug discovery process, i.e., target validation. Here potential targets are evaluated for suitability within new or established drug screens [5]. Once validated, targets are incorporated into primary drug screens that are typically high capacity and high throughput. Large compound libraries can be screened in a relatively short time, thus producing a plethora of "hits," i.e., combinations of compounds and target activity that meet certain minimum, usually crude, criteria. Due to recent emergent technologies for primary screening, increasingly larger numbers of hits have created another bottleneck at candidate optimization, where hits are qualified to leads through structure–activity relationship investigations, cytotoxicity, and secondary screening assays [5]. Thus, both bottlenecks have arisen as a consequence of advances in technology, especially miniaturization and automation, at their respective preceding steps in the drug discovery process. To break these bottlenecks, we have developed HCS to automate steps downstream of bottlenecks and to provide deeper biological information from cells. Our goal is to reduce the high failure rate of lead compounds by providing high biological content information at earlier stages in the drug discovery process. Such HCS information elaborates both temporal and spatial measurements of single or multiple target activities within cell populations at the level of the single cells. Although the details about HCS reagents, automated imaging analysis systems, and the bioinformatics support have been described elsewhere [5], some of the advantages of HCS are listed here (Table 1). It is important to stress that HCS is a platform for knowledge building; its advantages are derived from the unique combination of its component technologies.

HCS starts with live cells. Following compound treatment of live cells, two different HCS approaches can be taken. In one approach, cells are fixed and, in many cases, fluorescently labeled, prior to imaging analysis. The advantages of fixed-endpoint HCS include the flexibility to analyze samples without time constraints and the ability to optimize and augment analysis because fixed samples can be repeatedly processed and reanalyzed. Several single and multiparameter assays have been designed using fixed-endpoint assays. These assays, designed and validated by us and several pharmaceutical companies, include transcription factor activation and translocation [5,6], microtubule reorganization [7], G-protein-coupled receptor internalization [8], and apoptosis [5]. A second approach to

Table 1 Advantages of HCS in the Early Drug Discovery Process

---

Cell-Centric Physiological Context
- Target activities are measured within multiple living cell types
- Entry of drugs into specific cellular compartments is measurable
- Screening can be accomplished within mixed cell types
- No need to isolate and purify targets
- Effects of compounds on cell structure, communication, and development can be measured
- Cellular functions (e.g., division, endocytosis, motility) become quantifiable drug targets
- Signal detection is done within volumes on the order of a picoliter
- The entire screening process can be miniaturized (e.g., CellChip platform)

Multiparametric Approach to Screening
- Drug specificity is assessed by simultaneously measuring competing targets in the same cell
- Measures of toxicity are accompanied by target activity values
- Measurement of activities downstream of target activity is possible
- Unanticipated side effects of compounds can be measured

Automation of Complex Tasks
- Sample preparation uses optimized fluorescent reagent kits (e.g., HitKit existing automation technology)
- Imaging algorithms extract target activity values concurrent with data collection
- Automated kinetic assays that include automated liquid handling are possible

Generation of New Biological Knowledge
- New data management technology transforms enormous amounts of raw data into meaningful information
- Couple genomics, proteomics, and compound library databases with HCS data using the linking tools provided by the Cellomics Knowledgebase
- Discover complex cellular pathway interrelationships and the effect lead compounds have on them using the data-mining tools in the Cellomics Knowledgebase

---

HCS is the live cell kinetic assay. In this mode, temporal as well as high-content spatial data on target activities are collected and analyzed simultaneously.

Designed specifically for HCS, the ArrayScan® II system detects multiple fluorescence channels over the visible spectrum within living or fixed cells prepared with corresponding fluorophore-labeled targets. Importantly, the ArrayScan II system is distinguished from standard fluorescence microscopy systems by its fully automated acquisition, processing, and analysis of cell images with the capability of arraying cells in stacks of high-density microplates. The ArrayScan II system has a total magnification range from approximately 10× to 400×. This gives optical resolution ranges from less than 1 µm for subcellular spatial measurements to hundreds or thousands of micrometers for field-based measurements. During acquisition, fields of cells are automatically identified, focused upon, exposed, and imaged using a cooled charge-coupled device (CCD) camera. A high-capacity plate stacker enables "walk-away" operation of the system, and a live-cell environmental chamber maintains optimal temperature and atmospheric conditions for kinetic screening. Details of the unique multiparameter HCS capabilities of the ArrayScan II system are presented elsewhere [5] and are available on-line at *http://www.cellomics.com.*

The ArrayScan Kinetics HCS Workstation was designed to automate large-scale HCS of live cells, specifically facilitating drug-induced kinetic studies, by virtue of a 30-plate incubated plate stacker, on-board fluidics, and plate handling. Additional distinguishing features include eight excitation and eight emission channels, continuous focusing system, fluorescence polarization capability, and a higher HCS throughput capacity. Currently, no alternative automated HCS platform exists for live cells. The ArrayScan Kinetics HCS Workstation can be used as a standalone screening workstation or as a module within an integrated drug discovery platform comprising both high-throughput and high-content screening. Both fixed-endpoint and live-cell kinetic HCS assays provide a cellular context that in vitro assays of target activity do not match. The latest details on this inimitable drug discovery system can be obtained on-line at *http://www.cellomics.com.*

V. HCS OF DRUG-INDUCED MICROTUBULE CYTOSKELETON REORGANIZATION

As detailed above, HCS assays fall into two general classes: fixed endpoint and kinetic. Here we demonstrate both assay types in the quantification of microtubule targeted compounds. In the first assay, cells are treated with drugs, incubated for various times, fixed, and labeled to visualize microtubules. The labeling procedure involves immunofluorescence to visualize cytoplasmic microtubules. Figure 1 shows the results of an assay where mouse fibroblasts have been treated with several known microtubule-disrupting drugs. The effects of these standard drugs are being used in the development of imaging algorithms to automatically classify and quantify the effects of potential lead compounds on the microtubule cytoskeleton.

Apart from immunofluorescence-based reagents, live-cell kinetic HCS assays necessitate the use of molecular-based fluorophores, most notably among them the green fluorescent protein (GFP) from jellyfish [7] and other sources [9]. Protein chimeras consisting of mutant GFP molecules and a protein that interacts specifically with intracellular microtubules have been constructed and at least one has been reported [7]. We present here a chimera that has been transfected into cells and acts to provide live measurements of microtubule dynamics in living cells. Figure 2 shows cells transfected with this fluorescent chimera, which converts the cells into HCS reagents, and the effects of drugs on the microtubule

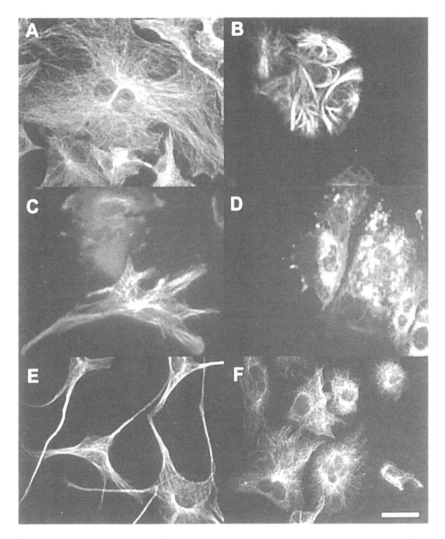

Figure 1 A fixed-endpoint, high-content assay of microtubule disruption. Mouse fibroblasts were treated with drugs followed by the visualization of the microtubule cytoskeleton using immunofluorescence techniques. The cells were treated as follows: A, no treatment; B, paclitaxel; C, curacin A; D, nocodazole; E, staurosporine; F, colchicine. Each drug had a distinct effect on cell morphology and microtubule organization. Scale bar = 20 μm.

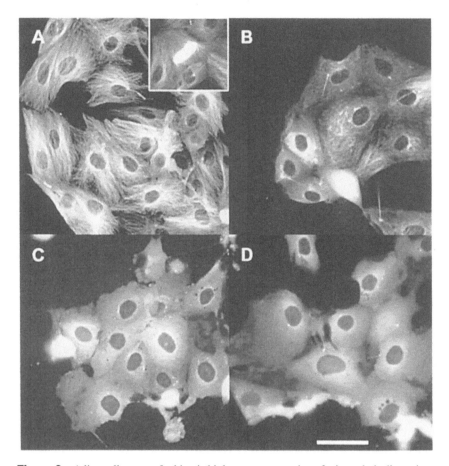

Figure 2 A live cell reagent for kinetic high-content screening of microtubule disruption. Porcine epithelial cells were transfected with a plasmid encoding a chimera composed of a protein that readily incorporates into cellular microtubules and a mutant green fluorescent protein. The cells in panel A show the distribution of microtubules in untreated cells with the inset depicting a brightly labeled spindle in a mitotic cell. The other panels show the effects of microtubule disrupting drugs that include B, vinblastine; C, curacin A; and D, colchicine.

cytoskeleton in these engineered sensor cells. In these cells, with this reagent, the microtubule-disrupting drugs had just as profound an effect on microtubules as they did in the fixed-endpoint assay described above. Although not shown here, we have measured the kinetics of microtubule disruption over periods ranging from seconds to hours using these chimeric HCS reagents. Nevertheless, the data shown here represent well the cytoskeletal reorganization and microtubule dissolution that these drugs induce in living cells. Imaging algorithms similar to those developed for the fixed-endpoint assay of microtubule reorganization are being developed for the live-cell assay, but they contain a kinetics component as an added dimension. Therefore, the reagents described above for the fixed-endpoint and kinetic assays can be used either alone or in conjunction with other reagents to form the basis of multiparameter assays, a powerful application of HCS [5].

VI. SPECIALIZED FLUORESCENT REAGENTS THAT FIND DUAL USE IN HCS AND HTS

In many cases, high-content screens involve intracellular spatial measurements (e.g., translocation of molecules between cellular compartments), yet there is a class of screens where the fluorescent reagents can be engineered to yield high-content data from a high-throughput read-out. That is, using the example of intracellular translocation as an illustration, a fluorescent reagent can be designed not only to translocate between cellular compartments in response to some molecular activity but to alter its fluorescence spectral properties upon translocation. Thus, a measurement of the spectral change of the reagent rather than a high-resolution measurement of spatial distribution is used as a reporter of an intracellular translocation. Such dual-use reagents that report both their dynamic distribution and activity within living cells are often designed from macromolecules and are termed fluorescent protein biosensors [10,11]. Careful design of HCS reagents therefore makes it possible to build powerful platforms where high-throughput and high-content screens can be coupled.

An example of a relatively simple fluorescent reagent that finds dual use in high-content as well as high-throughput assays is JC-1, a fluorescent dye that partitions preferentially into live mitochondria and acts as a reporter of membrane potential within the organelle [12,13]. JC-1 monomers (green fluorescent) are present in regions of mitochondria that exhibit relatively low membrane potential, whereas JC-1 aggregates (orange fluorescent) partition preferentially into regions of relatively high membrane potential. Figure 3 shows an orange fluorescent image of JC-1 (Molecular Probes Inc., Eugene, OR) in porcine epithelial cells. At the magnification shown, it was possible to resolve numerous mitochondria in a population of living cells. Furthermore, a heterogeneous distribution of JC-1 aggregates was measured single mitochondria. Thus, a high-content measurement of JC-1 monomers and aggregates in living cell mitochondria can be used not only to assess the effects of lead compounds on mitochondrial physiology but also to identify the mitochondrial compartment as a fiduciary marker for the colocalization of other fluorescent reagents in the same cell.

JC-1 also finds use as a fluorescent reagent for high-throughput live-cell screening. The fluorescence signals emanating from all cells a well can be mea-

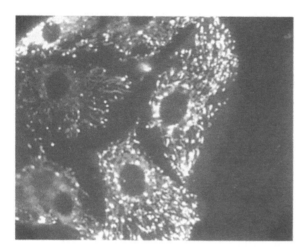

Figure 3 Porcine epithelial cells labeled with JC-1. LLCPK cells were labeled in culture with JC-1 and this micrograph depicts the intracellular distribution of the fluorescent probe. Once added to the extracellular medium, JC-1 rapidly crosses the plasma membrane and partitions specifically into mitochondrial membranes where it reports the electrical potential.

sured simultaneously for both the monomeric and aggregated forms of JC-1 using, for example, a fluorescence microplate reader. Unlike the ArrayScan II system, a microplate reader provides no cellular spatial information but rapidly assesses average cellular mitochondrial potential by measuring the ratio of green and orange fluorescence from an entire monolayer of labeled cells. Figure 4 shows an example of living cell mitochondrial potential measurements made with a fluorescence microplate reader. The kinetic data are presented as a fluorescence ratio (JC-1 aggregate/JC-1 monomer) that is independent of dye concentration but proportional to the mitochondrial potential averaged across an entire well. The kinetic trace for untreated cells exhibits a small decrease over the first minutes, which is likely due to the cooling of the cells within the microplate reader as well as the change in cell medium pH that occurs with the transfer of the microplate from an incubator (5% CO_2) to atmospheric conditions. Nevertheless, a significant decrease in mitochondrial potential was measured upon the addition of an inhibitor of oxidative energy production, valinomycin, to the living cells. Thus, a high-throughput assay of mitochondrial potential can be used to qualify promising lead compounds for more sophisticated high-content assays that may include spatially resolved mitochondrial potential measurements as well as macromolecular translocations [5,6] and organellar functional morphology changes within a population of the same cells [8]. Dual-use fluorescent reagents therefore will find

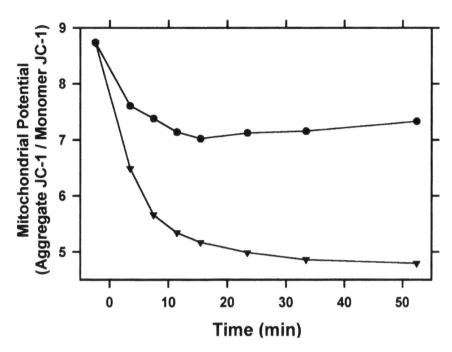

Figure 4 A prototype high-throughput assay for drugs that alter mitochondrial potential. LLCPK cells, labeled with JC-1, were either left untreated (*filled circles*) or treated with 10 nM valinomycin (*filled triangles*) at time = 0. Kinetic measurement of the JC-1 fluorescence ratio is used to quantify the loss of mitochondrial membrane potential induced by the ionophore valinomycin. A high-throughput assay using this approach would simultaneously measure mitochondrial potential changes in multiple wells of a microplate.

utility in many distinct aspects of the drug discovery process and become reagents that are even more powerful when used to couple high-throughput and high-content assays on the same drug discovery platform.

VII. COUPLING HIGH-THROUGHPUT AND HIGH-CONTENT SCREENING WITH MICROARRAYS OF LIVING CELLS: THE CELLCHIP™ SYSTEM

Miniaturization of assays is one of the major forces driving improved productivity in early drug discovery [14,15]. New drug development technologies and the explosion in genetic data as a result of the Human Genome Project have driven the development of miniaturized test beds or "biochips" for genetic analysis based on microarrays of nucleic acid sequences. These biochips encompass a very diverse array of technologies and applications. Imprinted with several hundred different nucleic acid sequences, biochips use electro-optical means of addressing applications ranging from expression analysis to genotyping and mutation screening [16,17]. Biochips integrated into sample processing, metering, measuring, mixing, and sorting systems have laid the foundation for miniaturized "sample to answer" systems. The first generation of biochips is focused on surface anchored oligonucleotides and oligopeptides whose information content is dictated by the four-character nucleotide language of the DNA or the 20-character language of amino acids. Furthermore, the single-stranded DNA oligonucleotides are limited in their information content and applications, as they do not provide information on DNA–protein and other interactions [18].

We believe that miniaturized cell arrays constitute the next logical frontier in early drug discovery. The multidimensional language of cellular physiology is only partly described by the combinatorial integration of nucleotide and amino acid languages. When high-content screens of living cells arrayed on miniaturized solid supports are used to dissect this complex language, they provide deep biological information on target distribution and activity in space and time. The CellChip system is a combinatorial of surface chemistries, cell and tissue types, and HCS fluorescent reagents. On the chip, single or multiple engineered cell types are microarrayed in predetermined spatial addresses (Fig. 5) on an optically clear polymer or glass solid phase support substrate [14]. The "footprint" of each cellular domain can be adjusted to accommodate either a single cell or a colony of

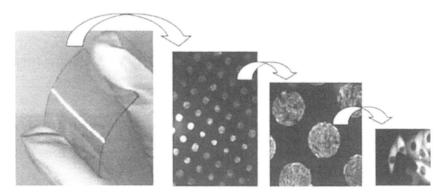

Figure 5   Colonies of cells microarrayed on polymer and glass solid-phase supports. Each domain is fluidically and optically isolated. This enables massive parallelization of assays on a single chip. Production of a library of chips, where the library encompasses multiple cell types and multiple biochemical pathways, enables high sample throughput coupled with high information output of the pharmacological profile of compound libraries.

cells. The cell adhesive domains can be populated either with a single cell type or with multiple cell types by adhesive cell sorting from a mixed-cell population, according to selective adhesive interactions with particular cell-specific ligands coupled to the individual domains [5].

HCS assays designed for microplates have been successfully transferred to the CellChip system. One of these assays—the cytoplasm-to-nucleus transloca-tion of intracellular molecules—is a class of cell-based screens that tests the abil-ity of candidate drug compounds to induce or inhibit transport of transcription fac-tors from the cytoplasm the nucleus. Sensor cells arrayed on CellChips are treated with a combination of chemical entities. The assays can be run as fixed-endpoint or live-cell kinetic assays. For example, in a fixed-endpoint assay, an array of sen-sor cells is treated with a chemical fixative and labeled with a fluorescent nucleic acid probe and an antibody against the transcription factor or stress-associated protein labeled with another fluorescent conjugate. The test consists of measuring the fluorescence from the antibody in the nucleus (the nucleus being defined by the nucleic acid probe), versus the cytoplasm defined by the cell domain outside of the nucleus. Proprietary algorithms facilitate quantitation of the kinetics and amount of transcription factor or stress protein translocation into the nucleus over time [6]. Using a polymer-based CellChip system, we have quantified the activa-tion-induced translocation of NF-κB, a transcription factor involved in cell stress molecular pathways, in response to tumor necrosis factor-α (TNF-α). Appropriate cellular domains on the CellChip platform were dosed with TNF-α; the cells were fixed, permeabilized, and labeled for the NF-κB p65 and nuclear domains (NF-κB Activation HitKit™; Cellomics, Inc.). As seen in Figure 6, there was a redistribu-tion of the transcription factor to the nucleus because of stimulation. There was up to a fourfold increase in both the normalized nuclear intensity and the normalized ratio between nuclear and cytoplasmic intensities post translocation. This increase is equivalent to the results obtained in the microplate platform [6].

The advantages offered by miniaturization of a drug discovery platform include (1) a combined HTS and HCS platform with a single-pass read of the HTS data from all "wells" prior to HCS "drill-down"; (2) higher throughput; (3) reduced processing time; (4) increased number of tests run in a massively parallel format on one substrate; (5) smaller reagent volumes; (6) conservation of new chemical entities (NCEs); and (7) reduced waste. The integration of such advan-tages translates into a dramatic reduction of cost and acceleration of productivity in candidate compound testing. For example, migration of assays from 96-well microplates to 1536-well microplates reduces the reagent cost by 100-fold. Migra-tion from the 96-well microplate format to microarrayed cells on chips will fur-ther drop the volume of reagents and the cost of plate handling. For example, a chip with microarrayed cells in a density format of 100 wells per cm^2 will reduce the reagent cost by 500-fold from the 96-well format. Furthermore, developing chips microarrayed with tissue-specific cells will have a tremendous impact in

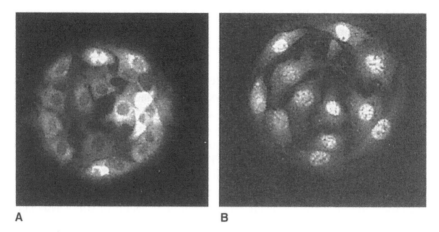

A   B

Figure 6 Mammalian cells contained within the CellChip system employed in a high-content screen for transcription factor activation. As a result of stimulation with a proinflammatory factor such as TNF-α, there is a spatial redistribution of NF-κB. There is a four-fold increase in normalized nuclear intensity post stimulation. (A) Unstimulated cells on the polymer based CellChip platform. (B) TNF-α stimulated cells on the polymer-based CellChip platform.

screening the potency, specificity, toxicity, and efficacy of test compounds against a "tissue-like" ensemble leading to higher predictive relevance of the live-cell data. Developing multiple cell-based test beds microarrayed in addressable biochips will facilitate the use of these "microscale tissues" as powerful indicators and predictors of the in vivo performance of the lead compound or toxin using HCS.

The evolution of a miniaturized cell-based drug discovery and identification platform, the CellChip system [5,14], a variant of the generic biochip, will march in tandem with other miniaturization technologies aimed at shrinking benchtop instruments into their hand-held miniaturized versions [19]. The integration of HTS and HCS onto a single platform (Fig. 7) will meet the high-sample-through-put and high-information-output needs of the pharmaceutical industry. This combined platform reduces the data capture, processing, and analysis times and provides a complete cell-based screening platform. Developing technologies to enable arrays of multiple cells on glass or plastic chips, with each cell carrying its own reagents in the form of single- or multiple fluorescence reagents including fluorescent protein biosensors [11], adds multidimensional power to a complete drug screening platform. Furthermore, reagent and assay technology developments made on platforms based on the present HCS technology or standard microplates will migrate directly to the CellChip system.

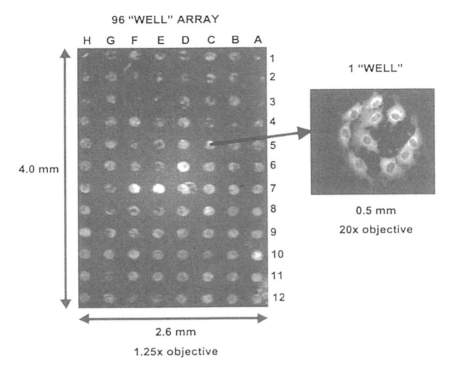

Figure 7 Combining high-throughput screening (HTS) and high-content screening (HCS) on the same platform. The massive parallelization achievable with miniaturization is shown in a simple simulation on this surface-modified plastic platform. The HTS is simulated here to detect "hits" on the miniaturized chip platform. Lack of fluorescence signals in wells E3, F3, A3, and B4, for example, indicate "non-hits." HCS measurements are then made only on the 'hit' wells to gain more in-depth information to produce more "highly qualified hits." Further depth and breadth of information can be obtained by arraying multiple organ-specific cells on a single chip and fluidically addressing each domain with a reagent of choice.

The future of biochips in early drug discovery is bright because enabling HTS technologies, such as biochip platforms for screening, have captured the attention of the biopharmaceutical market. The early biochips were designed for applications driven by genomics. These "gene chips" are projected to penetrate and capture a significant portion of a billion dollar HTS market over the next 2–4 years. Following close on the heels of the "gene chips" are "protein chips" that exploit the proteome as a tool for drug discovery. The CellChip system will build on present and future genomic and proteomic databases to provide multidimensional measures of cellular physiology. Furthermore, the integration of high sample throughput with high information output on the CellChip system will yield faster and more efficient winnowing of "leads" from "hits," thereby optimizing the selection of the compounds early in the process of drug discovery.

VIII. CELLOMICS KNOWLEDGEBASE EMBODIES A NEW PARADIGM FOR BIOINFORMATICS: CREATION OF KNOWLEDGE FROM HCS

Genomics, proteomics, and the knowledge base built from cellular information are critically important to the drug discovery process. The Cellomics Knowledgebase is the logical extension of genomics and proteomics because it defines the organization and analysis of cellular information based on new knowledge. The Cellomics Knowledgebase will contain all the knowledge related to cell structure and function. Pharmaceutical researchers will interact with this Cellomics Knowledgebase in a biologically intuitive way to explore cellular mechanisms to be able to select optimal targets for drug discovery and to screen potential lead compounds more effectively.

The Cellomics Knowledgebase captures the complex temporal and spatial interplay of all the components that compose the living cell. For example, the process of signal transduction relies on a highly coordinated network of intracellular ions, metabolites, macromolecules, and organelles. Most signal transduction processes are therefore a series of specific physical-chemical interactions. In this aspect, the functioning of a cell is conceptually similar to that of a computer neuronetwork. Computer neuronetworks are composed of simple subunits that perform rudimentary mathematical operations. However, there are many such units and, most importantly, these units are highly connected, using the output from one unit as the input to another. Cellular signal transduction offers a parallel strategy to the neuronetwork approach; the basic units of signal transduction are proteins and other cellular components. Each component can participate in one or more cellular functions while involved in a complicated interaction with one or more other cellular components in time and space. Therefore, the design of the Cellomics Knowledgebase reflects the functional significance of the interactions among the cellular constituents.

Figure 8 illustrates cellular interactions by showing a simplified fragment of the model for the Cellomics Knowledgebase. This fragment captures the core information of cellular pathways. This core is composed of a record of interactions of cellular constituents and the logical connections among these interactions. The cellular constituents are abstracted into the "functional unit" class in the model. A functional unit can be either a "component" or an "assembly." A component represents a single protein, metabolite, or other cellular constituent together with external stimuli. An assembly is composed of functional units, meaning that it can

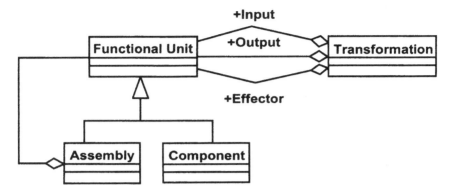

Figure 8 Fragment of the UML (unified modeling language) model for the Cellomics Knowledgebase.

be made up of individual components or other assemblies. Functional units, assemblies, and components record the interactions of cellular constituents. The logical connections of these interactions are recorded in the "transformation" class. A transformation can have many functional units acting as inputs, outputs, and effectors. For example, in the simple transformation depicted in Figure 9, the chemical conversion of a substrate into a product is catalyzed by an enzyme, a

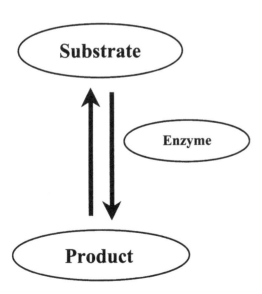

Figure 9 A transformation.

motif that is repeated for many of the hundreds of millions of chemical reactions that are occurring simultaneously in a living cell. In this model, for the transformation from the substrate to the product, the substrate acts as the input and the output is a chemically altered product. In this case, an enzyme acts as an effector. If we drill down on any of the components shown in the scheme, we find that each may be a complex assembly made up of more components that maintain their own temporal, spatial, and chemical properties within the living cell. For example, if the enzyme chosen in the model as an effector is pyruvate dehydrogenase, the enzyme that couples two major oxidative metabolic pathways, we find that it is itself a complex macromolecular assembly. The pyruvate dehydrogenase complex comprises multiple copies of three distinct enzymes that require five coenzymes for activity [20]. The pyruvate dehydrogenase complex is precisely assembled to optimize the oxidation of pyruvate to acetyl Coenzyme A and CO_2. In eukaryotes, the enzyme complex is further localized into a higher order structure, the mitochondrion, which in turn exhibits a temporal and spatial distribution of activities or transformations within the cell. Therefore, constituents of the transformation class exist as collections of cellular components in time and space from the continuum of ions, metabolites, macromolecules, and organelles.

Having captured cellular interactions, the design of the Cellomics Knowledgebase must also take into account the unique features of cell biological information, such as:

1. The flow of information from genomics to proteomics to the living cell. Any insight into the function of cell biology will require seamless integration of information across this continuum.
2. Cell biological information is often incomplete or in an unconfirmed state. For example, we need to be able to record the fact that a protein X interacts with an experimentally isolated assembly Y, although Y is not characterized well and the components of Y may be unknown. The database must be flexible enough to be rapidly and accurately updated as unknown components become characterized entities.

How might cellular knowledge be best visualized and probed by the user? One common way to represent cellular knowledge is through pathway diagrams. There are many well-defined metabolic and signaling pathways, but, in isolation, they have lost their physiological context. In reality, pathways often intersect with other pathways to form networks of molecular interactions. Within the Cellomics Knowledgebase, a pathway is a collection of transformations. This collection contains the same functional units and transformations as defined in a well-known pathway, and it can be generated de novo from a database query. Hence, we use the term "molecular wiring diagrams" instead of "pathway diagrams."

The Cellomics Knowledgebase will also provide a new generation of data mining capabilities. For example, the Cellomics Knowledgebase will provide functions for the analysis of complex cellular response patterns to drug candidates. Data mining tools will make possible automated comparison of these patterns with the patterns of successful and unsuccessful leads to guide the user further down the drug discovery process.

In summary, the Cellomics Knowledgebase is a knowledge management tool for cell biology and cell-based drug discovery. In the drug discovery process, knowledge is generated from "data" and "information." Data are the measured values from cellular events that have been acquired, such as from HCS. Information is the result of putting data into a relevant context. For example, an HCS value becomes information when related to a particular assay with specific parameters such as cell type, reagent or reagents used, and the structure and concentration of the drug used in the assay. Knowledge therefore is the understanding of the biological meaning of information. With this understanding, the acquisition of data can be modified and new information extracted to further improve the knowledge base. Knowledge is synthesized by forming connections between disparate pieces of information. Thus, the Cellomics Knowledgebase strives to provide tools for the analysis and visualization of these connections, such as the connection between screening results, compound structure, and biological context. This connection, and the knowledge built from it, will enable researchers from diverse backgrounds to interpret and utilize new and established information, thus unifying multiple screening projects from multiple laboratories.

The construction of complete cellular knowledge will be achieved with deliberate steps of discovery. Being able to incorporate these incremental discoveries into the context of the existing knowledge through the Cellomics Knowledgebase will become critical to a systematic understanding of cell biological functions. We believe that the pharmaceutical industry will be a primary beneficiary of this new level of understanding.

IX. PROSPECTUS

An epoch is rapidly approaching in which the sequence of many organismal genomes, including that of humans, will be deciphered and in which a genomics knowledge base will be built on the foundation of the voluminous data. Nevertheless, we envision this period in the near future as a prologue to the era of the cell where life science discovery, especially in the pharmaceutical industry, will be cell centric rather than focused on isolated genes and proteins. New thinking will be required to interpret the exceedingly complex web of molecular processes that compose life at the cellular level. How, then, will we begin to unravel the integration of living components in time and space within cells? We predict that an amalgamation of molecular biological, biochemical, and cell biological disciplines will be tapped to supplant cells into being reporters of their own molecular activities.

Furthermore, a novel approach to informatic and bioinformatic knowledge building integrated with a miniaturized platform for cellular data acquisition will become a major force in defining and shaping the molecular circuitry of the cell.

Several issues will be resolved during the evolution of the integrated technologies that will be required to define and structure cellular knowledge. First, new generations of luminescent reagents, including fluorescent protein biosensors, will be necessary to simultaneously measure multiple molecular processes in time and space within living cells. Innovative engineering of cells and the surfaces with which they interact will ensure that a wide range of cell types (e.g., adherent and nonadherent, mixtures of cell types, etc.) will be amenable to HCS. A fully automated system for extracting cellular data from images will speed the analysis of multiple cellular pathways and provide for computation concurrent with data acquisition. Finally, a fresh approach to informatics and bioinformatics will combine published data of cellular chemistry with HCS data into an unrivaled knowledge base of the multidimensional processes involved in the molecular basis of life. Therefore, the key to unlocking the door to this new era will be the intuitive integration of technologies that will be required to decipher the language of the cell.

ACKNOWLEDGMENTS

This work is supported in part by the DoD under a DARPA contract (N00014-98-C-0326), and a program project grant from the National Cancer Institute (P01 CA78039-01).

REFERENCES

1. Wilson EB. Introduction. In: Cowdry Ev, ed. General Cytology: A Textbook of Cellular Structure and Function for Students of Biology and Medicine. Chicago: University of Chicago Press, 1924:3–11.
2. Edström JE. Nucleotide analysis on the cyto-scale. Nature 1953;172:809.
3. Haynes PA, Gygi SP, Figeys D, Aebersold R. Proteome analysis: biological assay or data archive? Electrophoresis 1998;19:1862–1871.
4. Celis JE, Gromov P. 2D protein electrophoresis: can it be perfected? Curr Opin Biotechnol 1999;10(1):16–21.
5. Giuliano KA, DeBiasio RL, Dunlay RT, Gough A, Volosky JM, Zock J, Pavlakis GN, Taylor DL. High-content screening: a new approach to easing key bottlenecks in the drug discovery process. J Biomol Scr 1997;2:249–259.
6. Ding GJF, Fischer PA, Boltz RC, Schmidt JA, Colaianne JJ, Gough A, Rubin RA, Miller DK. Characterization and quantitation of NF-κB nuclear translocation induced by interleukin-1 and tumor necrosis factor-α. Development and use of a high capacity fluorescence cytometric system. J Biol Chem 1998;273:28897–28905.

7. Kain SR. Green fluorescent protein (GFP): applications in cell-based assays for drug discovery. Drug Disc Today 1999;4:304–312.

8. Conway BR, Minor LK, Xu JZ, Gunnet JW, DeBiasio R, D'Andrea MR, Rubin R, DeBiasio R, Giuliano K, Zhou L, Demarest KT. Quantification of G-protein coupled receptor internalization using G-protein coupled receptor–green fluorescent protein conjugates with the ArrayScan high-content screening system. J Biomol Scr 1999; 4:75–86.

9. Matz MV, Fradkov AF, Labas YA, Savitsky AP, Zaraisky AG, Markelov ML, Lukyanov SA. Fluorescent proteins from nonbioluminescent anthozoa species. Nat Biotechnol 1999;17(10):969–973.

10. Giuliano KA, Post PL, Hahn KM, Taylor DL. Fluorescent protein biosensors: Measurement of molecular dynamics in living cells. Annu Rev Biophys Biomol Struct 1995;24:405–434.

11. Giuliano KA, Taylor DL. Fluorescent-protein biosensors: New tools for drug discovery. Trends Biotech 1998;16:135–140.

12. Reers M, Smith TW, Chen LB. J-aggregate formation of a carbocyanine as a quantitative fluorescent indicator of membrane potential. Biochemistry 1991;30:4480–4486.

13. Smiley ST, Reers M, Mottola-Hartshorn C, Lin M, Chen A, Smith TW, Steele GDJ, Chen LB. Intracellular heterogeneity in mitochondrial membrane potentials revealed by a J-aggregate-forming lipophilic cation JC-1. Proc Natl Acad Sci USA 1991;88: 3671–3675.

14. Kapur R, Giuliano KA, Campana M, Adams T, Olson K, Jung D, Mrksich M, Vasudevan C, Taylor DL. Streamlining the drug discovery process by integrating miniaturization, high throughput screening, high content screening, and automation on the CellChip system. Biomed Microdev 1999;2:99–109.

15. Service RF. Coming soon: the pocket DNA sequencer. Science 1999;282:399–401.

16. Service RF. Miniaturization puts chemical plants where you want them. Science 1998;282:400.

17. Fodor SPA, Read JL, Pirrung MC, Stryer L, Lu AT, Solas D. Light-directed, spatially addressable parallel chemical synthesis. Science 1991;251:767–773.

18. Carlson R, Brent R. Double-stranded DNA arrays: next steps in the surface campaign. Nat Biotechnol 1999;17:536–537.

19. Marshall S. Fundamental changes ahead for lab instrumentation. R&D Mag 1999: 18–22.

20. Lehninger AL, Nelson DL, Cox MM. In: Principles of Biochemistry. New York: Worth Publishers, 1993:447–451.

14

Miniaturization Technologies for High-Throughput Biology

Walter D. Niles and Peter J. Coassin
Aurora Biosciences Corporation
San Diego, California

I. INTRODUCTION

A strategy is summarized for the integration of cellular biology with instrument systems to miniaturize fluid delivery, assay containment, and detection for high-throughput screening and biological research. Specific components of the process include the handling of microliter scale volumes of liquids (microfluidics), fluorescence detection, sample handling, and bioassay technology amenable to high-density formats. The components enable ultrahigh-throughput (e.g., 100,000 samples per day) biological assays. These systems provide the increased productivity required for determining gene functions in a whole-cell context. Miniaturization of these technologies is essential to achieve the goal of 100,000 samples per day.

A. Key Integrated Miniaturization Technologies

NanoWell assay plates (Aurora Biosciences)
Sample handling and liquid dispensing
    Piezo-based aspiration and dispensation
    Solenoid valve–based aspiration and dispensation
    Reagent dispensation—cells, dyes, media, etc.
Fluorescence Detection

B. Why Is miniaturization Critical to Ultrahigh-Throughput Screening Development?

Miniaturization of the assay reactions enables conservation of compounds, reagents, and biologicals, and makes facile the scale-up for parallel (simultaneous) screening of a large number of compounds. Ultimately, miniaturization of the assay reaction is a critical and essential aspect of achieving high-throughput sample processing. Materials handling, robotic speed, material cost, and other logistical aspects would ultimately prevent optimal deployment of a high-throughput (>100,000 samples per day) system without assay miniaturization and increased reaction well density in the assay plate. Successful miniaturization requires optimization of the assay, the cell density, the expression level of the active readout protein, and the fluorigenic substrate concentration inside the cells to provide sufficient signal intensity to facilitate rapid measurement of activity of the cellular process under study. Typical assays are staged with positive and negative controls run in separate assay wells such that end-point readings of fluorescence provide meaningful data and determination of kinetics is unnecessary. Kinetic or rate measurements are possible with the instrumentation but typically require additional time-based liquid additions or optical measurements in order to establish analyte concentration.

II. THE SCREENING PROCESS

A. Assay Development

Aurora is developing assays for cellular physiological processes based on fluorescence resonance energy transfer (FRET). In FRET, excitation energy is transferred from one fluorophore (the donor) to another fluorophore (the acceptor) when the two molecules are in close proximity (<10 nm) and in the optimal relative orientation, and the emission spectrum of the donor overlaps the absorption spectrum of the acceptor. Aurora has developed a variety of energy transfer fluorophore pairs that undergo efficient energy transfer when the donor is excited. Some of these FRET pairs are covalently bonded together and this bond is broken to detect molecular change. Other FRET pairs are spatially associated but not covalently linked. The FRET rate constant is quantifiably diminished after the critical association between the donor and acceptor fluorophores is disrupted. FRET can also be effected by the bringing together of a donor and an acceptor. Either method provides a clear readout of the molecular event. Aurora has commercially developed three different types of FRET-based fluorophores: Green Fluorescent Protein and its variants, a gene expression reporter that is intrinsically fluorescent; β-lactamase, an enzyme-based reporter that cleaves a FRET-based substrate; and the voltage-potential dyes, which make possible the detection of voltage potential across a cell membrane. The gene expression reporters can be introduced into the cell by transfection of the cell with a plasmid encoding its sequence. Regulatory elements incorporated upstream from the enzyme-coding sequence can be specified to enable linking expression of the reporter with cellular physiological processes and signal transduction cascades. Some of the fluorophore pairs under development by Aurora are as follows:

1. Pairs of mutated Green Fluorescent Proteins with overlapping fluorescence spectra. The proteins are covalently linked by an amino acid sequence tailored to be the substrate for specific proteases, phosphatases, and associative binding mechanisms.
2. Coumarin and fluorescein dyes linked by a cephalosporin moiety that is a substrate for bacterial β-lactamase. The combined dual-fluorophore compound is synthesized in a cell membrane–permeant acetoxyester form that can be passively loaded into cells and activated into fluorescent form by endogenous esterases. With this compound, cells are transfected with an expression plasmid encoding β-lactamase under control by transcription factor elements that are gene regulatory elements for the physiological signal transduction cascade that is of interest to the investigator.
3. Coumarin dye linked to the headgroup of phosphatidylethanolamine and bisoxonol cyanine dye is a lipophilic fluorophore pain that partitions to lipid bilayer membranes of cells from the aqueous phase. Since the distribution of the charged oxonol is determined by the membrane potential of the cell, this probe pair is suited to assay membrane ion channels.

Assays are developed by transfection of cells with the desired expression plasmid. Once a cell type is successfully transfected and the transfected cells are selected and propagated as a clonal cell line, the miniaturized assay is ready for staging. Assays are constructed by addition of the cells and the fluorigenic substrates in combination with either activators or inhibitors of the physiological process under study, together with the chemical compound under test in a reaction well. Fluorescence intensities of the donor and acceptor are measured under donor excitation. Aurora has constructed the Ultra-High-Throughput Screening System (UHTSS) as an industrial platform that automates the performance of miniaturized assays in a replicated format that can screen a large number of chemical compounds in a single pass through the platform (Fig. 1). The UHTSS has been developed to enable reliable miniaturization of the construction and measurement of FRET-based cellular assays.

B. Compound Distribution

Chemical compound libraries are screened, by introducing the compound in cellular physiological assays, to determine whether the compound exerts a pharmaco-

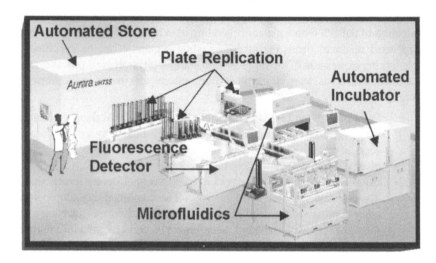

Figure 1 The Aurora Ultra-High-Throughput Screening System (UHTSS). The compounds are stored in industry-standard 96- and 384-well storage plates in the store. Compounds are screened for effects on physiological processes (probed in the assay cell lines) by automated selection from the store and conveyance of the compound plate to replication stations, where compounds are prepared for assay. Assays are staged by combining the compounds with assay reagents and cells in miniaturized reaction vessels at the microfluidic stations, incubating the reagents, and measuring fluorescence of donor and acceptor fluorophores at the detector.

logical effect and is of physiological interest. Library screening demands considerable precision of automation to handle the vast number of compounds in libraries and accurate liquid handling to preserve a stock of potentially valuable material for a large number of assays. A database is used to maintain the information regarding each compound, such as its location in the storage facility, its well location in a barcoded storage microplate, its stock concentration, and assay information such as the details of cellular assay experiments. Key automated steps are retrieval of storage plates and redistribution into assay plates (Fig. 2). High-throughput compound distribution is achieved with automated liquid handling to enable a large number of parallel assays to be run on a large number of compounds at the same time. This requires that liquids be distributed rationally by the automation system into arrays of reaction wells that provide for a scientifically significant screen to ensure that each chemical compound is tested in a physiological assay and to decrease the possibilities of false-positive or false-negative responses that necessitate retesting. Miniaturization demands that the very small quantities of material be delivered accurately and precisely to individual small reaction volumes.

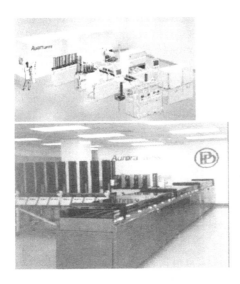

Store over 1,000,000 compounds

Access 1-400,000 per day for screening

Select 2,400 per day for retest

Figure 2 Automated chemical compound library. The compounds are stored individually in 96-well- or 384-well format bar-coded microplates. Compounds are tracked using a database that coordinates the automated actions performed on the compounds stored in each plate. The future portends further miniaturization of the compound storage to 1536-well and 3456-well format microplates.

C. Loading the Assay

To facilitate construction of parallel assays for large numbers of test compounds at a time, special high-density reaction well formats have been created that enable scaling of biological assays to the reduced volume required. To construct assays in small volumes requires confluence of accurate and precise fluid handling, automated positioning of fluid dispensers, and assay well design to avoid a series of potential pitfalls inherent in miniaturization. Thus, assays are constructed by bringing reaction wells that are formatted to evolving industry-standard designs under arrays of multiplexed fluid dispensers from which are ejected the constituents of the reaction. These include the engineered cells developed to serve as chemical and physiological platforms for the reaction, the cell culture medium, the buffers and any particular reagent requirements, the cell-permeant dual fluorophore, the traditional agonist (or antagonist) used to stimulate the transduction pathway, and the chemical compound under test. Each reaction requires a particular concentration of reagent or compound, and the delivery of each chemical may be constrained by particular physical properties such as solubility. Thus, loading an assay to a total final volume of 1–2 µl requires combining assay constituents that are dispensed in volumes that may range from 0.1 to 1 µl (i.e., a range of

10,000-fold). This range of volumetric liquid delivery requires dispenser modalities that are adapted and suitable for specific ranges of volumes such as 0.1–10 µl or 0.1–10 nl. Each range of dispensing is performed by a single modular platform that can be replicated for the different reagents or to improve speed of delivery. Typically at these volume ranges, noncontact dispensation methods have inherent advantages over contact-based methodologies. Contact-based dispensation can be particularly effective in a "touch-off" mode with larger volumes or in dry plates but becomes cumbersome in small volumes.

D. Incubation

With cellular physiological assays, biochemical action occurs predominantly inside the cells, even with cascades that are triggered at the cell surface, such as agonist binding to a receptor. Thus, once the assay is loaded into the reaction well, the cells are incubated to enable.

1. The generation of a steady-state level of the expressed readout enzyme. This is determined by the activation (or inhibition) of the signal transduction cascade under study by the added agonist (antagonist) and the concomitant effect of the test compound (if any) on the steady-state level of activation of the pathway. The steady-state level of the readout enzyme is a direct indicator of the level of pathway activation.
2. The membrane-permeable dual-fluorophore compound (chemical name CCF2/CCF4) permeating the cells and becoming fluorescent by the action of endogenous esterases on the acetoxy esters that facilitate membrane permeation.

This requires that the cells be incubated to achieve physiological steady state after assay loading. Assays are typically constructed in several steps:

1. The cells and medium or buffer are loaded and the cells are allowed to attach to the reaction well bottom in one step;
2. The physiological activators and test compound are loaded in other steps; and
3. The reagents necessary for the fluorescent readout are loaded.

Each step may be performed at a different temperature. The challenge for miniaturization in large formats is that both the high-density format array of (miniaturized) reaction wells and the incubator must be optimized for maintenance of physiological conditions. This includes maintenance of the atmospheric conditions of relative humidity and temperature, as well as buffer capacity (% CO_2), at levels propitious for cell survival and for avoidance of evaporation over the periods needed (up to 24 h) to stage the assay. In addition, this places demands on the plate material to be favorable for the growth of cells, i.e., no toxic constituents that interfere with cell survival, no materials that contribute to fluorescence background, and high thermal conductivity to enable uniform warmth.

E. Detection

Miniaturized assays impose stringent requirements on the sensitivity and gain of the detection system. All Aurora-based assays are FRET based, and so it is necessary to measure both the donor and acceptor emission intensities in well-separated wavebands with high sensitivity. With miniaturized, high-density format assays, the detector measures the fluorescence of each color and in each reaction well of the high-density format plate. Miniaturization forces the detector to provide the capacity to accurately measure the fluorescence signals arising from small numbers of cells (1000–10,000) within each small well. Thus, each cell must contain a sufficient number of fluorophores to contribute a detectable signal. Additional demands on sensitivity arise from heterogeneous responses in the population of cells within each well. Thus, the fluorescence detectors need to be relatively noise free and stable in order to accurately measure the fluorescence using a smaller number of spatial and temporal samples of each well. For high throughput, the detectors need high sensitivity and fast response to enable accurate measurement with a minimum of dwell or transit time over each well.

F. Results Database

To discover new therapeutic lead candidates in the compound library, the effect of each test compound on the physiological processes under study in the cell-based assays needs tabulation in the compound database. The initial step is rapid conversion of the raw output of the detectors into a format suitable for storage in a database and statistical analysis. Database records for each compound are linked to other databases that include spectroscopy and other data to provide the compendium of data for each compound. High-throughput, miniaturized, high-density format screening generates potentially a large number of individual data records that include (1) test compound concentration (2) physiological processes tested, (3) agonist identity and concentration for each assay, (4) presence of modulators in addition to the test compound, and (5) different physical and chemical conditions that may be used during an assay. Furthermore, in addition to these sets of data, the outcomes of various analytical procedures, such as EC_{50}, IC_{50}, inhibitor concentrations, competitive and noncompetitive K_m and V_{max}, and other types of analysis (Schild, Dixon, nonparametric indices of significance). The limitation imposed by miniaturization is that an extremely large dataset is produced for each compound. To fully understand the efficacy and potential effects of each compound, and to rapidly identify leads, large data reduction and visualization tools are used to enable the effect of a compound to be compared against other test compounds and standard agonists or modulators and across physiological assays.

III. PLATE DESIGN AND PERFORMANCE

Two criteria are important for the design of a miniaturized assay plate. The plate must provide a high-density array of identical reaction vessels to which reagents and cells can be readily added during assay construction. In addition, it must not contribute distortion to the fluorescence intensity signals being read. The high-density well array plate is constructed to be as nonreactive as possible and to provide an inert physical platform that physically stages the assay and the detection of the assay readout. Aurora has designed and manufactured specialty NanoWell assay plates that consist of a 48 × 72 well array that is scaled from the industry standard 96-well (8 × 12) format. The plate has the same footprint as 96- and 384-well plates, and is fitted with a custom-designed lid that prevents evaporation and contamination. Each reaction well in the NanoWell plate is capable of holding 2.5 µl of liquid. The scaled format of wells makes possible automated positioning to be effected by subdividing the ranges used in 96-well format motor placement systems.

The bottom of the NanoWell plate (Fig. 3) consists of a single <0.2-mm thin sheet of clear cyclo-olefin copolymer (COC) that provides both a chemically inert

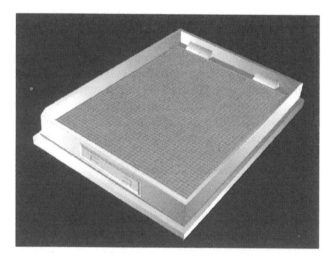

Figure 3   The Aurora Biosciences NanoWell assay plate. The plate is constructed to have the same total-size "footprint" as industry-standard microplates. The plate contains an array of 3456 reaction wells, each with a maximum volume of 2.7 µl. The reaction well arrangement comprised a 1.5-mm center-to-center distance and is scaled as a 6 × 6 well subdivision of the 9-mm center-to-center distance between the wells in the industry-standard 96-well microplate. The plate thickness is 3 mm. The plate is mounted in a custom-designed caddy. A close-fitting special lid covers the top of the plate and effectively seals each well against evaporation.

and an optically clear ($n = 1.65$) smooth surface. The plate can be brought down very close to the focusing optics of the fluorescence detector, so that bottom reading provides an unobstructed high numerical aperture sampling of the fluorescence emanating from each well. The circular well bottom is 0.95 mm in diameter, the diameter of the well at the top is 1.3 mm, and the well depth is 3 mm. The interstitial material between the wells consists of black dye mixed with COC polymer. The opacity minimizes the contamination of fluorescence measurements of each well by skew light originating from adjacent wells. The NanoWell plate bottom is optically planar to within 0.25 mm across its length, so that sphericity and astigmatism are reduced. Circular well, in contrast to square-shaped wells, provide for the uniform distribution of cells across the bottom of the wells.

Chemical inertness results in the surface at the bottom of each well being difficult to derivatize with typical covalent reagents. This has both advantages and drawbacks. The advantage is that the surface composition is always known. In addition, the material is essentially nontoxic to cells introduced into the wells. The drawback is that cells need to interact with the surface in some normal physiological manner for survival (i.e., expression of metabolic phenotype, entrance into a particular phase of the growth cycle). Chemical inertness thus requires some level of derivatization to facilitate cell–substrate adhesion (Fig. 4). The well bottoms are easily treated to create an artificial extracellular matrix (e.g., poly-L-lysine, collagen, gelatin, fibro-/vitronectins, etc). Nonpolarity of the well material favors adsorption of hydrophobic reagents, potentially reducing their bioavailability. This reduction in bioavailability is mitigated by indusion of extracellular serum factors that provide carrier capabilities. In general, bioavailability scales as the ratio of hydrophobic surface area to aqueous volume, which is approximately 50-fold greater for a well in the 96-well plate compared with a well in a NanoWell plate.

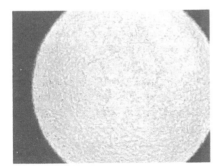

Figure 4 Phase contrast micrograph of Chinese hamster ovary (CHO) cells grown in single well of a NanoWell plate. The micrograph was obtained 6 h after seeding 2 μl of 10^6 cells/ml. The well bottom was coated with poly-L-lysine.

The inert plastic material also provides a very high electrical resistance. This effectively isolates each well from stray electrical currents created in ungrounded robotic positioning platforms. This also makes the plate susceptible to accumulation of static charge, which ultimately is not deleterious to the assay cells but may affect liquid dispensing.

IV. MICROFLUIDIC TECHNOLOGY

A. Sample Distribution Robot System

1. Piezo-actuated Dispensers and the Piezo Sample Distribution Robot

The Piezo Sample Distribution Robot (PSDR) is designed for delivery to assays of liquid volumes in the subnanoliter range. The conceptual framework within which the need for subnanoliter dispensing was developed is that the individual compounds the chemical library were synthesized in limited quantity and that replication of the synthetic run would not be efficacious if no useful leads were generated by the run. Hence, it is important to maximize the information derived from the limited quantity of each compound that is produced. The PSDR was designed to enable miniaturization of assays to submicroliter volumes by enabling delivery of materials present in only limited quantity, such as the constituents of chemical compound libraries, or those that are prepared in solutions with relatively high concentrations. The PSDR dispenses by piezo-actuated compression of a liquid–vapor interface. This results in the ejection of a single drop of liquid from the interface with a drop volume of 300–700 pl. The PSDR enables construction of microliter scale volumes by adding negligible quantities of concentrates.

To appreciate the value of the PSDR, it is useful to determine the number of molecules in a 2-μl reaction volume for various concentrations and then to calculate the stock concentration required if these molecules are delivered in a single bolus of liquid. For example, a 1 nM final concentration in 2 μl requires 1.2×10^9 molecules or 2 fmol. To contain this number of molecules in a single drop of 500 pl volume, the concentration of substance in the stock solution must be 4 μM. It is noteworthy that many compounds, such as small peptides and heterocyclic hydrocarbons, have aqueous solubility limits below this value. For a 1 μM final concentration, the situation is even more difficult in that the concentration of material in a single delivered drop must be 4 mM. The PSDR enables the delivery of these small amounts of compounds in extremely small volumes. This permits the use of stock concentrations within the solubility limit and overcomes one of the significant limitations to assay miniaturization.

Each piezo-actuated compression dispenser (Fig. 5) consists of a 1-mm-diameter vertical glass microcapillary with a small (<100 μm diameter) orifice at the bottom end. The top portion of the microcapillary is connected to a hydraulic

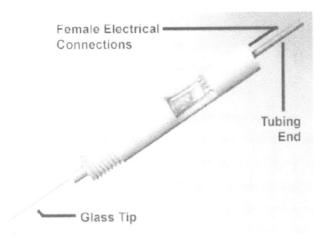

Figure 5 The piezo-actuated liquid dispenser. The glass tip is a microcapillary with an opening at the bottom end that serves as a discharge, orifice. The glass microcapillary extends all the way through the dispenser and at the top is connected with the liquid-filled pressure control system. The microcapillary is surrounded by an annular-shaped, radially-polled piezoelectric ceramic material in the portion covered by the housing. The electrical stimulating leads to the piezo are exposed to the external electrical control system at the connections.

system that allows liquid to be moved from the system into the dispenser micro-capillary during washes or into the microcapillary through the orifice when external liquid is aspirated prior to dispensing. About midway up, the glass tube is surrounded by an annular radially polled piezoelectric ceramic element. When a voltage pulse is applied between the inner and outer faces of the piezo annulus, the element increases in volume and radially compresses the liquid-filled glass tube. At the liquid–vapor interface that spans the discharge orifice of the glass tube, the compression creates a transient capillary wave. If the voltage pulse is of sufficient amplitude, the capillary wave possesses enough energy to move liquid from the microcapillary to a wave crest to create a forming drop. Because formation of a capillary wave requires a fixed energy, each generated drop has fixed energy. Thus, each drop generated has the same volume and is ejected with the same velocity. One square-wave electrical pulse to the piezo produces one drop. Since the amount of piezo-induced compression is contingent on the amplitude of the voltage pulse, the volume of a single drop is controlled by the pulse height. The number of pulses controls the total volume delivered to a well.

The PSDR consists of four parallel heads each consisting of 96 dispensers arrayed in the industry-standard 12×8 format (Fig. 6). In operation, the dispensers are filled with chemical compounds to be delivered to assay plates by removing a

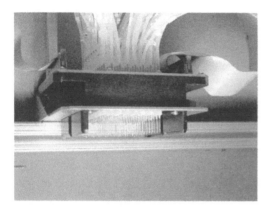

Figure 6 A single head consisting of a 12 × 8 format array of 96 piezo-actuated dispensers. The dispensers are oriented vertically with the discharge orifice of the glass microcapillary facing down. The stainless steel–covered top of each microcapillary is inserted into its own Teflon tube that is connected to the hydraulic pressure control system. The ribbon cables are electrical connections to the electrical pulse control circuitry. Each PSDR uses 4 of these 96-dispenser heads to paulitate simultaneous liquid delivery to 4 NanoWell plates.

96- or 384-well master compound plate from the store and transporting it to the PSDR. The plate is robotically placed under a 96-dispenser head and raised so that the microcapillary tips are submerged in the compound solutions. The pressure control system is used to aspirate several microliters of test compound into each dispenser. The master compound plate is then lowered and transported back to the store, and a 3456-well NanoWell plate, in which an assay is being staged, is brought up to the head. Each dispenser is filled with a single compound from a chemical library. A total of 36 wells can be addressed to create a formatted experimental grid in which the compound concentration is varied (by the number of drops delivered) and in which the experimental conditions are covered (e.g., test compound without agonist or modulator). The test compound is then dispensed to one or more of the 36 wells that can be addressed by each dispenser. Each dispenser contains more than enough material to deliver more than 20 nl of test compound to each of the addressable 36 wells. Dispensing is uniform across the 96 dispensers in each head (Fig. 7). The number of drops elicited in each visit of a dispenser tip to a well is controllable. Delivery to each well is reliably varied (Fig. 8).

Spatial accuracy of dispensing can be affected by static charge that attaches to the non-conductive plate material surrounding each well. The charge has the effect of attracting the small drops of ejected material because the liquid is fairly conductive and the liquid–vapor surface is a site of dielectric discontinuity. The

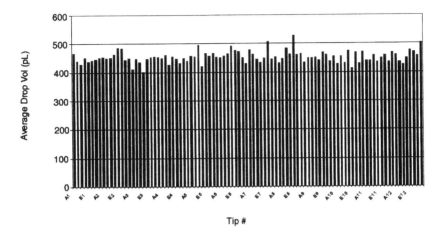

Tip #

Figure 7 Dispensing accuracy. A few microliters of 5 mM stock fluorescein was aspirated into each of 96 dispenser tips in a head and then 20 drops were delivered by each tip to a 96-well plate filled with 0.2 ml sodium borate buffer, pH 9.2. The height of each bar denotes the average volume of each drop. The average drop volume for the population of dispensers is 472 ± 46 pl.

effect of this static potential is to deflect the discharged drop toward the site of accumulated charge. This is avoided by bringing the plate to within 0.25 mm of the tip bottoms. In addition, the static charge can be neutralized by grounding the robotic element chassis and by deionization. These treatments decrease the plate potential difference down to about 20 V/cm^2. At this level, no spatial errors in dispensing are made when the dispenser tips are 0.5 mm above the well rims.

V. SOLENOID-BASED DISPENSER TECHNOLOGY

A. The Reagent Distribution Robot

1. Solenoid-Controlled Liquid Dispensing

For dispensing volumes that are larger than the subnanoliter volumes dispensed by the piezo-actuated dispensers, more traditional fluid-handling technologies have been miniaturized to deliver the microliter-sized liquid volumes. These dispensers, termed reagent dispensers (Fig. 9), utilize a solenoid-controlled valve to enact and disengage physical blockade of a hydraulic pathway in order to regulate liquid flow (Fig. 10). The dispensing tube (vertically oriented) is divided into two parts by a solenoid-controlled valve. At the lower end of the tube below the valve is the discharge orifice with a specially fabricated nozzle (<1 mm diameter).

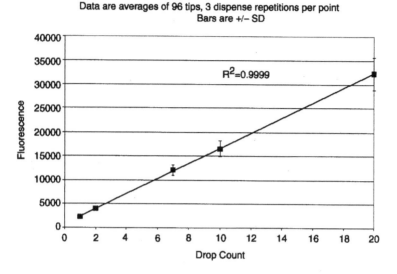

Figure 8 Linearity. In these experiments, three separate buffer-filled plates were used for each drop count. Each point shows the fluorescence of the borate buffer–diluted fluorescein averaged over all 96 dispenser tips in a head, and for all three plates. This confirms that each request for a delivered drop results in the subsequent dispensing of a drop. The implementation of the PSDR enables drop requests to range from 1 to 256 drops.

Above the valve, the entire hydraulic system is maintained at a fixed positive pressure of about 10 psi when the pathway is filled with liquid. The solenoid valve consists of a metal core wrapped by an insulated wire that is, in turn, surrounded over a portion by an annular conductor that is clamped at a fixed current (detent). When current flows through the wire wrapped around the core, the newly generated magnetic field forces the solenoid core into alignment with the field established around the annular conductor (active). The solenoid is mechanically fixed to obstruct the flow path in the detent field, so that when the solenoid is activated, the flow path toward the discharge orifice becomes contiguous with the pressurized hydraulic system and liquid moves out through the orifice. Because of the time course of the valve movement, the activating and deactivating electrical currents can only be incremented on a millisecond time scale. This confines the linear range of volumes to 0.1–5 µl, which can be achieved by varying the duration over which the valve remains open. At short times volume precision is limited by the inertia of the volume that must be moved in order to obtain any liquid dispensing into the target well, and at long times the volume moved is sufficient to cause a droop in system

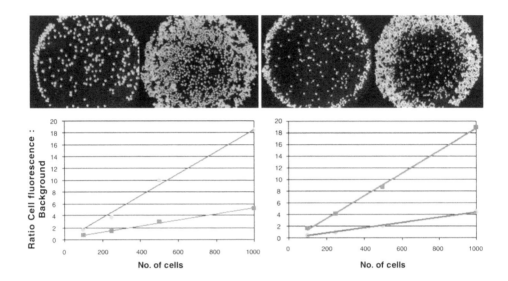

Figure 14.16 Isoproterenol stimulation of Jurkat cells transfected with NF-AT–β-lactamase vector. The upper panel shows fluorescence micrographs of individual wells seeded with Jurkat cells after 4 h incubation in the dual-FRET fluorophore CCF2. The pair of panels of green cells at the left show cells that were not treated with isoproterenol. The green fluorescence originates by direct excitation of the coumarin and sensitization of fluorescein fluorescence by FRET in the intact CCF2 molecule. The leftmost panel was obtained by seeding 250 cells in the well, whereas the adjacent panel to the right shows 1000 cells. The plot at bottom shows the quantitative relation between blue (coumarin) and green (fluorescein) fluorescence intensities as a function of cell density. In unstimulated cells, green fluorescence predominates. The pair of panels at the right shows Jurkat cells after stimulation with isoproterenol. The expressed β-lactamase has cleaved the dual-FRET fluorophore, relieving the quenching of the coumarin fluorescence.

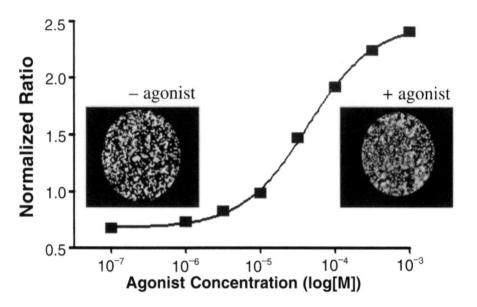

Agonist Dose Response in NanoWell™ Plate

Figure 14.17 Dose–response curve for Jurkat cells transfected with a β-lactamase reporter gene and stimulated with carbachol. The emission intensity ratio at 460–520 nm was normalized by the sensitization ratio obtained at 10^{-5} M agonist concentration.

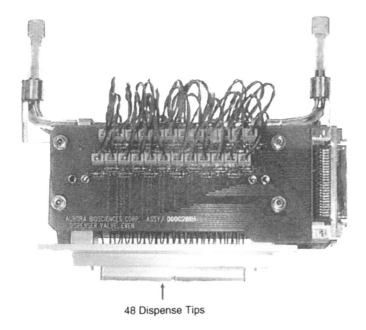

48 Dispense Tips

Figure 9 A single 48-channel solenoid valve-controlled microliter-volume reagent dispenser is shown. The linear array of 48 orifices is at the bottom. The electrical connections for control of the solenoid valve for each orifice are at the top. The upper left valve controls influx to the hydraulic line connecting all 48 orifices, whereas the valve at the upper right regulates efflux.

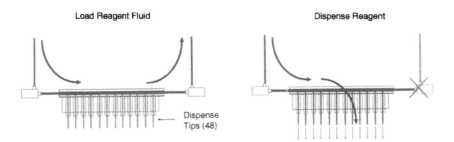

Load Reagent Fluid   Dispense Reagent

Dispense
Tips (48)

Figure 10 Filling and dispensing from the linear array. The common hydraulic line is connected to the supply volume of liquid to be dispensed at left while the right line goes to a disposal container. The common hydraulic line is subjected to a constant hydrostatic pressure. With both left and right valves open, the common line is filled with fluid to be dispensed. The outlet valve is closed to equalize pressure across the common line. The solenoid valves are then opened to enable dispensing. Volume is controlled by the duration for which the orifice valves are open.

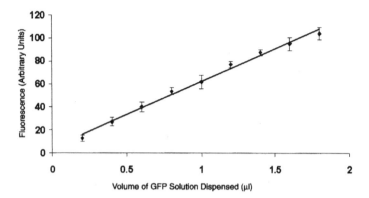

Figure 11 Linearity of dispensation of microliter volumes by solenoid-controlled dispensers. The supply line to a linear array of 48 orifices was filled with 10^5/ml green fluorescent protein-expressing CHO cells. A single NanoWell plate was passed under the orifice array and 8 sequential columns of 48 wells each received the same volume. Volume was set by adjustment of the duration for which the solenoid-gated valve was activated. The dispensed volume is directly proportional to valve open time for volumes between 0.2 and 2.0 μl.

pressure. Nonetheless, this range of volume is all that is required for dispensing reagent volumes to the miniaturized reaction wells (Fig. 11).

2. High-Throughput Liquid Dispensing to Multiple Reaction Wells

The reagent dispensers are used to deliver the major components of the assays to the reaction wells. These constituents typically consist of the dispersed assay cells in cell growth media, fluorigenic precursor substrates, and agonists and other physiological modulators. The reagent dispensers are arrayed linearly in a head assembly (Fig. 9) that enables reagent delivery to each well in a single row of 48 wells in a high-density NanoWell assay plate at a single positioning of the plate relative to the dispenser. Because each dispenser solenoid is individually addressable, discharge through each outlet can be individually controlled and each well could, in theory, receive entirely different reaction constituents (Fig. 12).

In practice, each linear array of 48 dispensers is fed by a common supply line at fixed pressure that, in turn, is connected to a single large-volume bottle of one reagent (Fig. 10). Assays are constructed using multiple linear arrays, each supplied with a different reagent. An assay is staged by sequential visits of each well to the dispensing position under each orifice serving a column of wells. Thus, each linear array dispenses a reagent to each of the 48 wells in a column at a time.

NanoWell Plate

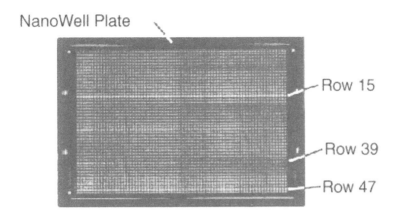

Row 15

Row 39

Row 47

Figure 12 Differential filling of NanoWell assay plate wells with different components using solenoid-controlled dispensers. The plate was passed under two different dispenser arrays. The supply bottle of the first array contained aqueous red food coloring. During passage under the red dispenser, all valves were opened except at positions 15, 39, and 47, so that all rows except these received 1 µl of red dye. The second array's liquid supply contained 100 µM fluorescein in borate buffer pH 9.2. When the plate was passed under the second set of dispensers, all valves were closed except over rows 15, 39, and 47. The open time of each valve was varied to dispense 1.5-, 1.0-, and 0.5-µl volumes, respectively. This reveals that the solenoid dispenser arrays can be used to deliver different components to different reaction wells on the same high-density plate, as is needed for the construction of controlled physiological assays.

The plate is moved under the dispenser head 72 times to position each of the 72 wells in a row under the orifice servicing the row. The plate is then moved to the next linear array of dispensers to receive the next reagent. In this way, reactions can be mixed directly in each well over a short time course. This avoids the necessity of mixing reagents together in the supply volumes with possible deleterious effects due to reaction, oxidation, and so forth.

In general, solenoid-based dispensers provide the major improvement to dispensing technology–over mechanical (plunger)–based delivery with respect to the construction of microliter scale volume assays. Solenoid-actuated valves are useful in regulating small diameter (0.1–1 mm) flow pathways due to the length scale over which relatively small electromagnets can produce forces sufficient to rapidly move the dead weight of the occlusion. Because the small outlets can be fixtured into arrays that match the formats of high-density reaction well arrays, the solenoid-based valves are one of the most important technologies enabling miniaturization and are used to deliver the bulk of the reagents to the assay wells.

VI. FLUORESCENCE DETECTION

The miniaturized assay technologies under development by Aurora all utilize measurement of FRET fluorescence. This requires measurement of the emission intensities of two fluorophores nearly simultaneously (or at least in close temporal sequence) in two reasonably well-separated spectral wavebands. This multiple-wavelength emission quantitation is thus a subset of the broader domain of multicolor measurement. Because only two fluorophores are needed in a FRET measurement, the selection of a single waveband for measurement of each dye that is relatively uncontaminated by fluorescence from the other probe (i.e., avoidance of "spillover") obviates the requirement for continuous spectrometry. Instead, miniaturization creates challenges at the level of the optical interface between the sample and light collection to enable the measurement of light from as few fluorophores in as few cells as possible. The NanoWell assay plate provides a useful cellular reaction platform that brings the cells to a distance from the optics that is essentially fixed. This enables maximization of numerical aperture in a way that depth of field includes the entire layer of cells settled on the bottom of the well. Thus, the observation optics can be brought very close to the well bottom and, moreover, each well is read with the same numerical aperture optics.

The major challenges of miniaturization are several in fluorescence detection:

1. Delivery of a sufficient excitation light to the donor fluorophore to produce significant acceptor sensitization, so that changes in donor and acceptor emission are meaningful
2. Collection of sufficient light from the sample from each fluorophore for measurement
3. Separation of the light into the relevant wavebands
4. Reproducibly replicating the excitation-emission optics at each assay well

Aurora fluorescence measurement has exploited the high internal reflectivity of fused-silica waveguides to accomplish delivery of light to and from the assay well bottom (Fig. 13). An objective lens is interposed between the well bottom and the front of the light guide. For excitation of the donor, light from a high-intensity arc-discharge lamp is directed through heat suppression and bandpass filters to select the proper wavelengths. This filtered light is then focused by a condenser onto one end of a resin-clad fiber bundle that is brought to a lens positioned very close to the bottom of the well. Excitation light can either be focused on the cells at the bottom of the well (confocality) or allowed to remain nonvergent (by using the condenser to focus the excitation beam at the back-focal plane of the objective lens). Confocal excitation delivers more light to fewer fluorophores. A duplicate paired set of light guides is used to collect the emitted light focused by the objective lens.

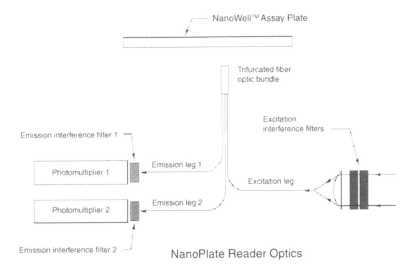

NanoPlate Reader Optics

Figure 13 Schematic of the optical pathway in the NanoPlate fluorescence plate reader. The assay plate is scanned by the optical reader head by moving the plate. Excitation light is delivered to each well, and emission light is collected from each well by an optical reader head and a trifurcated fiberoptic bundle. The emission filter stacks are used to separate the emission light into the two wavebands originating primarily from the donor and acceptor fluorophore probes. With two photomultiplier tubes, one for each emission waveband, both donor and acceptor fluorescence intensities are measured simultaneously.

One set leads to a stack of interference filters that isolates the light emitted by the donor fluorophores and the other set leads to a stack that isolates the acceptor emission. Each stack sits atop the photocathode faceplate of a photomultiplier tube. Thus, the emissions from both fluorophores are obtained simultaneously.

In order to maximize the throughput of the miniaturized, high-density format system, the NanoWell plate is scanned relative to the optical fluorescence detector (Fig. 14). At Aurora, the plate is moved by high-resolution motorized screws and the optical system is fixtured in place. This results in each well being represented as a set of discrete integrated intensities obtained for the scan. The interstitial material between the wells attenuates the fluorescence, so that the raw output of each photomultiplier resembles a periodic wave. Nearest-neighbor analysis is used to isolate the intensity peaks corresponding to the well centers in each scan of a row of wells. The well array format is used to isolate wells containing no fluorescent material. Furthermore, statistical analysis enables exclusion of the rare, extremely intense yet spatially small fluorescent objects that are dust particles. Data acquisition must keep up with the rate of plate scanning and the amount of data that the two photomultipliers are capable of generating. In any

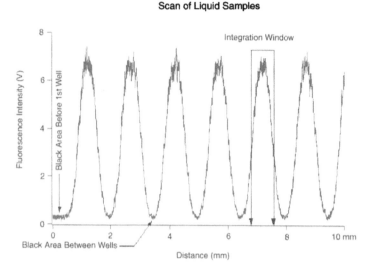

Figure 14 Raw data from the NanoWell plate reader illustrating the continuity of the digitized data. All 3456 wells are scanned in less than 2 min. The trace shows the digitized output of one photomultiplier tube during a scan of six wells in a single row. The raw data are processed to corrected fluorescence data originating from each well by averaging the fluorescence intensities in the integration window. The integration window is determined by the locations of local minimum and maximum fluorescence intensities and their values. The illustrated scan was obtained with 100 nM fluorescein in borate buffer pH 9.2 through the green emission channel.

case, fluorescence measurement requires a very small fraction of the time needed to construct and measure miniaturized cell-based physiological reactions in high density (Fig. 15).

VII. HIGH-THROUGHPUT FUNCTIONAL BIOLOGY

Ultrahigh-throughput screening utilizing microliter volume assays is made possible with the types of instrumentation described for manipulation of replicated small liquid volumes and for simultaneous two-color measurements repeated many times. This is demonstrated using a standard cell-based assay that is amenable for testing signal transduction pathways mediated by G-protein-coupled receptors. In this assay, Jurkat cells are transfected with an expression vector in which a gene encoding β-lactamase is under control of a set of NF-AT nuclear transcription activation sites. β2-Adrenergic receptor activation by isoproterenol

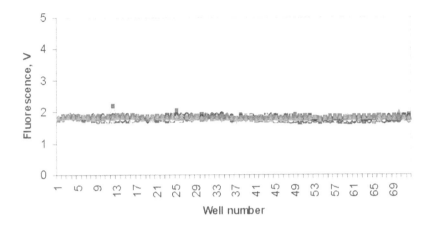

Figure 15 Performance of the NanoWell plate fluorescence reader. All 3456 wells were filled using a single 48-orifice array with 10 nM 6-carboxyfluorescein (CF) in 10 mM borate buffer pH 9.2. The integrated well fluorescence intensities are plotted for all 48 rows of 72 wells. The background fluorescence is too low to be shown on the ordinates but amounts to less than 3 mV of PMT output. The minimum detectable level of CF is 64 pM.

or muscarinic activation by carbachol results in the heterotrimeric G-protein-dependent activation of phospholipase C. The resulting inositol triphosphate–activated release of calcium ion from intracellular stores activates calcineurin, a phosphatase that activates the NFAT transcription regulator and promotes expression of β-lactamase. Activity of β-lactamase is determined by the use of the cephalosporin-linked coumarin-fluorescein dye pair (CCF2). Thus, the expression level of β-lactamase in these transfected Jurkat cells provides a direct indication of the extent of β-adrenergic activation. The enzyme activity is directly indicated by the amount of coumarin fluorescence, resulting from CCF2 cleavage and dequenching of the coumarin fluorescence by the disruption of FRET with fluorescein, relative to the amount of fluorescein fluorescence, which is sensitized by FRET with the directly excited coumarin. Distinguishing receptor activation in these cells is unambiguous (Fig. 16).

To construct the assays shown in Figure 17, the NanoWell assay plate well was seeded with 2000 detached (spinner culture) cells in serum-free growth medium using a single array of the solenoid-based reagent-dispensing robot (RDR). The plate was then incubated at 37°C for 6 to allow the cells to attach to the well bottom. The carbachol was added after a second pass through the RDR, and, after a 2-h incubation, the CCF2 fluorigenic reagent was added. Fluorescence was measured after 4 in CCF2 at room temperature. The receptor activation is clearly revealed as an inversion in the amount of blue fluorescence relative to

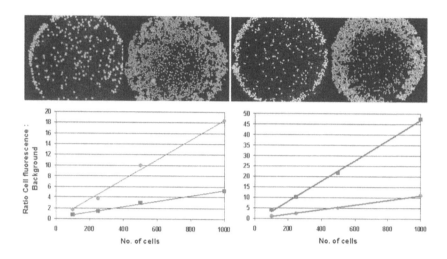

Figure 16 Isoproterenol stimulation of Jurkat cells transfected with NF-AT–β-lactamase vector. The upper panel shows fluorescence micrographs of individual wells seeded with Jurkat cells after 4 h incubation in the dual-FRET fluorophore CCF2. The pair of panels of green cells at the left show cells that were not treated with isoproterenol. The green fluorescence originates by direct excitation of the coumarin and sensitization of fluorescein fluorescence by FRET in the intact CCF2 molecule. The leftmost panel was obtained by seeding 250 cells in the well, whereas the adjacent panel to the right shows 1000 cells. The plot at bottom shows the quantitative relation between blue (coumarin) and green (fluorescein) fluorescence intensities as a function of cell density. In unstimulated cells, green fluorescence predominates. The pair of panels at the right shows Jurkat cells after stimulation with isoproterenol. The expressed β-lactamase has cleaved the dual-FRET fluorophore, relieving the quenching of the coumarin fluorescence. See color plate.

green. In quantitative studies, the donor–acceptor fluorescence intensity ratio depends on the agonist concentration, indicating the pharmacological validity of the FRET sensitization ratio.

This relatively simple fluorescent assay for receptor activation consists of a significant number of operations, such as cell seeding in medium, addition of agonist, addition of fluorigenic reagent, and several incubations at different temperatures. The steps needed to construct the assay must be performed within constraints of time and physical condition. Nonetheless, construction and measurement of the assay consists of relatively simple steps—fluid addition, incubation, or fluorescence reading—that are amenable to automation. The precision of the automation enables the assay to be miniaturized.

Agonist Dose Response in Nanowell™ Plate

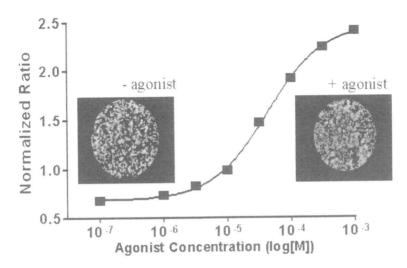

Figure 17 Dose–response curve for Jurkat cells transfected with a β-lactamase reporter gene and stimulated with carbachol. The emission intensity ratio at 460–520 nm was normalized by the sensitization ratio obtained at 10^{-5} M agonist concentration. See color plate.

Further utility of the miniaturized assay is provided by a different set of transformed Jurkat cells that are activated by carbachol and provide a convenient cell-based assay for screening chemical compounds for possible effect on signal transduction processes mediated by muscarinic receptors and heterotrimeric G-proteins (in addition to NFAT and NFκB-activated gene transcription). In Figure 18, the results of screening 100,000 compounds in 30-NanoWell plates are summarized by the extent to which test compound can overcome pirenzepine-mediated inhibition of carbachol-stimulated green-to-blue conversion. In these experiments, about 1–10 pmol of each test compound was added to each well in a NanoWell assay plate with the PSDR. The compounds were added to the seeded cells and incubated for 6 h, then the cells were stimulated with carbachol in the presence of pirenzepine and processed for assessment of β-lactamase activation.

VIII. SUMMARY

The technologies of liquid handling, assay construction, and fluorescence detection provide a set of operational modules that can be configured to perform a wide

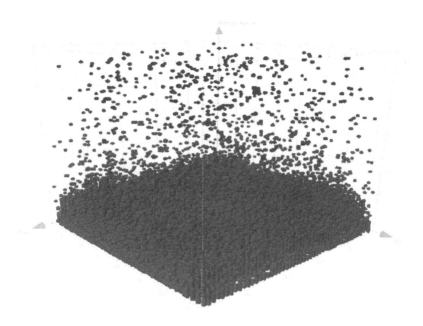

Figure 18   Lead candidates determined in a screen of carbachol-activated β-lactamase transcription. The compounds were tested for their ability to overcome pirenzapine-mediated inhibition of muscarinic activation by carbachol. The X-Y plane represents NanoWell plate position at which the compound was tested. The ordinate denotes the percentage increase in green-to-blue emission and, hence, lead candidacy of the tested compound.

variety of assays. The key features are that they enable cell-based fluorescence measurements and so are adapted to screening for effects on potentially intricate physiological pathways in intact, living cells. In addition, the liquid handling has been parceled so that a particular instrument is specialized for a range of volumes that are consistent with the physical methodologies used to obtain control of the dispensed volume. Solenoid-based hydrostatic delivery is required for the range and precision of control of microliter-volume dispensing. At the subnanoliter level, more transient pressure control mechanisms are necessary and so piezo technology is useful. These technologies are fully amenable to the design of new assays for new physiological pathways and for determination of gene product functions.

15
Data Management for High-Throughput Screening

Lee Amon
MarketQwest Associates
Fremont, California

I. INTRODUCTION

A. Background

Data management is an integral requirement of any high-throughput screening (HTS) effort. Ultimately, the purpose of any screening program is to acquire information that can be turned into knowledge in the drug discovery process. In order to achieve this goal, the results of all tests, along with all appropriate contextual information, must be reliably captured by a data management system and made available to researchers throughout an organization. The tracking of sample locations, test conditions, the capture of raw results, and the transformation of raw results into calculated and meaningful information requires robust and flexible information systems with effective user interfaces, as well as links to inventory and other information systems. This chapter will highlight some of the issues involved in developing and maintaining an informatics system to support HTS.

B. Issues in HTS Data Management

1. Large Volumes of Data

The introduction of automation to biological screening has resulted in an increase in the volume of data of many orders of magnitude. In the early 1990's a large pharmaceutical research organization might screen tens of thousands of samples in a year. By the late 1990's some large research organizations were screening as many as 22 million samples in a single year. Clearly in order to achieve this type of volumes, informatics systems must be a part of the overall strategy, both to aid with the logistics of HTS and to support decision-making.

2. Addition of Automation

The defining feature of HTS is the application of automated systems to biological testing, greatly increasing the number of samples that can be tested in any time period. The increase in the number of samples being tested has a number of complicating side effects. First, since the goal of increasing throughput is to gain knowledge regarding the interactions of molecules and targets, results data must be collected, analyzed, and made accessible to researchers. Information processes that are possible by hand with small volumes of data require automated systems when large volumes of data are involved. Second, the use of automation introduces the possibility of mechanical error. Finding the error and isolating the results is a major issue for HTS informatics systems.

3. Variability Inherent in Biological Experiments

Early in the days of HTS, many comparisons were made between the application of automation to biological screening and that in other industries, such as manufacturing. Many presentations and papers of the time talked about the "industrialization of research." While certain aspects of the process, particularly inventory and logistics, did become more industrialized, the predictions underestimated the rapid changes in the research process, as well as the variability inherent in biological systems. The nature of discovery research dictates rapid change. By comparison, the basic principles of double-entry accounting have not changed since the 1500s. While there have been, and will continue to be, changes in the details, such changes pale in comparison to those in scientific research, where even many of the leading scientists to today cannot tell you where the process will be going 5 years from now.

II. ACQUISITION OF DATA

In almost all cases, the end point of an HTS experiment is a change in the state of the contents of a well that may be detected by an automated device, typically referred to as a reader, or a plate reader. The change in state may be an increase in fluorescence, radioactivity, or absorption. The plate reader will measure the state of the sample at a set time or over a period of time. In some experiments, the detector takes multiple readings. In almost all cases, the output of the reader is a series of raw results, which must be either normalized or reduced, and combined with other information, in order to produce meaningful results.

A. Integration with Automation Equipment

Plate readers most often produce one or more text files, which contain the raw results of the experiment. These results are often expressed in terms of counts per minute (CPM), optical density (OD), or fluorescence. These results can be extremely difficult for scientists to interpret in their raw form for several reasons. An example of such a file is shown in Figure 1. There are several things that we can see regarding this file. First, we can see that besides the raw result, there is other potentially valuable information contained in header section, such as filters used and temperature. Next, we see the results in a "data block". These are the raw

```
Read time: 7/29/98 11:19
Plate ID:    SampPlat101
Barcode:
Method ID:            Galanin TRF Screen
Comment: tic tac stds type 1 green red plate 1
Max cps:  1.78E+07 cps
Min counts:     236        counts
Microplate format:   Packard White 96
Detection mode:    F
Excitation side:    Top
Excitation filter:    1        485-20 (Fluorescein)
Excitation polarizer filter:    o
Attenuator mode:    m
Emission side:    Top
Emission filter:    1        535-25 (Fluorescein)
Emission polarizer filter:    o
Z Height:  4      mm        Numeric
Conversion method:  Comparator
Integration time:     100000    us
Total integration time: 100000    us
Readings per well:  1
Time between readings:    100      ms
Shake Time:     0        s
Temperature:    23.8      °C
Instrument tag:     Application's Lab
Serial number:      AN0065
Data:      Intensity
Units:     cps
```

	1	2	3	4	5	6	7	8	9	10	11	12
A	15416754	16174624	17774608	16883962	15993355	16617787	15854868	15358044	17155580	16851530	17464322	49469
B	16749729	16732580	16919286	16919286	16883962	15901794	16649150	15505432	16764194	16706653	17259128	22175
C	15592631	16930910	16683497	16999124	16030343	15769842	16038291	15064792	16340762	15772406	16925004	18100
D	16147708	16193517	16715106	16051556	16285916	15757040	16482484	16706653	16925004	16810660	16580875	24924
E	15211197	16174624	21607	16883962	15993355	16617787	15854868	15358044	17155580	16851530	17464322	22933
F	16672032	16732580	16919286	16649150	15505432	15901794	16649150	15505432	16764194	16706653	17259128	65863
G	14889129	16930910	16683497	16999124	16030343	15769842	16038291	15064792	16340762	15772406	16925004	21038
H	16158464	16193517	16715106	16051556	16285916	15757040	16482484	15769842	17259128	16810660	16580875	72213

Figure 1 Raw output of an LJL Analyst plate reader. Automated plate readers can produce a great deal of information; however, the information is not always formatted in a way that is straightforward or easy for data systems to capture. Most modern plate readers can be programmed to produce data in desired formats. Here we see sample output from an LJL Analyst plate reader. The 8×12 block of numbers in the center contain the raw results for this plate. Other information, such as filters used, temperature, etc., may be included. It is typically up to the information system to parse the information out of this type of file, process the raw results; and store all information in appropriate fields in the database. Note also that ancillary information, such as sample ID or well type, is not included in this file.

results, but we can quickly surmise that reviewing the raw results would not be an efficient way to analyze the experiment. For one thing, there is no indication of what was in each well that was tested. While many readers today can accept input from a bar code and will include the bar code plate identifier in the reader file, there is no indication of what sample was in the plate, what concentration was used for the test, or other information required. In addition, to make sensible decisions on the basis of this data, the scientist must perform other analyses, such as stability of the controls, overall level of activity for the assay, etc. While looking at a single plate of raw results might give an indication of the answer, one would have to keep a fair amount of information in one's head. For example, where were the controls for this experiment located? What ranges of numbers indicate activity vs. inactivity? Are the results seen on this plate in line with what should be expected from this type of assay? While it may be possible for a scientist to manually analyze one plate worth of data, imagine trying to do this for 1000 plates run in a single day. It may be possible, but it certainly would not be a good use of the researcher's time.

B.   Integration with Other Information Systems

In order to present the data to the scientist in a format that can aid in efficient decision making, the raw results in the reader file must be parsed and brought into an information system, where the results will be integrated with information such as the sample tested, the kind of well (sample, control, reference, or other), and other conditions, then calculated and presented to the scientist so that decisions can be made. This integration can be challenging for a number of reasons.

- The plate read by the detection device is almost never the inventory plate. It is usually a copy made at the time of the test. Therefore, the information system must associate the ID of the assay plate with the inventory plate that was the source.
- The layout of the reader file can vary dramatically from one reader to the next. In fact, most readers have several programmable modes that allow them to create files with a number of different formats. Information systems must properly parse the information.
- The layout and configuration of the test plate is different for different experiments. In fact, sometimes within a single experiment multiple plate layouts may be used. The information system mist be able to associate the correct layout with each plate.
- Finally, when making decisions, the scientist will frequently want to see results from other tests for the same samples. This means that the system will here to have the capability to query other databases.

C. Well Types and Plate Layouts

One key piece of information that is not captured in either inventory systems or by the reader file is the plate layout. The plate layout describes the contents of each well in a plate. Plate layouts typically include information such as sample ID's concentration, and the location of control wells or standards. While this is typical information, plate layouts can include any variable that the scientist has under his or her control, such as pH or salinity. In some cases, the scientist will even place different targets (enzymes, receptors, or cell lines) in the wells. This information is crucial for a meaningful calculation and interpretation of the results. Most HTS information systems have specialized input screens to support the definition of plate layouts. The variety of plate layouts used for different types of experiments requires that any general-purpose information system be extremely flexible. In Figure 2a and b, we see two examples of commonly used plate layouts. In Figure 2a, there are 8 control wells in column 1, and 88 samples each at a single concentration in the rest of the plate. In Figure 2b, there are only 8 samples on the plate, but each is tested at 12 different concentrations. These are only two examples of possible plate layouts, which can vary widely from experiment to experiment

D. Calculation, Reduction, and Normalization of Data

Once the raw results are brought into the data system, some form of calculation is needed to make the data meaningful to the scientist. This is important because the raw numbers coming out of the reader file can vary widely based on the type of detection used as well as the specifics of the assay. Using just the raw numbers, it would be almost impossible for the scientist to quickly determine the quality of the assay run or to determine if any samples displayed unusual activity. Even within a single assay, results coming from plates taken at different times may vary substantially. So, unless the raw results are somehow normalized, the scientist can be easily misled. The most common calculated results are as follows:

- Percent Inhibition
- Percent of control
- IC_{50} or EC_{50}
- K_i
- Ratios

1. Percent Inhibition and Percent of Control

Percent inhibition and percent of control are perhaps the two most commonly used calculations in the HTS environment. In both cases, the calculations show the activity of the sample(s) being studied relative to the activity shown by a known

(A)

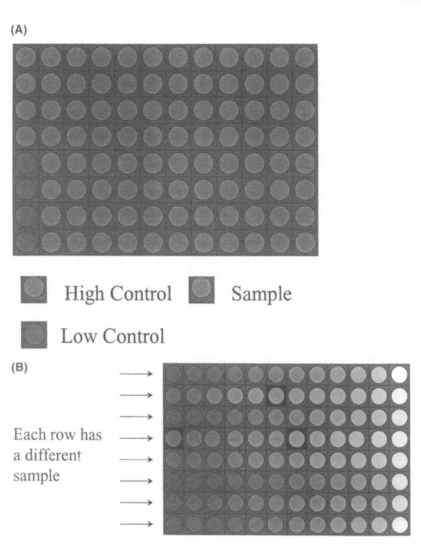

High Control   Sample

Low Control

(B)

Each row has a different sample

Logarithmic decrease in concentration

Figure 2 Here are two sample plate layouts. (A) shows the layout for a typical primary screen. In this layout, 4 high controls and 4 low controls are placed in the leftmost column. A different sample is placed in each of the other 88 wells. All samples are tested at the same concentration. (B) Only 8 different samples are tested, but each sample is tested at 12 different concentrations.

set of controls or standards after accounting for systematic noise as expressed in the low controls.

The percent inhibition calculation is

$$1 - [(\text{sample}) - (\text{average of low controls})]/[(\text{average of high controls}) - (\text{average of low controls})]$$

The percent of control calculation is

$$[(\text{sample}) - (\text{average of low controls})]/[(\text{average of high controls}) - (\text{average of low controls})]$$

Note that these two calculations are the inverse of the other. In many cases, researchers will calculate both and use the one that is most familiar to them. For the remainder of this chapter, we will use only percent Inhibition, but we will mean both.

a. Variations

Replicated Percent Inhibition. In many cases, experimentalists will attempt to reduce experimental error by using two or more wells to test each sample. The replicates are averaged and then the averages compared. If there is a high deviation within the sample responses (e.g., if one replicate shows an Inhibition of 80%, and the other replicate shows an inhibition of 5%), we have a pretty good indication that one of them is wrong. Sometimes the replicates are on the same plate, and sometimes the entire plate is replicated. Again, the information system needs to be able to tell where the samples are, find the replicate, and perform the appropriate calculation.

Controls on a Special Plate. In the most common application of percent inhibition tests, control wells are placed on each plate. However in many cases experimentalists will choose to place the control wells on a designated control, reference, or quality control plate. The controls from this plate are then used to calculate results of samples on other plates.

Percent inhibition tests represent a good first-pass indication of the activity of a sample. When dealing with a large number of samples, where you are looking for 10-fold or better differences in activity level, these tests give you a fast, reasonable indication of which samples are worth following up. However, there are several shortcomings to these measurements. First, they are single-point measurements, so we only learn the activity level of a compound at a certain concentration. It may be impossible to make reasonable comparisons regarding the relative activity of different samples if they were tested at different concentrations. In addition, these measurements give no indication of the nature of the activity. To obtain this type of information, other types of tests have to be run. The most common of these tests are the dose–response and the kinetics tests, described in the following sections *b. Dose–Response Tests.* All dose–response tests measure the activity of a sample over a range of concentrations. The results of these tests are usually computed using one of many nonlinear curve fitting algorithms to find a measure called either the IC_{50} or the EC_{50}. In both cases, these measures tell us the concentration at which the compound shows an activity level of 50%. This measure is superior to percent inhibition for several reasons. First, it allows reasonable comparisons between different compounds. Second, it is a much finer measure of activity because it also shows information about the nature of the activity. For example, how rapid is the response to changes in concentration? What is the concentration level at which activity maximizes? At what concentration is there no activity? (See Fig. 3.)

c. Kinetics Experiments. Kinetics experiments measure the rate of change in activity of a sample over time. The usual measure of activity for a kinetics experiment is K_i, the maximum rate of change. There are a wide variety of models used to calculate K_i. One of the most popular models is the Michealis—Menten model, which typically takes the form

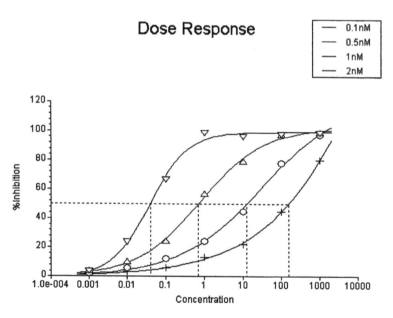

Figure 3 This figure shows a set of fitted dose–response curves. The dotted line shows the concentration of the IC_{50} (the concentration level where 50% of the inhibition activity is observed). Farthest to the left is the sample with the lowest IC_{50}, and in most cases would be indicative of the most potent sample.

$$\frac{v = V[A]}{K_{mA} + [A]}$$

where V and K_{mA} are constants at a given temperature and a given enzyme concentration. A deeper explanation of kinetics and other calculations used in biochemical screening is available from *Symbolism and Terminology in Enzyme Kinetics, Recommendation 1981*, Nomenclature Committee of the International Union of Biochemistry (NC-IUB). The web version, prepared by G. P. Moss, can be found at *http://www.chem.qmw.ac.uk/iubmb/kinetics/*.

d. Ratios. A large number of experiments require that several results be compared. For example, in some tests we are interested in both protein growth and cell survival. In other tests the exact level of activity is not considered as important as the change in activity from a baseline. In these and several other types of test, the results are typically reported as a ratio.

III. VALIDATION OF EXPERIMENTAL RESULTS

A. Detection of Experimental Error

In any experiment, there is a chance of error. The addition of automation and the increased number of samples tested at any given time increase the probability of error. So, before the scientist even begins to look for meaning in the results of an experiment, he or she must determine if the results are useful at all, or if experimental error means that the results are invalid.

B. False Positives vs. False Negatives

There are two types of experimental error that are generally to be accounted for: false positives and false negatives. False positives look like hits but aren't, whereas false negatives are hits that are never revealed. In many cases, scientists care very little about these errors if they are random occurrences, impacting a small number of samples. The assumptions are that false positives will be found with relatively inexpensive follow-up tests, and that there is enough overlap in the chemical space that for any false negative there will be other similar compounds tested that will yield the correct answers. In short, given the nature of biological systems, the assumption is that there will be some level of random error, and most scientists will deal with that. The bigger concern for most HTS scientists is the detection of systematic error, which may invalidate the entire experiment or a large portion of the experimental results. These errors can be very expensive and difficult to recover from. Typically, most scientists depend on the use of controls, or known positives and negatives, to avoid experimental errors.

C. Sources of Error

1. Automation Equipment Failure

Equipment failure is one of the most common sources of experimental error in the automated environment. Typical automation failures include improper dispensing of reagents, physical mishandling of plates, and the failure of incubators and detection devices. Computer systems and software that control the automation equipment are also subject to failure. It should be noted that each increase in throughput and/or plate density comes with a period of increased automation error. This is to be expected, as many of the issues become more problematic, and tolerances become tighter. As an example, a typical well in a 96-well plate can contain 200 ul. On a 1536–well plate, a typical well contains 10 ul. A variation of 1 ul will be 0.5% of a 96-well plate but 10% of a 1536-well plate.

2. Stability of Reagents or Targets

Many HTS tests involve the use of radioactive labels, which are subject to decay. Most involve the use of enzymes, receptors, proteins, or live cells, all of which are subject to degradation or contamination. Needless to say, if an enzyme breaks down, or if the cells die before the test, the results of the test are invalid.

3. Environmental Issues

a. Temperature/humidity. Most biological tests are designed to be performed within some range of conditions. Failure to maintain these conditions may result in invalid test results. As an example, in low-humidity environments, evaporation can be an extreme problem. If the liquid in a well evaporates before the test is completed, clearly the results will not be valid.

IV. DECISION SUPPORT

A. Finding Systematic Error

Given the possibility of some kind of systematic error and the dramatic effect that such errors can have on the results of a test, it makes sense for the scientist to validate that the experiment ran properly before searching for active compounds. The major methods of detecting systematic error are (1) the use of controls and standards, and (2) the search for patterns within the data.

1. Use of Controls and References

The most common way to detect systematic error is by the use of control wells on each plate. Control wells contain samples with a known activity or no sample at all. At the conclusion of the test, the scientist's first action will typically be to check the controls. Did they run as expected? How tightly did the results cluster? Was there wide variation in the results over time? Was there an acceptable difference in activity between the high and low controls (Signal-to-noise ratio)?

2. Search for Patterns

The results of most HTS experiments should be random, with a small number of hits randomly distributed over the library tested. If the results indicate that one area (such as a specific row, column, or well location) had an unusual level of activity, it is usually indicative of some kind of systematic error. As with almost anything else in HTS, there are exceptions to this. For example, if screening a combinatorial library, where all members of a row contain a common substructure, increased activity for an entire row would not be uncommon, and might be exactly what you are looking for.

B. Locating Hits Quickly

In most HTS environments, the difference between a hit and other samples is somewhat dramatic, often on the order of 10-fold. Under these circumstances, it is fairly straightforward to locate the hits and move forward. There are a number of methods for locating hits, ranging from graphical display of the data (Fig. 4) to simple database queries, such as "find the top $x\%$ in terms of activity." Many organizations use standard deviation, looking for samples that are 2σ more active than average. In many cases, locating the most active samples and producing a list of the identifiers is all that is required. This list is sent to a sample room (or back to the automation equipment) for replating and confirmation or secondary tests.

1. Evaluating a Single Run or an Entire Campaign

Often, the HTS lab will run an organization's entire library of compounds through a screen over a period of several weeks to several months. This is often referred to as a campaign. Many organizations will wait until the entire campaign is completed before evaluating samples. They do this because they have found that their libraries have sections (sublibraries), which are more or less active than the norm. If one of these sublibraries is run early, the threshold for activity may be set improperly. Therefore, it is more effective to wait until the entire library has been tested to make threshold evaluations.

C. Integration of Other Data

Sometimes it is desirable to consider information other than the results. Most often this information is used to narrow the number of hits down and to eliminate hits

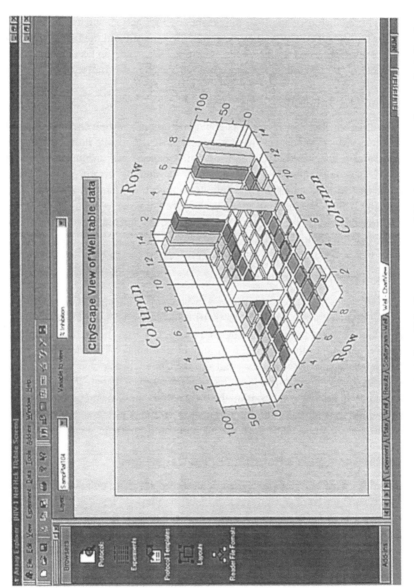

Figure 4 Assay Explorer offers a graphical view. This allows users to quickly detect patterns that may be indicative of systematic problems in the assay or quickly isolate interesting data.

that are not worthy of further study. Some of the key information used to eliminate hits includes the following:

- *Results from other tests.* If a compound is found to be active against a number of other targets, the compound is likely to have undesirable side effects.
- *Physicochemical data.* The most common filtering method is the Lipinski rule of 5. This set of rules looks for compounds that are likely to have reasonable absorption characteristics and eliminates those that don't.

At this point, some people ask, "Why run those compounds in the first place?" If, after all, they are just going to be eliminated after the primary screen, doesn't it make sense to remove them in the first place? There are two reasons why these compounds are typically run in primary screens. First, many companies maintain their entire libraries in 96-well plates. It is easier and less expensive to simply test everything than to pick out certain compounds. Second, in some cases these may be the only active compounds in a screen. While none of them will be drugs, the information gathered will give medicinal chemists a starting point in terms of how to develop compounds further.

D. Graphical Display vs. Tabular Display

There are many fine books on the subject of human interaction with and comprehension of data, and a detailed discussion of the subject is beyond the scope of this chapter. For now, we will simply say that both tabular and graphical displays of data have their place, and most systems provide a combination of displays. We will discuss some of the common graphical displays used, as well as some of the basic requirements for effective tabular displays.

1. Tabular Display

A tabular display is basically a spreadsheet, showing the data in columns and rows. The most common spreadsheet in use today is that of Microsoft Excel. Most systems specifically designed for HTS data management try to offer an "Excel-like" spreadsheet capability. Commercial examples of these systems include CSAP from Oxford Molecular and Assay Explorer from MDL Information Systems, (Fig. 5A). A very popular HTS package, ActivityBase from IDBS (Fig. 5B) uses Excel as the front end. Tabular displays are useful in that they give scientists a detailed and precise view of specific results. Typically, tabular displays will need to sort and filter the results so that a meaningful subset can be displayed. It is unrealistic to assume that any scientist can find meaningful data in a tabular display of 100,000 records; however, scientists can do a query such as, "Show me the 50 most active compounds from this test," and a tabular report can be useful. Tabular reports could also be useful for statistical summaries of a large experiment.

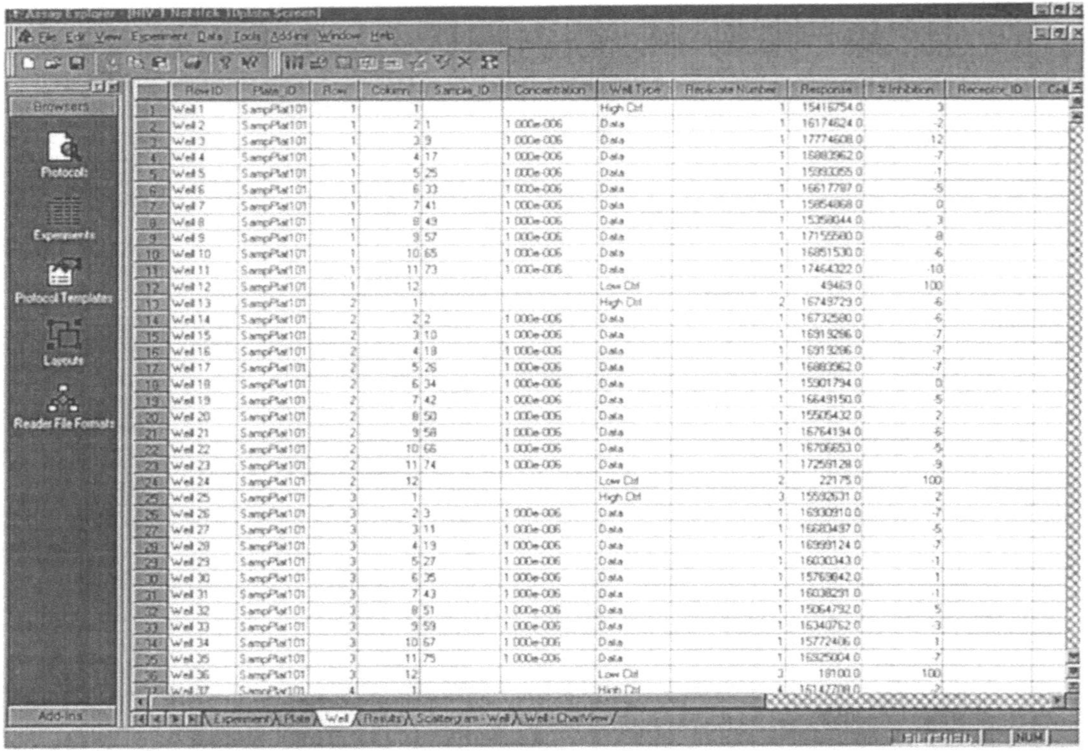

(A)

Figure 5 Tabular formats. Here are tabular presentations of results from two popular commercial systems: Assay Explorer, (MDL Information Systems) (A) and Activity Base (ID Business Solutions) (B) In each of these examples a table of data from an assay is presented to the user. Note that the tables contains fields such as concentration, sample ID, and well type, as well as the calculated value for the sample. This information is not contained in a typical reader file, as seen in Figure 1, and must be extracted from inventory systems or input directly

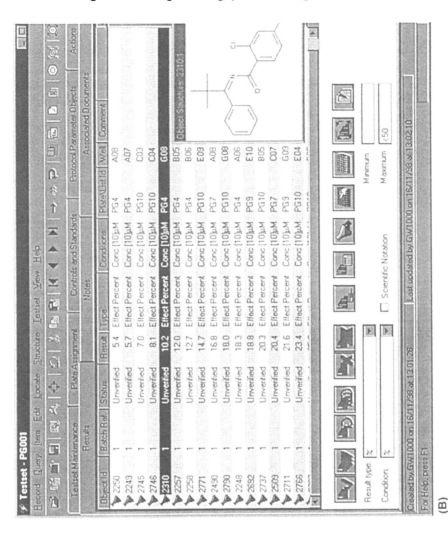

(B)

Figure 5 Continued

2. Graphical Display

Properly designed graphical displays allow scientists to quickly analyze large amounts of data, as well as to spot trends and outliers. Some of the typical graphs used in HTS include scatter charts and control charts. Scientists would generally request that any graphical display be interactive so that it can be used as a query device. Typical graphical displays are seen in Figures 4 and 6.

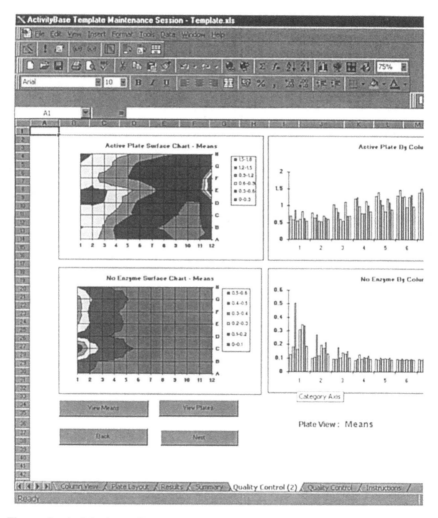

Figure 6   Activity base offers users a number of graphical views. This allows users to quickly detect patterns that may be indicative of systematic problems in the assay or quickly isolate interesting data.

E. Reporting

In addition to display of the data, most organizations will want a hard copy of at least a summary of the results. Often the hard copy contains statistical data regarding the experiment and a summary of interesting results. These reports are usually stored in a laboratory notebook. Again, it is unlikely that anyone would want to create a hard-copy report showing the results of hundreds of thousands of compounds, 99% of which are inactive.

V. DATA ANALYSIS AND MINING

Up to now, we have been discussing display and reporting of the results for a single experiment. The key decisions made at the single-experiment level include the following: (1) Did this experiment run as expected? (2) Were there any hits, or interesting compounds? While these are interesting and useful questions to ask, other questions can require even deeper analysis and place an increased strain on information systems. For example: (1) Of the compounds that were active in this test, which were active (or not active) in other tests? (2) Are there structural components of the hits that would account for the activity? (3) Do any of the hits have physicochemical properties that would indicate that bioavailability, solubility, or potential toxic effects?

A. Cross-Assay Reports

1. Pivoted Data

In most data management systems, results data are stored in some variant of a long skinny table. This means that a single column in the table can hold multiple result types and that other columns are required to describe the results. An example of a simplified long skinny table is shown in Table 1. Long skinny tables make for efficient and flexible data storage because they do not require new columns or other modifications to define new variables. However, they do not present the data in a manner that is intuitive to the scientist. Most scientists prefer to see data in a short and wide format, in which each variable associated with a compound is represented as a column. An example of a short wide table is given in Table 2. Note that each test is now a column, so the scientist can quickly answer questions such as, "Which compounds were active in this test, but not in others?" or, for the compounds of interest, "Are there tests that were not run?" Converting data representation from tall/skinny, as it is stored, to short/wide is known as pivoting the data. The data pivot can take place in many different ways, and many biological information management systems have a data-pivoting function built in.

In Table 2, note how easy it is to tell which samples have been run in which tests, and which samples were active in one test but inactive in other tests. Unfor-

Table 1 A Simplified Tall Skinny Table

Sample Number	Test Number	Result
SLA-0019	Test 4	80
SLA-0011	Test 7	71
SLA-0015	Test 9	93
SLA-0022	Test 5	28
SLA-0014	Test 8	95
SLA-0013	Test 3	37
SLA-0002	Test 1	49
SLA-0006	Test 5	90
SLA-0013	Test 6	39
SLA-0021	Test 4	80
SLA-0011	Test 2	37
SLA-0004	Test 2	63
SLA-0002	Test 3	38
SLA-0001	Test 8	45
SLA-0001	Test 9	0
SLA-0010	Test 9	52
SLA-0012	Test 8	66
SLA-0016	Test 7	69
SLA-0023	Test 2	55
SLA-0003	Test 5	58
SLA-0023	Test 8	95
SLA-0009	Test 8	3
SLA-0010	Test 6	46
SLA-0021	Test 7	28
SLA-0007	Test 6	97
SLA-0005	Test 9	48
SLA-0017	Test 1	95
SLA-0023	Test 6	91
SLA-0019	Test 3	2
SLA-0001	Test 4	0
SLA-0011	Test 3	4
SLA-0006	Test 4	17
SLA-0003	Test 8	84
SLA-0020	Test 5	52
SLA-0003	Test 2	92
SLA-0021	Test 9	82
SLA-0006	Test 9	78
SLA-0013	Test 1	78
SLA-0012	Test 5	99
SLA-0001	Test 3	87
SLA-0009	Test 2	43
SLA-0013	Test 9	100
SLA-0015	Test 7	66

Table 1 Continued

Sample Number	Test Number	Result
SLA-0010	Test 1	62
SLA-0020	Test 9	8
SLA-0001	Test 2	73
SLA-0017	Test 5	2
SLA-0002	Test 8	21
SLA-0012	Test 9	27
SLA-0021	Test 3	40
SLA-0012	Test 7	54
SLA-0022	Test 9	52
SLA-0022	Test 4	23
SLA-0015	Test 5	63
SLA-0008	Test 6	99
SLA-0011	Test 5	73
SLA-0010	Test 8	55
SLA-0008	Test 3	61
SLA-0006	Test 3	55
SLA-0014	Test 2	86
SLA-0019	Test 1	74
SLA-0003	Test 1	35
SLA-0020	Test 1	10
SLA-0018	Test 3	79
SLA-0008	Test 9	61
SLA-0019	Test 6	23
SLA-0020	Test 8	50
SLA-0009	Test 5	1
SLA-0016	Test 1	5
SLA-0002	Test 5	3
SLA-0021	Test 1	35
SLA-0015	Test 6	39
SLA-0004	Test 8	31
SLA-0004	Test 4	42
SLA-0019	Test 8	99
SLA-0019	Test 9	100
SLA-0007	Test 1	11
SLA-0001	Test 6	25
SLA-0008	Test 5	32
SLA-0005	Test 2	35
SLA-0003	Test 7	18
SLA-0018	Test 9	68
SLA-0007	Test 7	92
SLA-0005	Test 8	61
SLA-0023	Test 1	11
SLA-0012	Test 6	5

Table 1 Continued

Sample Number	Test Number	Result
SLA-0014	Test 5	62
SLA-0002	Test 2	62
SLA-0017	Test 4	48
SLA-0009	Test 3	59
SLA-0003	Test 6	23
SLA-0001	Test 5	71
SLA-0004	Test 7	94
SLA-0022	Test 2	37
SLA-0003	Test 3	76
SLA-0023	Test 9	24
SLA-0011	Test 8	50
SLA-0001	Test 1	87
SLA-0008	Test 7	73
SLA-0015	Test 8	46
SLA-0011	Test 1	90
SLA-0014	Test 7	100
SLA-0009	Test 7	10
SLA-0012	Test 2	54
SLA-0004	Test 3	76
SLA-0013	Test 8	71
SLA-0018	Test 5	97
SLA-0007	Test 4	90
SLA-0019	Test 7	99
SLA-0022	Test 7	38
SLA-0018	Test 8	91
SLA-0016	Test 2	42
SLA-0010	Test 3	37
SLA-0017	Test 9	24
SLA-0023	Test 5	95
SLA-0002	Test 4	66
SLA-0018	Test 7	91
SLA-0018	Test 6	7
SLA-0001	Test 7	23
SLA-0020	Test 6	15
SLA-0014	Test 1	15
SLA-0013	Test 4	84
SLA-0016	Test 6	91
SLA-0010	Test 4	76
SLA-0022	Test 8	92
SLA-0016	Test 4	7
SLA-0016	Test 3	22
SLA-0017	Test 2	39
SLA-0015	Test 2	82

Table 1 Continued

Sample Number	Test Number	Result
SLA-0021	Test 8	54
SLA-0017	Test 6	62
SLA-0006	Test 8	11
SLA-0023	Test 7	33
SLA-0012	Test 4	24
SLA-0022	Test 3	58
SLA-0004	Test 5	95
SLA-0005	Test 4	13
SLA-0015	Test 1	20
SLA-0005	Test 5	87
SLA-0010	Test 7	85
SLA-0012	Test 1	91
SLA-0013	Test 5	25
SLA-0019	Test 2	2
SLA-0002	Test 9	64
SLA-0010	Test 5	5
SLA-0007	Test 3	26
SLA-0006	Test 7	99
SLA-0008	Test 2	52
SLA-0009	Test 6	71
SLA-0022	Test 6	38
SLA-0010	Test 2	4
SLA-0015	Test 4	31
SLA-0009	Test 4	68
SLA-0023	Test 4	42
SLA-0007	Test 2	14
SLA-0011	Test 9	73
SLA-0011	Test 4	32
SLA-0008	Test 1	78
SLA-0008	Test 8	95
SLA-0005	Test 7	34
SLA-0002	Test 6	73
SLA-0013	Test 2	51
SLA-0017	Test 3	68
SLA-0014	Test 4	4
SLA-0002	Test 7	30
SLA-0015	Test 3	4
SLA-0022	Test 1	89
SLA-0007	Test 5	83
SLA-0008	Test 4	25
SLA-0013	Test 7	38
SLA-0018	Test 4	3
SLA-0009	Test 9	65

Table 1 Continued

Sample Number	Test Number	Result
SLA-0014	Test 6	85
SLA-0021	Test 6	88
SLA-0018	Test 1	16
SLA-0020	Test 4	77
SLA-0007	Test 9	100
SLA-0005	Test 6	42
SLA-0023	Test 3	18
SLA-0014	Test 3	86
SLA-0007	Test 8	58
SLA-0014	Test 9	89
SLA-0006	Test 6	2
SLA-0003	Test 4	17
SLA-0011	Test 6	68
SLA-0009	Test 1	51
SLA-0017	Test 7	12
SLA-0021	Test 5	63
SLA-0021	Test 2	66
SLA-0020	Test 7	64
SLA-0020	Test 2	18
SLA-0019	Test 5	43
SLA-0004	Test 9	39
SLA-0016	Test 5	1
SLA-0016	Test 8	48
SLA-0006	Test 1	25
SLA-0018	Test 2	22
SLA-0003	Test 9	76
SLA-0005	Test 3	22
SLA-0016	Test 9	92
SLA-0020	Test 3	67
SLA-0017	Test 8	22
SLA-0004	Test 6	12
SLA-0006	Test 2	38
SLA-0012	Test 3	47
SLA-0005	Test 1	22
SLA-0004	Test 1	81

Table 2 A Simplified Short Wide Table

	Test 1	Test 2	Test 3	Test 4	Test 5	Test 6	Test 7	Test 8	Test 9
SLA-0017	95	39	68	48	2	62	12	22	24
SLA-0012	91	54		24	99	5	54	66	27
SLA-0011	90	37	4	32		68	71	50	73
SLA-0022	89	37	58	23	28	38		92	52
SLA-0001	87	73	87	0	71	25	23	45	0
SLA-0004	81	63	76	42	95	12	94	31	39
SLA-0008	78	52	61	25	32	99	73	95	61
SLA-0013	78	51	37	84	25	39	38	71	100
SLA-0019	74	2	2	80	43	23	99	99	100
SLA-0010	62	4	37	76	5	46	85	55	52
SLA-0009	51	43	59	68	1	71	10	3	65
SLA-0002	49	62	38	66	3	73	30	21	64
SLA-0021	35	66	40	80	63	88	28	54	82
SLA-0003	35	92	76	17	58	23	18	84	76
SLA-0006	25	38	55	17	90	2	99	11	78
SLA-0005	22	35	22	13	87	42	34	61	48
SLA-0015	20	82	4	31	63	39	66	46	93
SLA-0018	16	22	79	3	97	7	91	91	68
SLA-0014	15	86	86	4	62	85	100	95	89
SLA-0023	11	55	18	42	95	91	33	95	24
SLA-0007	11	14	26	90	83	97	92	58	100
SLA-0020	10	18	67	77	52	15	64	50	8
SLA-0016	5	42	22	7	1	91	69	48	92

tunately, this type of table makes for very inefficient storage, especially if there are sparsely populated columns. Also, this type of table is also very inflexible, since the addition of a new test requires the addition of new columns.

2. Classical Structure Activity

One of the goals of pharmaceutical research has been to find the relationship between small-molecule chemical structure and biological activity. One simple, but widely used, method of analysis is the structure–activity relation report. This report shows a chemical structure and pieces of information describing the activity on each row. An example of a structure–activity report is shown in figure 7. The addition of quantitative measures of physicochemical properties is called QSAR and is the province of molecular modelers. Structure–activity relationship reports

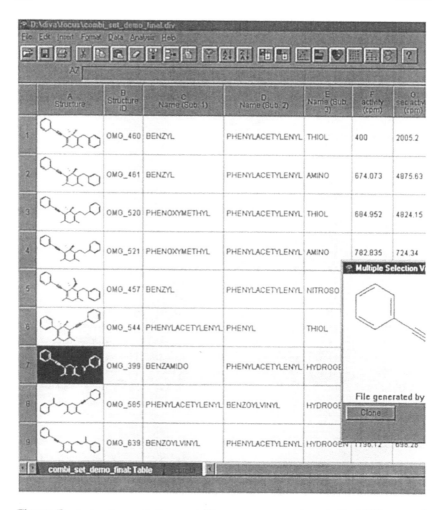

Figure 7 A structure–activity report. Here we see a report created in DIVA, a popular analysis and reporting tool from Oxford Molecular Ltd. Each row contains information regarding one compound, along with the structure, and a number of physicochemical properties.

are very useful, particularly for small numbers of compounds; however, the amount of data rapidly becoming available in most large life science companies will completely overwhelm the cognitive ability of most scientists to view and analyze the data. As we move into higher volumes of data, data reduction and visualization techniques become more important.

B. Visualization of Data

When working with large volumes of data, humans tend to respond to visual cues much more rapidly than textual displays of the data. Several data visualization tools in use today allow users to simultaneously view multiple attributes. It has been established that by using a combination of size, shape, color, position, and texture, it is possible to perceive up to eight dimensions simultaneously. We show an example of a popular data mining tool, Spotfire Pro from Spotfire Inc., in Figure 8. In this example, the results of multiple tests are displayed as dimensions, and physicochemical properties of the samples are displayed as colors, shapes and sizes. Spotfire allows the user to graphically reduce the dataset to the results of interest.

VI. LOGISTICS

A. Plate Handling

HTS is almost entirely performed in microplates, each containing between 96 and 3456 wells. During the past several years, the 384-well plate has supplanted the 96-well plate as the primary HTS vehicle. Tracking the contents of each well in each plate and associating the results with the proper sample is of crucial importance for an HTS system, but several factors must be overcome.

The detected plate (the assay plate) is rarely the plate stored in inventory. Often, the process of detection itself is destructive. Whether detection is destructive or not, the addition of the biological reagents would make the assay plate unusable for future tests. The usual process has the automation equipment copy a plate taken from inventory to create the new assay plate. Reagents are then added to the assay plate, and the detection is performed. At some point, the data management system must be told what is in the assay plate or told how to associate the assay plate with the information in an inventory plate. This can be done in several different ways. Two examples follow. (1) The liquid-handling device, which actually makes the assay plate, keeps a running list of the assay plates that it makes as well as the inventory plates from which it makes each one. In this case, the data management system will have to look up the inventory plate for each assay plate and the get the appropriate inventory information. (2) When making an assay

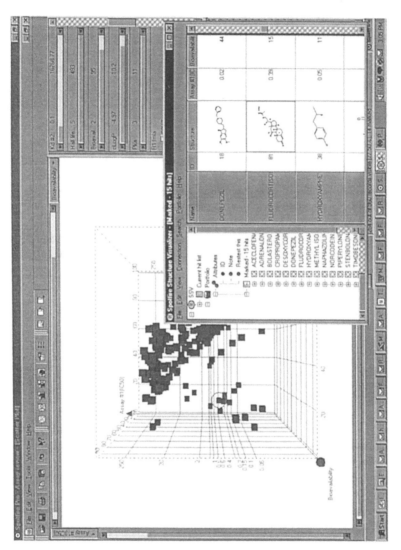

Figure 8 The sheer volume of data being produced by high-throughput screening is overwhelming users' ability to interpret results using conventional means. Spotfire, from Spotfire, Inc., is one of a number of programs designed to help users mine the data and extract information. In this example, we see the results of several different assays combined in a multidimensional display. Users manipulate the slide bars to further select interesting results. A small cluster of interesting results is identified in the lower left corner, and the results for

plate, the liquid handler applies a bar code identifier that includes the inventory plate ID plus an extension. When the data system reads the plate ID (usually in the reader file), it needs to parse out the inventory plate ID and retrieve appropriate inventory information.

B. Special Cases

1. Consolidation

An increasing percentage of HTS experiments are being performed on 384-well plates. However, most storage is still done in 96-deep-well plates. During the process, four 96-well plates are typically combined into a single 384-well plate. So, as sample is transferred from each of the 96-well plates to a different location on the 384-well plate, the information system must be informed about the new location of the sample.

2. Format Changes

Often, samples are purchased from outside suppliers or are stored in inventory in a format that is not compatible with the format used for the test. For example, many suppliers provide compounds in 96-well plates with all wells filled; however, most tests require that one or two columns of wells be left blank for controls. In these cases, once again, samples must be moved to different locations on the new plates, and the information system must keep track of which samples are moved where.

3. Pooling/Deconvolution

Some laboratories, in an effort to increase throughput, intentionally mix 8–12 samples per well. When a well displays activity, the samples contained in that well are tested individually to find the "hot" sample. Assuming that 1% or less of all samples are active, this will result in a dramatic decrease in the number of wells tested, thus increasing throughput and decreasing costs. A special case of pooling is called orthogonal pooling. In this case each sample is put into two wells, but the combination of samples is unique in each well, and any two wells will only have one sample in common. Therefore, when any two wells are active, the common sample can be located and retested for confirmation.

VII. CONCLUSION AND FUTURE TECHNOLOGIES

Predicting the future in any case is a perilous thing to do. In the case of a rapidly changing field, such as HTS, it is downright foolhardy, but that won't keep us from trying. Most of the predictions we are making are just extrapolations of technologies under way. There is always the possibility that a major technological innovation will change the course of screening dramatic changes in HTS processes, or perhaps even obviating the need for HTS. Even in the absence of such dramatic discontinuities, we can see several new technologies that will have an impact on the practice of screening.

A. Higher Densities and Ultrahigh-Throughput Screening

First, the drive toward higher and higher densities will continue. The economics of HTS make a compelling case. Increases in speed of throughput are a secondary issue to reduction in the cost of reagents used. We fully expect the HTS standard to move from 96-well plates to 384, on to 1536, and possibly as high as 3456. The effect that this will have on informatics systems is fairly obvious. First, as noted earlier, smaller wells require much tighter tolerances; hence, the need for the capability to detect systematic errors will become even more acute. In addition, as we move to higher densities, new visualization tools will become a requirement, as many of the visualizations designed for 96- and 384-well plates will simply not be usable for 3456-well plates. Finally, the need for users to be able to quickly locate information for single samples will become more acute. Higher densities and faster instrumentation together are allowing throughput to increase dramatically. The increased throughput levels, referred to as ultrahigh-throughput screening, will put additional strain on information systems, forcing the systems to process more information at a higher rate.

B. Wider Use of HTS Techniques

One of the effects of the adoption of HTS throughout the pharmaceutical industry has been to move the bottleneck in the discovery pipeline downstream. Essentially, this means that HTS labs are producing hits at a faster rate than the therapeutic areas and development can absorb them. One strategy for dealing with this new bottleneck is to adapt HTS style techniques for metabolism, toxicity, and other secondary and development assays. This change will have a dramatic effect on information systems, as the data produced by these tests are usually far more complex than these produced in classical HTS assays. For one thing, these tests can often have more than one end point. For example, some toxicity tests measure the effects of exposing the a specific type of cell to different samples. The scientist may want to record the percentage of cells that died (or survived), the reproduction rate, the growth rate, and if any specific types of proteins were expressed. Some tests go as far as measuring specific types of damage to the cell. The challenge to the information system is to be able to collect all of the relevant information so as to allow the scientist to declare all of the appropriate variables for the experiment and record the appropriate contextual information (e.g., how was the test run?).

C. HTS Kinetics and High-Content Screening

Until recently, the goal of all HTS programs was simply to increase throughput, the sheer number of samples processed, and hence the volume of data produced. Many HTS scientists believe that this goal has been largely accomplished and that further investment in increasing throughput will bring diminishing returns. The next goal is to increase the quality of the data produced. Essentially, this means that the goal is no longer to simply test more samples but rather to learn more about each sample tested. Some organizations call this "high-content screening" (HCS). HCS involves tests where multiple end points are achieved for each sample. In addition, many kinetics experiments (where multiple readings are taken for each sample over a course of time) have been adapted for automation. Now, instead of a single reading for a well, there can be up to 100 readings for each well. There is a great debate concerning what to do with this raw data. Should it be stored at all? Can it be archived? Should it be available for on-line queries? Most organizations have (to date) decided that it is impractical to attempt to store all the raw data on line but that it can be archived in off-line storage, such as zip drives, and the reduced data (such as K_i) can be stored on-line.

D. Conclusion

While it may not be possible to predict what HTS will look like in the future, several points are clear.

- The volume of data will continue to increase. Whether it is from higher throughput, higher content, or both, more data will be available to scientists. The challenge to the information system designer, then, is to create tools that allow the scientist to store all the relevant data and then retrieve it in such a way that information can be extracted quickly. The goal is to help the scientist find "actionable" data, or data that cause the scientist to make a decision, such as "this sample is worthy of further study" or "the results of this test should be rejected."
- As the volume of data increases, data storage systems will come under increasing pressure. Currently, most major pharmaceutical companies store all chemical or biological data in Oracle databases from Oracle Corporation. Oracle is migrating technology to object orientation, which can provide increased performance. It will be up to the developers of chemical and biological information management systems to utilize advances in the underlying core technologies as they become available.

- Data-mining tools are being developed for industries ranging from retail to financial services. While the volume of data being produced by HTS and related technologies calls for data mining and statistical solutions, and there is a great deal of work going on in this area, it is unclear at the time of writing whether general-purpose data-mining tools can be adapted for drug discovery.
- Science will continue to evolve, and information systems must also continue to evolve to support the science.

16

Combinatorial Chemistry: The History and the Basics

Michal Lebl
Illumina, Inc.
San Diego, California

I. DEFINITION

What is combinatorial chemistry? There have been several opinions, some formulated very sharply, but most expressing what combinatorial chemistry is not. At the end of the conference "Combinatorial Chemistry 2000" in London, we organized a discussion session because we wanted to answer this question and make sure that our understanding of the term reflects the fact that at least some operations in the synthesis of the group of chemical compounds is performed in combinatorial fashion. Unfortunately, when it came to the public vote, the scientists in the audience voted for a much broader definition of combinatorial chemistry. The majority expressed the opinion that combinatorial chemistry is defined by the design process, i.e., that compounds designed by the combination of building blocks (and synthesized by whatever means) are the subject of combinatorial chemistry. In the literature, the term combinatorial chemistry is used very often; however, the definition is found rarely. Seneci [1] says that "combinatorial chemistry refers to the synthetic chemical process that generates a set or sets (combinatorial libraries) of compounds in simultaneous rather than a sequential manner." *Journal of Combinatorial Chemistry* defines combinatorial chemistry as "a field in which new chemical substances—ranging from pure compounds to complex mixtures—are synthesized and screened in a search for useful properties."

But do we really need to define combinatorial chemistry before discussing the history of this branch of science? Must we have consensus about the term combinatorial chemistry before we start the new journal with the term in its title? (There are already several journals with the term combinatorial chemistry on their cover.) Apparently not, and the precise definition is probably not as important as the fact that the novel techniques are being widely accepted and applied as needed for a variety of projects, starting from finding new drug candidates and ending in discovery of new inorganic materials.

II. HISTORY

Maybe the best introduction to combinatorial chemistry is through its brief history. In 1959, the young chemist Bruce Merrifield, had the idea that it would be extremely beneficial to modify the sometimes unpredictable behavior of growing peptide chain intermediates by attaching the chain to the polymeric matrix, the properties of which would be very uniform from step to step [2–5]. His invention of solid-phase synthesis, for which he was awarded the Nobel Prize [4], changed the field of peptide synthesis dramatically. Synthesis of oligonucleotides followed immediately [6]; however, solid-phase synthesis of organic molecules was pursued basically only in the laboratory of Professor Leznoff [7,8]. Even though solid-phase synthesis was more or less accepted in the chemical community, it took another 20 years before the new ways of thinking about generation of a multitude of compounds for biological screening brought combinatorial chemistry to life. Pressure from biologists motivated the development of combinatorial chemistry. Chemists could not keep up with the demand for the new chemical entities. Big pharmaceutical companies started to screen their entire collections of chemical compounds against new targets, and the rate at which these collections grew seemed unsatisfactory. Ronald Frank in Germany [9], Richard Houghten in California [10], and Mario Geysen in Australia [11] devised ways to make hundreds of peptides or oligonucleotides simultaneously by segmenting the synthetic substrate–solid support. Frank used cellulose paper as the support for the synthesis of oligonucleotides. Cutting the circles of the paper and reshuffling the labeled circles for each cycle of the coupling was a very simple way to generate hundreds of oligos. Houghten enclosed classical polystyrene beaded resin in polypropylene mesh bags, later called "tea-bags" or "T-bags," and used them for parallel synthesis of hundreds of peptides. The principle was the same: combine the bags intended for coupling the same amino acid and resort the bags after each cycle of coupling. Geysen used functionalized polypropylene pins arranged in the fixed grid. Each pin was then immersed in a solution of activated amino acid pipetted into the individual wells of microtiter plate. Pins were not resorted after each step, but the common steps of the synthesis (washing, deprotection) were done by introduction of the pins into the bath containing appropriate solvent. These techniques cleared the way for the arrival of real combinatorial techniques applied to general organic chemistry and not only to the specific arena of peptides and oligonucleotides.

For biologists and biochemists, working with mixtures was absolutely natural—well, it was natural also for natural products chemists—however, organic chemists were (and still are) horrified when mixtures were mentioned. Therefore, development of specific binders selected from the astronomically complex mixtures of RNA by selective binding and amplification of selected molecules by polymerase chain reaction (PCR) was accepted enthusiastically, and papers describing it were published in *Science* [12] and *Nature* [13,14]. (Larry Gold and his colleagues were adventurous enough to build a company around this technology—NeXstar—now merged with Gilead, in Colorado.) Relatively fast acceptance was given to the techniques generating specific peptides on the surface of the phage, panning for the binding sequences and amplification of the phage [15,16], described by Smith. Again, the approach was basically biological. However, earlier attempts to publish papers describing the use of synthetic peptide mixtures for determination of epitopes in *Nature* were unsuccessful; the world was not ready for chemical mixtures. Geysen's seminal paper was eventually published in *Molecular Immunology* [17] and did not find a large audience. In this paper the mixture of amino acids was used for the coupling at the defined positions, thus generating large mixtures of peptides. Mixtures showing significant binding were "deconvoluted" in several steps to define the relevant binding peptide sequence at the end.

The pioneer in development of the methods for creating the equal mixtures (of peptides) was Arpad Furka in Hungary. His method of "portioning-mixing" was invented in 1982 (*http://szerves.chem.elte.hu/Furka/index.html*) and presented as posters in 1988 and 1989 [18,19]. The method was not noticed until 1991, when it was reinvented and published in *Nature* by two independent groups, Lam et al. in Arizona ("split-and-mix" method) [20] and Houghten et al. in California ("divide–couple–recombine" method) [21]. Technology of deconvolution of mixtures was the basis of formation of Houghten Pharmaceuticals, Inc., later renamed Trega Biosciences, Inc. (Leon, Germany). Finding the active molecule requires synthesis of the second (and third, and fourth etc.) generation mixtures of lower complexity based on the activity evaluation of the most active mixture from the first round of screening. An alternative method is positional scanning in which mixtures of the same complexity with defined building blocks in all positions of the sequence are screened and the importance of individual blocks is ascertained. The combinations of all "important" residues are then assembled in the possible "candidate sequences," which are then tested individually [22]. The use of mixture-based libraries was reviewed recently [23].

Portioning-mixing (split-and-mix, divide–couple–recombine) is a simple but powerful method that not only allows generation of equimolar mixtures of compounds but is also the basis of one-bead-one-compound technology for the screening of individual compounds (as recognized by Lam [20,24,25]). In this modification, the synthetic compounds are not cleaved from the resinous bead, and binding is evaluated by assay performed directly on the bead. The structure of a compound residing on positively reacting bead is then established by direct methods or by reading "the code" associated with that particular bead. The one-bead-one-compound technique can be modified for the release of the compound to solution [26], or to semisolid media [27], to allow for the use of assays not compatible with solid-phase limitation. Again, this technology jump-started the first combinatorial chemistry company, Selectide Corporation, in Tucson, Arizona (now part of Aventis).

III. SMALL ORGANIC MOLECULES

Libraries of peptides and oligonucleotides were relatively easy to handle both in the mixture and in the individual one-bead-one-compound format. Determination of structure of peptide and/or oligonucleotide is made relatively easy by sequencing requiring picomolar or even lower amounts of material. At the same time synthetic methodologies for their synthesis are well developed. However, a good candidate for new successful drug is being sought between "small organic molecules." Libraries containing nonoligomeric organic compounds were obviously the next step in the development of combinatorial chemistry. Jonathan Ellman recognized this need and developed a method for solid-phase parallel synthesis of benzodiazepines [28]. His publication, together with published results from Parke-Davis [29] and Chiron [30,31], started a flood of communications about application of solid-phase synthesis to preparation of enormous numbers of different categories of organic compounds, with the major focus on heterocyclic molecules. (Numerous compilations of solid-phase syntheses were published; see, for example, [32–35], and a dynamic database of all relevant publications is available on the Internet (*http://www.5z.com/divinfo*).).

Transformation of one-bead-one-compound libraries to the arena of small organic molecules requires methods allowing simple and unequivocal determination of the structure from the individual bead containing picomolar amounts of analyzable material. This problem was addressed by inclusion of "tagging" into the synthetic scheme [36–39]. The structure of the relevant molecule is determined by reading the "tag." The most elegant method for tagging was developed by Clark Still [37]. Again, as a rule in this field, the result was formation of a new company, Pharmacopeia. In this method, the tagging of the organic molecule is achieved by a relatively small set of halogenated ethers attached to the bead as a defined mixture in each step of the synthesis, forming digital code (each molecule of the tagging substance is either present—digit 1—or absent—digit 0), evaluated after detachment from the bead by gas chromatography.

It did not take long before the combinatorial techniques were applied to material science [40–44]. These libraries are produced usually in a spatially addressable form and were used to find new supraconductive, photoluminescent, or magnetoresistive materials.

IV. SYNTHETIC TECHNIQUES

Although the pressure to produce more compounds was visibly coming from pharmaceutical companies, most of the new techniques were developed at academic institutions. Big companies still did not embrace the new techniques possibly due to the fact that they are quite simple and inexpensive to implement. Pharmaceutical companies do not want simple solutions; they would rather invest in enormous automation projects. In the end the managers are judged by the budget they were able to invest, and a big room full of robotic synthesizers definitely looks impressive. Another major factor is the "visibility" of the compound produced. Production of 100 nmoles of the compound (about 50µg of an average organic compound), which can make 100 ml of 1 µM solution (enough for 1000 biological assays), is unacceptable—simply because it is not "visible." Companies usually require 5–50 mg of the compound (more than enough for 1 million assays) just to "have it on the shelf." And techniques providing 100 nmoles are definitely cheaper and require less automation than techniques needed to make milligram quantities of the compound.

A very elegant technique for synthesizing numerous organic compounds in parallel was introduced by Irori in San Diego. This company was based on the idea that it is possible to label individual polymeric beads with the readable radiofrequency tag, which will be built during the split-and-mix synthesis of any type of molecule. Even though this very ambitious goal has not yet been achieved, the technique of "Microkans"—small containers made from polymeric mesh material containing inside beads used for solid phase synthesis together with radiofrequency tag [45,46]—is used in numerous laboratories [47]. The most recent incarnation of this technique (based on the original principle of "tea-bag" synthesis of Houghten [10]), is the labeling of small disks containing 2–10 mg of synthetic substrate, called "NanoKans," by a two-dimensional bar code on a small ceramic chip [48].

On the other hand, thousands of compounds can be synthesized relatively inexpensively in polypropylene microtiter plates using either "surface suction" [49] or "tilted centrifugation" [50]. However, nothing can be more economical and versatile for synthesis of up to couple of hundred compounds than disposable polypropylene syringes equipped with polypropylene frits, as introduced by Krchnak [51]. A syringe is charged with the solid support of choice, and all steps of the synthesis are performed by aspirating appropriate reagents using needles and (if needed) septum-closed bottles. The operation of syringes can be simplified by the use of domino blocks [52].

V.   PHILOSOPHY AND CRITERIA

The different approaches to the synthesis of libraries illustrate the different philosophies of laboratories and companies. The same difference in thinking can be found in the value given to the purity of prepared compounds. Different companies apply different criteria. However, in the end you will always hear: "We do not accept anything worse than 80 (75, 85, 70)% purity." Well, what purity is being talked about? High-performance liquid chromatography with ultraviolet detector? All compounds would have to have the same absorbtion coefficient. Or evaporative light-scattering (ELS) detector? Slightly better. Or mass spectroscopic (MS) purity? There is nothing like MS purity! Maybe nuclear magnetic resonance (NMR), but who can evaluate several hundreds or thousands of NMR spectra each day? Anyway, what does this number tell you? Only a rough approximation of how many potentially good leads you will miss by not looking at the samples at all. The only really important information that the chemist should provide to the biologist is whether he or she can guarantee the preparation of the same sample tomorrow or a year from now. Does he or she have the stable, well-rehearsed protocol and reliable source of starting materials? If yes, every biologist should be happy to screen his or her compounds. If the biological activity is found in the impure sample, the likelihood that the active component of the mixture can be found after isolation of all components is pretty high. By the way, the probability that the activity is higher than observed in the mixture is also high. And, as a free bonus, the active species might not be the one that was targeted but rather the side product of unexpected (and hopefully novel) structure. This would make the patent people happy. For a long time I did not meet a combinatorial chemist who did not have a story about active compound being a side product.

We could go on discussing combinatorial chemistry, but because this text is intended to be an introduction to the history of the fields, we will stop here and refer readers to the published literature. The histories and personal recollections of the pioneers in this field were compiled in the inaugural issue of *Journal of Combinatorial Chemistry* [53], and a similar format was used for a history of solid-supported synthesis [54,55]. In addition to books on the subject of combinatorial chemistry and solid-phase synthesis [56–74], we recommend attendance at biannual symposia on solid-phase synthesis and combinatorial techniques [75], organized by Roger Epton. Reading of recent review articles [32–35,76–88] is also helpful. We also direct readers to the Internet site compiling all papers published in this exciting and rapidly growing field, which can be found at *http://www.5z.com/divinfo.*

REFERENCES

1.   Seneci P. Solid-Phase Synthesis and Combinatorial Technologies. New York: John Wiley & Sons, 2001.

2. Merrifield B. Concept and early development of solid-phase peptide synthesis. Meth Enzymol 1997;289:3–13.

3. Merrifield RB. Solid phase peptide synthesis. I. The synthesis of a tetrapeptide. J Am Chem Soc 1963;85:2149–2154.

4. Merrifield RB. Solid phase synthesis (Nobel lecture). Angew Chem Int Ed 1985;24:799–810.

5. Merrifield RB. Life During a Golden Age of Peptide Chemistry: The Concept and Development of Solid-Phase Peptide Synthesis. Washington, DC: American Chemical Society, 1993.

6. Letsinger RL, Mahadevan V. Stepwise synthesis of oligodeoxyribonucleotides on an insoluble polymer support. J Am Chem Soc 1966;88:5319–5324.

7. Leznoff CC, Wong JY. The use of polymer supports in organic synthesis. The synthesis of monotrityl ethers of symmetrical diols. Can J Chem 1972;50:2892–2893.

8. Leznoff CC. 1999 Alfred Bader Award Lecture: From early developments in multi-step organic synthesis on solid phases to multi-nuclear phthalocyanines. Can J Chem 2000;78(2):167–183.

9. Frank R, Heikens W, Heisterberg-Moutsis G, Blocker H. A new general approach for the simultaneous chemical synthesis of large numbers of oligonucleotides: segmental solid supports. Nucl Acid Res 1983;11:4365–4377.

10. Houghten RA. General method for the rapid solid-phase synthesis of large numbers of peptides: specificity of antigen-antibody interaction at the level of individual amino acids. Proc Natl Acad Sci USA 1985;82:5131–5135.

11. Geysen HM, Meloen RH, Barteling SJ. Use of peptide synthesis to probe viral antigens for epitopes to a resolution of a single amino acid. Proc Natl Acad Sci USA 1984;81:3998–4002.

12. Tuerk C, Gold L. Systematic evolution of ligands by exponential enrichment: RNA ligands to bacteriophage T4 DNA polymerase. Science 1990;249:505–510.

13. Ellington AD, Szostak JW. In vitro selection of RNA molecules that bind specific ligands. Nature 1990;346:818–822.

14. Ellington AD, Szostak JW. Selection in vitro of single-stranded DNA molecules that fold into specific ligand-binding structures. Nature 1992;355:850–852.

15. Smith GP. Filamentous fusion phage: novel expression vectors that display cloned antigens on the virion surface. Science 1985;228:1315–1317.

16. Smith GP, Petrenko VA. Phage display. Chem Rev 1997;97(2):391–410.

17. Geysen HM, Rodda SJ, Mason TJ. A priori delineation of a peptide which mimics a discontinuous antigenic determinant. Mol Immunol 1986;23:709–715.

18. Furka A, Sebestyen F, Asgedom M, et al. Highlights of Modern Biochemistry. Proceedings of the 14th International Congress of Biochemistry, held in Prague, 1988. Ultrecht: VSP, 1988; 13, Cornucopia of peptides by synthesis. p. 47.

19. Furka A, Sebestyen F, Asgedom M, Dibo G. More peptides by less labour. 1988. Poster presented at Xth International Symposium on Medicinal Chemistry, Budapest, 1988.

20. Lam KS, Salmon SE, Hersh EM, Hruby VJ, Kazmierski WM, Knapp RJ. A new type of synthetic peptide library for identifying ligand-binding activity. Nature 1991; 354:82–84.

21. Houghten RA, Pinilla C, Blondelle SE, Appel JR, Dooley CT, Cuervo JH. Generation

and use of synthetic peptide combinatorial libraries for basic research and drug discovery. Nature 1991;354:84–86.

22. Dooley CT, Houghten RA. The use of positional scanning synthetic peptide combinatorial libraries for the rapid determination of opioid receptor ligands. Life Sci 1993;52:1509–1517.

23. Houghten RA, Pinilla C, Appel JR, Blondelle SE, Dooley CT, Eichler J, Nefzi A, Ostresh JM. Mixture-based synthetic combinatorial libraries. J Med Chem 1999;42(19):3743–3778.

24. Lam KS, Lebl M, Krchnak V. The "one-bead one-compound" combinatorial library method. Chem Rev 1997;97(2):411–448.

25. Lebl M, Krchnak V, Sepetov NF, Seligmann B, Strop P, Felder S, Lam KS. One-bead-one-structure combinatorial libraries. Biopolymers (Pept Sci) 1995;37(3):177–198.

26. Salmon SE, Lam KS, Lebl M, Kandola A, Khattri PS, Wade S, Patek M, Kocis P, Krchnak V, Thorpe D, et al. Discovery of biologically active peptides in random libraries: solution-phase testing after staged orthogonal release from resin beads. Proc Natl Acad Sci USA 1993;90(24):11708–11712.

27. Salmon SE, Liu-Stevens RH, Zhao Y, Lebl M, Krchnak V, Wertman K, Sepetov N, Lam KS. High-volume cellular screening for anticancer agents with combinatorial chemical libraries: a new methodology. Mol Diver 1996;2(1–2):57–63.

28. Bunin BA, Ellman JA. A general and expedient method for the solid phase synthesis of 1,4-benzodiazepine derivatives. J Am Chem Soc 1992;114:10997–10998.

29. DeWitt SH, Kiely JS, Stankovic CJ, Schroeder MC, Cody DMR, Pavia MR. "Diversomers": an approach to nonpeptide, nonoligomeric chemical diversity. Proc Natl Acad Sci USA 1993;90:6909–6913.

30. Simon RJ, Kaina RS, Zuckermann RN, Huebner VD, Jewell DA, Banville S, Ng S, Wang L, Rosenberg S, Marlowe CK, et al. Peptoids: a modular approach to drug discovery. Proc Natl Acad Sci USA 1992;89:9367–9371.

31. Zuckermann RN, Martin EJ, Spellmeyer DC, Stauber GB, Shoemaker KR, Kerr JM, Figliozzi GM, Goff DA, Siani MA, Simon RJ, et al. Discovery of nanomolar ligands for 7-transmembrane G-protein-coupled receptors from a diverse N-(substituted)-glycine peptoid library. J Med Chem 1994;37:2678–2685.

32. Dolle RE. Comprehensive survey of combinatorial library synthesis: 1999. J Comb Chem 2000;2(5):383–433.

33. Franzen RG. Recent advances in the preparation of heterocycles on solid support: a review of the literature. J Comb Chem 2000;2(3):195–214.

34. Guillier F, Orain D, Bradley M. Linkers and cleavage strategies in solid-phase organic synthesis and combinatorial chemistry. Chem Rev 2000;100(6):2091–2057.

35. Sammelson RE, Kurth MJ. Carbon–carbon bond-forming solid-phase reactions. Part II. Chem Rev 2001;101(1):137–202.

36. Kerr JM, Banville SC, Zuckermann RN. Encoded combinatorial peptide libraries containing non-natural amino acids. J Am Chem Soc 1993;115:2529–2531.

37. Nestler HP, Bartlett PA, Still WC. A general method for molecular tagging of encoded combinatorial chemistry libraries. J Org Chem 1994;59:4723–4724.

38. Nielsen J, Brenner S, Janda KD. Peptides 94, Proc.23.EPS; Maia HLS (ed); Leiden: ESCOM; 1995;Implementation of encoded combinatorial chemistry. pp. 92–93.

39. Nikolaiev V, Stierandova A, Krchnak V, Seligmann B, Lam KS, Salmon SE, Lebl M. Peptide-encoding for structure determination of nonsequenceable polymers within libraries synthesized and tested on solid-phase supports. Pept Res 1993;6(3): 161–170.

40. Briceno G, Chang H, Sun X, Schulz PG, Xiang XD. A class of cobalt oxide magnetoresistance materials discovered with combinatorial synthesis. Science 1995;270: 273–275.

41. Sun XD, Gao C, Wang JS, Xiang XD. Identification and optimization of advanced phosphors using combinatorial libraries. Appl Phys Lett 1997;70(25):3353–3355.

42. Takeuchi I, Chang H, Gao C, Schultz PG, Xiang XD, Sharma RP, Downes MJ, Venkatesan T. Combinatorial synthesis and evaluation of epitaxial ferroelectric device libraries. Appl Phys Lett 1998;73(7):894–896.

43. Wang J, Yoo Y, Gao C, Takeuchi I, Sun X, Chang H, Xiang XD, Schultz PG. Identification of a blue photoluminescent composite material from a combinatorial library. Science 1998;279(5357):1712–1714.

44. Xiang XD, Sun X, Briceno G, Lou Y, Wang KA, Chang H, Wallace-Freedman WG, Chen SW, Schultz PG. A combinatorial approach to materials discovery. Science 1995;268:1738–1740.

45. Nicolaou KC, Xiao XY, Parandoosh Z, Senyei A, Nova MP. Radiofrequency encoded combinatorial chemistry. Angew Chem Int Ed 1995;34:2289–2291.

46. Moran EJ, Sarshar S, Cargill JF, Shahbaz MM, Lio A, Mjalli AMM, Armstrong RW. Radio frequency tag encoded combinatorial library method for the discovery of tripeptide-substituted cinnamic acid inhibitors of the protein tyrosine phosphatase PTP1B. J Am Chem Soc 1995;117:10787–10788.

47. Xiao XY, Nicolaou KC. Combinatorial Chemistry: A Practical Approach; Fenniri H (ed); Oxford: Oxford University Press; 2000;4, High-throughput combinatorial synthesis of discrete compounds in multimilligram quantities: nonchemical encoding and directed sorting. pp. 75–94.

48. Xiao X, Zhao C, Potash H, Nova MP. Combinatorial chemistry with laser optical encoding. Angew Chem Int Ed 1997;36(7):780–782.

49. Lebl M, Krchnak V, Ibrahim G, Pires J, Burger C, Ni Y, Chen Y, Podue D, Mudra P, Pokorny V, et al. Solid-phase synthesis of large tetrahydroisoquinolinone arrays by two different approaches. Synthesis-Stuttgart 1999;(11):1971–1978.

50. Lebl M. New technique for high-throughput synthesis. Bioorg Med Chem Lett 1999;9(9):1305–1310.

51. Krchnak V, Vagner J. Color-monitored solid-phase multiple peptide synthesis under low-pressure continuous flow conditions. Pept Res 1990;3:182–193.

52. Krchnak V, Padera V. The domino blocks: A simple solution for parallel solid-phase organic synthesis. Bioorg Med Chem Lett 1998;8(22):3261–3264.

53. Lebl M. Parallel personal comments on "classical" papers in combinatorial chemistry. J Comb Chem 1999;1(1):3–24.

54. Hudson D. Matrix assisted synthetic transformations: a mosaic of diverse contributions. I. The pattern emerges. J Comb Chem 1999;1(5):333–360.

55. Hudson D. Matrix assisted synthetic transformations: a mosaic of diverse contributions. II. The pattern is completed. J Comb Chem 1999;1(6):403–457.

56. Bannwarth W, Felder E, Mannhold R, Kubinyi H, Timmerman H (eds). Combinatorial Chemistry: A Practical Approach. Methods and Principles in Medicinal Chemistry. Weinheim: Wiley-VCH, 2000.

57. Burgess K (ed). Solid-Phase Organic Synthesis. New York: John Wiley & Sons, 2000.

58. Dorwald FZ (ed). Organic Synthesis on Solid Phase: Supports, Linkers, Reactions. New York: Wiley-VCH, 2000.

59. Fenniri H (ed). Combinatorial Chemistry: A Practical Approach. Oxford: Oxford University Press, 2000.

60. J Jung G (ed). Combinatorial Chemistry: Synthesis, Analysis, Screening. Weinheim: Wiley-VCH, 1999.

61. Miertus S, Fassina G (eds). Combinatorial Chemistry and Technology. Principles, Methods, and Applications. New York: Marcel Dekker, 1999.

62. Moos WH, Pavia MR (eds). Annual Reports in Combinatorial Chemistry and Molecular Diversity, Vol. 2. Dordrecht: Kluwer, 1999.

63. Bunin BA (ed). The Combinatorial Index. San Diego: Academic Press, 1998.

64. Gordon EM, Kerwin JFJ (eds). Combinatorial Chemistry and Molecular Diversity in Drug Discovery. New York: John Wiley & Sons, 1998.

65. Terrett NK (ed). Combinatorial Chemistry. New York: Oxford University Press, 1998.

66. Cabilly S (ed). Combinatorial Peptide Library Protocols. Totowa: Humana Press, 1997.

67. Czarnik AW, DeWitt SH (eds). A Practical Guide to Combinatorial Chemistry. Washington, DC: American Chemical Society, 1997.

68. Devlin JP (ed). High Throughput Screening: The Discovery of Bioactive Substances. New York: Marcel Dekker, 1997.

69. Fields GB, Colowick SP (eds). Solid-Phase Peptide Synthesis. San Diego: Academic Press, 1997.

70. Wilson SR, Czarnik AW (eds). Combinatorial Chemistry. Synthesis and Applications. New York: John Wiley & Sons, 1997.

71. Abelson JN (ed). Combinatorial Chemistry. San Diego: Academic Press, 1996.

72. Chaiken IM, Janda KD (eds). Molecular Diversity and Combinatorial Chemistry. Libraries and Drug Discovery. ACS Conference Proceedings. Washington, DC: Americal Chemical Society, 1996.

73. Cortese R (ed). Combinatorial Libraries: Synthesis, Screening and Application Potential. New York: Walter de Gruyter, 1996.

74. Jung G (ed). Combinatorial Peptide and Nonpeptide Libraries: A Handbook. New York: VCH, 1996.

75. Epton R (ed). Innovation and Perspectives in Solid Phase Synthesis and Combinatorial Libraries. Birmingham: Mayflower Scientific Limited, 1999.

76. Kassel DB. Combinatorial chemistry and mass spectrometry in the 21st century drug discovery laboratory. Chem Rev 2001;101(2):255–267.

77. Reetz MT. Combinatorial and evolution-based methods in the creation of enantioselective catalysts. Angew Chem Int Ed 2001;40(2):284–310.

78. An H, Cook PD. Methodologies for generating solution-phase combinatorial libraries. Chem Rev 2000;100(9):3311–3340.

79. Barnes C, Balasubramanian S. Recent developments in the encoding and deconvolution of combinatorial libraries. Curr Opin Chem Biol 2000;4(3):346–350.

80. Brase S. New linkers for solid phase organic chemistry. Multidirectional (multifunctional), backbone amide, and traceless linker. Chim Oggi 2000;18(9):14–19.

81. Brase S, Dahmen S. Traceless linkers: only disappearing links in solid-phase organic synthesis? Chem Eur J 2000;5(11):1899–1905.

82. Domling A, Ugi I. Multicomponent reactions with isocyanides. Angew Chem Int Ed 2000;39(18):3169–3210.

83. Enjalbal C, Martinez J, Aubagnac JL. Mass spectrometry in combinatorial chemistry. Mass Spectrom Rev 2000;19(3):139–161.

84. Gauglitz G. Optical detection methods for combinatorial libraries. Curr Opin Chem Biol 2000;4(3):351–355.

85. Hewes JD. High throughput methodologies: a new paradigm for chemicals and materials research. Chim Oggi 2000;18(9):20–24.

86. Kopylov AM, Spiridonova VA. Combinatorial chemistry of nucleic acids: SELEX. Mol Biol 2000;34(6):940–954.

87. Nestler HP. Combinatorial libraries and molecular recognition: match or mismatch? Curr Org Chem 2000;4(4):397–410.

88. Porco JA Jr. Organic synthesis using chemical tags: the third leg of parallel synthesis. Comb Chem High Throughput Screening 2000;3(2):93–102.

17
New Synthetic Methodologies

Tasir S. Haque, Andrew P. Combs, and Lorin A. Thompson
Bristol-Myers Squibb Company
Wilmington, Delaware

The synthesis of libraries of diverse drug-like molecules is dependent on the avail-ability of reliable and general synthetic methods. This chapter is intended to give the reader an overview of the latest developments in solid-phase and solution-phase syntheses directed to constructing libraries of compounds for biological screening. The brevity of this review with respect to some of the more established synthetic methods is by no means meant to diminish their importance, but rather to maintain the focus of this chapter on the most recent synthetic methodology advances. The reader is encouraged to consult the extensive literature referenced at the end of the chapter for complete details of these new synthetic methods.

I. INTRODUCTION

The development of high-throughput screening (HTS) technology in the late 1980s and early 1990s and the dramatic increases in the number of biological targets available from the Human Genome Project has fueled the desire of pharma-ceutical companies for larger numbers of compounds to screen against these new biological targets. The solid-phase synthesis of benzodiazepines was first demon-strated in 1977 by Camps Diez and coworkers [1]. Around this same time, several other organic chemists, including Leznoff and Frechet, also synthesized small molecules on solid supports [2–4]. However, little general notice was taken of these accomplishments until the early 1990s when Ellman and Hobbs-Dewitt pub-lished their syntheses of benzodiazepines, and solid-phase synthesis was recog-nized as an ideal method for the construction of large compound libraries [5,6]. Multiple parallel synthetic techniques first described by Geysen (using multipin arrays [7]) and Houghten (using "tea-bag" methods [8]) and combinatorial synthesis by the split-and-mix method initially described by Furka et al. made possible the synthesis of vast numbers of diverse compounds for biological screening [9,10]. The rapid medicinal chemistry optimization of lead compounds discovered from these collections by analogous parallel synthesis methods promised to shorten the time required to advance these compounds to clinical trials. Although in 1992 it was clear that solid-phase synthesis methods could significantly enhance the drug discovery process, the lack of robust solid-phase synthetic methodologies severely limited its utility. The race was then begun to discover new synthetic methods, invent new robotics and instrumentation, develop computer-assisted library design and analysis software, and integrate these tools into the drug discovery process. The plethora of recent publications in combinatorial organic synthesis (COS) and the establishment of three new journals dedicated to combinatorial chemistry (*Journal of Combinatorial Chemistry, Molecular Diversity, Combinatorial Chemistry and High Throughput Screening*) demonstrates the commitment of the synthetic organic community to these endeavors [11–39].

A. Strategies for Combinatorial Library Syntheses

The efficient combinatorial synthesis of quality compound libraries can be reduced to a few basic principles: (1) Compound libraries must be amenable to HT synthesis. (2) Scope of chemistry must be sufficiently broad. (3) Building blocks must be readily available. (4) Library purities must be excellent (>85% on average). (5) Yield must be adequate (>25% on average). The ideal library synthesis thus consists of short chemical sequences composed of highly optimized synthetic reactions to ensure adequate yields and high purities of the library members. A variety of building blocks used in the synthesis would be available from commercial sources or one- to two-step syntheses, allowing for the rapid synthesis of large compound libraries.

Solid-phase synthesis is one of the most powerful methods for construction of large compound libraries. It is amenable to "split-and-pool" methods for extremely large (>10^4–10^7 member), single-compound-per-bead libraries, mixture libraries, or discrete compound syntheses. The ability to drive reactions to completion using excess reagents and simple removal of impurities from the crude reactions by washing the resin permits multistep synthesis of complex scaffolds in excellent purities and yields. Recent advances in solution-phase scavenging and solid-supported reagents are also proving to be effective in multistep synthesis of libraries. A comparison of the advantages and disadvantages of solid-phase versus solution-phase synthesis described by Coffin in a recent article by Baldino is provided in Table 1 [39] (please refer to the article for clarification of the "issues" discussed in the table). The obvious synergies of these two methods are apparent from the table. A proficient combinatorial chemistry lab is capable of utilizing either solution-phase or solid-phase HT methods, and the decision of which

Table 1   Advantages and Disadvantages of Solution-Phase vs. Solid-Phase Parallel
Synthesis[a]

Issues	Solution phase	Solid phase
1. Range of accessible reactions	++	−
2. Production of congeneric sets of compounds in SAR. ordered arrays	++	−
3. Use of in-process controls	+	−
4. Effort required to "combinatorialize" a synthetic reaction or scheme	+	−
5. Linker attachment sites	N.A.	−
6. Larger scale resynthesis of bioactive library members	++	−
7. Choice of solvents	+	−
8. Operating temperatures	+	−
9. Heterogeneous reagents	+	−
10. Scavenger resins	+	−
11. Cost of reagents and materials	+	−
12. Abundance of literature precedents	++	−
13. Location-based sample identification	++	−
14. Tagging-based sample identification	−	+
15. Capital investment required	−	+
16. Maintaining inert conditions	−	+
17. Mass-action reagent excess	−	++
18. Library transformations with no change in diversity	−	+
19. Protecting groups	−	+
20. Multistep synthesis	−	+
21. Use of bifunctional reagents	−	+
22. Access to split-and-pool amplification	−	++

[a]See original article for detailed discussion [39].

method to use is based on a variety of factors. These factors include the type of
chemistry to be performed, the size and scale of the library, and the intended use
of the library (i.e., lead discovery library versus lead optimization or structure–
activity relationship library).

II.   SOLID-PHASE SYNTHESIS METHODOLOGIES

Numerous advances in solid-phase synthesis methodologies have been published
in the literature in the past decade. In fact, most solution-phase synthetic transfor-

mations have now been performed in some form on solid supports. This section presents brief descriptions of many of the most recent solid-phase synthesis advances and attempts to explain the importance of these methods for the rapid synthesis of compound libraries. The reader can expect to gain from this section a good overview of the current state of the art and where the field of solid-phase synthesis is headed at the beginning of the 21st century.

A. Introduction to Polymer-Supported Synthesis

1. Pros and Cons of Synthesis on Support

The concept of polymer-supported synthesis was popularized by Bruce Merrifield with the publication in 1963 of his seminal paper describing the solid-phase synthesis of peptides [40]. In this work, Merrifield covalently attached an amino acid to an insoluble polymer bead made from polystyrene cross-linked with 1–2% divinylbenzene (Fig. 1). When placed in a reaction solution, the polystyrene beads swell and allow solvent to penetrate the bead, permitting a dissolved reagent access to the linked amino acid. Because the beads do not dissolve they can be isolated from the solution by simply filtering them on a fritted funnel. The power of this method is the trivial isolation of the polymer (and thus the polymer-bound compound) from a reaction solution by filtration after the addition of each new reagent. This method completely eliminates the need for isolation and purification of the intermediate products, each of which usually requires an aqueous extraction and chromatographic purification. This procedure is particularly useful in the synthesis of peptides, where the addition of each amino acid in solution requires two chemical steps (deprotection and coupling), as well as a separate time-consuming purification after the addition of each new amino acid (for more details, see Figure 15 and the section on peptide synthesis on solid support). Using the solid-phase procedure an entire peptide can be assembled while attached to the polymer bead, and only a single purification step at the end of the synthesis is necessary. Peptides of unprecedented length and purity were synthesized in a much shorter

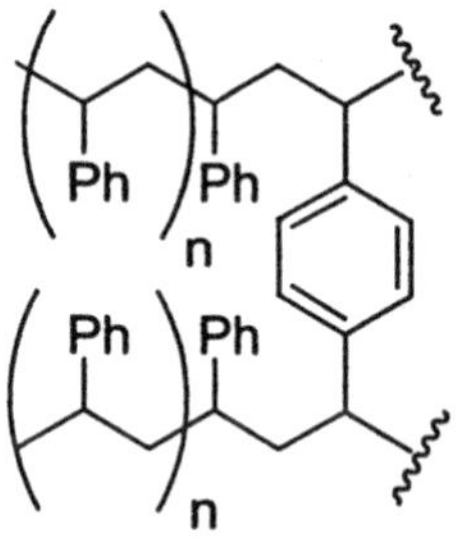

Figure 1 Structure of cross-linked polystyrene.

time using the Merrifield procedure than was previously possible using traditional solution-phase peptide synthesis methods. The success of polymer-bound peptide synthesis also resulted in the development of similar technology for the construction of other biopolymers, including oligonucleotides, which are now routinely constructed in a completely automated fashion.

The concept of polymer-supported synthesis for molecules other than peptides was investigated in the late 1960s and early 1970s by a number of investigators who helped to define the scope and limitations of polymer-bound synthesis of organic molecules [2,3]. There are a number of advantages to polymer-bound synthesis. As mentioned above, the main advantage of an insoluble polymer support is that the insoluble polymer may be isolated from a reaction solution by filtration, making conventional purification of the desired compound unnecessary. This simplified purification procedure allows the use of a large excess of reagents to drive a reaction to completion while minimizing the time needed to purify and isolate the desired product from the complex reaction solution.

Linkage of a molecule to a polymer support also facilitates encoding; an identifying tag of some kind can be linked to the polymer bead containing a particular molecule. Systems have been developed to allow screening of millions of compounds followed by identification of active structures by decoding tags attached to the polymer bead during the synthesis of the particular compound [41].

Although solid-phase organic synthesis (SPOS) remains one of the most powerful techniques for parallel synthesis, it has drawbacks. Disadvantages of this method may include diminished reaction rates for certain reactions, formation of support-bound impurities that are released along with the desired molecule during cleavage, and the necessity of developing a method for linkage of the desired compound to the support. The analysis of resin-bound intermediates can also be complicated, and additional time is often required to develop robust and versatile chemistry for multistep syntheses on solid support. A variety of tools have been developed or adapted to aid in the analysis of compounds on a solid support, including solid-state nuclear magnetic resonance (NMR), Fourier transform infrared (IR) and mass spectroscopies, as a number of color tests for the presence or absence of certain functional groups [42–46]. New technologies have been designed to try to retain the benefits of solid-phase chemistry while minimizing the drawbacks (see section on solution-phase polymer-supported synthesis).

B. Synthetic Transformations on Solid Supports

1. Carbon–Heteroatom Coupling Reactions on Solid Supports

Carbon–heteroatom coupling reactions are the most widely used synthetic transformations for the construction of compound libraries. *N*-Acylation, *N*-alkylation, *N*-arylation, *O*-acylation, *O*-alkylation, and *O*-arylation are just a few examples of these ubiquitous reactions performed on solid supports (Scheme 1). Nearly all

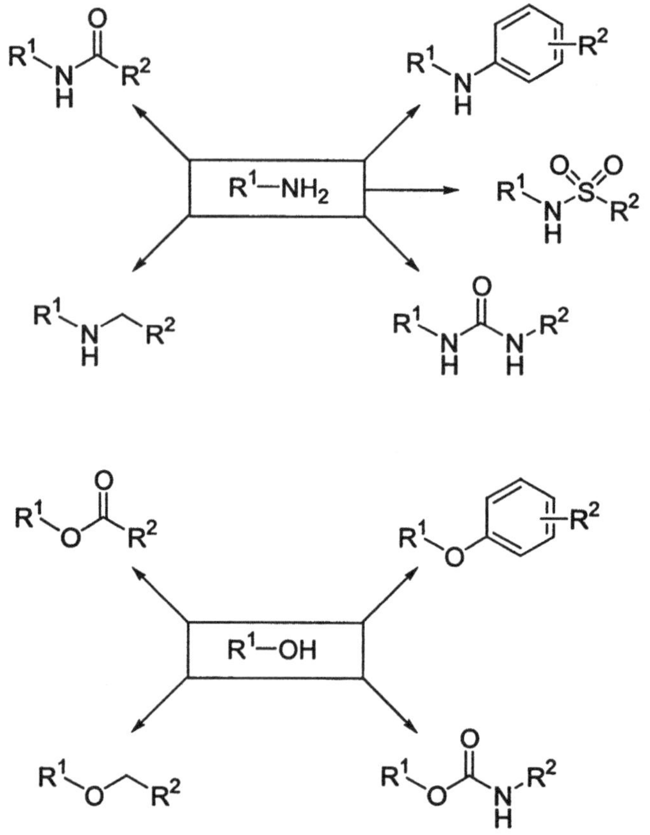

Scheme 1

reported multistep solid-phase syntheses incorporate one or more of these reactions. In general, these reactions tend to be easily optimized, occur at or near room temperature, and are not particularly sensitive to air or moisture. These mild reaction conditions simplify tremendously the automation of the library synthesis since reagents and reactions do not need to be cooled, heated, or kept under an inert atmosphere. Recent engineering advances in instrument design do permit the HT synthesis of compound libraries under these more demanding conditions. Thousands of the reagents used in these syntheses are available from commercial sources. Diverse or focused sets of reagents can therefore be readily purchased for incorporation into diversity-oriented or target-directed compound libraries.

a. N-Acylation, N-Alkylation, and N-Arylation. Many synthetic methods for the derivatization of resin-bound amines have been optimized for the construction of diverse compound libraries. The ease of amine incorporation and subsequent derivatization, along with the large and diverse set of amine building blocks that are commercially available, has driven the exploitation of this functionality. A wide variety of resin-bound amines are thus readily available, since they can be incorporated onto the support in high yields and purities via standard amino acid chemistry, reductive amination of aldehyde-functionalized resins, or amine displacement of resin-bound halides, to name just a few synthetic methods (Fig. 2).

Derivatization of resin-bound amines can be accomplished by many different synthetic transformations, thus allowing the generation of diverse product libraries. Several examples are given in Scheme 1. *N*-Acylation is a particularly useful diversity forming reaction, since thousands of building blocks (acids, acid chlorides, sulfonyl chlorides, isocyanates, chloroformates, carbamoyl chlorides, and more) are commercially available and each can be performed in high yield (Scheme 1). *N*-Alkylation of resin-bound amines is another useful reaction sequence, since it affords basic secondary or tertiary amine products with dramatically different chemical and physical properties. The aldehyde, alkyl halide, or alcohol building blocks necessary for the synthesis of these *N*-alkylamine compounds (via reductive amination or *N*-alkylation respectively) are also readily available, allowing large, diverse libraries of these compounds to be synthesized. A general method for the *N*-arylation of resin-bound amines is a relatively new addition to the optimized solid-phase reactions [47–50]. A complete description of

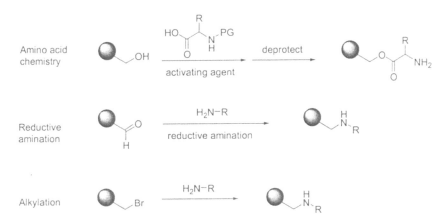

Figure 2 Examples of resin-bound amines.

these transformations can be found in the section on transition metal–mediated coupling reactions.

    b. O-Acylation, O-Alkylation, and O-Arylation. The carbon–oxygen bond is a ubiquitous motif found many drugs. Therefore, solid-phase synthetic methods for carbon–oxygen bond formation (*O*-acylation, *O*-alkylation, and *O*-arylation) have been utilized many times in compound library synthesis (Scheme 1). The robust nature of this chemistry with respect to the ease of synthesis and variety of building blocks that undergo efficient chemical reaction make these methods very attractive for diverse compound library construction. While the resultant esters can be somewhat unstable to proteases under physiological conditions, the ether and carbamate linkages are typically stable.

    The hydroxyl functional group also offers a handle for linking a scaffold to a suitable polymer support. This technique has been a useful synthetic strategy for those libraries where a free hydroxyl group is desired in all members of the library. The solid-phase synthesis of hydroxyethylamine aspartyl protease inhibitor libraries and prostaglandin libraries are excellent examples of this strategy (Fig. 3) [51–53]. The hydroxyl group is an integral part of the aspartyl protease inhibitor

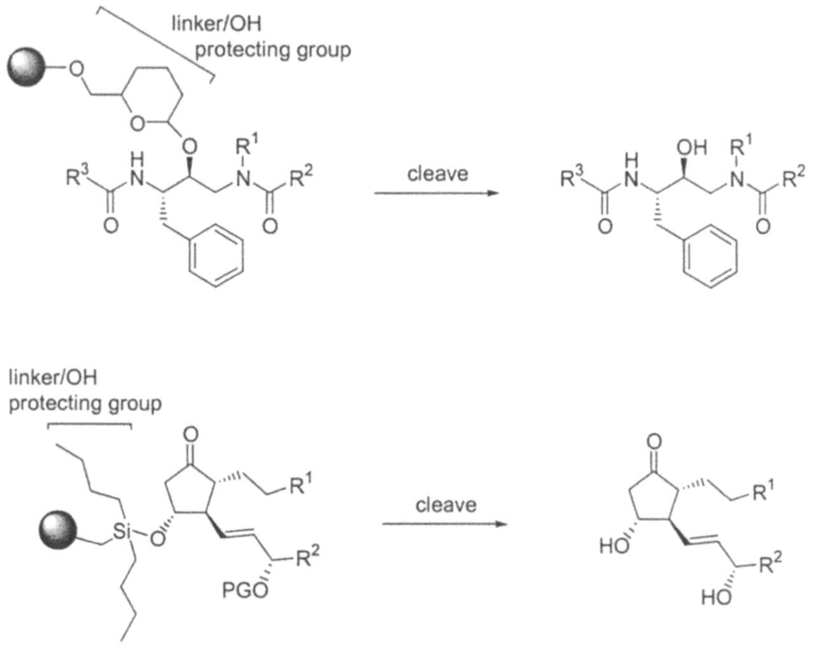

Figure 3 Use of support/linker as hydroxyl protecting group in synthesis of hydroxyethylamines (*top*) and prostoglandins (*bottom*).

and prostaglandin pharmacophores. The linkage at the conserved hydroxyl group not only binds the core to the resin for subsequent derivatization but also protects the hydroxyl from undesired reactions during the library synthesis. The free hydroxyl group is only revealed upon cleavage of the final products from the solid support.

2. Carbon–Carbon Bond–Forming Reactions on Solid Supports

The biopolymer syntheses described in a following section involve the formation of a carbon–heteroatom bond (an amide bond for peptides, a glycosidic ether linkage for oligosaccharides, and a phosphate ester bond for oligonucleotides). While the ability to form these bonds is crucial to the synthesis of biopolymers, an expanded set of reactions is required to allow chemists to access more complex organic structures. A key tool for synthetic organic chemists is the ability to synthesize carbon–carbon (C—C) bonds. There are numerous methods available for the generation of C—C bonds in normal solution chemistry (which in most cases translate well to soluble polymer chemistry). However, these methods must often be modified for reactions in the presence of a solid support, where factors such as polymer solubility (or "swelling" ability), reagent solubility, and compatibility of any linker or previously existing functionality must be taken into consideration. Extensive effort has gone into developing conditions for a variety of C—C bond–forming reactions on solid supports, a number of which are now available to the chemist for use in the parallel synthesis of small organic molecules [54]. Several examples of these reactions are shown below. Numerous other C—C bond–forming reactions have been described, including metal-mediated coupling reactions (such as Stille, Suzuki, and Heck reactions) [27] and multiple-component condensations (Passerini, Ugi, and Biginelli reactions, for example) [55]. Many of these other reactions are described briefly elsewhere in this chapter, and in-depth discussions can be found in several recent reviews of solid-phase synthesis [14,17,26,27,29,54,56].

The Grignard reaction involves the attack of a carbon nucleophile (for Grignard reactions, a carbon-magnesium halide salt) on an electrophilic carbon such as an imine, Weinreb amide, or ketone, as shown in the examples in Figure 4 [57]. While the examples above show classical magnesium bromide Grignard salts acting as nucleophiles, similar reactions have been demonstrated on support using organolithium and organocuprate reagents. (Cuprates are traditionally used to introduce a carbon nucleophile to an α,β-unsaturated carbonyl group at the β position of the double bond.) When performing reactions with strong nucleophiles/bases such as Grignard reagents, consideration must be given to factors such as the other functional groups present on support, whether the linker can withstand reaction conditions involving strong nucleophiles, and so on. There exist in the literature numerous examples of Grignard reagents being successfully applied in a library format to a support-bound reactant.

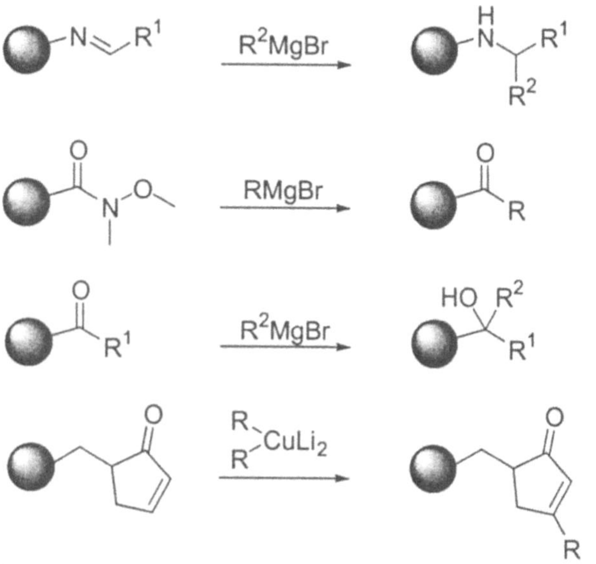

Figure 4 C—C bond formation on solid support: carbon nucleophiles (Grignard and cuprate additions).

The Wittig and Horner–Emmons reactions (Fig. 5) are often used to install C—C double bonds into a target molecule and have been readily applied to support-bound synthesis. The Baylis–Hillman reaction (Fig. 5) involves the coupling of an aldehyde to an electron-poor alkene. Unlike most other C—C bond–forming reactions, it does not require an inert atmosphere and can usually be conducted at room temperature. These mild reaction conditions make the Baylis–Hillman reaction well suited for combinatorial and parallel synthetic applications [58]. In an enolate alkylation, the enolate is generated by reaction of a carbonyl-containing compound with a strong base (shown in Fig. 5). The enolate is then reacted with an electrophile, resulting in formation of the C—C bond. There have been various reports of enolates being generated and alkylated on support to install a C—C bond adjacent to a carbonyl group. Chiral auxiliaries have been attached to support adjacent to the reacting center to influence the stereochemistry of the chiral center that is formed, with diastereoselectivites that were found to be comparable to those obtained via the analogous solution-phase reaction.

3. Transition Metal–Mediated Coupling Reactions

Transition metal–mediated coupling reactions have been utilized extensively in solid-phase syntheses [27]. Palladium-mediated Heck, Suzuki, and Stille reactions

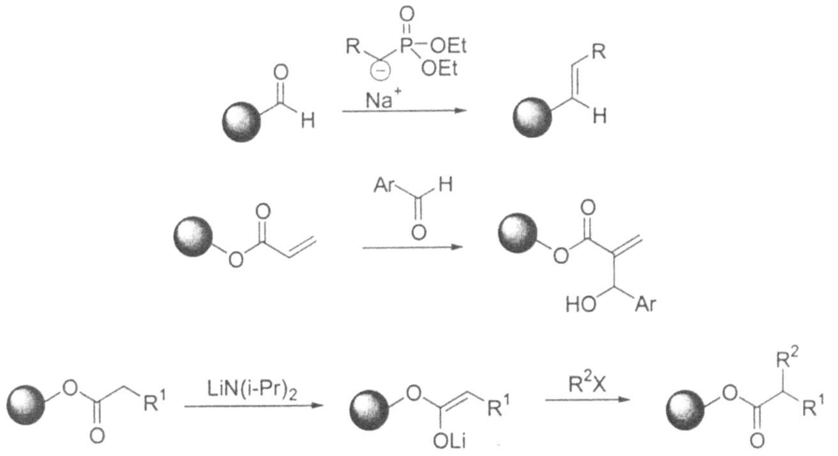

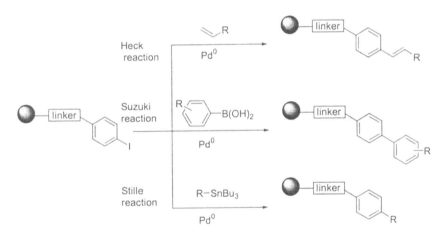

Figure 5 C—C bond formation on solid support: Horner–Emmons reaction (*top*), Baylis–Hillman reaction (*middle*), and enolate formation and reaction (*bottom*).

Figure 6 Support-bound Heck, Suzuki, and Stille reactions.

are particularly useful for diversifying compound libraries due to their generality and efficiency of coupling (Fig. 6). These biaryl- and arylalkene-forming reactions have been effected in high yield with either the metallated arene/alkene or the arylhalide bound to the solid support.

The recently developed transition metal–mediated olefin metathesis has been utilized in a number of solid-phase syntheses for the construction of rings of

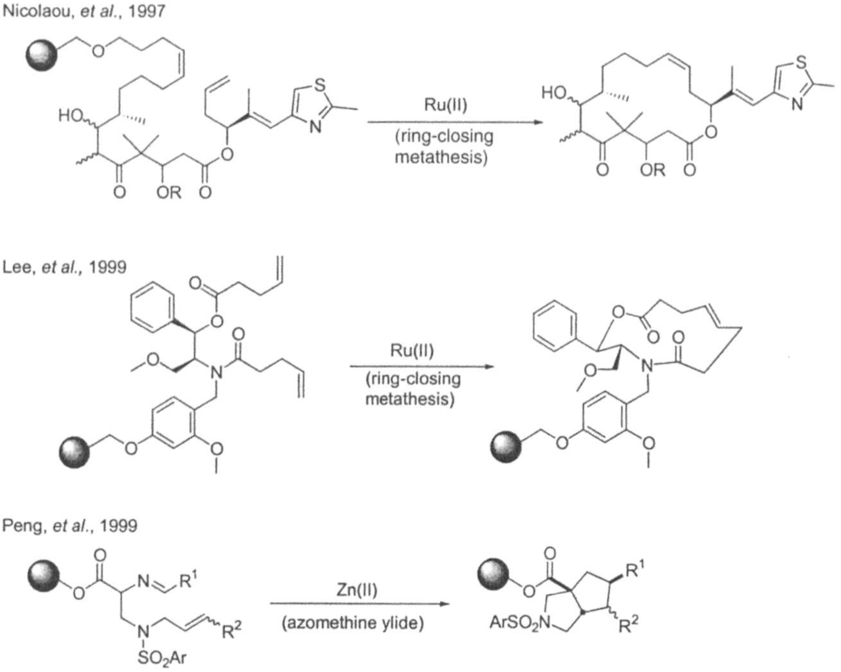

Nicolaou, *et al.*, 1997

Lee, *et al.*, 1999

Peng, *et al.*, 1999

Figure 7 Three examples of transition metal–catalyzed ring closing reactions on solid support.

various sizes, including several examples of macrocycles that would be inaccessible by other solid-phase synthetic methods (Fig. 7) [59–61]. The generality of the method has made olefin metathesis a useful tool for the synthesis of various macrocycles. The resulting cyclic scaffolds are preferred over their linear counterparts since they often bind more tightly to proteins, due in part to their reduced entropy of binding. Medicinal chemists also glean additional structural information from leads discovered from these compound libraries, since their mode of binding can be predicted with greater precision due to decreased conformational flexibility of the molecules.

Recent advances in palladium-mediated and copper-mediated *N*-arylation reactions have been demonstrated on solid supports (Fig. 8) [47–50]. These new synthetic methods are particularly useful due to the omnipresent nature of the *N*-aryl bond in biologically active compounds. *N*-Arylation of support-bound amines by copper-acetate-mediated coupling of boronic acids afford *N*-arylated amines, while suitably substituted arylhalides on solid supports can be *N*-arylated with a variety of primary and secondary amines using palladium catalysis. These com-

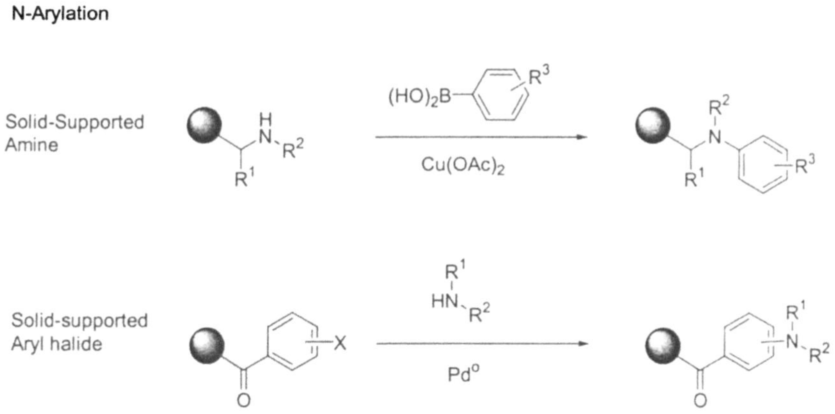

N-Arylation

Figure 8 Two examples of N-arylation chemistry on a solid support.

plementary reactions provide new synthetic avenues for the generation of diverse structures not previously available to the combinatorial chemist.

4. Intramolecular Cyclization–Resin–Cleavage Strategies

When conducting syntheses on a support, whether that support is a soluble polymer or an insoluble ("solid") phase, it is desirable to minimize the number of reaction steps required to obtain the final products. The time and material saved in such combinations of steps (e.g., by not having to wash a library on solid support between reactions) is often worth the price of a small decrease in yield or purity. The two steps of cyclization to form a ring and cleavage of product from support have been combined in a number of reaction sequences. In the situation where cyclization directly results in cleavage from support, product purity is excellent. Typically, only the desired completed sequence is capable of cleavage, whereas any incomplete sequences remain on the support. When the cyclization and cleavage reactions occur sequentially (such as in the cyclopentapiperidinone case shown below, where acidic cleavage and cyclization are not necessarily simultaneous), and the cyclization does not proceed to 100% completion, both the cyclized and uncyclized material are released into solution. Both cyclization to release product and "one-pot" cleavage followed by cyclization of product have been successfully applied to a number of small-molecule syntheses on polymeric support, as shown in Figures 9 and 10.

Three examples of syntheses where cleavage from support occurs as a direct result of cyclization (such that only the desired cyclized material is isolated) are shown in Figure 9 [62,63]. In all three cases, *only* the cyclized product is obtained in high purity, though varying yields, after the cyclization/cleavage step. All impu-

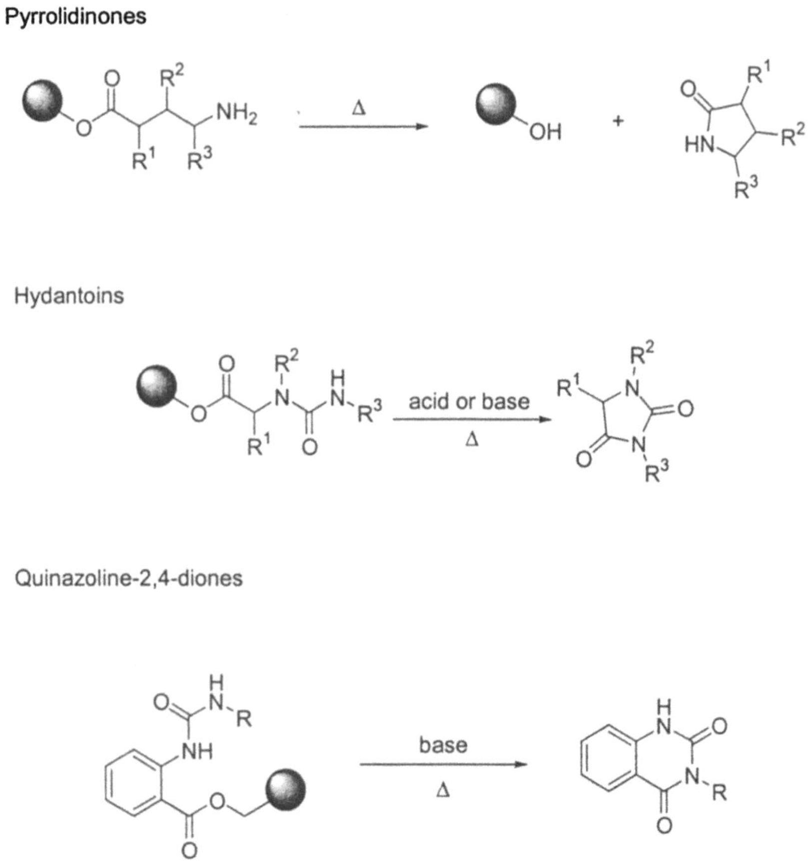
Pyrrolidinones
O
R2
NH2
R1
R3
Δ
OH
+
R1
R2
HN
R3
Hydantoins
acid or base
Δ
Quinazoline-2,4-diones
base
Δ

Figure 9 Three examples of simultaneous cyclization and cleavage reactions.

rities either are washed from the resin prior to the final step or remain attached to the solid phase.

Two examples where cleavage and cyclization are not necessarily linked events are shown in Figure 10. The reaction conditions result in cleavage of material from support, whether or not cyclization occurs. In the dihydrobenzodiazepine-2-one case, the product ester is generated after reaction with sodium methoxide at the terminal carboxylic acid/ester, while cyclization takes place via amine attack at the unsaturated carbon adjacent to the amide [64]. In the cyclopentapiperidinone case, trifluoroacetic acid (TFA) cleaves the free amine from the resin, then subsequently catalyzes the observed cyclization [65]. In these two cases, if cyclization could not occur, the molecules are still cleaved from support

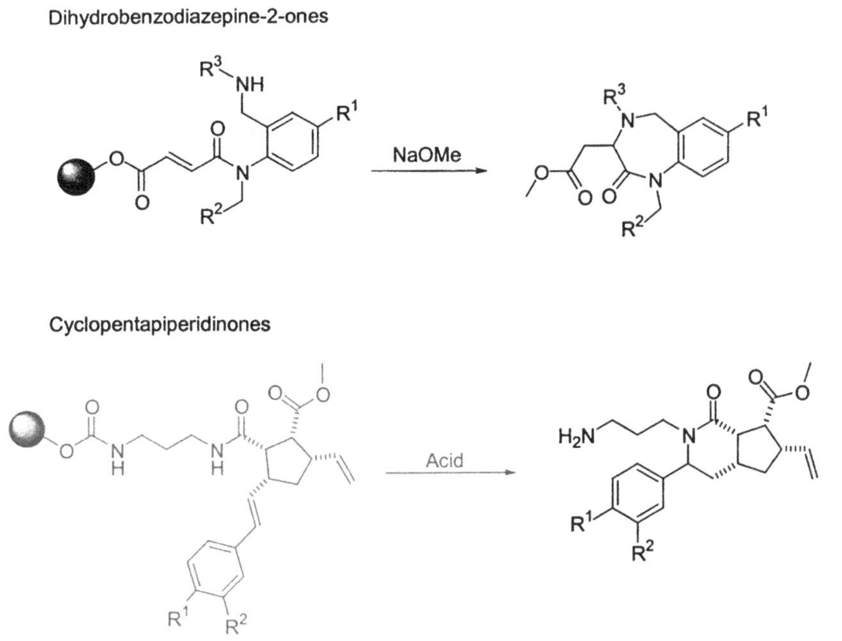

Dihydrobenzodiazepine-2-ones

Cyclopentapiperidinones

Figure 10 Two examples of cleavage from support, followed by nonsimultaneous cyclization.

and hence an additional impurity (the uncyclized material) may be present in the final product.

5. Cycloadditions

Carbocyclic and heterocyclic cores are frequently used to display pharmaceutically interesting functional groups. The cyclic core allows for the specific orientation of functional group side chains, often resulting in improved binding affinity or specificity versus more flexible linear cores. One method for obtaining cyclic and heterocyclic cores that has been exploited to a great extent in parallel and combinatorial synthesis is the cycloaddition reaction. Cycloadditions are very attractive to the chemist synthesizing a compound library, since in one step multiple bonds can be formed, introducing a carbocycle or heterocycle while concurrently installing one or more side chains in specific positions on the cyclic core. Strategies have also been developed whereby cyclization to provide the desired molecule and cleavage from solid support occur simultaneously (see previous section on intramolecular cyclization/cleavage strategies). A number of different support-bound cycloadditions have been reported, usually resulting in formation of four-, five-, and six-membered rings with varying displays of side chains around the cores [17,29,36,54,66]. Several examples of cycloadditions on solid support are shown in Figure 11.

6. Multiple-Component Reactions on Solid Supports

Multiple-component (MC) reactions simultaneously condense three or more components to generate new complex molecules in a single synthetic transformation (Fig. 12). Relatively few such synthetic transformations are known when compared with bimolecular reactions. Even so, these unique reactions are particularly desirable for generating libraries of complex molecules since only a single step need be optimized and performed to bring together as many as five different components. These solid-phase syntheses thus require substantially less time to optimize reaction conditions and are easier to perform in an HT manner for large-compound-library construction. Many of these reactions are also tolerant of a variety of functionalities on the individual components and thus allow the combinatorial chemist to synthesize structurally diverse compound libraries. Although MC reactions offer substantial efficiencies in the time and effort required to construct single-compound-per-well libraries, they do not allow for "split-and-pool" synthesis strategies due to the inherent nature of the MC condensation process.

The first MC reaction to be performed both in solution and on a solid support was a three-component Passerini reaction, affording a library of azinomycin analogs (Fig. 13) [21,55,67–69]. A variety of MC reactions have since been effected where one of the components is bound to the solid support, including the Ugi reaction, Mannich reaction, Biginelli reaction, Grieco three-component reaction, and a thiazolidinone synthesis, to name a few [55,70]. Recent advances in the use of MC reactions have focused on the subsequent synthetic manipulation of the generic MC scaffold to reduce the peptide-like nature of the products. The solid-phase or solution-phase synthesis of lactams [71], pyrroles [72], imidazoles [73,74], imidazolines [75], and ketopiperazines [76] from Ugi products are a few examples of such MC reactions and subsequent synthetic elaboration to afford libraries of heterocycles (Fig. 14).

C. Resin-to-Resin Transfer Reactions

A synthetic method that would enable a chemist to synthesize a novel reagent on one resin and subsequently transfer it to another derivatized resin (i.e., resin-to-resin transfer) would be a useful tool for the convergent construction of diverse compound libraries. A recent report by Scialdone et al. demonstrates such a transformation, where an isocyanate was generated from one resin, then diffused into

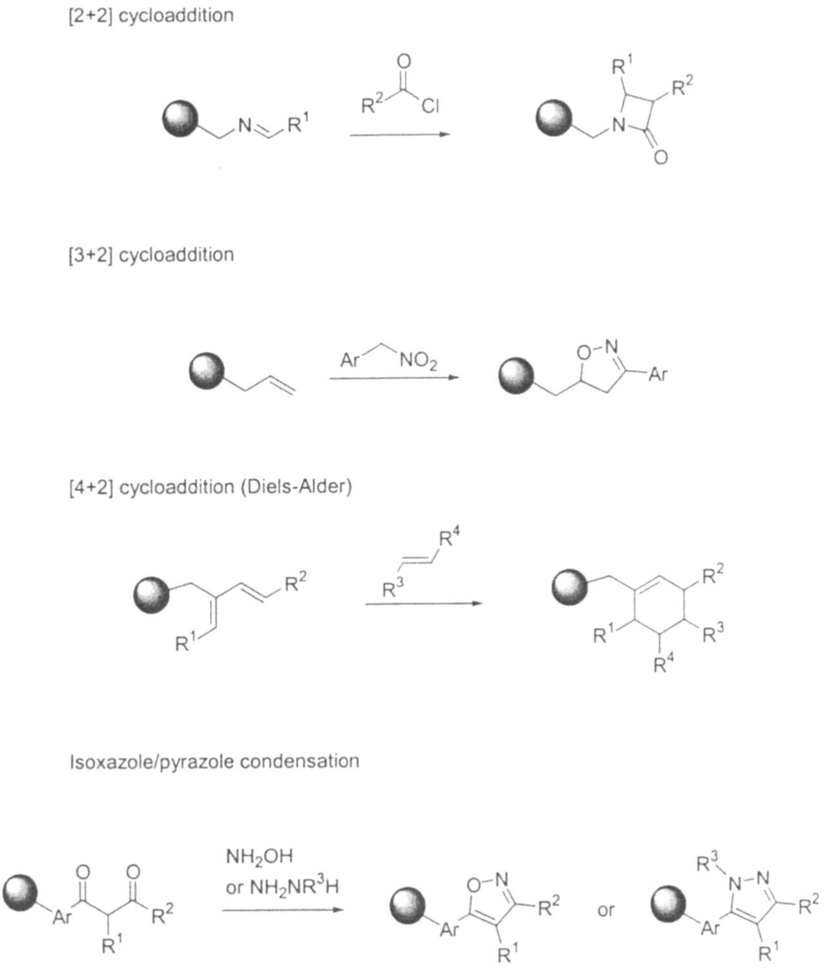

[2+2] cycloaddition

[3+2] cycloaddition

[4+2] cycloaddition (Diels-Alder)

Isoxazole/pyrazole condensation

Figure 11 C—C bond formation: cycloaddition and heterocyclic condensation reactions.

and reacted with another appropriately functionalized resin to generate novel ureas (Scheme 2) [77].

Another example of resin-to-resin transfer, used in a Suzuki reaction, has been reported. In this case, the support-bound boronic ester is released from one resin via mild hydrolysis and reacted with a resin-bound aryl iodide to yield the biaryl product on support (Scheme 3) [78]. The ability to synthesize increasingly complex building blocks by solid-phase methods and subsequently utilize them as

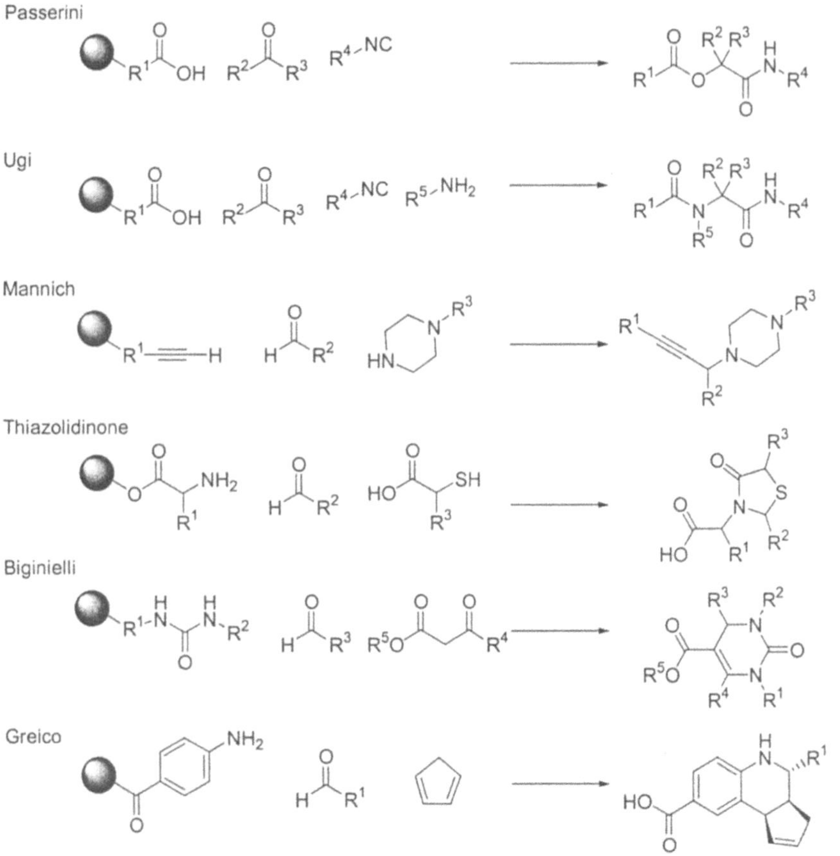

Figure 12 Representative multiple-component reactions performed on solid supports.

building blocks for a new solid-phase synthesis is an important step toward the construction of structurally complex compound libraries.

III. COMPLEX MULTISTEP SYNTHESIS ON SOLID SUPPORTS

A. Oligiomers—Natural and Unnatural

Many of the synthetic techniques used for the synthesis of libraries of small organic molecules were originally developed for the chemical synthesis of biopolymers. Extensive research has gone into the required activating protocols and the wide array of protecting groups needed to synthesize large (20–100 steps)

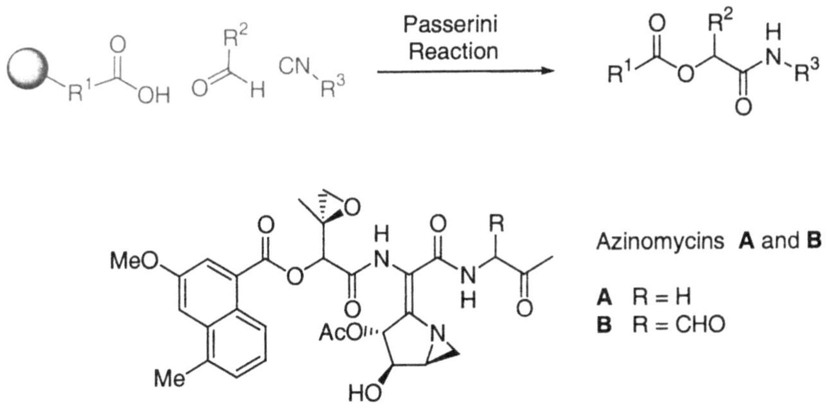

Figure 13 Passerini's three-component condensation to afford azinomycin library.

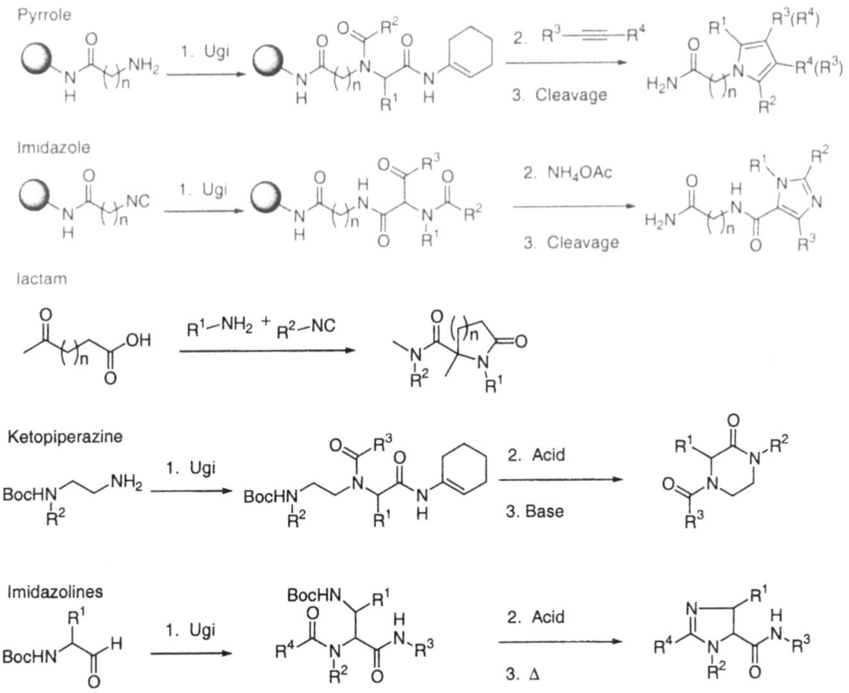

Figure 14 Examples of multiple-component reactions for both solid-phase and solution-phase synthesis of heterocycles.

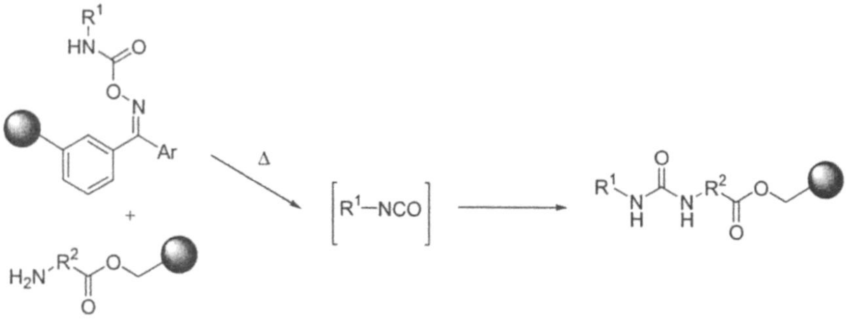

Scheme 2

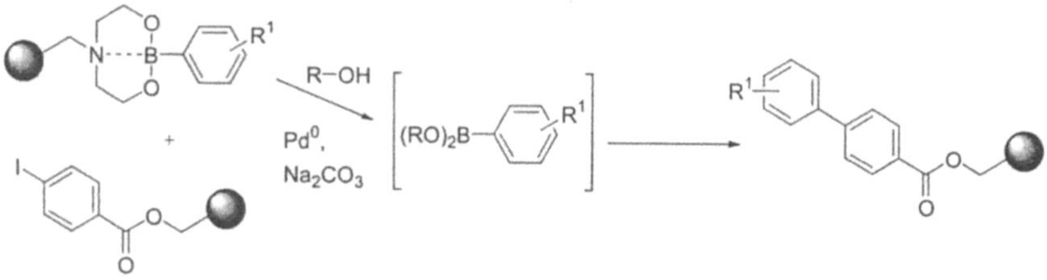

Scheme 3

biopolymers in high yields and purities. The three major classes of biopolymers, peptides, oligosaccharides, and oligonucleotides, have all been chemically synthesized on support, and each of these classes is discussed below.

1. Peptide Synthesis on Solid Support

The chemical synthesis of peptides was performed by Merrifield in 1963 and represents the original application of solid-phase synthesis of organic molecules [79]. Whereas very large peptides and proteins are often synthesized by biochemical methods (e.g., overexpression in *Escherichia coli.* [80]), synthesis on solid support is frequently used when peptides (typically lower than 50 amino acids) or peptides containing unnatural amino acids are desired (Fig. 15). (Peptides containing unnatural amino acids can be expressed using Schultz's modified tRNA technique [81]. However, for short peptides or in cases where a significant amount of peptide is desired, chemical synthesis is still preferred.) While there have been a number of different routes developed for support-bound peptide synthesis, two techniques are used most frequently. One of these is the 9-fluorenylmethoxycarbonyl (Fmoc)–based approach, using amino acids that are protected at the back-

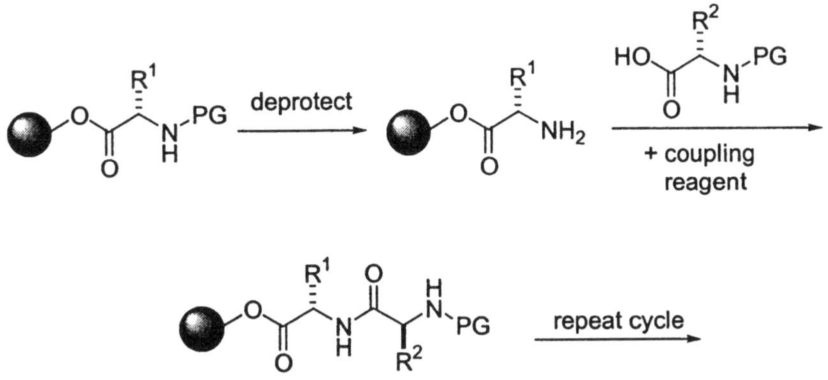

Figure 15 Solid-phase peptide synthesis. Side chains are represented by R groups, and PG indicates a protecting group.

bone nitrogen with the base-labile Fmoc group and at side-chain functional groups with acid-labile protecting groups. In the Fmoc–amino acid approach, side chain nitrogens are protected using *t*-butyloxycarbonyl (t-Boc) groups. Amino acids are coupled to the amino terminus of the growing peptide on solid support via use of an activating agent to boost the reactivity of the reacting carboxylate [82,83]. After each coupling step, the amino terminus is prepared for the next reaction by removal of the Fmoc protecting group. When completed, the peptide is removed from support by a strong acid cleavage step, which simultaneously removes all of the acid-labile side-chain protecting groups, resulting in the desired peptide. Coupling conditions and reagents have been refined to provide high efficiency while minimizing racemization of the amino acid stereocenters.

Peptide libraries numbering in excess of 1 million compounds have been generated using standard Fmoc-based chemistry in a split-and-mix library synthesis format. For example, a 6.25 million member mixture-based library of tetrapeptides synthesized using Fmoc-based chemistry was used to identify several 0.4- to 2.0-nM agonists of the mu opioid receptor [84]. Synthesis of peptides on solid support via the Fmoc-based strategy is easily automated, and a variety of peptide synthesizers that apply this chemistry have been developed. Many of the concepts and reagents that have been applied to Fmoc–amino acid peptide synthesis are used in combinatorial organic small-molecule synthesis as well, including various resins and linkers, coupling reagents, and protecting groups. In particular, a wide variety of the coupling reagents used to make amide and ester linkages in peptides have found extensive application in the generation of small-molecule libraries.

The second frequently applied support-bound peptide synthesis strategy is the *t*-butoxycarbonyl (t-Boc)–protected amino acid approach, where the acid-labile t-Boc-protecting group protects peptide backbone amines during coupling [85]. In this approach, side chains are protected using benzyl groups. These protecting groups are stable to the mildly acidic conditions used during deprotection of the peptide terminus. The support-bound t-Boc-protected amino terminus is deprotected by exposure to acid (typically trifluoroacetic acid in dichloromethane), and the next residue is added to the peptide via use of an activating agent, as described above. The completed peptide is cleaved from support by a very strong acid, usually hydrofluoric acid (HF) or trifluoromethane sulfonic acid (TFMSA). A variation of the t-Boc–amino acid strategy is widely applied for solution-phase synthesis of small peptides (i.e., free of polymeric support). The t-Boc–amino acid peptide synthesis technique is often used in industrial settings. However, it is applied less frequently than the Fmoc–amino acid strategy in academic or research settings. This most likely is due to the special equipment and extraordinary care that must be used with the t-Boc–amino acid strategy as a result of the extremely harsh cleavage conditions required to cleave the finished peptide.

2. Oligonucleotide Synthesis on Solid Support

The synthesis of oligonucleotides on a solid support has been developed to such an extent that it is now readily automated; the synthetic steps are typically high yielding, and extremely long oligonucleotides can be synthesized. The protection and reactivity of only four different nucleotides had been considered in the optimization of DNA synthesis [86]. Molecular biology techniques, such as polymerase chain reaction (PCR), have increased the need for chemically synthesized oligonucleotides (e.g., to act as primer sequences in PCR). The demand for methods to chemically synthesize oligonucleotides is especially strong when synthetic, or "unnatural," nucleotides are to be incorporated, when milligram quantities of a oligonucleotide are needed, or when a library of relatively short oligonucleotides (less than 30 nucleotides) is desired. The technique most commonly used for oligonucleotide synthesis on support is the phosphoramidite coupling method, a general outline of which is shown in Figure 16. In this technique a nucleotide is coupled to the free hydroxyl of a support-bound nucleotide, forming a phosphite triester. The phosphite is then oxidized to a phosphate triester, the protecting group (PG^2) is removed from the primary hydroxyl of the terminal nucleotide, and the coupling process is repeated. This method has been successfully applied in automated oligonucleotide synthesizers due to the high yields and purity of products typically observed for each step of the sequence.

3. Oligosaccharide Synthesis on Solid Support

Oligosaccharides remain one of the last biopolymers to succumb to automated solid-phase or solution-phase chemical synthesis. They present a special challenge to chemical synthesis, either on support or in solution, due to both the number of

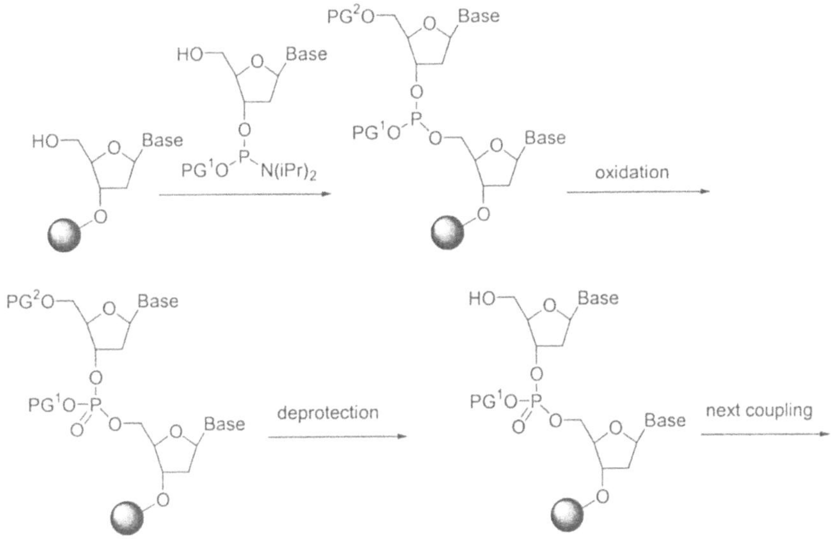

Figure 16 Support-bound oligonucleotide synthesis. PG^1 and PG^2 indicate two different protecting groups.

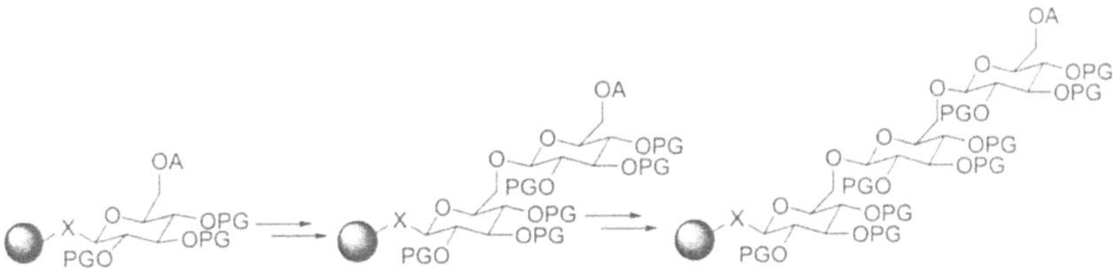

Figure 17 Representation of oligosaccharide synthesis using a support-bound glycosyl acceptor. PG indicates protecting groups, and OA indicates the glycosyl acceptor in the elongation reaction.

hydroxyl groups of similar reactivity that must be protected and the selective deprotection of a specific hydroxyl group that is required for glycosidic bond formation (Fig. 17). Added to these issues is the requirement that glycosidic bond formation proceed in a stereospecific manner, ideally with accessibility to either stereoisomer. The synthetically demanding requirements of obtaining regiospecific and stereospecific bond formation at each coupling step balances the advantages of support-bound synthesis (ease of purification of intermediates, ability to drive reactions to completion using excess reagents). While the oligosaccharide area of biopolymer synthesis is not as fully developed as the areas of peptides or oligonucleotides, many significant advances have been made in recent years [87–89].

The parallel synthesis of oligosaccharides has been accomplished using both soluble and insoluble polymers. Glycoside elongation has been accomplished by either chemical or enzymatic bond formation. Glycopeptides have also been synthesized on support, where the peptide is elongated after glycosylation; then the saccharide is attached to a peptide side chain and elongated, or, alternatively, the completed oligosaccharide is attached to the completed support-bound peptide [88,90,91]. Glycopeptides fall into two classes; *O*-linked glycopeptides and *N*-linked glycopeptides (examples of which are shown in Fig. 18).

Oligosaccharides have been synthesized on polymeric support using two approaches: either the glycosyl donor is on support and the acceptor is in solution, or the glycosyl acceptor is on support and the donor is in solution. An example of a support-bound glycosyl donor strategy applied to the synthesis of a β-linked oligosaccharide is shown in Figure 19 [92].

The advances in techniques for the chemical synthesis of the three major classes of biopolymers discussed above have allowed scientists to explore hybrids of the biopolymers. As mentioned above, glycopeptides have been synthesized on a solid phase, with the oligosaccharide segment being elongated after coupling to a support-bound peptide. A related approach, where the completed oligosaccharide is coupled to the support-bound peptide, has also been reported. Likewise, peptide-DNA hybrids, or peptide nucleic acids (PNAs), have been synthesized [93,94]. In a PNA, the phosphate-sugar backbone of the oligonucleotide has been replaced by a peptide amide backbone (Fig. 20). PNAs have received considerable attention as potential antisense and antigene drugs, as well as tools for probing DNA structure and helix stability [95,96].

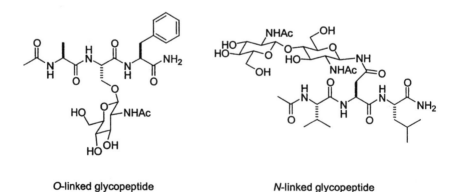

           O-linked glycopeptide   *N*-linked glycopeptide

Figure 18   Examples of *O*-linked and *N*-linked glycopeptides.

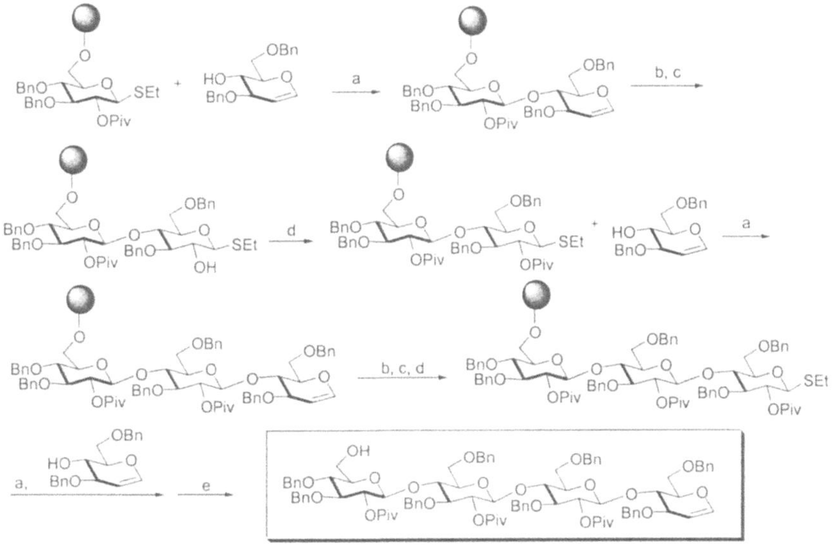

a) Methyl triflate, 2,6-di-tertbutylpyridine, 4Å sieves, CH_2CL_2, 0 °C to rt, 8 h. b) Dimethyldioxirane, CH_2Cl_2, 0 °C. c) 1:1 ethanedithiol and CH_2Cl_2, trace of trifluoracetic acid. d) Pivaloyl chloride, 4-dimethylaminopyridine, CH_2Cl_2. e) Tert-butylammonium fluoride/acetic acid (2:1), THF, 40 °C, 18h.

Figure 19 Tetrasaccharide synthesis using a support-bound glycosyl donor, as described by Zhang et al. Bn indicates a benzyl protecting group, and Piv indicates a pivaloyl protecting group.

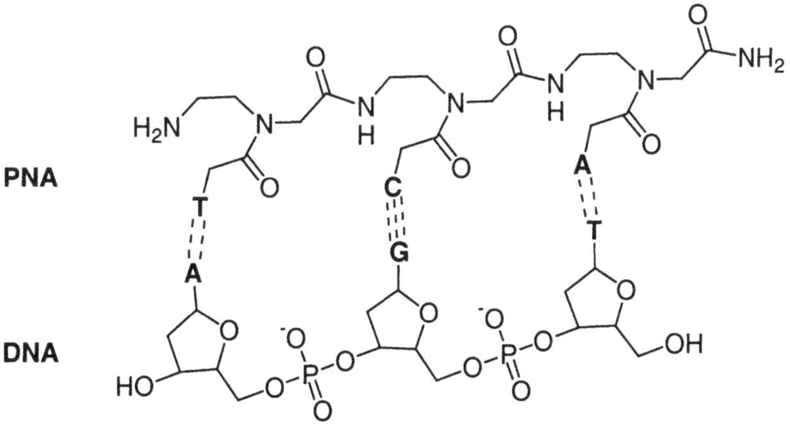

Figure 20 Base pairing of a segment of a DNA molecule with a PNA molecule, where C, G, A, and T represent the corresponding nucleic acids.

4. Unnatural Oligomers

The proper orientation of pharmacologically important side chains around a central core is fundamental to medicinal chemistry. Nature accomplishes this orientation in peptides and proteins by displaying amino acid side chains around the peptide backbone. Libraries of peptides are often used to identify the proper side chains and orientation for binding to a receptor or enzyme active site. However, peptides (amino acid oligomers) have significant pharmacological drawbacks that typically make them unsuitable as orally bioavailable drugs. A number of unnatural oligomers have been reported in recent years, many of which have been synthesized on a solid-phase or soluble polymer support. In their attempts to mimic the display of side chains by a normal peptide backbone, chemists have developed these various oligomers, while endeavoring to overcome some of the liabilities of peptides (i.e., susceptibility to proteolysis, poor bioavailability, etc.). Several examples of unnatural oligomers are shown in Figure 21, along with a natural peptide backbone for comparison [97–105]. This figure is not meant to represent an inclusive set, as several other unnatural oligomers (e.g., the peptide nucleic acids mentioned in the previous section) have also been synthesized.

B. Heterocycle/Pharmacophore Synthesis

As the number of different chemical transformations available to chemists has expanded, the complexity of molecules that may be synthesized in parallel has likewise increased. Chemists have taken advantage of the new tools available to them to synthesize molecules of significant complexity. Several interesting examples of solid-phase small-molecule synthesis are shown in Figures 22–27.

Relatively early yet significant examples of small molecule combinatorial synthesis are the 1,4-benzodiazepine libraries, synthesized on a solid phase in the early 1990s [5,106,107]. Benzodiazepines are known to have a wide range of biological activities. The 1,4-benzodiazepine scaffold represents a versatile pharmacophore (or core structure), off of which multiple diverse elements may be displayed. The synthesis shown in Figure 22 allows for the incorporation of four diverse elements (represented as R^1-R^4) around the central benzodiazepine core. Another example of the synthesis of an important pharmacophore on a solid phase is that of the quinolones (Fig. 23) [108]. Quinolones compose a class of broad-spectrum antibiotics discovered relatively recently. In their demonstration of quinolone solid-phase synthesis, MacDonald and coworkers included the known antibiotic ciprofloxacin in order to highlight the ability of their quinolone library to generate pharmaceutically relevant compounds.

Four recent pharmacophore syntheses on support are shown in Figures 24–27. In all four cases, at least three diversity elements may be displayed around a central core. The bicyclic guanidines derive their diversity elements from amino

Peptide

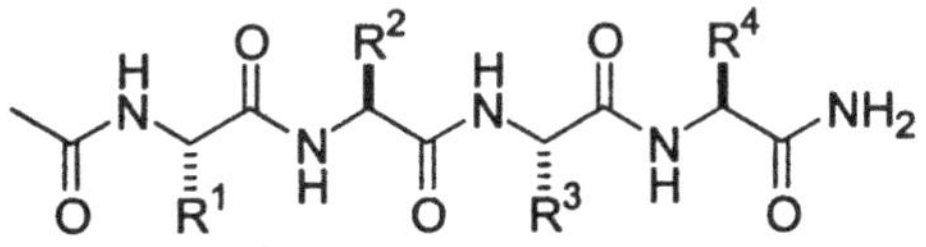

Reduced oligopeptide

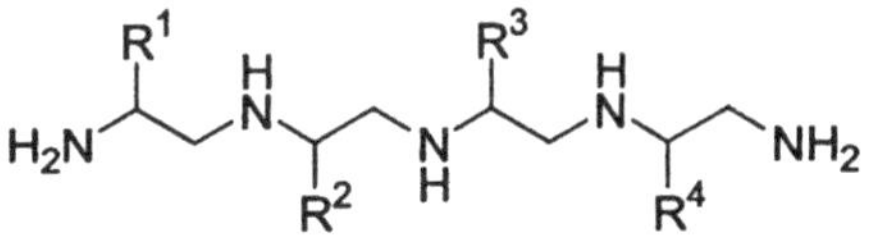

Oligo-β-peptide

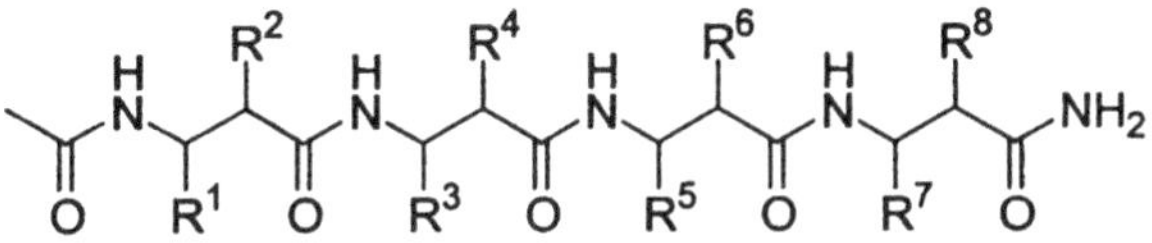

Oligopeptoid

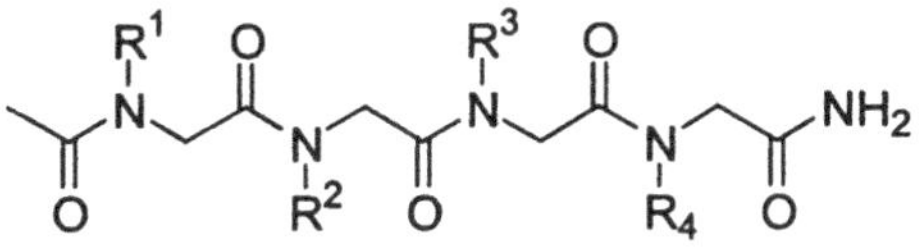

Azatide

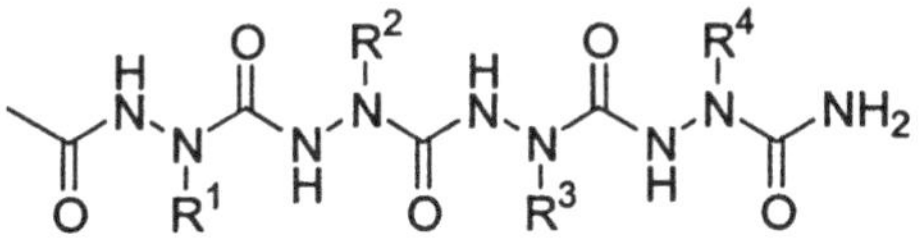

Oligocarbamate

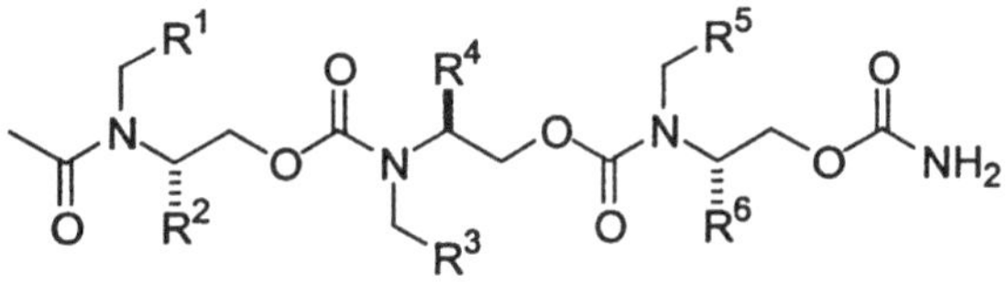

Oligourea

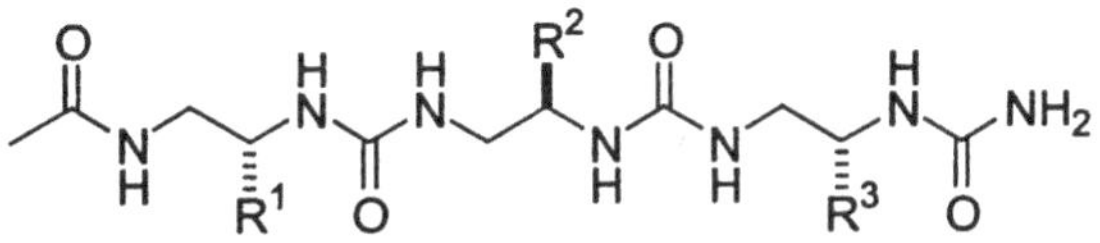

Oligopyrrolin-4-ones

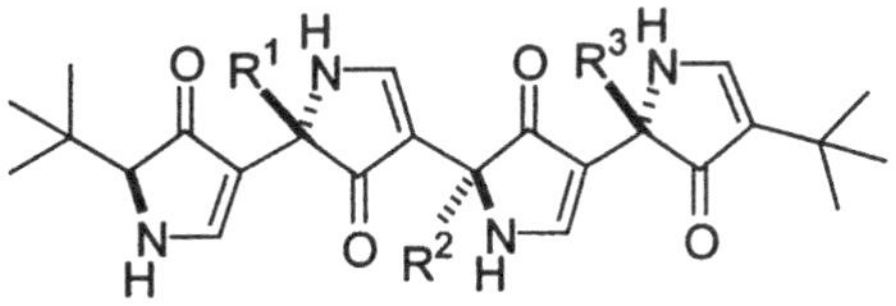

Vinylogous polypeptide

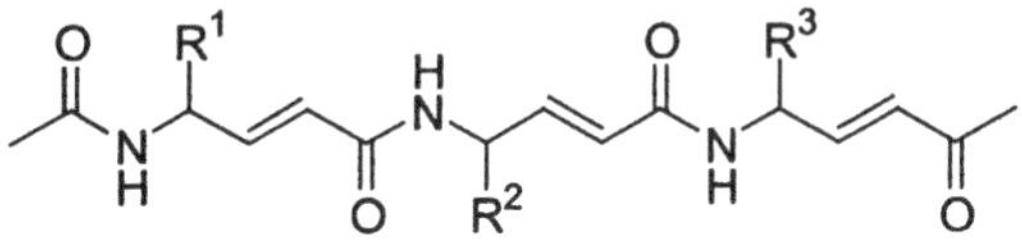

Figure 21 Peptide backbone, followed by various unnatural oligomer structures, indicating display of side chains (R groups).

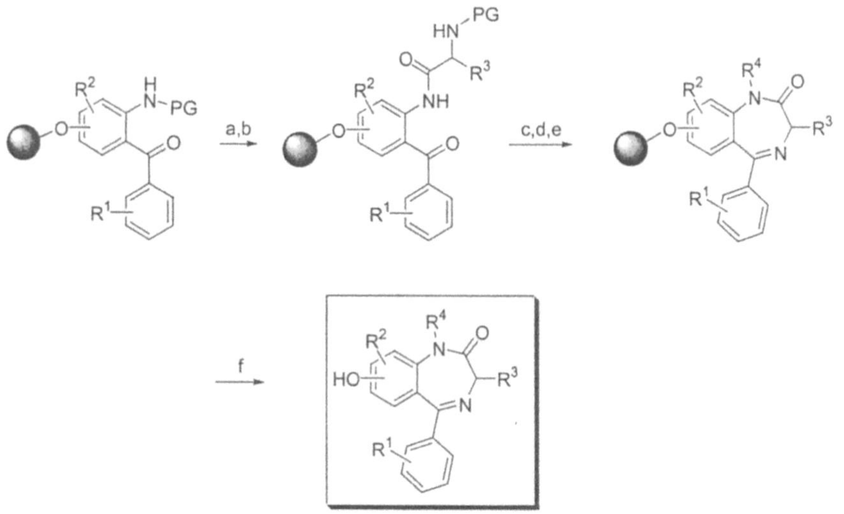

a) Fmoc ("PG") deprotection. b) N-protected amino acid fluoride coupling. c) Fmoc ("PG") deprotection at 60 °C, resulting in cyclization. d) Amide deprotonation. e) Alkylation of amide nitrogen (introduction of R⁴). f) Acidic cleavage from support.

Figure 22   Solid-phase synthesis of 1,4-benzodiazepines.

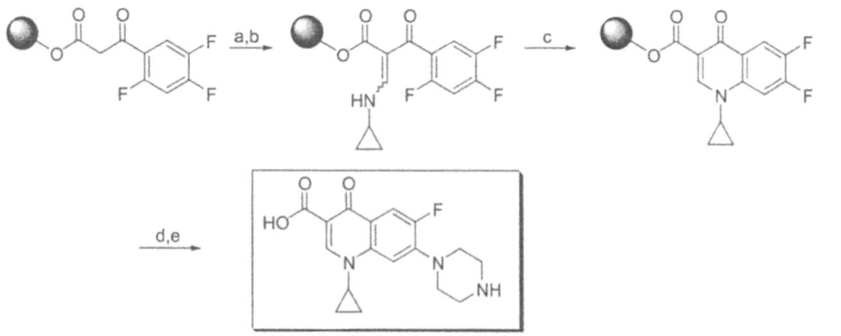

a) Activation with dimethylformamide dimethyl acetal. b) Cyclopropylamine addition. c) Cyclization with tetamethylguanidine, 55 °C. d) Nucleophilic substitution with piperazine. e) Acidic cleavage from support.

Figure 23   Solid-phase synthesis of quinolones (ciprofloxacin is shown in the box as the final product).

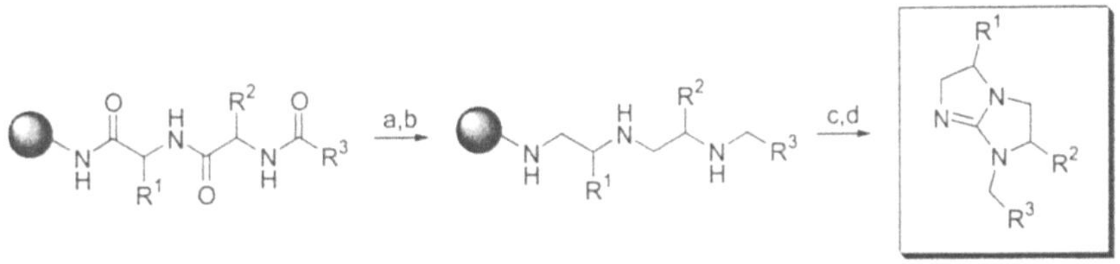

a) Amide reduction with borane-THF. b) Dissociation of amine-borane complexes with piperidine. c) Cyclization with thiocarbonyldiimidazole. d) Acidic cleavage from support.

Figure 24 Solid-phase synthesis of bicyclic guanidines.

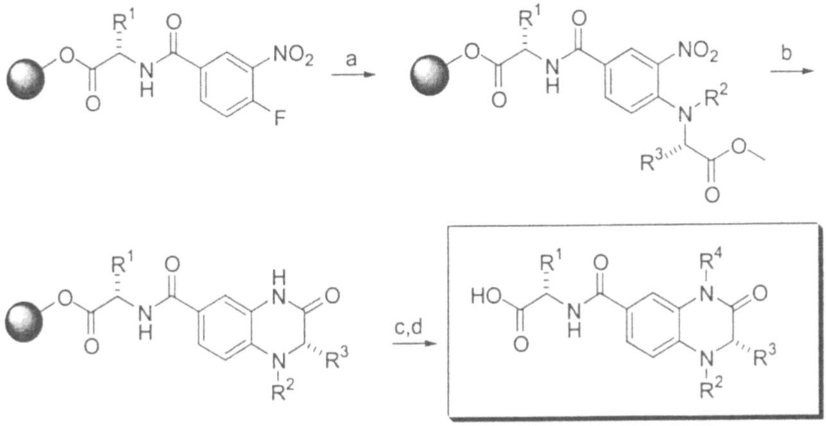

a) Aryl fluoride displacement with amino acid ester. b) Nitro group reduction with tin chloride, with concomitant cyclization. c) Introduction of R^4 via alkylation. d) Acidic cleavage from support.

Figure 25 Solid-phase synthesis of benzopiperazinones.

acids; an acylated dipeptide is synthesized on support, the amide carbonyl groups are reduced, and the resulting triamine is then cyclized (Fig. 24) [109]. The benzopiperazinones (Fig. 25) also derive side-chain diversity (at two positions) from amino acids, and a postcyclization alkylation on support introduces functionality at the R^4 position [110]. The oxopiperazine core is assembled via a tandem N-acyliminium ion cyclization–nucleophilic addition, resulting in the construction

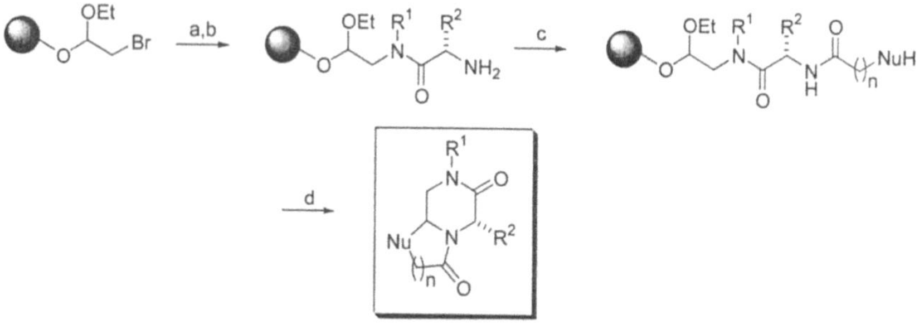

a) Amine displacement of bromide to install R[1]. b) Acylation with Fmoc-protected amono acid, followed by Fmoc deprotection with piperidine. c) Acylation with carboxylic acid containing a nucleophile ("NuH"). d) Acidic cleavage and nucleophillic cyclization via N-acyliminium ion.

Figure 26 Solid-phase synthesis of oxapiperazines.

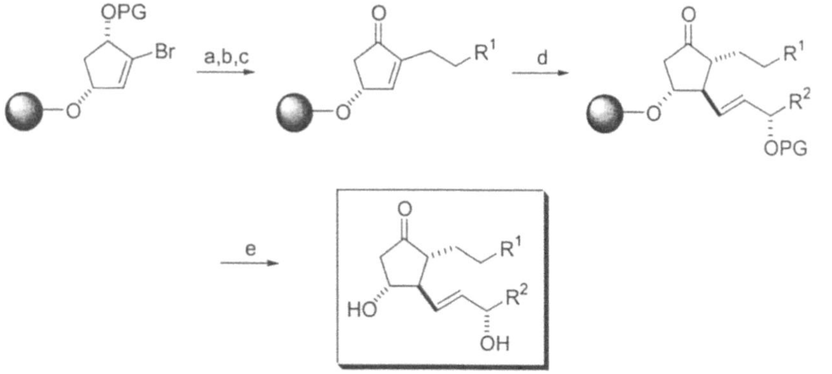

a) Acidic deprotection of alcohol. b) Suzuki cross-coupling reaction (C-C bond formation) to introduce R[1] side chain. c) Oxidation of alcohol to ketone with Dess-Martin periodinane. d) Vinyl cuprate addition (C-C bond formation) to install lower, R[2] side chain. e) Acidic cleavage from support and simultaneous alcohol deprotection.

Figure 27 Solid-phase synthesis of prostaglandins.

of both rings in a single step (Fig. 26) [111]. Finally, the prostaglandin synthesis shown in Figure 27 is an excellent example of the application of a variety of solid-phase reactions, including enantioselective C—C bond formation and oxidation of an alcohol to a ketone [53,112].

The Schreiber group has recently undertaken the development of "complexity-generating" reactions to access diverse compounds. One example of this approach is shown in Figure 28, where the 7-5-5-7 ring system was generated in six steps on support. The synthesis involves two key complexity-generating steps: an Ugi reaction (followed by an intramolecular Diels–Alder reaction) and a ring-closing metathesis. The final product contains five stereocenters and was isolated as a single stereoisomer. The aurthors report that optimization of the support-bound reactions is underway, with the goal of generating a library via split-pool synthesis.

C. Natural Product Total Syntheses on Solid Support

The total synthesis of complex natural products offer formidable synthetic challenges even without the added difficulties involved with the optimization of solid-phase synthesis [113]. These challenges have been met by several different research labs with the recent completion of such natural products as epothilones A and B [59], the fumiquinazoline alkaloids [114], and analogs of indolactam V [115] (Fig. 29). The degree of difficulty of these syntheses and proficiency with which they have been achieved are evidence that solid-supported synthesis has matured into an applicable method for the generation of complex molecules.

Ganesan's solid-phase synthesis of (+)-glyantrytpine and several close analogs (fumiquinazoline alkaloids) from readily available starting materials demonstrate the potential of this technology to rapidly access natural product structures [114]. The synthesis began with Fmoc-protected L-tryptophan on solid support. Subsequent elongation to a linear tripeptide was followed by a cyclative cleavage from support, resulting in the desired fumiquinazoline alkaloids. The versatility of this approach was demonstrated by the synthesis of 17 unnatural fumiquinazoline analogs, where L-alanine, L-leucine, and L-phenylalanine were used in place of L-tryptophan. The final products were obtained in moderate to good yields and high purity.

Nicolaou's total synthesis of epothilones A and B reveals the potential synergies between solution and solid-phase synthesis [59]. Complex subunits were synthesized in solution and then combined on the solid support to achieve a highly convergent method for the rapid construction of the uncyclized scaffold (Scheme 4). A strategic olefin linkage of the acyclic precursor to the solid support allowed for simultaneous macrocyclization and cleavage of the reaction product from the resin via ring-closing metathesis. A subsequent epoxidation in solution, followed by resolution of diastereomers, led to the desired natural product. This type of hybrid solution-phase and solid-phase approach is particularly attractive to the medicinal chemist, since it allows for the rapid generation of analogs of these biologically active natural products.

Schreiber and coworkers have described the synthesis of a library of "natural product–like" compounds. The library contained over 2 million compounds and was derived from two cores that vary in the nature of the R group in the tem-

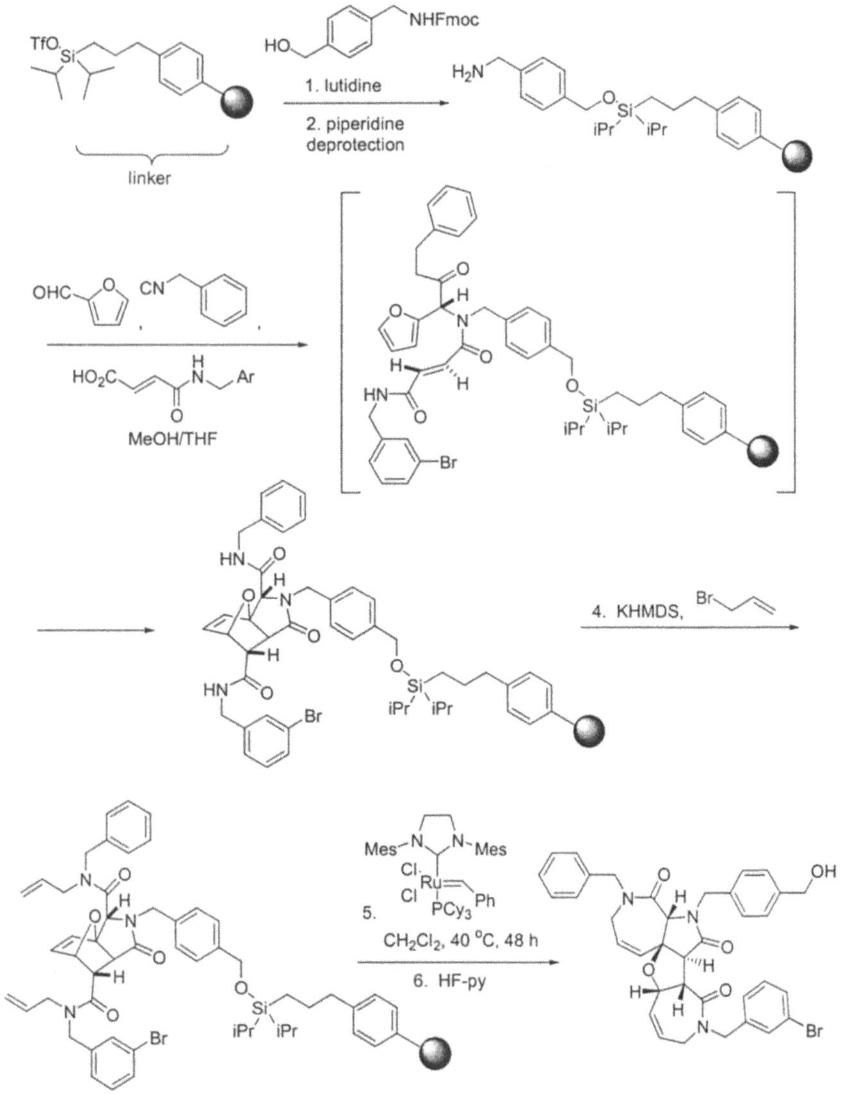

Figure 28   Solid-phase synthesis using "complexity-generating" reactions to produce a 7-5-5-7 ring system.

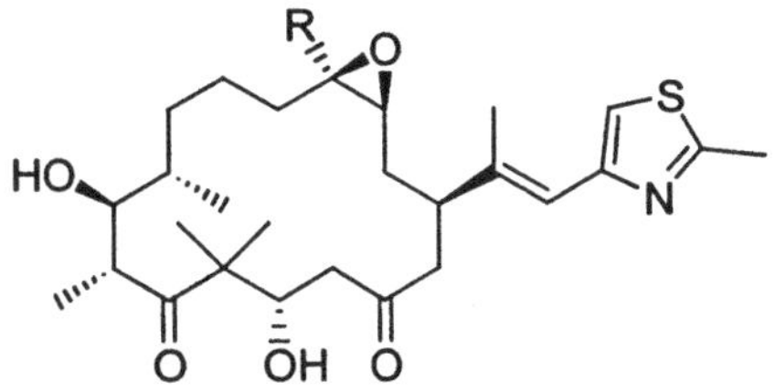

R = H   Epothione A

R = Me Epothione B

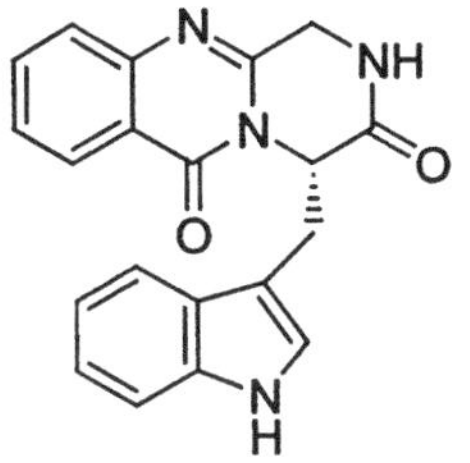

(+)-glyantrypine (fumiquinazoline alkaloid) 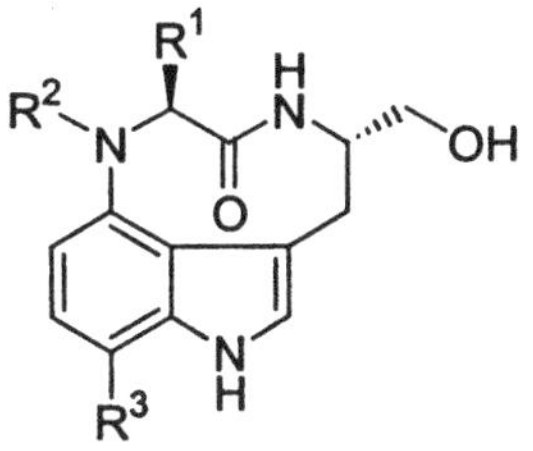   Indolactam V analogues

Figure 29 Natural products and natural product analogs synthesized on solid support.

plate (Fig. 30) [116]. Several other groups are also looking at cores related to natural products in order to access structural classes that were previously inaccessible by parallel synthesis [60,117]. This application of solid-phase synthesis begins to bridge the gap between the relatively simple small molecules traditionally made via combinatorial methods and very complicated natural products, as chemists seek more sophisticated cores for their libraries.

IV. SOLUTION-PHASE SYNTHESIS METHODOLOGIES

A. Solution-Phase Polymer-Supported Synthesis

While the majority of reports of parallel and combinatorial synthesis still involve the attachment of reactants (either reagent or substrate) to an insoluble support, there have been numerous publications describing parallel synthesis using soluble polymers [20,37,38]. The major advantage that use of a soluble polymer holds over a "classical" insoluble polymer (e.g., polystyrene beads) is that reactions occur entirely in the solution phase, so that little or no modification of a traditional non-polymer-supported synthesis is necessary. A second advantage is that reaction kinetics are often faster with the soluble polymer than with a two-phase system. Upon completion of the reaction, the desired product (attached to the soluble polymer) is isolated by precipitation of the polymer, by extraction (e.g., into a fluorous

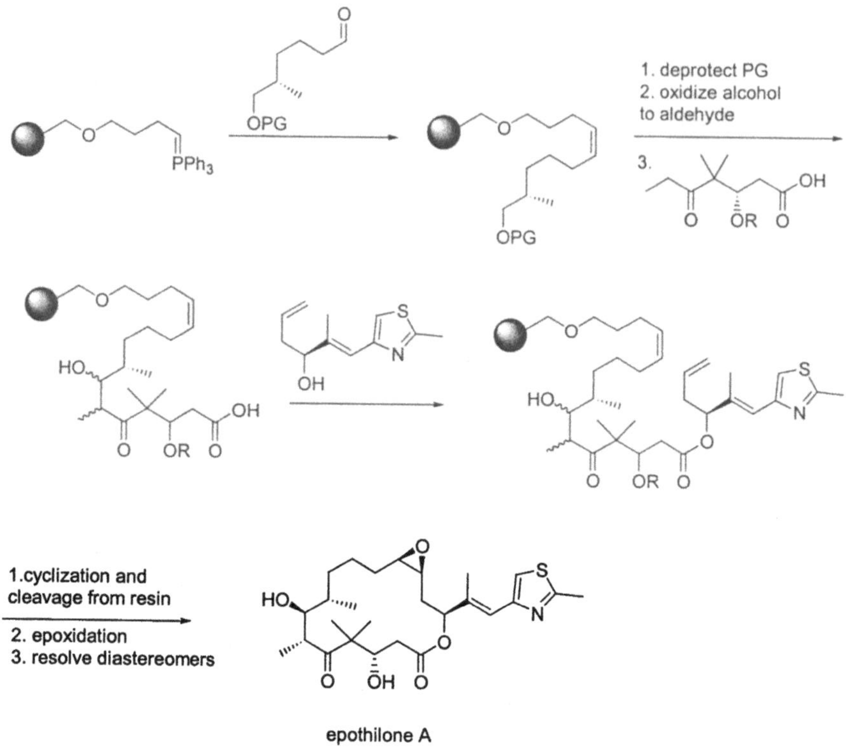

Scheme 4

solvent when using a fluorous polymer), or by means of separation based on molecular weight (such as equilibrium dialysis or size exclusion chromatography). Some examples of soluble polymers include polyethylene glycol (PEG), polyvinyl alcohol, non-cross-linked polystyrene, and polyacrylic acid (Fig. 31). Since the polymer-bound component can be separated from the other reagents at the end of the reaction, excess reagents may still be used to drive reactions to completion, affording high yields and purities of products.

When using soluble polymer supports, such as PEG, consideration must be given to the size and solubility properties of the polymer to be used, as well as to the size of the desired product molecule. As the size of the attached molecule increases, its solubility properties can often moderate or dominate the solubility properties of the polymer, potentially resulting in loss of product due to incomplete crystallization or extraction. A number of different polymers have been applied to solution-phase parallel synthesis, as selected for their solubilizing characteristics and compatibility with reaction chemistry.

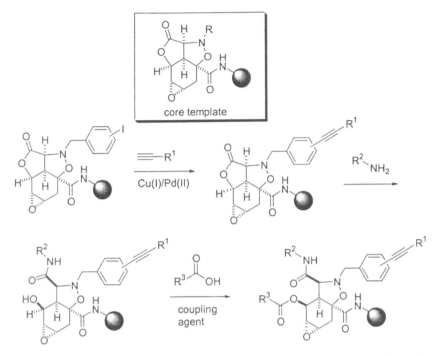

Figure 30 Core template (in box) and representative synthesis of the "natural-product-like" library from the benzyl-derived core and alkyne, amine, and carboxylic acid building blocks. For the core template, R represents either benzyl or phenyl side chains.

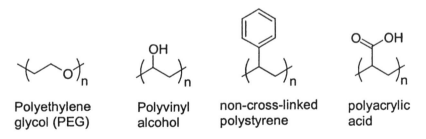

| Polyethylene glycol (PEG) | Polyvinyl alcohol | non-cross-linked polystyrene | polyacrylic acid |

Figure 31 Examples of soluble polymer supports.

Chemistry has been developed to take advantage of the unique properties of highly fluorinated hydrocarbons. It has been recognized that solvents comprising these fluorinated hydrocarbons are immiscible with water and with many organic solvents, resulting in a "fluorous" phase [118]. Compounds attached to highly fluorinated "tags" may be reacted in solution in pure organic solvents or solvents containing a fluorous cosolvent, then extracted into a fluorous phase upon completion of the reaction. Likewise, reagents may be attached to highly fluorinated tags and extracted into a fluorous phase and away from the product. A third option is to use a fluorinated solid phase, such as silica, with a fluorinated bonded phase to selectively bind and separate the fluorous-tagged material from the reaction mixture. Techniques involving the use of fluorinated tags have the advantages of allowing reactions to be run in solution, followed by straightforward separation of product or reactant (depending on which contained the fluorous tag). No translation of solution-phase procedures is necessary. However, such fluorous tagging has yet to find widespread use in parallel and combinatorial chemistry, due in part to the poor commercial availability of several of the required reagents.

Dendrimers have been suggested for use as soluble polymer supports for combinatorial libraries (Fig. 32) [119]. Separation from reactants is accomplished by methods such as size exclusion chromatography or ultrafiltration, where the larger dendrimer is isolated from the smaller reactants. Dendrimers typically have considerably higher loading (more molecules of product per gram of support) than insoluble polymers, and again there is no need to translate solution-phase procedures for use with dendrimer supports. While it would appear that there are several advantages for the use of dendrimers over insoluble polymer supports, there have been relatively few reports of dendrimer-supported parallel or combinatorial syntheses. Only a few dendrimers are commercially available, and the methods of purification required between steps (size exclusion chromatography or ultrafiltration) have not yet been developed in a readily accessible HT format.

B. Solution-Phase Reactions Involving Scavenging Resins

It was first recognized by Kaldor and coworkers that solid-supported nucleophiles and electrophiles could be used for rapid purification of compound libraries synthesized in a standard solution-phase reaction [18,120]. The advantages of this

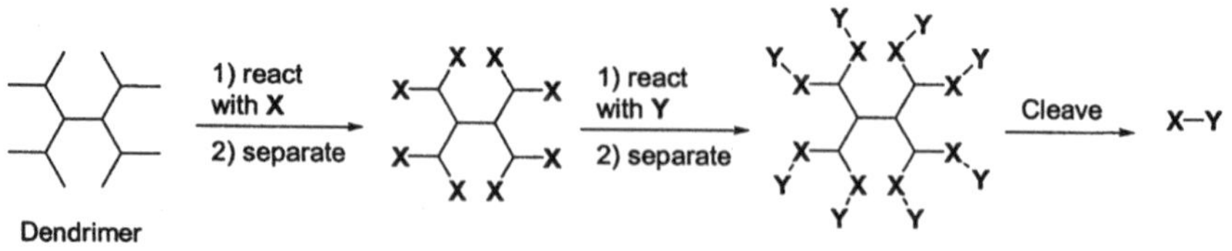

Dendrimer

Figure 32   Dendrimer-supported synthesis.

technique include standard solution-phase kinetics, easy analysis of reactions using conventional methods, and no need for the development of linker chemistry. The largest incentive to pursuing this methodology is that the development time for the synthesis of new compounds can be much shorter than the time necessary to develop a new solid-phase synthesis. This reduction in time is critical particularly when medicinal chemists are developing methods for exploration of structure–activity relationships (SARs) in the intensely competitive pharmaceutical industry. Sequestering agents allow the most straightforward type of parallel synthesis; standard reactions are carried out in solution in parallel, and replacement of the normally time-consuming workup by simply mixing the reaction solutions with an appropriate scavenger on support and filtering to provide the pure products eliminates purification.

There are several potential drawbacks to solution-phase synthesis involving either scavenging resins or resin-bound reagents (discussed in a later section). For example, it is not possible to design split-and-pool syntheses, as the reaction products are free in solution and not associated with any tag or bead to separate. This can limit the size of the library (number of compounds) produced. In addition, while several examples of longer syntheses involving scavenging or resin-bound reagents are shown below, reaction sequences using these reagents are typically very short, on the order of one to three steps. This is in contrast to syntheses on solid support, which are often five or six steps long, and occasionally much longer. (For examples of longer sequences, see the preceding sections on complex multistep synthesis on solid supports.)

Support-bound scavengers have been developed for a variety of common reagents. There are two common varieties of scavengers: ionic reagents that remove impurities by forming salts, and reaction-based scavengers that react chemoselectively with an undesired excess reagent. Ionic reagents were the first such resins to be reported [120]. Amines can be removed by forming salts with support-bound sulfonic or carboxylic acids (sulfonic acid resins such as Dowex are common), and acids can be removed with support-bound amines, such as high-loading trisamine resins. Acid-functionalized resins are also commonly employed to scavenge excess metals and metal alkoxides from organometallic reactions, including Grignard and alkyllithium additions [121]. These reactions are relatively selective, as the unreacted polar reagents are usually removed from uncharged products. Although conceptually simple, these procedures are extremely powerful and are used routinely in parallel synthesis.

Chemists have also used ion exchange resins to "trap" products instead of impurities. In this inverse application of scavenger resins (often termed "catch and release" purification), the charged product is captured by an appropriate ion exchange resin. The reaction impurities are then washed away, and the pure product is released from the ion exchange resin by elution with an appropriate buffer (Fig. 33). This technique has also been applied in cases where the product is selectively reacted with a resin-bound reagent to form a covalent link to the support.

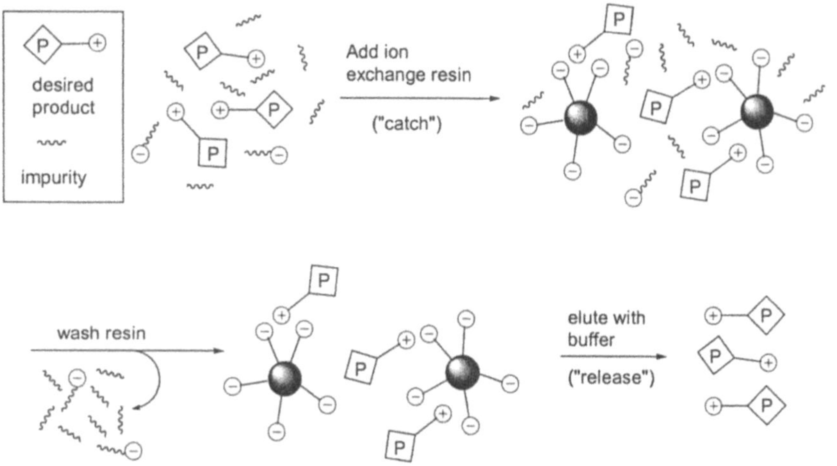

Figure 33 Cartoon of "catch and release" purification; a cationic product is captured on an anionic ion exchange resin. The neutral and anionic impurities are washed away, and the pure product is eluted from the resin.

The impurities are then washed away, and the product is released via a second reaction or cleavage step.

Most reactivity-based scavengers are functionalized polystyrene resins. Nucleophilic impurities such as amines or thiols can effectively be removed by the use of electrophilic resins. Some examples of these reagents include polymer-bound isocyanates, sulfonyl chlorides, anhydrides, aldehydes, and chloroformates. Excess electrophiles, such as acid chlorides, isocyanates, aldehydes, alkyl halides, α,β-unsaturated carbonyl compounds, and sulfonyl chlorides, can be sequestered using polymer-bound nucleophiles such as amines and thiols [122–124]. Examples of several different classes of reactivity-based scavengers are shown (being used for purification of products) in Figure 34 [122–126]. The large number of different reagents available for these purification techniques allows "tuning" of the reactivity of a scavenger. For example, a thiol can be removed from a solution containing an amine by use of an α-iodoamide resin as an electrophile. This reagent will selectively react with the more nucleophilic thiol over the desired amine-containing product [125]. The loading levels of polymer-bound scavengers are important; the swelling of resins requires the use of large solvent volumes, such that higher resin loading levels of scavenger are desirable to minimize dilution of the reaction mixture and amount of resin required. The following section highlights some more advanced scavengers that have been developed to remove specific impurities and demonstrate the power of this technique.

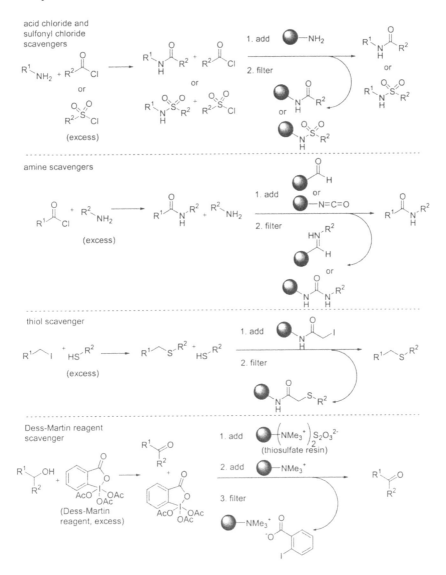

Figure 34 Reactivity-based scavenger resins.

Parlow and coworkers have developed a scavenging method for the versatile Dess–Martin oxidation procedure [126]. Reaction of a primary or secondary alcohol with an excess of the Dess–Martin reagent in solution produces an aldehyde or ketone. The excess reagent is usually removed in solution-phase reactions by reduction of the unreacted reagent with sodium thiosulfate followed by aqueous extraction. Parlow and coworkers have developed a thiosulfate resin by simply washing commercial chloride-form Amberlyst A-26 ion exchange resin with thiosulfate (Fig. 34). Treating a crude reaction solution from a Dess–Martin oxidation with the thiosulfate resin reduces the unreacted Dess–Martin reagent to o-iodobenzoic acid, which can then be efficiently sequestered by any of a number of basic resins. This chemistry was demonstrated on a number of alcohols to produce the corresponding aldehydes or ketones in good yields and excellent purities (>99% in almost all cases as measured by GC/MS and ^{1}H NMR).

Ion exchange sequestering is an efficient procedure to remove excess impurities from reaction mixtures; however, in the pharmaceutical industry the use of sulfonic acid resins is limited by the presence of basic amines on a large number of desired products. Parlow and coworkers have devised a strategy to make possible the sequestration of a reactive amine from a solution containing a desired basic but nonnucleophilic amine [127]. By adding tetrafluorophthalic anhydride (TFPA) to such a reaction mixture, the excess reactive amine is consumed, leading to formation of the phthalamide with a pendant carboxylic acid (Scheme 5). Both the

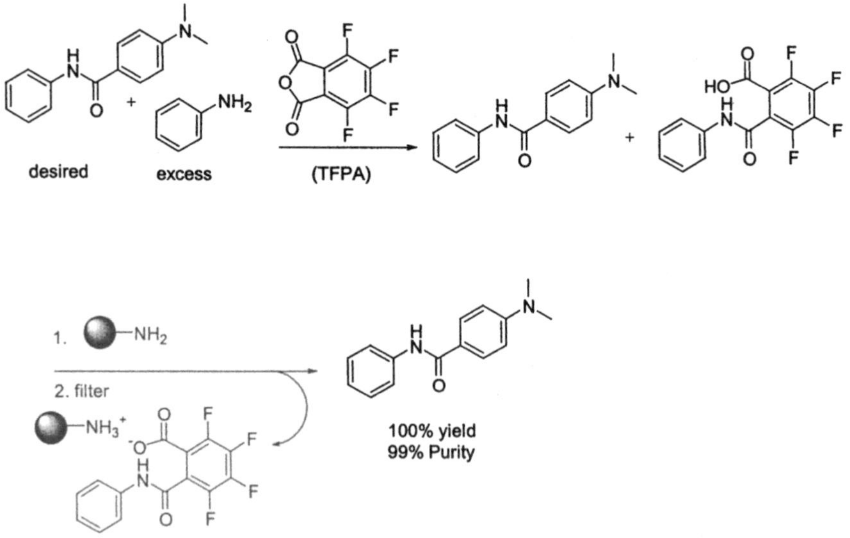

Scheme 5

resulting carboxylic acid and any excess anhydride can be sequestered using a basic resin, leaving only the desired basic amine in the reaction solution. This procedure is effective for removing relatively poor nucleophiles, such as anilines, that do not react completely with most support-bound electrophiles.

In another example of material design, Kirkland and coworkers prepared functionalized porous silica microspheres for use as scavengers in combinatorial chemistry [128]. The silica microspheres are more than 99.995% pure and have a uniform particle size and shape that provides superior mass transfer properties. The microsphere beads are easy to handle, do not swell, and are efficient scavengers in both polar and nonpolar solvents. The microspheres can be functionalized with the same functional groups as polystyrene beads and therefore can be used in many of the same situations as conventional scavengers. These silica-based materials have been evaluated for the ability to sequester a number of acids, acid chlorides, and amines from typical reaction solutions.

C. Solution-Phase Reactions Involving Resin-Bound Reagents

A complementary approach to removing excess reagents from a reaction solution using a support-bound sequestering agent is to immobilize the reagent on an appropriate solid phase. Addition of an excess of this solid-supported reagent to a suitable substrate in solution provides a product that can be purified by simple filtering off of the support-bound reagent. This approach is conceptually relatively old but has been recently revitalized as is evident by the vast number of support-bound reagent classes that have been developed for solution-phase parallel synthesis. There are now commercial resins available that deliver support-bound equivalents of many types of reagents, including acids, bases [tertiary amine, 4-dimethyl-aminopyridine (DMAP), phosphazine, etc.], acylating agents (see below), coupling agents (carbodiimides), reducing agents (borohydride, cyanoborohydride, silylhydrides), oxidizing agents (permanganate, chromium, ruthenium, osmium), catalysts (palladium, asymmetrical catalysts), a wide variety of protecting groups, and many other reagent classes. A discussion of *all* of the reagents currently available is beyond the scope of this chapter. The interested reader is directed to the review articles mentioned in the introduction to the solution-phase chemistry section and listed at the end of the chapter [18,33,123]. Several classes of these reagents are described in detail below.

Amide formation is a reaction of fundamental importance in medicinal chemistry, consequently, many techniques to form amides using polymer-assisted solution-phase (PASP) chemistry have been developed. A convenient method is to utilize a support-bound alcohol that is functionalized using either a carboxylic acid and coupling agent or an acid chloride to provide a support-bound activated ester. These reagents can then be stored and are typically stable for months. Simply stirring an excess of the support-bound activated ester with an amine provides (after a filtration step to remove the support) a high yield of a desired amide. Adamczyk and coworkers have developed an *N*-hydroxysuccinimide-functional-ized resin for this purpose, utilizing a Michael addition of a support-bound thiol to *N*-hydroxymaleimide to provide the functionalized resin **2** (Fig. 32) [129].

A resin similar to that discussed above has been reported by Salvino and coworkers whereby reaction of aminomethyl resin with 4-carboxytetrafluorophe-nol provides a support-bound pentafluorophenyl (PFP)–ester equivalent **3** (Fig. 35) [130]. Loading of the resin with a carboxylic acid or sulfonyl chloride pro-vides a support-bound activated ester. This tetrafluorophenyl alcohol resin has the advantage that solid-phase ^{19}F NMR can be utilized to quantitatively determine the loading level of the polymer-bound active ester reagents [131]. Other support-bound reagents for transformations of this type have been previously reported, including support-bound 1-hydroxybenzotriazole (HOBt) equivalents, a polymer-bound *o*-nitrophenol (o-NP) equivalent **4** (Fig. 35) [132], and the Kaiser oxime resin [133]. Chang and Schultz have recently analyzed resins **2,** the *o*-nitrophenyl

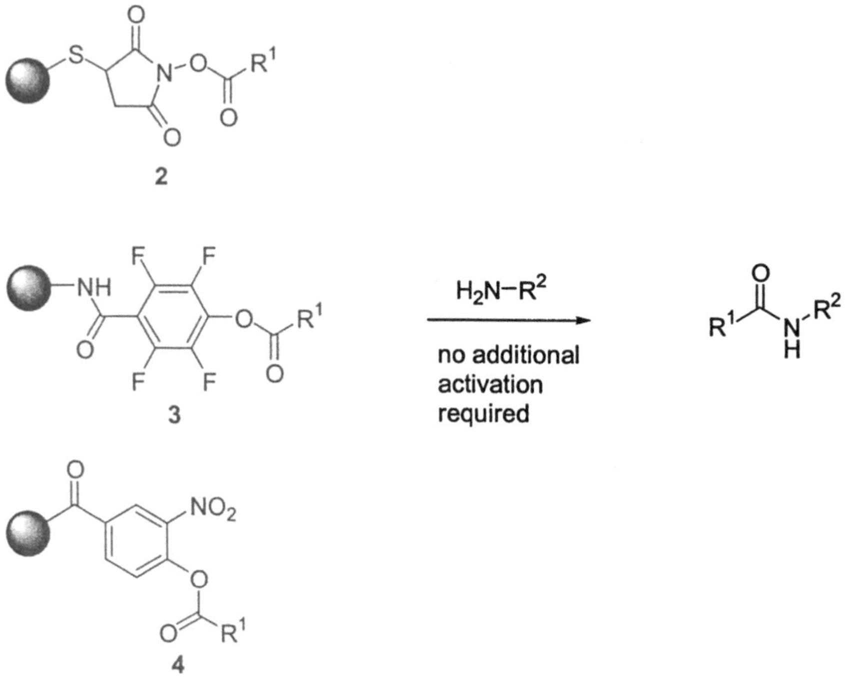

Figure 35 Support-bound activated esters that can be directly reacted with an amine nucleophile.

ester resin, the Kaiser oxime resin, and commercial HOBt resin for their relative abilities to act as support-bound acylating agents [134]. By acylating all four resins with a carboxylic acid containing a dye and monitoring the rate of amide formation with benzylamine, the relative order of reactivity of the resins was determined to be as follows: P-HOBt >> P-N-hydroxysuccinimide > P-o-nitro-phenyl >> P-oxime.

Several groups have developed "safety catch" linkers whereby the linking unit is stable to a variety of acidic and basic conditions. The term "safety catch" arises from the fact that the resins normally must be activated prior to release of the product (so the linker is "safe" until intentionally modified to provide an acti-vated ester equivalent). Kenner and Ellman have reported sulfonamide-based link-ers that are stable under most reaction conditions [135–137]. Upon chemical acti-vation, the linker serves as an activating group, and the product can be released by reaction with amines or alcohols to produce amides or esters (Fig. 36). Scialdone and coworkers have published several applications of phosgenated oxime (phoxime) resin (**5**) [138]. The phoxime resin also serves as a reactive equivalent, requiring thermal rather than chemical activation. This polymer-bound reagent traps amines as support-bound urethanes that are thermally labile and can be cleaved by thermolysis to provide isocyanates. The released isocyanate reacts with amines present in the cleavage solution producing highly substituted ureas (Scheme 6) (see also the previous section on resin-to-resin transfer).

A number of laboratories have investigated the synthesis and use of poly-mer-bound 1H-benzotriazole as both a support-bound reagent and traceless linker for library synthesis. It is fitting that the Katritzky group published the first report of such a reagent for the synthesis of amine libraries, as that same group has pio-

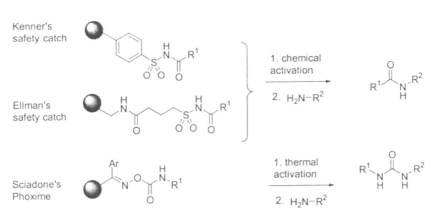

Figure 36 Support-bound reactants requiring activation prior to reaction with an amine nucleophile.

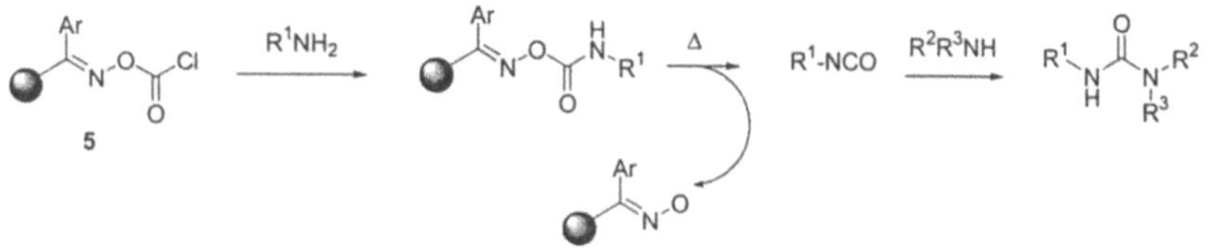

Scheme 6

neered the use of this reagent in traditional solution-phase chemistry [139]. Treatment of any of the benzotriazole resins with an aldehyde and an amine under conditions suitable for formation of the Schiff base produces the polymer-bound benzotriazole–Schiff base adduct **7** (Scheme 7). Cleavage is then effected by substitution with a suitable nucleophile, such as a hydride, Grignard, or Reformatsky reagent, to produce a new, substituted amine **8** in good yield. Given the utility of benzotriazole in the synthesis of substituted heterocycles, it is certain that polymer-supported benzotriazole equivalents will be useful for many different heterocycle syntheses in the future.

Cycloaddition reactions utilizing support-bound substrates are popular due to the large increase in complexity of the final products afforded by these reactions. Smith has utilized a commercially available alkyldiethylsilane-functionalized polymer (PS-DES resin) activated as the triflate to prepare resin-bound silyl enol ethers of enones (Scheme 8) [140]. These resin-bound intermediates then provide access to a variety of cycloaddition products. Smith has investigated the Diels–Alder chemistry of these intermediates, and Porco and coworkers [141] have demonstrated the utility of these precursors in providing functionalized esters from Claisen rearrangement chemistry. Given the utility of trimethylsilyl triflate (TMS-OTf) and related silyl triflate catalysts in a variety of traditional solution-phase transformations, such as glycosylation, PS-DES triflate is likely to be a useful reagent for many transformations in library synthesis.

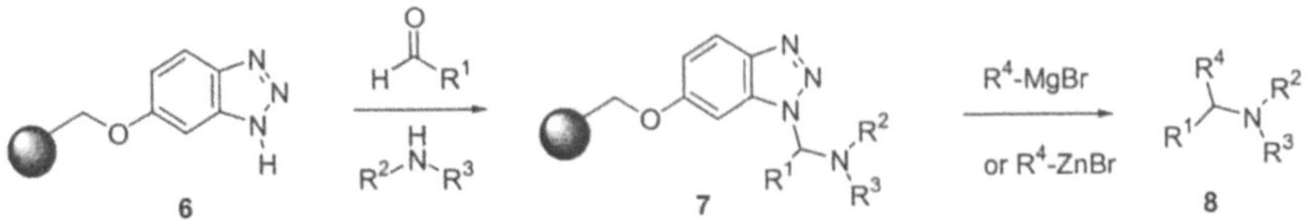

Scheme 7

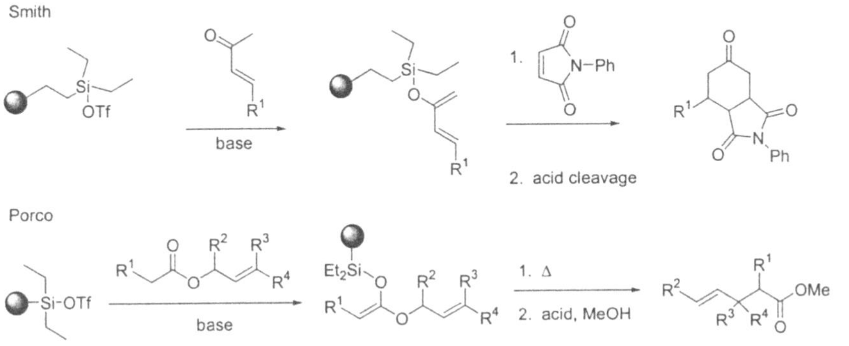

Smith

Porco

Scheme 8

D. Multistep Synthesis with Resin-Bound Scavengers and Reagents

The development of a large number of strategies for PASP chemistry has allowed the synthesis of increasingly complex molecules using only fast PASP purification. This section details some of these advances, which provide a strong base for the future of the field.

One important synthetic target for the Ley group has been the hydroxamate inhibitors of the matrix metalloproteinases (MMPs) [142]. Inhibitors similar to the known inhibitor CGS-27023A (Scheme 9, **13**, R^1 = i-Pr, R^2 = 4-MeO-phenyl, R^3 = 3-pyridyl) were prepared from amino acid *t*-butyl esters. The synthesis involved the use of support-bound amines to scavenge excess sulfonyl chloride and alkyl halide reagents, use of a support-bound base in an alkylation, and use of support-

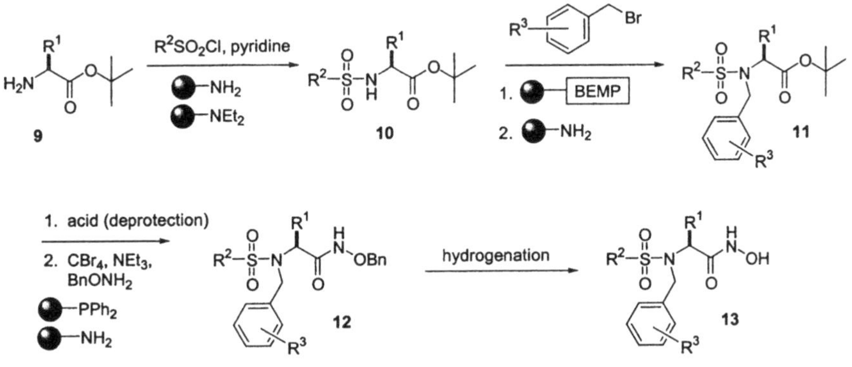

Scheme 9

bound triphenylphosphine to generate an acid bromide in solution. Condensation with aromatic sulfonyl chlorides followed by workup with P-NH$_2$ and desalting with ion exchange resin provides the sulfonamides **10**. Alkylation of the sulfon-amide with P-BEMP (a resin-bound base) and a benzyl halide yields compounds **11** after removal of excess halide with P-NH$_2$. The *t*-butyl ester is cleaved with acid and the hydroxamic acid functionality is introduced by preparing the acid bromide, followed by condensation with *O*-benzylhydroxylamine hydrochloride in the presence of base. Hydrogenation provides the final products **13** (27 examples). No chromatography was necessary, and products were isolated in high (90–98%) overall purity and variable (39–100%) yields.

The Ley group has extended these concepts to include the multistep synthesis of natural products as well as the solution-phase preparation of libraries. The synthesis of racemic oxomaritidine and epimaritidine (Scheme 10) was accomplished starting with 3,4-dimethoxybenzyl alcohol [143]. All six steps of the reaction sequence involve the application of a resin-bound reagent. Oxidation with polymer-supported perruthenate to the aldehyde followed by reductive amination with amine **16** using P-borohydride (a resin-bound reducing agent) gave the secondary amine **17,** which was then trifluoroacetylated using P-DMAP. Oxidative spirocyclization to **19** was achieved using polymer-bound (diacetoxyiodo)benzene. After removal of the trifluoroacetate protecting group with P-carbonate, the resulting amine spontaneously undergoes 1,4-addition to provide racemic crystalline oxomaritidine. Reduction with polymer-supported borohydride provides

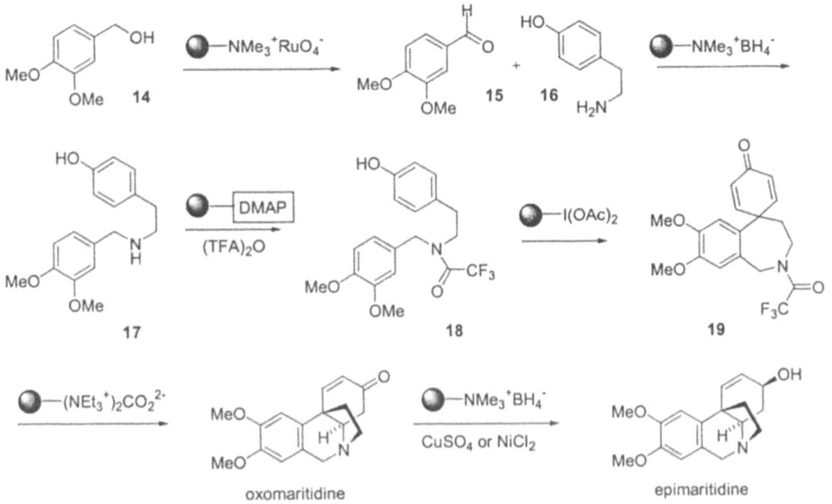

Scheme 10

epimaritidine. Both natural products were prepared in excellent overall yield and purity.

A final example is the multistep synthesis of the analgesic natural product epibatidine, an alkaloid isolated from the Ecuadoran poison dart frog *Epipedobates tricolor* [144]. The 10-step synthesis involves support-bound reagents being used in oxidations, reductions, basic catalysis, and catch-and-release purification of the final product. The sequence begins with reduction of the acid chloride **20** with support-bound borohydride followed by oxidation with polymer-bound perruthenate to afford the aldehyde **21** (Scheme 11). Henry reaction catalyzed by basic resin is followed by elimination to styrene **23**. Diels–Alder reaction with the diene **24** occurs smoothly in a sealed tube to yield the cyclohexanone **25**, which is then reduced with support-bound borohydride to the alcohol. Mesylation with P-DMAP affords the mesylate. Reduction of the nitro group without concomitant dehalogenation proved to be difficult; however, the modification of polymer-bound borohydride with nickel(II) chloride provided an impressive solution to this

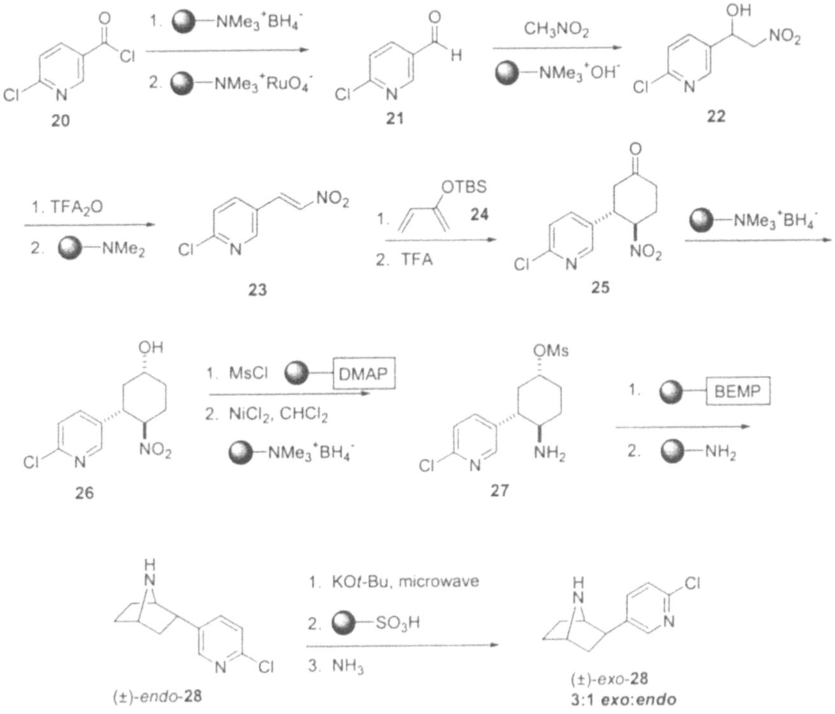

Scheme 11

problem, and the desired product **27** was isolated in 95% yield as a 7:1 mixture of diastereomers. The critical transannular cyclization of **27** to *endo*-epibatidine occurred in 71% yield upon treatment with P-BEMP, and the unreacted cis isomer of **27** could be removed by reaction of the remaining mesylate using P-NH$_2$ (a nucleophilic support–bound amine). Finally, the natural product was prepared by isomerization to the desired exo isomer followed by catch and release purification using a polymer-bound sulfonic acid. The natural product **28** was released from the support by eluting with ammonia in methanol and was isolated as a 3:1 exo endo mixture in more than 90% purity by ^{1}H NMR and LC MS analysis.

V. CONCLUSION

Since Furka's and Geysen's seminal work in peptide library synthesis in the late 1980s, combinatorial chemistry has matured into its own discipline. Today combinatorial chemistry encompasses an extremely broad range of technologies and methodologies that have brought many seemingly unrelated scientific fields together. The meshing of high-throughput synthesis, computational design, robotics, and informatics has provided a framework for modern research. The combinatorial chemistry lab is now highly automated, allowing hundreds of reactions to be performed in parallel. This new paradigm for discovery is transforming the way scientists think about setting up experiments. The basis of the scientific method is being retooled for the 21st century chemists who are equipped to solve problems by asking not one question at a time but many. The development of new synthetic methods to create the desired libraries of molecules for the study of their specific function is critical and will continue to determine one's ultimate success. Recent advancements in the field of combinatorial organic synthesis (COS) on solid phase and in solution phase are providing powerful tools to the chemist seeking to apply these new principles. The continued development of novel methodologies and technologies in combinatorial chemistry promises a new and bright future for science in general.

REFERENCES

1.   Camps Diez F, Castells Guardiola J, Pi Sallent J. Solid phase synthesis of 1,4-benzodiazepine derivatives. Span. ES: (Patronato de Investigacion Cientifica y Tecnica "Juan de la Cierva", Spain)., 1977.
2.   Leznoff CC. Use of insoluble polymer supports in organic chemical synthesis. Chem Soc Rev 1974;3:65–85.

3. Leznoff CC. The use of insoluble polymer supports in general organic synthesis. Acc Chem Res 1978;11:327–333.
4. Frechet JMJ. Synthesis and application of organic polymers as supports and protecting groups. Tetrahedron 1981;37:663–683.
5. Bunin BA, Ellman JA. A general and expedient method for the solid-phase synthesis of 1,4-benzodiazepine derivatives. J Am Chem Soc 1992;114:10997–10998.
6. DeWitt SH, Kiely JS, Stankovic CJ, Schroeder MC, Cody DMR, Pavia MR. "Diversomers": an approach to nonpeptide, nonoligomeric chemical diversity. Proc Natl Acad Sci USA 1993;90:6909–6913.
7. Geysen HM, Meloen RH, Barteling SJ. Use of peptide synthesis to probe viral antigens for epitopes to a resolution of a single amino acid. Proc Natl Acad Sci USA 1984;81:3998–4002.
8. Houghten RA. General method for the rapid solid-pase synthesis of large numbers of peptides: specificity of antigen-antibody interaction at the level of individual amino acids. Proc Natl Acad Sci USA 1985;82:5131–5135.
9. Furka A, Sebestyen F, Asgedom M, Dibo G. General method for rapid synthesis of multicomponent peptide mixtures. Int. J. Pept. Protein Res. 1991;37:487–493.
10. Sebestyen F, Dibo G, Kovacs A, Furka A. Chemical synthesis of peptide libraries. Bioorg. Med. Chem. Lett. Vol. 3, 1993:413–418.
11. Balkenhohl F, von dem Bussche-Hünnefeld C, Lansky A, Zechel C. Combinatorial synthesis of small organic molecules. Angew Chem Int Ed Engl 1996;35:2288–2337.
12. Gordon EM, Gallop MA, Patel DV. Strategy and tactics in combinatorial organic synthesis. Applications to drug discovery. Acc Chem Res 1996;29:144–154.
13. Thompson LA, Ellman JA. Synthesis and applications of small molecule libraries. Chem Rev 1996;96:555–600.
14. Hermkens PHH, Ottenheijm HCJ, Rees D. Solid-phase organic reactions: a review of the recent literature. Tetrahedron 1996;52:4527–4554.
15. Früchtel JS, Jung G. Organic chemistry on solid supports. Angew Chem Int Ed Engl 1996;35:17–42.
16. Czarnik AW, DeWitt SH (eds). A Practical Guide to Combinatorial Chemistry. Washington, DC:American Chemical Society, 1997.
17. Hermkens PHH, Ottenheijm HCJ, Rees DC. Solid-phase organic reactions II: a review of the literature Nov 95-Nov 96. Tetrahedron 1997;53:5643–5678.
18. Kaldor SW, Siegel MG. Combinatorial chemistry using polymer-supported reagents. Curr Opin Chem Biol 1997;1:101–106.
19. Wilson S, Czarnik AW. Combinatorial Chemistry: Synthesis and Application. New York: Wiley, 1997.
20. Gravert DJ, Janda KD. Organic synthesis on soluble polymer supports: liquid-phase methodologies. Chem Rev 1997;97:489–509.
21. Ugi I, Dömling A, Gruber B, Almstetter M. Multicomponent reactions and their libraries - a new approach to preparative organic chemistry. Croat Chem Acta 1997;70:631–647.
22. Flynn DL, Devraj RV, Naing W, Parlow JJ, Weidner JJ, Yang S. Polymer-assisted solution phase (PASP) chemical library synthesis. Med Chem Res 1998;8:219–243.

23. Czarnik AW. Combinatorial chemistry. Anal Chem 1998;70:378A–386A.
24. Dolle RE. Comprehensive survey of chemical libraries yielding enzyme inhibitors, receptor agonists and antagonists, and other biologically active agents: 1992 through 1997. Mol Diversity 1998;3:199–233.
25. Flynn DL, Devraj RV, Parlow JJ. Recent advances in polymer-assisted solution-phase chemical library synthesis and purification. Curr Opin Drug Disc Dev 1998;1:41–50.
26. Brown RCD. Recent developments in solid-phase organic synthesis. J Chem Soc Perkin Trans 1 1998:3293–3320.
27. Andres CJ, Whitehouse DL, Deshpande MS. Transition-metal-mediated reactions in combinatorial synthesis. Curr Opin Chem Biol 1998;2:353–362.
28. Nefzi A, Dooley C, Ostresh JM, Houghten RA. Combinatorial chemistry: from peptides and peptidomimetics to small organic and heterocyclic compounds. Bioorg Med Chem Lett 1998;8:2273–2278.
29. Booth S, Hermkens PHH, Ottenheijm HCJ, Rees DC. Solid-phase organic reactions III: a review of the literature Nov 96–Dec 97. Tetrahedron 1998;54:15385–15443.
30. Merritt AT. Solution phase combinatorial chemistry. Comb Chem High Throughput Screening 1998;1:57–72.
31. Houghten RA, Pinilla C, Appel JR, Blondelle SE, Dooley CT, Eichler J, Nefzi A, Ostresh JM. Mixture-based synthetic combinatorial libraries. J Med Chem 1999;42:3743–3778.
32. Dolle RE, Nelson Jr. KH. Comprehensive survey of combinatorial library synthesis: 1998. J Comb Chem 1999;1:235–282.
33. Drewry DH, Coe DM, Poon S. Solid-supported reagents in organic synthesis. Med Res Rev 1999;19:97–148.
34. Hall SE. Recent advances in solid phase synthesis. Mol Diversity 1999;4:131–142.
35. Kobayashi S. New methodologies for the synthesis of compound libraries. Chem Soc Rev 1999;28:1–15.
36. Nuss JM, Renhowe PA. Advances in solid-supported organic synthesis methods, 1998 to 1999. Curr Opin Drug Disc Dev 1999;2:631–650.
37. Coe DM, Storer R. Solution-phase combinatorial chemistry. Mol Diversity 1999;4:31–38.
38. Wentworth Jr. P, Janda KD. Liquid-phase chemistry: recent advances in soluble polymer-supported catalysts, reagents, and synthesis. Chem Commun 1999:1917–1924.
39. Baldino CM. Perspective articles on the utility and application of solution-phase combinatorial chemistry. J Comb Chem 2000;2:89–103.
40. Merrifield RB. Solid-phase peptide synthesis. I. The synthesis of a tetrapeptide. J Am Chem Soc 1963;85:2149–2154.
41. Nestler JP, Bartlett PA, Still WC. A general method for molecular tagging of encoded combinatorial chemistry libraries. J Org Chem 1994;59:4723–4724.
42. Kaiser E, Colescott RL, Bossinger CD, Cook PI. Color test for detection of free terminal amino groups in the solid-phase synthesis of peptides. Anal Biochem 1970;34:595–598.
43. Vojkovsky T. Detection of secondary amines on solid phase. Pept Res 1995;8:236–237.

44. Gallop MA, Fitch WL. New methods for analyzing compounds on polymeric supports. Curr Opin Chem Biol 1997;1:94–100.

45. Yan B. Monitoring the progress and the yield of sold-phase organic reactions directly on resin supports. Acc Chem Res 1998;31:621–630.

46. Fitch WL. Analytical methods for quality control of combinatorial libraries. Mol Diversity 1999;4:39–45.

47. Combs AP, Saubern S, Rafalski M, Lam PYS. Solid supported aryl/heteroaryl C-N cross coupling reaction. Tetrahedron Lett 1999;40:1623–1626.

48. Rafalski M, Saubern S, Lam PYS, Combs AP. Cupric acetate-mediated N-arylation by arylboronic acids: Solid-supported C-N cross-coupling reaction. Book of Abstracts, 218th ACS National Meeting, New Orleans, Aug. 22–26, 1999:ORGN-342.

49. Tadesse S, Rafalski M, Lam PYS, Combs AP. Copper acetate-mediated N-arylation of cyclic and acyclic secondary amines on solid support. Book of Abstracts, 218th ACS National Meeting, New Orleans, Aug. 22–26, 1999:ORGN-343.

50. Combs AP, Rafalski M. N-Arylation of sulfonamides on solid supports. J Comb Chem 2000;2:29–32.

51. Kick EK, Ellman JA. Expedient method for the solid-phase synthesis of aspartic acid protease inhibitors directed toward the generation of libraries. J Med Chem 1995;38:1427–1430.

52. Haque TS, Skillman AG, Lee CE, Habashita H, Gluzman IY, Ewing TJA, Goldberg DE, Kuntz ID, Ellman JA. Potent, low-molecular-weight non-peptide inhibitors of malarial aspartyl protease plasmepsin II. J Med Chem 1999;42:1428–1440.

53. Thompson LA, Moore FL, Moon Y-C, Ellman JA. Solid-phase synthesis of diverse E- and F-series prostaglandins. J Org Chem 1998;63:2066–2067.

54. Lorsbach BA, Kurth MJ. Carbon-carbon bond forming solid-phase reactions. Chem Rev 1999;99:1549–1581.

55. Dax SL, McNally JJ, Youngman MA. Multi-component methodologies in solid-phase organic synthesis. Curr Med Chem 1999;6:255–270.

56. Corbett JW. Recent progress in solid phase heterocycle syntheses. A review. Org Prep Proc Int 1998;30:491–550.

57. Franzén RG. Utilization of Grignard reagents in solid-phase synthesis: a review of the literature. Tetrahedron 2000;56:685–691.

58. Kulkarni BA, Ganesan A. Solid-phase synthesis of β-keto esters via sequential Baylis-Hillman and Heck reactions. J Comb Chem 1999;1:373–378.

59. Nicolaou KC, Winssinger N, Pastor J, Ninkovic S, Sarabia F, He Y, Vourloumis D, Yang Z, Li T, Giannakakou P, Hamel E. Synthesis of epothilones A and B in solid and solution phase. Nature 1997;387:268–272.

60. Peng G, Sohn A, Gallop MA. Stereoselective solid-phase synthesis of a triaza tricyclic ring system: a new chemotype for lead discovery. J Org Chem 1999;64:8342–8349.

61. Lee D, Sello JK, Schreiber SL. A strategy for macrocyclic ring closure and functionalization aimed toward split-pool syntheses. J Am Chem Soc 1999;121:10648–10649.

62. Boeijen A, Kruijtzer JAW, Liskamp RMJ. Combinatorial chemistry of hydantoins. Bioorg Med Chem Lett 1998;8:2375–2380.

63. Shao H, Colucci M, Tong SJ, Zhang HS, Castelhano AL. A practical solid phase synthesis of quinazoline-2,4-diones. Tetrahedron Lett 1998;39:7235–7238.

64. Bhalay G, Blaney P, Palmer VH, Baxter AD. Solid-phase synthesis of diverse tetrahydro-1,4-benzodiazepine-2-ones. Tetrahedron Lett 1997;38:8375–8378.

65. Cuny GD, Cao JR, Hauske JR. Ring opening cross-metathesis on solid support. Tetrahedron Lett 1997;38:5237–5240.

66. Franzén RG. Recent advances in the preparation of heterocycles on solid support: a review of the literature. J Comb Chem 2000;2:195–214.

67. Combs AP. Synthesis and structure–activity relationship analysis of dehydroamino acid derivatives related to the azinomycins. Department of Chemistry, University of California–Los Angeles, 1995.

68. Ugi I. Fast and permanent changes in preparative and pharmaceutical chemistry through multicomponent reactions and their "libraries." Proc Estonian Acad Sci Chem 1995;44:237–273.

69. Armstrong RW, Combs AP, Tempest PA, Brown SD, Keating T. Multiple-component condensation strategies for combinatorial chemistry synthesis. Acc Chem Res 1996;29:123–131.

70. Kiselyov AS, Armstrong RW. Solid support synthesis of tetrahydroquinolines via the Grieco three component condensation. Tetrahedron Lett 1997;38:6163–6166.

71. Harriman GCB. Synthesis of small and medium sized 2, 2-disubstituted lactams via the "intramolecular" three component Ugi reaction. Tetrahedron Lett 1997;38:5591–5594.

72. Mjalli AMM, Sarshar S, Baiga TJ. Solid phase synthesis of pyrroles derived from a four component condensation. Tetrahedron Lett 1996;37:2943–2946.

73. Sarshar S, Siev D, Mjalli AMM. Imidazole libraries on solid support. Tetrahedron Lett 1996;37:835–838.

74. Zhang C, Moran EJ, Woiwode TF, Short KM, Mjalli AMM. Synthesis of tetrasubstituted imidazoles via α-(N-acyl-N-alkylamino)-β-ketoamides on Wang resin. Tetrahedron Lett 1996;37:751–754.

75. Hulme C, Ma L, Romano J, Morrissette M. Remarkable three-step-one-pot solution phase preparation of novel imidazolines utilizing a UDC (Ugi/de-Boc/cyclize) strategy. Tetrahedron Lett 1999;40:7925–7928.

76. Hulme C, Peng J, Louridas B, Menard P, Krolikowski P, Kumar NV. Applications of N-BOC-diamines for the solution phase synthesis of ketopiperazine libraries utilizing a Ugi/de-BOC/cyclization strategy. Tetrahedron Lett 1998;39:8047–8050.

77. Hamuro Y, Scialdone MA, DeGrado WF. Resin-to-resin acyl- and aminoacyl-transfer reactions using oxime supports. J Am Chem Soc 1999;121:1636–1644.

78. Gravel M, Bérubé CD, Hall DG. Resin-to-resin Suzuki coupling of solid supported arylboronic acids. J Comb Chem 2000;2:228–231.

79. Merrifield RB. Solid-phase peptide synthesis (Nobel lecture). Angew Chem Int Ed 1985;24:799–810.

80. Baneyx F. Recombinant protein expression in Escherichia coli. Curr Opin Biotechnol 1999;10:411–421.

81. Liu DR, Magliery TJ, Pasternak M, Schultz PG. Engineering a tRNA and aminoacyl-tRNA synthetase for the site-specific incorporation of unnatural amino acids into proteins in vivo. Proc Natl Acad Sci USA 1997;94:10092–10097.

82. Bodansky M. Peptide Chemistry: A Practical Textbook. New York: Springer-Verlag, 1988.

83. Pennington MW, Dunn BM. Peptide synthesis protocols. In: Walker JM, ed. Methods in Molecular Biology, Vol. 35. Totowa, NJ: Humana Press, 1994.

84. Dooley CT, Ny P, Bidlack JM, Houghten RA. Selective ligands for the μ, δ, and κ opioid receptors identified from a single mixture based tetrapeptide positional scanning combinatorial library. J Biol Chem 1998;273:18848–18856.

85. Stewart JM, Young JD. Solid Phase Peptide Synthesis. Rockford: Pierce Chemical Company, 1984.

86. Marshall WS, Boymel JL. Oligonucleotide synthesis as a tool in drug discovery research. Drug Disc Today 1998;3:34–42.

87. Ito Y, Manabe S. Solid-phase oligosaccharide synthesis and related technologies. Curr Opin Chem Biol 1998;2:701–708.

88. Osborn HMI, Khan TH. Recent developments in polymer supported syntheses of oligosaccharides and glycopeptides. Tetrahedron 1999;55:1807–1850.

89. Seeberger PH, Haase W-C. Solid-phase oligosaccharide synthesis and combinatorial carbohydrate libraries. Chem Rev 2000;100:4349–4393.

90. Arsequell G, Valencia G. Recent advances in the synthesis of complex N-glycopeptides. Tetrahedron: Asymmetry 1999;10:3045–2094.

91. Hojo H, Nakahara Y. Recent progress in the solid-phase synthesis of glycopeptides. Curr Protein Pept Sci 2000;1:23–48.

92. Zheng C, Seeberger PH, Danishefsky SJ. Solid support oligosaccharide synthesis: construction of β-linked oligosaccharides by coupling of glycal derived thioethyl glycosyl donors. J Org Chem 1998;63:1126–1130.

93. Nielsen PE, Egholm M, Berg RH, Buchardt O. Sequence-selective recognition of DNA by strand displacement with a thymine-substituted polyamide. Science 1991;254:1497–1500.

94. Egholm M, Buchardt O, Nielsen PE, Berg RH. Peptide nucleic acids (PNA). Oligonucleotide analogues with an achiral peptide backbone. J Am Chem Soc 1992;114:1895–1897.

95. Nielsen PE. Peptide nucleic acid. A molecule with two identities. Acc Chem Res 1999;32:624–630.

96. Dean DA. Peptide nucleic acids: versatile tools for gene therapy strategies. Adv Drug Deliv Rev 2000;44:81–95.

97. Smith AB, III, Keenan TP, Holcomb RC, Sprengeler PA, Guzman MC, Wood JL, Carroll PJ, Hirschmann R. Design, synthesis, and crystal structure of a pyrrolinone-based peptidomimetic possessing the conformation of a β-strand: potential application to the design of novel inhibitors of proteolytic enzymes. J Am Chem Soc 1992;114:10672–10674.

98. Hagihara M, Anthony NJ, Stout TJ, Clardy J, Schreiber SL. Vinylogous polypeptides: an alternative peptide backbone. J Am Chem Soc 1992;114:6568–6570.

99. Gennari C, Salom B, Potenza D, Williams A. Synthesis of sulfonamido-pseudopeptides: new chiral unnatural oligomers. Angew Chem Int Ed Engl 1994;33:2067–2069.

100. Hamuro Y, Geib SJ, Hamilton AD. Novel molecular scaffolds: formation of helical secondary structure in a family of oligoanthranilamides. Angew Chem Int Ed Engl 1994;33:446–448.

101. Moree WJ, van der Marel GA, Liskamp RJ. Synthesis of peptidosulfinamides and peptidosulfonamides: peptidomimetics containing the sulfinamide or sulfonamide transition-state isostere. J Org Chem 1995;60:5157–5169.

102. Paikoff SJ, Wilson TE, Cho CY, Schultz PG. The solid phase synthesis of N-alkyl-carbamate oligomers. Tetrahedron Lett 1996;37:5653–5656.

103. Soth MJ, Nowick JS. Unnatural oligomers and unnatural oligomer libraries. Curr Opin Chem Biol 1997;1:120–129.

104. Hamper BC, Kolodziej SA, Scates AM, Smith RG, Cortez E. Solid phase synthesis of β-peptoids: N-substituted β-aminopropionic acid oligomers. J Org Chem 1998;63:708–718.

105. Appella DH, Christianson LA, Karle IL, Powell DR, Gellman SH. Synthesis and characterization of trans-2-aminocyclohexanecarboxylic acid oligomers: an unnatural helical secondary structure and implications for β-peptide tertiary structure. J Am Chem Soc 1999;121:6206–6212.

106. Bunin BA, Plunkett MJ, Ellman JA. The combinatorial synthesis and chemical and biological evaluation of a 1, 4-benzodiazepine library. Proc Natl Acad Sci USA 1994;91:4708–4712.

107. DeWitt SH, Czarnik AW. Combinatorial organic synthesis using Parke-Davis's Diversomer method. Acc Chem Res 1996;29:114–122.

108. MacDonald AA, DeWitt SH, Hogan EM, Ramage R. A solid phase approach to quinolones using the Diversomer technology. Tetrahedron Lett 1996;37:4815–4818.

109. Ostresh JM, Schoner CC, Hamashin VT, Nefzi A, Meyer J-P, Houghten RA. Solid-phase synthesis of trisubstituted bicyclic guanidines via cyclisation of reduced N-acylated dipeptides. J Org Chem 1998;63:8622–8623.

110. Morales GA, Corbett JW, DeGrado WF. Solid-phase synthesis of benzopiperazi-nones. J Org Chem 1998;63:1172–1177.

111. Vojkovský T, Weichsel A, Pátek M. Solid-phase synthesis of heterocycles containing an 1-acyl-3-oxopiperazine skeleton. J Org Chem 1998;63:3162–3163.

112. Dragoli DR, Thompson LA, O'Brien J, Ellman JA. Parallel synthesis of prostaglandin E_1 analogues. J Comb Chem 1999;1:534–539.

113. Wessjohann LA. Synthesis of natural-product-based compound libraries. Curr Opin Chem Biol 2000;4:303–309.

114. Wang H, Ganesan A. Total synthesis of the fumiquinazoline alkaloids: solid-phase studies. J Comb Chem 2000;2:186–194.

115. Meseguer B, Alonso-Diáz D, Griebenow N, Herget T, Waldmann H. Natural product synthesis on polymeric supports: synthesis and biological evaluation of an indolactam library. Angew Chem Int Ed 1999;38:2902–2906.

116. Tan DS, Foley MA, Shair MD, Schreiber SL. Stereoselective synthesis of over two million compounds having structural features both reminiscent of natural products and compatible with minaturized cell-based assays. J Am Chem Soc 1998;120:8565–8566.

117. Lindsley CW, Chan LK, Goess BC, Joseph R, Shair MD. Solid-phase biomimetic synthesis of carpanone-like molecules. J Am Chem Soc 2000; 122:422–423.

118. Curran DP. Parallel synthesis with fluorous reagents and reactants. Med Res Rev 1999;19:432–438.

119. Kim RM, Manna M, Hutchins SM, Griffin PR, Yates NA, Bernick AM, Chapman

KT. Dendrimer-supported combinatorial chemistry. Proc Natl Acad Sci USA 1996;93:10012–10017.

120. Kaldor SW, Siegel MG, Fritz JE, Dressman BA, Hahn PJ. Use of solid supported nucleophiles and electrophiles for the purification of non-peptide small molecule libraries. Tetrahedron Lett 1996;37:7193–7196.

121. Flynn DL, Crich JZ, Devraj RV, Hockerman SL, Parlow JJ, South MS, Woodard S. Chemical library purification strategies based on principles of complementary molecular reactivity and molecular recognition. J Am Chem Soc 1997;119: 4874–4881.

122. Parlow JJ, Devraj RV, South MS. Solution-phase chemical library synthesis using polymer-assisted purification techniques. Curr Opin Chem Biology 1999;3:320–336.

123. Thompson LA. Recent applications of polymer-supported reagents and scavengers in combinatorial, parallel, or multistep synthesis. Curr Oping Chem Biol 2000;4: 324–337.

124. Booth RJ, Hodges JC. Solid-supported reagent strategies for rapid purification of combinatorial synthesis products. Acc Chem Res 1999;32:18–26.

125. Sucholeiki I, Perez JM. New high loading paramagnetic support for solid phase organic chemistry. Tetrahedron Lett 1999;40:3531–3534.

126. Parlow JJ, Case BL, Dice TA, South MS. High-throughput purification of solution-phase periodinane-mediated oxidation reactions utilizing a novel thiosulfate resin. Book of Abstracts, 218th ACS National Meeting, New Orleans, Aug 22–26, 1999:ORGN-424.

127. Parlow JJ, Naing W, South MS, Flynn DL. In situ chemical tagging: tetrafluorophthalic anhydride as a "Sequestration Enabling Reagent" (SER) in the purification of solution-phase combinatorial libraries. Tetrahedron Lett 1997;38:7959–7962.

128. Thompson LA, Combs AP, L. Trainor G, Wang Q, Langlois TJ, Kirkland JJ. Functionalized porous silica microspheres as scavengers in parallel synthesis. Combi Chem High Throughput Screening 2000;3:107–115.

129. Adamczyk M, Fishpaugh JR, Mattingly PG. Preparation and use of N-hydroxysuccinimidyl active ester resins. Tetrahedron Lett 1999;40:463–466.

130. Salvino JM, Groneberg RD, Airey JE, Poli GB, McGeehan GM, Labaudiniere RF, Clerc F-f, Bezard DNA. Fluorophenyl resin compounds. Vol. 99/67288 A1. WO, 1999:113.

131. Drew M, Orton E, Krolikowski P, Salvino JM, Kumar NV. A method for quantitation of solid-phase synthesis using ^{19}F NMR spectroscopy. J Comb Chem 2000;2: 8–9.

132. Hahn H-G, Kee HC, Kee DN, Bae SY, Mah H. Synthesis of trifluoromethylated dihydro-1,4-oxathiin-3-carboxanilides through polymer-bound activated ester. Heterocycles 1998;48:2253–2261.

133. Smith RA, Bobko MA, Lee W. Solid-phase synthesis of a library of piperazinediones and diazepinediones via Kaiser oxime resin. BioMed Chem Lett 1998;8: 2369–2374.

134. Chang Y-T, Schultz PG. Versatile fluorescence labeling method using activated esters on solid support. BioMed Chem Lett 1999;9:2479–2482.

135. Kenner GW, McDermott JR, Sheppard RC. The safety catch principle in solid phase peptide synthesis. Chem Commun 1971:636–637.

136. Backes BJ, Virgilio AA, Ellman JA. Enhanced activation of Kenner's safety-catch linker: applications to solid-phase synthesis. J Am Chem Soc 1996;118:3055–3056.
137. Backes BJ, Ellman JA. An alkanesulfonamide "safety-catch" linker of solid-phase synthesis. J Org Chem 1999;64:2322–2330.
138. Scialdone MA, Shuey SW, Soper P, Hamuro Y, Burns DM. Phosgenated p-nitro-phenyl(polystyrene)ketoxime or Phoxime resin. A new resin for the solid-phase synthesis of ureas via thermolytic cleavage of oxime-carbamates. J Org Chem 1998;63:4802–4807.
139. Katritzky AR, Belyakov SA, Tymoshenko DO. Preparation of polymer-bound 1H-benzotriazole, a new potential scaffold for the compilation of organic molecule libraries. J Comb Chem 1999;1:173–176.
140. Smith EM. A polymer-supported silyl triflate and subsequent functionalization: synthesis and solid-phase Diels-Alder reactions of silyloxydienes. Tetrahedron Lett 1999;40:3285–3288.
141. Hu Y, Porco JA, Jr. Ester enolate Claisen rearrangement using a polymer-supported silyl triflate. Tetrahedron Lett 1999;40:3289–3292.
142. Caldarelli M, Habermann J, Ley SV. Synthesis of an array of potential matrix metalloproteinase inhibitors using a sequence of polymer-supported reagents. Bioorg Med Chem Lett 1999;9:2049–2052.
143. Ley SV, Schucht O, Thomas AW, Murray PJ. Synthesis of the alkaloids (±)-oxo-maritidine and (±)-epimaritidine using an orchestrated multi-step sequence of polymer supported reagents. J Chem Soc, Perkin Trans 1 1999:1251–1252.
144. Habermann J, Ley SV, Scott JS. Synthesis of the potent analgesic compound (±)-epibatidine using an orchestrated multi-step sequence of polymer supported reagents. J Chem Soc, Perkin Trans 1 1999:1253–1256.

18
Supports for Solid-Phase Synthesis

Christophe Fromont
Ribo Targets Ltd.
Cambridge, United Kingdom

Vincent Pomel
Serono Pharmaceutical Research Institute
Grand-Lancy, Switzerland

Mark Bradley
University of Southampton
Southampton, United Kingdom

Since the introduction by Merrifield of support-based peptide synthesis [1], insoluble polymer supports have been widely used for numerous synthetic processes to accelerate synthesis and product purification [2,3]. The original small-molecule solid-phase efforts by Leznoff [4], and more recent efforts, have demonstrated the synthetic advantages of solid-phase methods and have lead to solid-phase chemistry now playing a substantial role within most pharmaceutical companies, in part due to the ease of automation but also due to the inherent advantages of solid-phase chemistry. The increasing familiarity of synthetic chemists with solid-phase synthesis has led research groups to investigate a wide variety of supports in combinatorial synthesis [5,6]. The main purpose of this chapter is to review the different types of supports used in solid-phase synthesis, a crucial issue if any synthesis is ever to be successful and an area often ignored in a solid-phase campaign.

   The recent activity in solid-phase organic chemistry has focused almost entirely on gel-type resins due to their prior impact in solid-phase peptide synthesis. However, the more diverse chemistry that must be achieved nowadays has persuaded many groups and companies to investigate a wider range of solid supports compatible with different reaction conditions. Automation within pharmaceutical companies is also an issue in combinatorial chemistry in so far as solid-phase supports must be developed to facilitate automation and handling issues.

I. RESIN BEADS

A. Polystyrene Gel–Based Resins

In practice, gel-based, spherical resin beads of 50–200 μm diameter are commonly used in solid-phase organic chemistry (SPOC). These can be easily synthesized or bought from a range of commercial suppliers. The size, shape, and uniformity are important features, and the uniformity of cross-linked polymer particles is vital for reproducible SPOC. Robust spherical beads with a uniform size are preferred for reproducible chemistry, with irregularly shape particles being much more sensitive to mechanical destruction, often falling apart in the course of the chemistry. Bead size is also important since reaction rates are inversely proportional to bead size. The technique of suspension polymerization is almost universally used for resin synthesis and provides regular particles in a highly reproducible manner. Typically, styrene and divinylbenzene (DVB) mixtures are dispersed as spherical droplets in an excess of an immiscible phase (water) containing the polymerization initiator. The aqueous phase generally contains a low level of some dissolved suspension stabilizer, a surface-active species, which prevents the organic monomer droplets from conglomerating. In the course of the polymerization, these droplets are converted to the hard glassy beads. Then the resin particles can be collected by filtration; unreacted monomers, initiator, and other byproducts removed by solvent extraction; and the beads vacuum dried and sieved. The introduction of functionality onto a polymer support is usually achieved by direct chloromethylation to give the classical Merrifield resin. However, an alternative approach is to use a co-monomer that already bears the desired functionality in the free polymerization mixture or some precursor that can subsequently be transformed. This second strategy can be useful in producing a structurally well-defined resin network with control of functional group ratios (Fig. 1). So-called Merrifield resin and related PS-based analogues (e.g., aminomethyl resin) are the most widely used resins in SPOS today. They are characterized as being a gel-type polymer typically containing 1–2% cross-linking agent DVB which provides the links between the linear PS chains, with the whole polymer solvated and with reactions taking place throughout the polymer network, controlled by diffusion into the bead.

The percentage of DVB used in bead synthesis is very important for the mechanical strength and insolubility of the support but should not prevent the swelling of the resin beads when immersed in an organic solvent. Indeed, swelling is an essential feature of gel resins. At low cross-linkings, sufficient swelling occurs in so-called good solvents to allow the diffusion of reagents within the PS network. Merrifield resin swells in solvents with a solubility parameter similar to the polymer, e.g., toluene, with swelling inversely related to the ratio of DVB. On

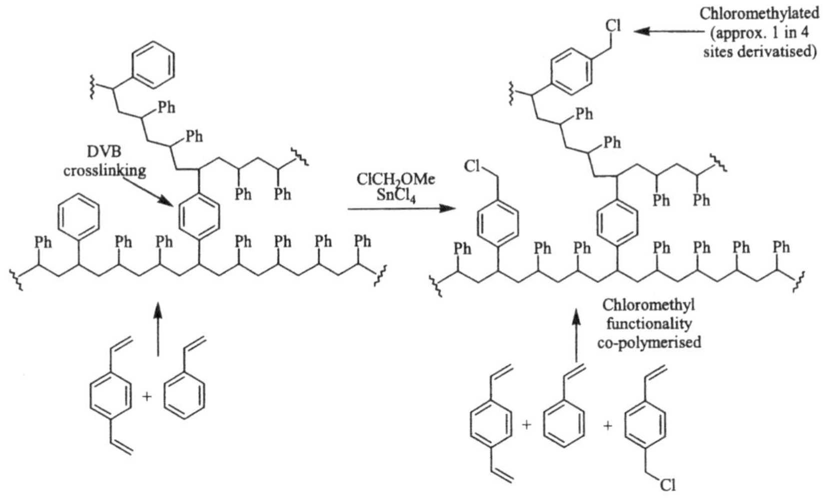

Figure 1 Synthesis of DVB-cross-linked PS resins and derivatization.

the other hand, Merrifield resins are not compatible with highly polar solvents such as water and methanol. The swelling and shrinking process always occurs from the outside to the inside of the resin network; thus, very low levels of DVB (< 1%) give mechanically weak networks that can be damaged by heating, handling, or solvent shock. On the other hand, highly cross-linked resin network may not swell even in a "good swelling solvent" but clearly will offer much greater mechanically stability. If a polystyrene network is fully swollen in a so-called good solvent and then shrunk in a bad solvent, e.g., during resin washing steps, mechanical shock takes place and the bead may disintegrate. This effect (osmotic shock) [6] and the degree of cross-linking must thus be considered in any solid-phase synthesis where many cycles of swelling and deswelling may be involved to reduce mechanical damage to the beads. Besides osmotic shock, PS supports have limitations when used with highly electrophilic reagents and at excessive temperatures (200°C). Impurities from commercially available Merrifield resin can arise from incomplete polymerization and/or from trapped solvents, which contaminate the final products or decrease the actual loading. It should also be borne in mind that very high levels of initiator (sometimes 5%!) are used in bead synthesis, which depending on the initiator used will undoubtedly have an influence on bead structure and chemistry. Although various methods have been investigated [7] to overcome the resin-based impurities, such as prewashing of resin beads, the main method appears to be based on final library purification as being the best way to readily remove impurities from library compounds, although perhaps not ideal [8].

B. Macroporous Resins

Macroporous resins have been used for many years in ion exchange applications, as polymeric adsorbents and for reverse-phase chromatography purifications. Macroporous resins are defined as a class of resin having a permanent well-developed porous structure even in the dry state (if they survive in this form). These resins are typically prepared by suspension polymerization of Styrene-DVB mixtures containing a porogen or diluent (an organic solvent in general) at a well-defined ratio providing resin beads with a defined pore structure. Removal of the porogen at the end of the polymerization provides a heterogeneous PS matrix with some areas completely impenetrable and others free of polymer. Macroporous resins are characterized by a hard, rough surface having a defined total surface area. Unlike Merrifield resin, these materials do not need to swell to allow access of reagents through the PS network as they possess a permanent porous structure that can be accessed by essentially all solvents; even solvents such as water can penetrate the macroporous PS-DVB matrix. When a solvent penetrates a macroporous resin, the polymer matrix tends to swell to some extent and often rapidly because the permanent holes provide rapid access through the network. However, due to the nature of the beads swelling takes place in the pores and little swelling of the beads takes place. Due to the nature and speed of diffusion, macroporous resins show much better resistance to osmotic shock during swelling and deswelling processes.

Comparisons between macroporous resins and a 2% cross-linked gel-based Merrifield resin have been undertaken [9]. Resin washing efficiency is, not unexpectedly, much more efficient with macroporous resins due to the rigid pores speeding up migration of material from the interior of the polymer to the bulk solvent. The kinetics for esterification between standard Merrifield resin and three macroporous resins from Rohm & Haas are shown in Table 1. This seems to show that more sites are more accessible in the gel-based resins, while reaction rates are comparable. However, since reaction rates are bead size dependent for the gel-based resins, it is hard to draw any real conclusions from these data.

Table 1 Kinetics for Esterification between Standard Merrifield Resin and Three Macroporous Resins

Resin (%) (48 h = 100%)	Loading (mmol/g)			Relative loadings	
	t = 4h	t = 20h	t = 48h	t = 4h	t = 20h
XAD 16	0.09	0.46	0.62	14	74
XAD 2010	0.16	0.54	0.61	26	88
XAD 1180	0.14	0.47	0.55	25	85
PS-CM (1%)	0.23	0.71	1.14	20	62

C. Poly(ethylene glycol)–Containing Resins

The development of polymer supports having both polar and nonpolar features has been of great interest for peptide synthesis. Although Merrifield resin has been widely used in solid-phase peptide synthesis (SPPS), the rate of incorporation of particular amino acid residues was found to decrease with increasing chain length. This decrease in yield was thought to be due to the unfavorable conformation adopted by the growing peptide chain and peptide aggregation. Thus to improve the physicochemical compatibility of PS supports, polar hydrophilic acrylamide-based copolymers were introduced as an attractive alternative to all PS-DVB supports, most notably by Atherton and Sheppard [10]. However, an alternative approach, which leads to the second most popular support type in solid-phase chemistry, after the PS gel–based resins, is modification of PS resin by the addition of PEG to generate PS-PEG-based materials. These hydrophilic solid supports were developed in theory to remove the reaction sites from the bulk "rigid" PS matrix to give a more solution-like environment as well as to broaden the solvent compatibilities of the support. However, another driving force was the need to prepare a solid support for continuous solid-flow solid phase peptide synthesis, which did not undergo dramatic volume changes during synthesis and arose at least in part from the early soluble PEG-based chemistries in the 1970s and 1980s. Various popular poly(ethyleneglycol)–containing synthetic polymers as solid supports are summarized in Table 2.

Table 2 Some Poly(ethyleneglycol)–Containing Resins

Support	Description
Grafted PS-PEG	
PS PEG [11]	Preformed PEG covalently attached onto the PS. Chemistry takes place on the end of the PEG.
TentaGel [12]	PEG polymerised onto 1% cross-linked hydroxymethyl-poly(styrene-*co*-divinylbenzene) resin beads.
ArgoGel [13]	PEG polymerized onto a malonate-derived 1,3-dihydroxy-2-methylpropane poly(styrene-*co*-divinylbenzene) resin beads.
NovaGel [14]	Methyl-PEG coupled onto 25% of resin sites. Chemistry takes place on the PS, not on the end of the PEG.
Copolymers	
PEGA [15]	Poly(dimethylacrylamide-*co*-bis-acrylamido-PEG)-*co*-monoacrylamido PEG.
TTEGDA-PS [16]	Poly(styrene-*co*-tetra(ethylene glycol)diacrylate).
CLEAR [17]	Poly(trimethylolpropane ethoxylate triacrylate-*co*-allylamine).

1. PS-PEG Supports

A preliminary approach to the synthesis of PS-PEG supports relied on covalent anchoring via amide linkages of defined PEGs onto amino-functionalized PS resins [11]. Later, a new version of PS-PEG was introduced by Bayer and Rapp [12], obtained by ethylene oxide grafting to give the material now known as TentaGel (Fig. 2). Optimized TentaGel grafted resins generally have PEG chains of about 3 kDa ($n = 68$ units; 70–80% by weight). PS-PEG beads display uniform swelling properties in a variety of solvents from medium- to high-polar media ranging from toluene to water.

The solution-like environment has an impact on reaction kinetics, allowing rapid access of reagents through the swollen resin to active sites. Rapp [18] has demonstrated that the kinetics of certain reactions on PS-PEG beads were similar to those in solution. However, TentaGel resin is far from being the perfect solid support due to (1) low loading capacity, (2) Lewis acid complexation onto the PEG chain, and (3) instability of the PEG chain to acidic media generating PEG contamination after TFA cleavage. To overcome these problems new families of PS-PEG resins with higher loading capacities, good acid stabilities, and low linear PEG impurities have been developed [13]. Thus, assuming that the acid instability of TentaGel resin was due to the benzylic ether PS-graft linkage, improved stability was obtained by using a longer linkage, while improved loading capacity has been obtained via bifurcation of functional groups prior to ethylene oxide grafting (Fig. 2) and reduced PEG graftings.

It is worth noticing that at the end of the polymerization material must be contaminated by linear or cyclic PEG, and this removal may be the source of repeated claims of contamination. A series of graft copolymers have been elaborated by varying the ethylene oxide/initiator ratio, providing well-defined graft lengths with predictable loadings (0.3–0.55 mmol/g). Some swelling properties of PS and PS-PEG resins are summarized in Table 3.

2. CLEAR Resins

CLEAR resins (cross-linked ethoxylate acrylate resin), introduced by Barany [17], are a unique family of supports that are highly cross-linked polymers (>95%

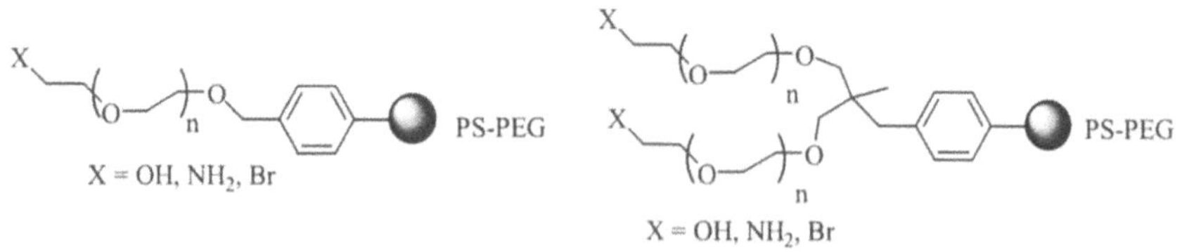

Figure 2 The two main PS-PEG supports used in solid-phase synthesis.

Table 3 Swelling Properties of PS and PS-PEG (ml/g)

Solvent	Water	THF	DCM	DMF	MeOH
PS-NH$_2$[a]	8.0	8.9	8.0	2.8	2.1
TentaGel-NH$_2$[b]	3.9	5.5	4.0	3.0	3.0
ArgoGel-NH$_2$[c]	6.4	8.6	5.0	4.9	4.0

[a]Obtained from Bachem.
[b]Obtained from Rapp Polymer.
[c]Obtained from Argonaut Technologies.

by weight of cross-linker) yet show excellent swelling properties, contrary to the general expectation of the time. These supports are prepared by radical polymerization of the tribranched cross-linker trimethylolpropaneethoxylate-triacrylate (1), with various amino-functionalized monomers, such as allylamine (2), or 2-aminoethyl methacrylate (3) (Fig. 3). The CLEAR supports differ from other polymers in that they are synthesized from a branched cross-linker used in a high molar ratio. The fact that the amino functionality can be introduced into the bead in the polymerization process ensures that the required substitution level can be obtained.

A number of different formulations were tested and prepared by bulk suspension to give the optimal material. These supports swell in a wide range of hydrophobic and hydrophilic solvents, such as water. Although these materials showed great chemical and mechanical stability in acidic and weakly basic conditions, the resins will dissolve in the presence of ammonia or aqueous bases due to the ammonolysis of the three ester linkages in the cross-linker.

3. Tetraethylene Glycol Diacrylate Cross-linked Polystyrene Support (TTEGDA-PS)

A number of groups [16,19] have developed resins based on varying the cross-linker to change the properties of the resin but maintaining the excellent chemical

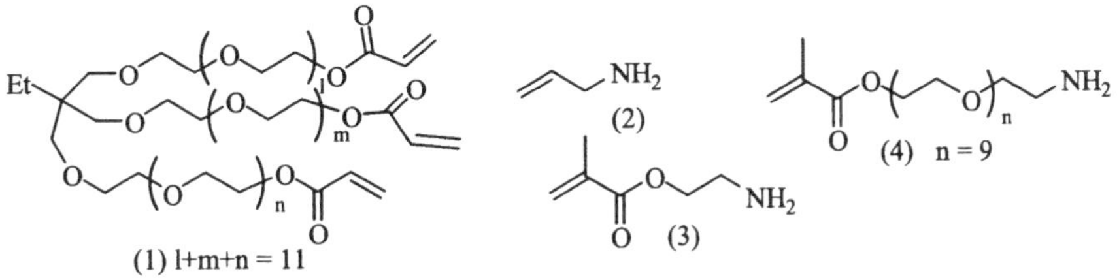

Figure 3 Monomers used in the highly cross-linked yet highly swelling CLEAR resins.

nature of the PS support. Pillai [16] investigated the use of polyacrylamide (PA) and PS supports cross-linked with *N,N*-methylenebisacrylamide (NNMBA), tetraethylene glycol diacrylate (TTEGDA), and DVB. It was shown that the polymer derived from TTEGDA-PA had a significant increase in reaction kinetics when compared with NNMBA-PA and DVB-PA supports. Gel-phase reaction kinetics with PA-DVB supports showed that the first 90% reaction sites were homogeneously distributed throughout the bead and had equal reactivity, while the remaining 10% were less available to external reagents. The major problems with PA supports is the lack of mechanical stability when compared to PS and chemical reactivity when used in an organic chemistry sense, although there is an optimal hydrophobic–hydrophilic balance. TTEGDA-PS provides these two essential features in a single matrix with a hydrophobic PS backbone and a flexible hydrophilic cross-linker (TTEGDA) [16], thus being insoluble but highly solvated. PS supports with 4% TTEGDA (Fig. 4) show good mechanical properties

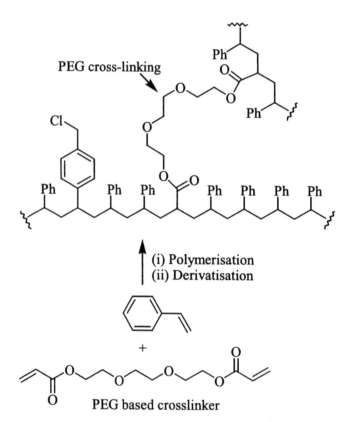

Figure 4   Hydrid PS- and PEG-based resins via PEG-based cross-linkers.

but with good swelling characteristics, rendering this support suitable for long-chain peptide synthesis.

As mentioned earlier, the swelling properties of a solid support are a crucial feature in SPS and a measure of the scope of a new support. The difference between 1% DVB-PS and 4% TTEGDA-PS was investigated. As expected, TTEGDA-cross-linked PS had enhanced swelling properties in polar solvents compared with DVB-PS support (Table 4) which renders maximal accessibility of reagents throughout the hydrophobic network.

4. PEGA (Polyethylene glycol-poly-(*N*,*N*-dimethylacrylamide) Copolymer

Polar acrylamide supports were introduced successfully by Sheppard [10] and coworkers as an alternative to polystyrene resin and used as a versatile cross-linked support for peptide syntheses. Meldal [15] introduced PEGA, a similar resin that contains a PEG component. PEGA is superior to many other existing supports for peptide synthesis in terms of the solution-like nature of the structure, although it is associated with handling problems and lacks chemical inertness. The PEG chain is the major constituent providing a highly flexible and biocompatible matrix. The polymer backbone was designed to allow macromolecules, such as enzymes, to penetrate the polymer network thereby facilitating solid-phase enzymatic reactions.

Typically, preparation of PEGA resins is carried out by an inverse suspension polymerization reaction in a mixture of *n*-heptane and carbon tetrachloride (6:4 v/v) due to the water solubility of the monomers (Fig. 5). Meldal and coworkers anticipated that PEGA 1900 ($n = 45$) had pores large enough to allow enzymes up to 50 kDa to penetrate the PEGA network [20]. In order to identify new enzyme inhibitors for matrix metalloproteinase 9 (MMP-9), which in its proform has a molecular weight of 92 kDa, longer cross-linked PEGs were used (4000–8000 Da,

Table 4 Comparison of DVB-PS and TTEGD-PS Swelling Properties (ml/g)

Solvent	1% DVB-PS	4% TTEGDA-PS
Chloroform	4.3	6.5
Tetrahydrofuran	5.2	8.7
Toluene	4.7	6.9
Pyridine	4.2	6.0
Dioxane	3.5	8.8
Dichloromethane	4.3	8.8
DMF	2.8	5.5
Methanol	1.8	2.2

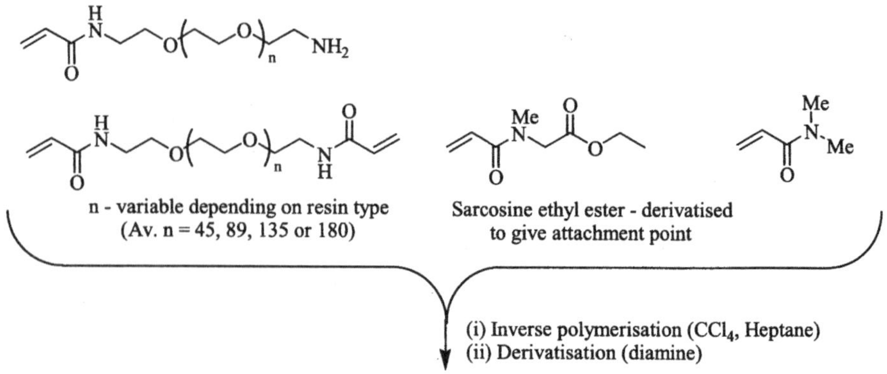

Figure 5   Monomers used for PEGA resin synthesis.

$n = 89, 135, 180$) were developed to increase the apparent "pore size" of these supports. Bisamino-PEGs were used to form partially or bis-*N*-acryloylated PEG as a macromonomer. These resins have high swelling properties and are suited for enzyme reactions despite initially low loading capacities (0.08–0.13 mmol/g). Introduction of acryloyl sarcosin with the bisacrylamido-PEG-1900, 4000, 6000, 8000, and dimethylacrylamide resulted in PEGA copolymer–type resins with a much higher loading capacity.

5. Enhancing Bead Loading: Dendrimers as Powerful Enhances of Functionality

One of the most powerful tools available to the combinatorial chemist is the process of split and mix in terms of the numbers of compounds that can be made and the economics of synthesis, with resin beads being used as the ultimate microreactor in synthesis. However, this method results in tiny amounts of compound being available with less than 1 nmol bead typically being available. This might be enough to identify an active bead, but it is not enough to conduct numerous biological assays or to validate the compound as a lead. More importantly, it is insufficient to determine the compound's structure using conventional techniques such as ^{1}H nuclear magnetic resonance (NMR). Such a low loading requires a tagging system to identify the compound and necessitates resynthesis on a larger scale either in solution or on the solid phase for rescreening. However, though elegant the introduction of a tag during the library synthesis is very time consuming. One solution to this problem is to increase the size of the beads. A larger bead will obviously bear more sites, although size is limited by bead stability, susceptibility to fracturing, and bead synthesis as well as poor reaction kinetics. Another approach is to multiply the functionalities on a bead by dendrimerization, using the hyperbranched nature of the dendrimer to amplify loading. Solid-phase lysine-based dendrimers were published by Tam [21] as a means of generating a high density of peptide functionality for antigen presentation (multiple antigen presentation system; MAPS), but resins with low loading were deliberately used to avoid possible steric problems. However, the development of solid-phase PAMAM dendrimers has provided a powerful tool to increase the loading of single beads [22]. The development of highly symmetrical dendrimers allows an extremely high loading to be obtained on the resin beads.

The efficiency of synthesis for the PAMAM dendrimers (Michael addition onto methyl acetate and ester displacement with a diamine) is achieved by using large excess of reagent compared to the loading of the resin as in any normal solid-phase synthesis and produces dendrimers cleaner than those from the solution approach. The multiplication of the terminal amino functionalities makes possible the analysis of compound cleaved from single beads [23]. Using a Tris-based monomer [24], a loading of 230 nmol per bead was obtained for a generation 2 dendrimer, which becomes a very acceptable loading for using the beads in a split-and-

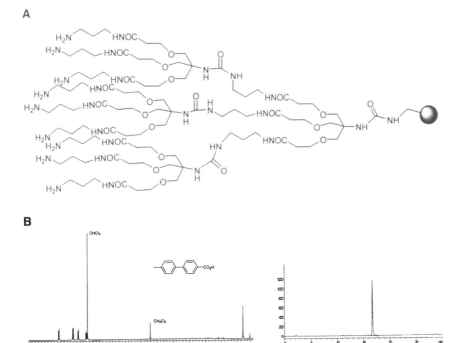

Figure 6 (**A**) Resin amplification via dendrimerization. (**B**) Single-bead cleavage analysis.

mix manner (Fig. 6). The NMR spectrum and high-performance liquid chromatography (HPLC) data of material from one bead are shown. This is the Suzuki product formed between 4-methylphenylboronic acid and resin-attached 4-iodobenzoic acid. Using this method, dendrimers have been synthesized on a range of other solid supports, either to be used as such or to modify the surface properties of the support.

II. SYNTHESIS ON SURFACES

A. Pins and Crowns

The limitations of linear "solitary" peptide synthesis were first overcome by Houghten [25] with the use of tea-bag methodology and Geysen with "pin" methodology [26]. The pin method was a revolutionary approach to peptide synthesis and moved away from traditional PS-based resins, allowing the synthesis of peptides on the surface of polyethylene (PE) supports [rod-like materials termed pins (4 mm diameter × 40 mm)] in a multiple parallel manner. These derivatized materials were prepared by radiation grafting in which the pins were placed in a γ-radiation source in the presence of an aqueous solution of acrylic acid. Radiation (initially 1 million rad) activated the surface by radical formation to a depth of several micrometers, which reacted with the acrylic acid to give rise to a polyacrylic

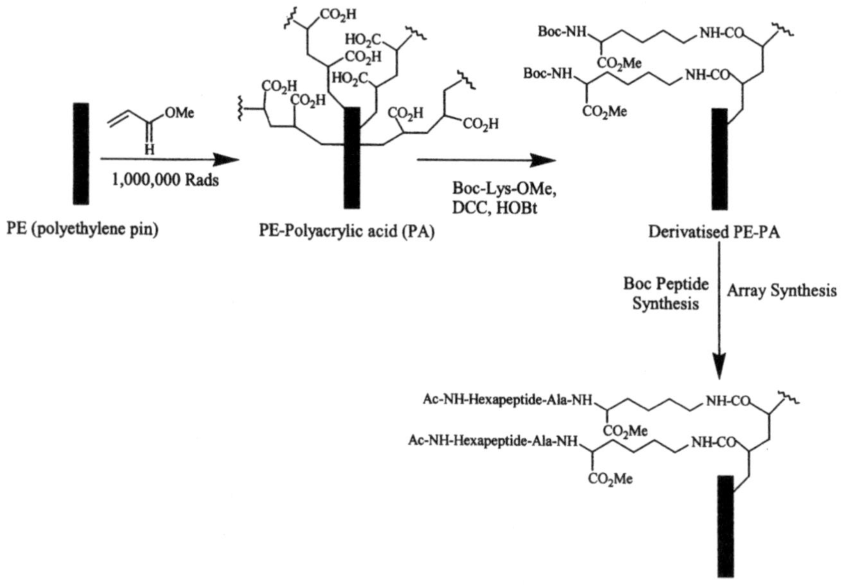

Figure 7 Initial method used for pin derivatization.

acid derivatized pin (Fig. 7). It was this (immobilized) graft that could then be used as a support for peptide synthesis, initially by coupling to a suitably protected lysine residue (Boc-Lys-OMe). Due to the discrete and handlable nature of the pins they could be arranged in an array format akin to the microtiter plates used for biological screening with synthesis taking place by dipping the tips of the pins into the appropriate solutions. Although the whole pin was derivatized, only the tip was actually used synthetically. The major problems were thus logistical, due to compound numbers, rather than chemical. This basic procedure allowed the synthesis in 1984 of 208 overlapping peptides covering the entire peptide sequence of the coat protein VP1 of foot-and-mouth disease virus (FMDV). This was accomplished using Boc chemistry with the peptide directly attached to the pin as shown in Figure 7. Two assumptions made by the authors in this original work were that an initial loading of at least 1 nmol would be sufficient for even a low-efficiency synthesis to allow antibody binding and that high purity was not necessary.

Developments and improvements on this original method took place at the end of the 1980s and in the 1990s, with three main driving forces: (1) development of linkers to allow cleavage from the pins [27]; (2) an improvement in their loading [28]; and (3) alterations in the grafting polymer to alter the physical and accessibility properties of the graft [29] (Fig. 8). Thus, in 1990 and 1991 derivatization of the pin by acrylic acid was followed by saturation coupling with Boc-1,6-diaminohexane and coupling to the most accessible sites with a limited amount of Fmoc-β-Ala-OH followed by capping of the remaining sites to give a loading of 10–100 nmol per pin [30]. Linkers could then be added to the derivatized pins. The first approach was to use DKP formation as a driving force for peptide release

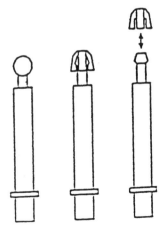

Figure 8   Radiation-grafted materials: Chiron crowns and removable pin heads. (From Ref. 29, reproduced with permission.)

allowing a "safety catch"–based cleavage from the solid support. The second method used hydroxymethylbenzoic acid as a linker, which allowed the peptide to be subsequently cleaved from the pin with ammonia vapor [31]. Both methods allowed release and analysis of peptides by HPLC and MS.

Subsequent developments led to the removable crown (although confusingly also called pins or detachable pinheads in the literature) (Fig. 8) [32]. Crowns were prepared by injection molding of granular polyethylene. They were 5.5 mm high and 5.3 mm in diameter, but importantly had a surface area of 1.3 cm^2, much improved over that of the pins. The second improvement involved the use of alternative monomers (Fig. 9). Variations in the vinylic monomer allowed alterations in the properties of the graft. Thus, changing from acrylic acid to hydroxyethyl methacrylate (HEMA) allowed much higher grafts weights to be obtained (graft weight increased from 1% to 15%) [32]. Thus, these materials could be esterified under normal DCC/DMAP coupling conditions with Fmoc-β-Ala-OH and controlled reaction timings, allowing only the most reactive/accessible sites to be derivatized before the capping of all remaining sites. This procedure allowed crowns with loadings of 1.0–2.2 μmol per crown to be prepared for solid-phase peptide synthesis. Later papers used a variety of monomers, including methacrylic acid and dimethylacrylamide [31], while PS grafts also became available. The crowns/pins thus became available with aminomethyl-PS functionali-

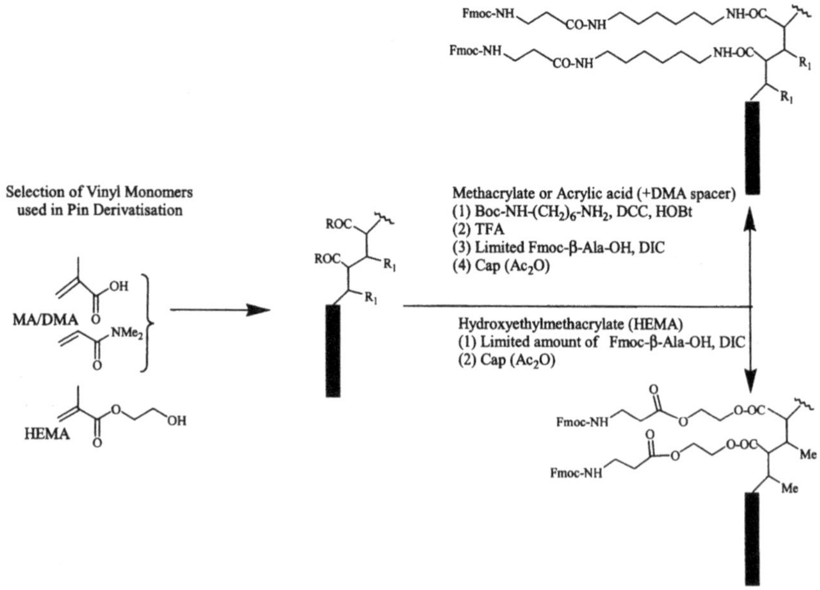

Figure 9 Second-generation pin/crown derivatization and loading.

ties, thus allowing a wide range of linkers, including the acid-labile Wang and Rink type of linkers, to be introduced onto these supports via the aminomethyl group, thus permitting the straightforward cleavage, analysis, and screening of micromolar quantities of compound. The ease of handling these small discrete crowns, which could be prepared in a variety of different colors as an inbuilt coding mechanism, and a broad range of loadings available (1–40 µmol) obviously made them very user friendly to the synthetic chemist for MPS.

The potential of these crowns was demonstrated in a series of papers from Chiron Mimotopes [33] and Ellman [34] including reductive aminations and Mitsunobu chemistries, and a large series of β-turn mimetics (using pins with a loading of 5.9 µmol) and 1680 1,4-benzodiazepines were prepared. Numerous groups have now used these materials in either an MPS- or a transponder-encoded defined split-and-mix synthesis. An addition to this area has been reported by Irori [47]. Radiation grafting was carried out as in the case of Chiron crowns, although in this case it was done on so-called microtubes (small plastic tubes) made of either polypropylene or a more chemically resistant fluoropolymer. However, they have not found widespread use.

B. Sheets

Sheet-type materials have been used for many years in the area of oligoucleotide and peptide synthesis. Early examples include the use of radiation-grafted polyethylene sheet, akin to Geysens pins, polypropylene membranes coated with cross-linked polyhydroxypropylacrylate, and derivatized glass or paper. Planar surfaces have a big advantage over beads used in combinatorial manner in that the structure of the compound can be directly deduced by its location on the support. The first of these methods used low-density polypropylene sheet that was γ-irradiated while immersed in a solution of styrene, a method commonly used at the time for the radiation grafting of surfaces [35]. Graft weights of some 440%, were obtained with the PS attached to the surface having a molecular weight of some 6×10^6 g/mol. Aminomethylation of the PS graft allowed linker attachment and peptide synthesis in good yield, with the sheet having a loading of about 29 µmol/cm^2. However, as far as we are aware, no more has been reported on the use of this material.

At the same time another approach was reported, although in this case the potential applications suggested were epitope mapping, affinity purification, and diagnostic testing as well as continuous-flow synthesis. The membrane used in this case was polypropylene coated with cross-linked hydroxypropylacrylate, which had a pore size of 0.2 µm [36]. Unfortunately, no details of the coating process or the materials loading were given, but four peptides were prepared on this membrane with good purities. More recently amino-functionalized polypropylene sheets have been used in DNA array synthesis, but the nature of the derivatization was not given [37].

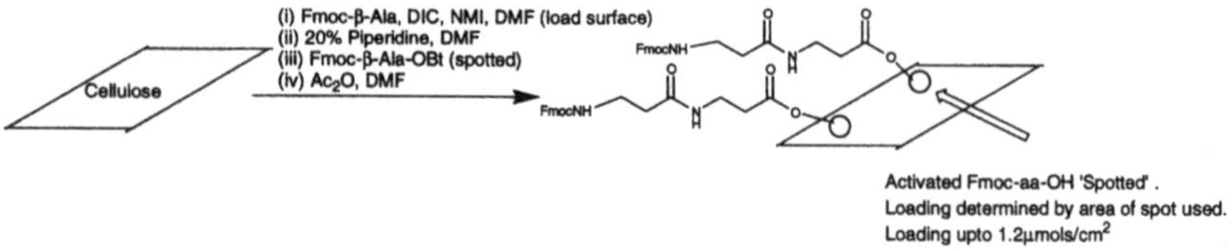

(i) Fmoc-β-Ala, DIC, NMI, DMF (load surface)
(ii) 20% Piperidine, DMF
(iii) Fmoc-β-Ala-OBt (spotted)
(iv) Ac$_2$O, DMF

Activated Fmoc-aa-OH 'Spotted' .
Loading determined by area of spot used.
Loading upto 1.2μmols/cm^2

Figure 10   Spot array synthesis on paper.

In 1990, Frank [37] introduced the concept of spot array synthesis of peptides. The basic premise being the suitability of cellulose paper as a support for standard Fmoc/tBu peptide synthesis (Fig. 10). Numerous peptides could be rapidly prepared by manual spotting of reagents, with up to 100 peptides prepared on an area of 4 cm^2, although 96 peptides based around a microtiter type of format became a standard format. Peptides were either screened on the paper, e.g., when looking for continuous epitopes, or released by DKP formation, analogous to the Chiron method, for solution screening, analysis, and characterization. Synthesis and screening of peptides was subsequently also carried out on Inimobilon-AV from Millipore in an identical spot manner.

A new material and concept were developed by Kobylecki [44] in which 1% PS resin beads were sandwiched between two layers of polypropylene sheet, giving a loading of approximately 5–10 nmol/cm^2. This material was used in a defined split-and-mix synthesis, using three sheets of material. Thus, in the first step a different amino acid was added to each sheet. The material was then cut into three strips and one strip from each sheet appended together. A different amino acid was added to each bundle of strips. The strips were lined up again as in the original three sheets and cut into squares with nine squares per sheet. The squares from each row were joined together and again functionalized with another amino acid. Thus this method uses the spatial nature of the material to define the synthetic sequence and prepare in this case 27 (3^3) peptides.

Other sheet-like materials have been used in peptide/DNA synthesis [45]. Thus, amino-functionalized sintered polyethylene (Porex X-4920 nominal pore size 30 μm) has either been used directly for DNA synthesis (loading 0.07 mmol/g) or derivatized with a chloromethylated styrene-based colloid having a diameter of 0.46 μm, to increase the loading to 9–12 μmol/g in an approach similar to that of the dendrimer methods described above. Another approach was described by Luo [46] in which porous polyethylene disks were oxidized to generate carboxylic acids on the surface that were subsequently derivatized with a diamine followed by carboxymethyl dextran. The acid sites were then loaded with diamines ready for synthesis. Thus, the polyethylene surface was in essence coated with derivatized dextran, making it highly hydrophilic and suitable for biological screening. However, accessibility to proteins might be very limited on these materials depending on the pore size of the polyethylene used. However, these last two methods are anecdotal.

C. Glass

In 1991, an extension of "spot" peptide synthesis was reported with the introduction by Affymax of peptides and oligonucleotides synthesis on glass [38]. In this process, light-based protecting groups were used for synthesis in conjunction with photolithographic masks, similar to those used in chip manufacture. The basic principle for photolithographic chemistry relies on a functionalized solid surface (glass/silica) which is treated with a photocleavable-protected linker or spacer to coat the surface (Fig. 11). A laser or photolithographic mask allows the light-induced deprotection of a well-defined (size and position) portion of the slide (Fig. 12). The disadvantage of this method is that it requires a relatively complex instrumentation and the development of a new array of synthesis tools.

In the reported cases a binary masking strategy was used, although later the permutational "stripe" masking strategy was used to increase library size. Using

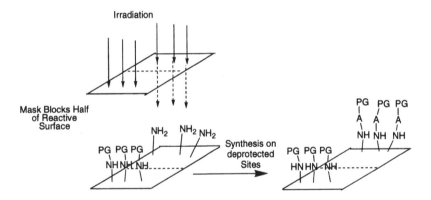

Figure 11 The concept of synthesis on glass using light-based protecting groups.

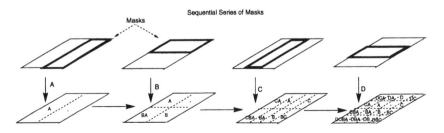

Figure 12 Masks for use in array synthesis.

this method, peptide arrays of 1024 peptides could be prepared in an area of 1.28 cm^2, which could then be screened directly (each peptide site being 400 nm^2). In a similar way, oligonucleotides could be prepared. Thus synthesis of short oligonucleotide probes and hybridization onto glass was published in 1994 by Fodor and coworkers who demonstrated the synthesis of a 1.28 × 1.28 cm array of 256 nucleotides and hybridized it toward the sequence 5′-GCGTAGGC-fluorescein [39]. The sequence specificity of the target hybridization was demonstrated by the fabrication of complementary probes differing by only one base, with the targets hybridizing almost totally specifically to its complementary sequence. However, a concern with all this chemistry, especially for oligonucleotide synthesis, is the efficiency of protecting group removal.

In 1996, MeGall [40] published the preparation of DNA arrays (using standard solid-phase oligonucleotide synthesis) using polymeric photoresist film as a physical barrier to mask selected region of the surface; exposure to light reveals the surface and allows the coupling of the first nucleoside. However, the harsh conditions required for deprotection could damage the library, and a bilayer process was developed. An inert polymeric film was introduced prior to the photoresist coat with the underlayer functioning as both a barrier to the chemical deprotection step and a protective layer to insulate the substrate surface from the photoresist chemistry and processing conditions. This was a direct application borrowed from the microelectronics industry allowing, it was claimed, more precise deprotection of the surface, thereby permitting creation of denser arrays. An array of 256 decanucleotides was synthesized and tested. For additional information, Wallraff and Hinsberg [41] published an overview of the lithographic imaging techniques. Southern [42] also reported using a physical masking approach to prepare DNA arrays with chemistry taking place on activated glass (Fig. 13), with areas being masked or separated from each other by physical "gaskets," in this case silicon rubber. The advantage with this method is that well-developed chemistry could be used, the limitations being the number of positions available for synthesis, which is limited by the accuracy of masking. In 1994, the stripped method was replaced by the regular shape of a diamond or disk mask in which linear translation of the mask allows the generation of a well-defined library [43], since a small translation of the mask allows defined parts of the slide to be deprotected and reacted.

A library of decamers was synthesised as an application of the technique and was used to study the hybridisation behavior of the corresponding synthetic deca-nucleotide in solution. However, the approach is much less practical and much more cumbersome than the light-based masking strategy.

In conclusion, a wide range of materials have been used and continue to be used for solid-phase synthesis. A number of these are very specific in application, such as synthesis on glass for DNA array synthesis. However, supports such as polystyrene resin are undoubtedly the workhorse of the industry, with others, such as the pins and PS-PEGs, having a much narrower role. There is clearly much

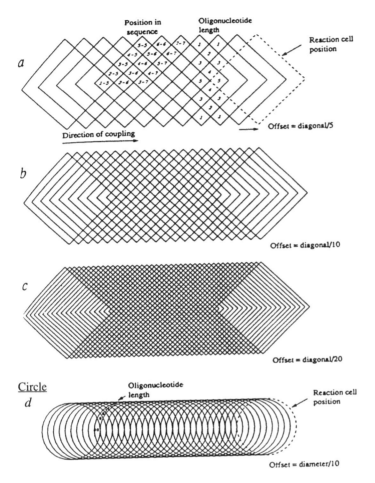

Figure 13 Physical masks for oligo array synthesis. (From Ref. 42, 43 with permission.)

scope for improved resin design and the generation of new supports for solid-phase synthesis.

REFERENCES

1. Merrifield RB. J Am Chem Soc 1963, 85, 2149.
2. Gallop MA, Barrett RW, Dower WJ, Fodor SPA, Gordon EM. J Med Chem 1994, 37, 1233.

3. Thompson LA, Ellman JA. Chem Rev 1996, 96, 555; Balkenhopl F, vondemBus-scheHunnefeld C, Lansky A, Zechel C. Angew Chem Int Edn Engl 1996, 35, 2288.

4. Leznoff CC. Acc Chem Res 1978, 11, 327.

5. Hodge P. Chem. Soc Rev 1997, 26, 417.

6. Sherrington DC. Chem Commun 1998, 2275.

7. MacDonald AA, Dewitt SH, Ghosh S, Hogan FM, Kieras L, Czarnik AW, Ramage R. Mol Div 1996, 1, 183.

8. The advent of automated HT purification means that low levels of impurities can be readily removed from the cleaved compounds at the end of the synthesis.

9. Hori M, Gravert DJ, Wentworth P, Janda KD. Bioorg Med Chem Lett 1998, 8, 2363.

10. Atherton E, Sheppard RC. Solid Phase Peptide Synthesis: A Practical Approach, Oxford: IRL Press 1985; Arshady R, Atherton E, Clive DLJ, Sheppard RC. J Chem Soc Perkin Trans 1 1981, 529.

11. Zalipsky S, Chang JL, Albericio F, Barany G. React. Polymers 1994, 22, 243.

12. Bayer E. Angew. Chemie., Int. Ed., 1991, 30, 113–129 and references therein; Bayer E, Albert K, Willish H, Rapp W, Hemmasi B. Macromolecules 1990, 23, 1937.

13. Gooding OW, Baudart S, Deegan TL, Heisler K, Labadie JW, Newcomb WS, Porco JA, Van Eikeren PJ. Comb Chem 1999, 1, 113.

14. NovaBiochem Catalogue, 2000.

15. Meldal M. Tetrahedron Letters, 1992, 33, 3077–3080; Meldal M, Auzanneau FI, Hindsgaul O, Palcic MM. J Chem Soc Chem Commun 1994, 1849.

16. Renil M, Nagaraj R, Pillai VNR. Tetrahedron., 1994, 50, 6681; Renil M, Pillai VNR. J Appl Polym Sci 1996, 61, 1585.

17. Kempe M, Barany G. J Am Chem Soc 1996, 118, 7083.

18. Rapp W. Chapter 16 in Combinatorial Libaries, Ed. G. Jung, Weinheim: VCH.

19. Willson ME, Paech K, Zhou W-J, Kurth MJ. J Org Chem 1998, 63, 5094.

20. Renil M, Meldal M. Tetrahedron Lett, 1995, 36, 4647–4650; Renil M, Ferreras M, Delaisse JM Foged NT, Meldal M. J. Pep. Sci., 1998, 4, 195.

21. Tam JP. Proc Natl Acad Sci USA 1988, 85, 5409.

22. Swali V, Wells NJ, Langley GJ, Bradley M. J Org Chem 1997, 62, 4902.

23. Wells NJ, Davies M, Bradley M. J Org Chem 1998, 63, 6430.

24. Fromont C, Bradley M. Chem Commun 2000, 283.

25. Houghten RA. Proc. Natl. Acad. Sci. USA 1985, 82, 5131.

26. Geysen HM, Meloen RB, Barteling SJ. Proc Natl Acad Sci USA 1984, 81, 3998, Geysen HM, Barteling SJ, Meloen RB. Proc Natl Acad Sci USA 1985, 82, 178.

27. Bray AM, Maeji NJ, Geysen HM. Tetrahedron Lett 1990, 31, 5811; Bray AM, Maeji NJ, Jhingran AG, Valerio RM. Tetrahedron Lett 1991, 32, 6163.

28. Maeji NJ, Valerio RM, Bray AM, Campbell RA, Geysen HM. Int. React. Polym. 1994, 22, 203.

29. Valerio RM, Bray AM, Campbell RA, Dipasquale A, Margellis C, Rodda SJ, Geysen HM, Maeji NJ. Int J Pept Protein Res 1993, 42, 1.

30. Bray AM, Maeji NJ, Valerio RM, Campbell RA, Geysen HM. J Org Chem, 1991, 56, 6659.

31. Bray AM, Jhingran AJ, Valerio RM, Maeji NJ. J Org Chem 1994, 59, 2197.

32. Valerio RM, Bray AM, Maeji NJ. Int J Pept Protein Res 1994, 44, 158.

33. Bray AM, Chiefari DS, Valerio RM, Maeji NJ. Tetrahedron Lett 1995, 36, 5081–5084; Valerio RM, Bray AM, Patsiouras H. Tetrahedron Lett 1996, 37, 3019.

34. Virgilio AA, Ellman JA. J Am Chem Soc 1994, 116, 11580; Bunin BA, Plunkett MJ, Ellman JA. New J. Chem., 1997, 21, 125; Virgilio AA, Bray AA, Zhang W, Trinh L, Snyder M, Morrissey MM, Ellman JA. Tetrahedron, 1997, 1994, 91, 4708; Bunin BA, Ellman JA. Am Chem Soc 1992, 114, 10997; Bunin BA, Plunkett MJ, Ellman JA. Proc Natl Acad Sci USA 1994, 91, 4708.

35. Berg RH, Almdal K, Pederson WB, Holm A, Tam JP, Merrifield RB. J Am Chem Soc 1989, 111, 8024.

36. Daniels SC, Bernatowicz MS, Coull JM, Köster H, Tetrahedron Lett., 1989, 30, 4345; Gao B, Esnouf MP. J Immunol 1996, 183.

37. Frank R. Tetrahedron, 1992, 48, 9217–9232; Gao B, Esnouf MP. J Biol Chem 1996, 271, 24634.

38. Fodor SPA, Read JL, Pirrung MC, Stryer L, Lu AT, Solas D. Science, 1991, 767; Pirrung MC. Chem Rev 1997, 97, 473.

39. Pease AC, Solas D, Sullivan EJ, Cronin MT, Holmes CP, Fodor SPA. Proc Natl Acad Sci USA 1994, 91, 5022.

40. McGall G, Labadie J, Brock P, Wallraff G, Nguyen T, Hinsberg W. Proc Natl Acad Sci USA 1996, 93, 13555; Pirrung MC, Fallon L, McGall G. J Org Chem 1998, 63, 241.

41. Wallraff GM, Hinsberg WD. Chem Rev 1999, 99, 1801.

42. Maskos U, Southern EM. Nucleic Acids Res 1993, 21, 2267 and 2269.

43. Southern EM, Case-Green SC, Elder JK, Johnson M, Mir U, Wang L, Williams JC. Nucleic Acids Res 1994, 22, 1368.

44. Terrett NK, Gardner M, Gordon DW, Kobylecki RJ, Steele J. Chem Eur J 1997, 3, 1917.

45. Devivar RV, Koontz SL, Peltier WJ, Pearson JE, Guillory, TA, Fabricant JD. Bioorg Med Chem Lett 1999, 9, 1239.

46. Luo KX, Zhou P. Lodish HF. Proc Natl Acad Sci USA 1995, 92, 11761.

47. Zhao C, Shi S, Mir D, Hurst D, Li, R, Xiao X-y, Lillig J, Czarnik AW. J. Comb. Chem 1999, 1, 91.

19

The NMR "Toolkit" for Compound Characterization

Paul A. Keifer
CST Associates
Omaha, Nebraska

I. INTRODUCTION

This chapter discusses the application of various nuclear magnetic resonance (NMR) spectroscopy techniques to the process of drug discovery. To make it easier to understand how drug discovery incorporates NMR data, all drug discovery–related activities have been categorized into one of the following six disciplines: (1) natural products research; (2) medicinal chemistry; (3) rational drug design (protein structure and modeling); (4) metabolism; (5) combinatorial chemistry, and; (6) drug production and quality control. Although this classification process may initially appear to be somewhat artificial, its use makes it easier to understand the applications and advantages of each NMR technique. However, readers should recognize that most drug discovery programs involve a blend of these six disciplines and therefore usually benefit from using a combination of different NMR techniques.

Most advances in NMR technology have occurred when someone tried to address a particular limitation in one of these six disciplines. However, once a new tool is developed, it can sometimes solve a different problem in a different discipline or spawn a whole new field of NMR. An example of the former is the use of magic-angle spinning first for solid-state NMR, then for small-volume solution-state NMR for natural products, and then for solid-phase synthesis resin NMR for combinatorial chemistry. An example of the latter is the development of indirect detection, which helped spawn the use of isotopically labeled proteins and triple-resonance NMR for determining the structures of biomolecules in rational drug design programs.

In addition to the simple migration of NMR techniques from one discipline to another, two or more NMR techniques can often be synergistically combined. A good example of this is the combination technique of (HP)LC-NMR. Its current implementation involves the use of indirect detection, shaped pulses, broadband decoupling, pulsed-field gradient (PFG) sequences, PFG shimming, automation, and small-sample probe design.

The purpose of this chapter is to examine some of these NMR tools and to see how they have influenced drug discovery programs. First we will see how they were initially used to solve a particular problem. Then we will see how some have been used to solve problems in other disciplines. Last, we will see how others have been synergistically combined to develop much more powerful tools.

Section II covers the basic tools in NMR, which include multidimensional NMR, high-field NMR, broadband decoupling, spin locks, shaped pulses, indirect detection, and PFGs. Section III introduces some additional applications of NMR and the more specialized tools in use, most of which are based on the technologies introduced in Section II. These include protein structure determinations and the multiple-channel indirect-detection experiments they spawned (Section III.A), water suppression techniques (Section III.B), and hardware and probe developments (Section III.C). The probe developments that are covered include small-volume probes and HR-MAS probes in Section III.C.2.a and b, as well as flow probes and cryogenic probes, which are sufficiently important to have been treated separately, in Sections III.E and III.G, respectively. Detailed information about combinatorial chemistry applications can be found in the discussions on solid-phase resin analysis using MAS (Section III.D) and the analysis of libraries stored in titer plates using flow NMR (Section III.E.2 and 3) Lastly, there are individual discussions on analyzing mixtures, combined NMR techniques, quantification by NMR, and the automation of NMR in the last parts of Section III.

II. BASIC NMR TOOLS

A. 1D, 2D, 3D, and *n*D NMR

One of the first tools to be developed was multidimensional NMR. The first NMR spectra to be observed contained only one frequency axis and so were called "one-dimensional" (even though they actually contain two dimensions of NMR information: frequency and amplitude). One-dimensional (1D) spectroscopy was the only real option for the early generations of continuous-wave (CW) spectrometers, but with the advent of pulsed Fourier transform NMR (FT-NMR) spectrometers some 20 years later, it was soon recognized that additional dimensions of NMR information could be obtained. Because some 1D NMR spectra had a crowded frequency axis (especially large molecules like proteins) or had coincidental or overlapping chemical shifts (especially poorly functionalized molecules like some steroids), methods to simplify these spectra were needed.

In the early 1970s, the first papers on two-dimensional NMR spectroscopy (2D NMR) began to appear [1]. Because 2D NMR allowed the NMR information to be spread in two dimensions, each of which could encode different kinds of information, most kinds of spectral overlap could be resolved. As an example, one dimension could contain chemical shift data, while the other dimension could encode information about spin-spin couplings.

Different pulse sequences were then developed to select all different kinds of information. The 2D correlations could arise from homonuclear or heteronuclear couplings, through-bond (scalar) or through-space (dipolar) couplings, or single-quantum or multiple-quantum couplings. They could also be designed either to detect the presence of or to actually measure the magnitude of a given kind of coupling. Experiments exploiting all of the various combinations of these possibilities were eventually developed and remain in use today. These include experiments that generate 2D data to measure: the presence of homonuclear scalar coupling [homonuclear correlation spectroscopy (COSY) and total correlation spectroscopy (TOCSY)], the magnitude of homonuclear scalar couplings [homonuclear 2D J spectroscopy (HOM2DJ)], the presence of heteronuclear scalar couplings [heteronuclear correlation spectroscopy (HETCOR), heteronuclear multiple-quantum correlations (HMQC), and heteronuclear multiple-bond correlations (HMBC)], the magnitude of heteronuclear scalar couplings [heteronuclear 2D J spectroscopy (HET2DJ)], the presence of homonuclear dipolar coupling [nuclear Overhauser effect (NOE) spectroscopy (NOESY)], the presence of heteronuclear dipolar coupling [heteronuclear NOE spectroscopy (HOESY)], and double-quantum, double-quantum-filtered, and multiple-quantum-filtered homonuclear scalar coupling correlation experiments (DQ-, DQF-, and MQF-COSYs). Many good books and reviews about 2D NMR can be found [2–4].

It is useful to understand that a 2D pulse sequence generates data that contain both a direct (F_2) and an indirect (F_1) dimension. The direct dimension, sometimes called the "real-time" dimension, consists of a series of one-dimensional experiments; each spectrum is completely acquired during one intact time interval, usually within a few minutes. However, the indirect dimension is generated by a "t_1" delay in the pulse sequence that is incremented many hundreds of time during a 2D experiment. A direct-dimension spectrum is acquired for each of these several hundred delay times, then the data are subjected to Fourier transformation a second time—along this indirect dimension—to produce the 2D dataset. Each spectrum along the indirect dimension is reconstructed from hundreds of direct-dimension spectra, and each datapoint in an indirect-dimension spectrum arises from a different direct-dimension spectrum. This means that each indirect-dimension spectrum is composed of datapoints acquired over many minutes (or hours or days). Any time-dependent instabilities (in the spectrometer, the environment, the sample, the electrical power, etc.) can cause a corruption of datapoints and therefore cause noise; since this noise runs parallel to the t_1 axis, it is called "t_1 noise." We will see later how t_1 noise, which is ubiquitous, can be troublesome enough that some NMR techniques, such as PFG, were developed to suppress it.

After a wide range of 2D NMR pulse sequences were developed, it was recognized that they could be effectively combined to create 3D, 4D, and even higher "nD" spectroscopies [5,6]. Each additional dimension is created by appending to the pulse sequence certain pulse-sequence elements (that contain an incrementing delay) that generate the desired effect. A 3D pulse sequence has one direct dimension and two incrementing delays, whereas a 4D dataset has three incrementing delays. Each dimension of an nD dataset usually encodes for different information, so a 3D HETCOR-COSY would have three distinct chemical shift axes (one ^{13}C and two ^1H) and three distinct faces. (If the data within the 3D cube are projected onto each of the three distinct faces, they would display 2D HETCOR, 2D COSY, and 2D HETCOR-COSY data, respectively.) These hyphenated experiments, combined with the power of 3D and 4D NMR, are proving to be very useful for elucidating the structures of large molecules, particularly for large (150–300 residue) proteins [7].

Since a 2D dataset contains three dimensions of information (two frequency axes and a signal amplitude), a contour-plot presentation is usually used to represent the data on paper. A 3D dataset is a cube in which each datapoint contains amplitude information. Since all this information is difficult to plot simultaneously, 3D data are usually plotted as a series of 2D planes (contour plots). Four (and higher) dimensional experiments are easy to acquire (aside from the massive data storage requirements), but plotting and examining the data becomes increasingly difficult, so that 3D is often the upper limit for routine NMR. We will see later how multidimensional NMR can be combined with multinuclear (triple-resonance) NMR experiments.

Although multidimensional NMR can provide more information, it also has some disadvantages. Its experimental time is longer; it usually requires more sample; setup of the experiment and processing and interpretation of the data require more expertise; it requires more powerful computer hardware and software; and it requires additional hard disk space. This means that a user should normally run the lowest dimensionality experiment that answers the question at hand. It is usually found in practice that the six disciplines of drug discovery use these multidimensional NMR techniques differently. Medicinal chemists, combinatorial chemists, drug production and quality control groups, and, to a lesser extent, metabolism groups usually use 1D NMR data to get most of their structural information. Medicinal chemists usually need only to confirm a suspected structure and rarely use 2D NMR. The drug production and quality control groups will use 2D techniques if they encounter a tough enough problem. Combinatorial chemists might like to have 2D NMR data but they don't have the time to acquire it, whereas metabolism chemists would often like to get 2D NMR data but often don't have enough sample. Natural products chemists routinely depend on 2D NMR techniques to unravel their total unknowns. Rational drug design groups use 2D and 3D (and sometimes 4D) NMR techniques routinely.

B. High-Field NMR

Multidimensional NMR was developed to simplify complex NMR spectra. Another way to simplify a complex or overlapped NMR spectrum is to place the samples in higher-field-strength magnets to generate more dispersion along each axis. This helps resolve overlapping signals and simplifies second-order multiplets, while at the same time increasing NMR sensitivity. These benefits have driven magnet technologies to improve to the point where magnets having proton resonance frequencies of 800 MHz (18.8 Tesla) are now routinely available. The disadvantage of these very high-field magnets is that they are much more expensive. (They primarily cost more to purchase, but they also have higher installation and operational costs, especially for cryogens, and they require bigger rooms with more sophisticated environmental controls.) These additional costs must be weighed against the time that can be saved by the improved performance, and both factors are balanced against the difficulties of the problems encountered. In practice, field strengths of 14.1 Tesla (600 MHz) and above are routinely used in rational drug design programs and occasionally in metabolism programs (due to their limited sample sizes). Natural products groups, and some drug production and quality control groups, usually use 400- to 600-MHz systems, while combinatorial chemistry, and especially medicinal chemistry groups, tend to use 300- to 500-MHz systems.

Improvements in magnet and shim coil technologies are also allowing the homogeneity of the magnetic field to be improved. This has allowed lineshape specifications to be cut in half over the last decade, and has improved the quality of solvent suppression in the NMR spectra of samples dissolved in fully protonated solvents.

C. Broadband Decoupling

Another way to simplify spectra is to use heteronuclear decoupling [8]. This both collapses a coupled multiplet into one single frequency, and (through other mechanisms) produces taller resonances. Decoupling can also increase the sensitivity of certain X nuclei (like ^{13}C) through nuclear Overhauser enhancements. In some triple-resonance experiments (discussed later), heteronuclear decoupling improves sensitivity by eliminating some undesirable relaxation pathways.

Although decoupling is generally desirable, the first available methods caused too much sample heating to be of routine use. More efficient decoupling schemes were eventually developed that produced a wider bandwidth of decoupling for a given amount of power. Starting from continuous wave (CW; unmodulated) decoupling, wider decoupling bandwidths were obtained with the development of noise-, WALTZ, MLEV, XY32, TYCKO, GARP, and DIPSI decouplings (not necessarily in order) [8,9]. These modulation schemes allowed decoupling to become quite routine and allowed new techniques, such as indirect detection (discussed below), to become practical. As knowledge of shaped pulses improved (discussed below), ever more efficient decoupling schemes like MPF1-10 [10], WURST [11], and STUD [12] were developed; the latter two by using advanced pulse shapes called adiabatic pulses [13]. No decoupling scheme is perfect for all applications or even for all field strengths. Each scheme provides a different balance of performance in terms of bandwidth per unit power, minimum linewidth, sideband intensity, complexity of the waveform (what hardware is needed to drive it), and tolerance of misset calibrations ("robustness"). The advantage of all these developments is that there is now a large set of different decoupling tools that are available to be used as needed.

D. Spin Locks

Better theories and understandings of spin physics resulted from the developments in broadband decoupling, and this allowed better spin locks to be developed. Spin locks were initially designed for experiments on solid-state samples, but in the 1980s it was shown that spin locks could also be used for solution-state experiments. Bothner-By and coworkers used a CW spinlock to develop the CAMEL-SPIN experiment (later known as ROESY; Rotating frame Overhauser Enhancement SpectroscopY) to get dipolar coupling (through-space) information [14]. Other groups subsequently reported the use of both lower rf field strengths [15] and pulsed spinlocks [16] to improve the quality of the ROESY data. Braunschweiler and Ernst used a spinlock to develop the HOmonuclear HArtmann-HAhn experiment (HOHAHA; later known as TOCSY) which provides a total scalar-coupling correlation map [17]. Bax and Davis showed that the MLEV-16 modulation scheme, used for broadband decoupling (discussed above), improved the quality of TOCSY data [18]. Kupce and coworkers built on their experience with adiabatic pulses to improve decoupling schemes to develop a spinlock using adiabatic pulses [19]. As discussed later, these spinlocks are proving useful in obtaining TOCSY data on MAS samples. This is helping combinatorial chemists acquire better data on solid-phase synthesis (SPS) resins. The hardware required to run spinlocked experiments is now routinely available, and these experiments usually provide better and more complete data than alternative experiments like COSY.

The typical use of a spinlock is as a mixing scheme to allow the spins to exchange information. This is how they are used in TOCSY and ROESY experiments. However, spinlocks have also been used, to destroy unwanted magnetization. For this application, the pulse sequence is usually written so that the spinlock only affects resonances at a specific (selective) frequency [20]. This allows them to be used to perform solvent suppression experiments for samples dissolved in protonated solvents (like H_2O). Non-frequency-selective spinlocks have also been used to destroy unwanted magnetization [21]. This use of a spinlock as a general purge pulse is a viable alternative to the use of homospoil pulses [22] and is in routine use.

The spin physics of the decoupling and spinlock sequences are related, and any given modulation scheme can often serve both purposes. In general, however, the sequences are usually optimized for only one of the two applications. Hence, MLEV-16, MLEV-17, and DIPSI are most commonly used as spinlock sequences, whereas WALTZ, GARP, WURST, and STUD are most commonly used as decoupling schemes [8].

E. Shaped Pulses

In addition to new decoupling and spinlock schemes, shaped rf pulses have also been developed. They are called "shaped pulses" because all of these pulses change amplitude, phase, or frequency (or some combination) as a function of time [23]. In doing so, the pulse can be designed to be more frequency selective, more broadbanded in frequency, more tolerant of misset calibrations, or capable of multifrequency or off-resonance excitation. Different applications require different balances of these characteristics.

If a pulse is made more frequency selective, it can be used in a variety of new applications. One application is "dimensionality reduction," in which a selective 1D experiment is used in place of a 2D experiment, or a selective 2D experiment is used in place of a 3D experiment. Selective experiments let you obtain a selected bit of NMR information faster and with higher signal-to-noise—but only if you already know what you are looking for. This can be useful for studying smaller amounts of samples (or more dilute samples) as is often required for natural products. Examples include the use of 1D COSY [24], 1D TOCSY [25], 1D NOE [26], DPFGSE-NOE (also sometimes erroneously called GOESY) [27,28], 1D HMQC (called SELINCOR) [29], 1D HMBC (called SIMBA) [30], and 1D INADEQUATE [31]. These sequences are less useful if you have many questions to be answered or don't know what you are looking for. Then it is usually advantageous to go ahead and run the complete 2D or 3D experiment and analyze it as completely as is required to solve the problem at hand.

Another use of selective pulses is to perform frequency-selective solvent suppression. Presaturation is the simplest example of the use of a frequency-selective pulse for solvent suppression (although the pulse used in presaturation is typically not shaped). Examples of frequency-selective shaped pulses that are used in solvent suppression include the S and SS pulses [32], Node-1 [33], and WET [34]. Note that although many commonly used water suppression sequences, such as 1331 [35] and WATERGATE [36], are frequency selective, they achieve that selectivity by using a train of nonshaped pulses, in the so-called DANTE technique [37], instead of using shaped pulses. (The DANTE technique permits the use of simpler hardware but results in a less accurate frequency profile.)

Historically, the primary application of solvent suppression was to obtain spectra of biomolecules (proteins, RNA, etc.) dissolved in $H_2O:D_2O$ mixtures. However, more recent work, especially on direct-injection NMR (discussed below), indicates that it is now practical to obtain ^1H NMR spectra of organic samples dissolved in fully protonated nonaqueous solvents. This is being used especially in combinatorial chemistry to obtain ^1H NMR spectra on samples dissolved in DMSO-h_6, $CHCl_3$, and aqueous solutions of CH_3CN and CH_3OH.

Frequency-selective pulses can also be used for narrowband selective decoupling. Such pulses can be placed in evolution periods to simplify spectra [38].

Not all shaped pulses are frequency selective (narrow bandwidth). In recent years there have been many fine examples of the use of both band-selective and broadband-shaped pulses. Sometimes these are used as single rf pulses, but more typically they have been used in decoupling schemes designed to hit either a selected, controlled, moderately wide region, or a very broadbanded region. A well-known example of band-selective pulses is the use of pulses [39] or decoupling schemes [40,41] to treat carbonyl-carbon resonances differently from aliphatic-carbon resonances in triple-resonance experiments (discussed below). Here, band-selective pulses are pulsing or decoupling regions of the spectrum that are from 1 to 4 kHz in width. Applications using adiabatic pulses that are region selective have also been described [42,43].

The use of shaped pulses that affect very wide (broadband) regions of a spectrum is also becoming more popular. Most of these examples exploit adiabatic pulses [13]. There are three advantages to using adiabatic pulses. First, they are uniquely capable of creating a good excitation profile over a wide frequency region. Second, they deposit less power into a sample (and hence cause less sample heating) for a given bandwidth than most other pulses. Third, they are quite tolerant of misset calibrations. This feature was originally exploited in applications that used surface coils—to compensate for the characteristically poor B_1 homogeneity of these coils—but some groups use this feature to simply make routine solution-state NMR spectroscopy more robust and less sensitive to operator calibration errors. Adiabatic rf pulses are being used in high-field ^1H-^{13}C correlation experiments (like HSQC) to achieve wider and more uniform inversion over the wide ^{13}C spectral width [11,44]. Adiabatic pulses are also being heavily used to create more efficient and wider bandwidth decoupling schemes (as discussed above in the decoupling section). Both of these applications are being used to facilitate high-field NMR spectroscopy of biomolecules.

One of the final tools in the shaped-pulse toolbox are the shifted laminar pulse (SLP) pulses [45], which are sometimes (imprecisely) called phase-ramped pulses. These pulses deliver their effects off resonance without changing the transmitter frequency. (It is undesirable to change the frequency of a frequency synthesizer during a pulse sequence because this affects the phase of the transmitter.) SLP pulses that affect only one off-resonance frequency change phase linearly as a function of time; hence, the alternative name "phase-ramped pulses." SLP pulses that affect two (or more) off-resonance frequencies are both phase and amplitude modulated due to the interaction of the two different phase ramps. SLP pulses can be created to affect any number of frequencies (as long as enough power is available). They can also be created using any pulse shape or duration (or combination of shapes and durations). This means, for example, that an SLP pulse can be made to hit three different frequencies, each with a different pulse width, and each with a different pulse shape (or phase) if desired. We will see later (in the discussion of LC-NMR) how SLP pulses are being used to obtain multiple-frequency solvent suppression using only one rf channel.

F. Indirect Detection

The development of indirect detection has probably had a bigger impact on all stages of drug discovery than any other NMR technique. Indirect detection is one of two methods for acquiring heteronuclear correlation data. The conventional method for acquiring 2D heteronuclear correlation data—called "direct detection" and exemplified by the HETCOR experiment described above—measures a series of X-nucleus spectra (typically ^{13}C) and extracts the frequencies of the coupled nuclei (typically ^1H) by using a Fourier transform in the t_1 dimension. The concept of indirect detection, first published in 1979 [46], inverts the process by acquiring a series of ^1H spectra, then Fourier-transforming the t_1 dimension of this dataset to (indirectly) obtain the X (^{13}C) frequencies [2,3]. The major benefit of using indirect detection is improved sensitivity—up to 30-fold or more, depending on the nuclei involved.

In hindsight, indirect detection seems like an obvious development, but because the instrumental requirements of running indirect detection are more demanding (two-scan cancellation, broadband X-nucleus decoupling, indirect-detection probes designed for water suppression), the method did not become truly routine until more than a decade later. They do not completely replace X-detected correlation experiments (which have superior X-nucleus resolution), but these ^1H-detected experiments are now the default for most users. When sensitivity is an issue, the indirect detection version of an experiment is usually used.

There are three classic indirect-detection experiments: HMQC, HMBC, and HSQC. (These acronyms stand for heteronuclear multiple-quantum correlation, heteronuclear multiple-bond correlation, and heteronuclear single-quantum correlation, respectively.) HMQC and HSQC detect one-bond H-X couplings, whereas HMBC detects long-range H-X scalar couplings. HMQC uses a multiple-quantum coherence pathway, while HSQC uses single-quantum coherence. HMQC was technically easier to run in the early days, but because the B_1 homogeneity of most NMR probes has improved since then, HSQC is now a better tool for most applications. Virtually all modern biomolecular experiments, and many natural-product experiments, currently use HSQC-style (rather than HMQC-style) coherence pathways [47,48]. HMBC is the primary tool for de novo structure elucidations of small molecules, particularly for natural products [49–53].

A big advantage of indirect detection is its increased sensitivity. A big disadvantage is its cancellation noise. Because only the ^{13}C satellites of a ^1H resonance are of interest in a $^1H\{^{13}C\}$ HSQC, the rest of the ^1H signal (98.9%) must be eliminated. In conventional pulse sequences this is accomplished by using a two-step phase cycle in which the ^{13}C satellites are cycled differently from the central ^1H-^{12}C resonance. Unfortunately, many spectrometer installations are not stable enough to provide clean cancellation (this is heavily dependent on the local environment), and the poorly canceled central-resonance signal ends up creating excessive t_1 noise in the spectrum. This is most visible in the study of unlabeled compounds, i.e., those that have natural abundance levels of ^{13}C (or ^{15}N). It becomes even more problematical in long-range HMBC-style experiments. Here the t_1 noise is often larger than the signals of interest, and more experiment time is spent signal-averaging to raise the signals of interest above the t_1 noise than to raise them above the thermal noise.

G. Pulsed-Field Gradients

In 1973 Paul Lauterbur discovered that linear gradients of B_0 (the magnetic field) could be used in NMR experiments to generate spatial information about what was located in the magnet [54]. This ultimately gave rise to the technique called magnetic resonance imaging (MRI), currently used in many hospitals and clinics. As imaging technology developed, it became possible to generate pulses of linear B_0 gradients, of different strengths, in a controlled fashion. Barker and Freeman were the first to demonstrate that these pulsed magnetic field gradients could be used for coherence selection to acquire 2D NMR data [55]. This capability was expanded and popularized by Hurd and coworkers in the early 1990s, who showed that pulsed-field gradients (PFGs) could be used in a number of different NMR experiments [56–58]. Thus, the PFG revolution was born.

PFGs can be used in several ways [58,59]. The original application was for imaging, and while this is usually used for clinical purposes, imaging techniques are also being used in drug discovery, primarily to study the metabolism of drugs [60]. PFGs are also useful in automating the shimming of high-resolution NMR samples [61,62]. Both ^{1}H and ^{2}H gradient shimming are in routine use for research samples as well as for samples being analyzed by routine automation. PFG techniques also allow old experiments to be run in different ways, and allow entirely new pulse sequences to be developed (discussed below).

PFGs embody experiments with a number of desirable attributes. One is that they allow some experiments to be acquired without phase cycling. This allows the data to be acquired much faster, as long as the quantity of sample is sufficient. This is especially useful for indirect detection, as well as for COSY experiments.

PFGs also allow data to be acquired with less t_1 noise. This is useful for experiments in which the quality of the data acquired with conventional methods is significantly degraded by the presence of t_1 noise. A classic example of this is indirect detection. Conventional (phase cycled) indirect-detection experiments use a two-step phase cycle to cancel the large signals from protons not bound to ^{13}C (or ^{15}N) nuclei, which is 98.9% of the signal in unlabeled samples (discussed above). Any imperfections in the cancellation leave residual signals that cause the t_1 noise. In HMBC in particular, because it detects the long-range multiple-bond correlations, which are often small, this t_1 noise may be bigger than some of the desirable signals [63,64]. Since the PFG versions of HMBC select the desired signals (coherences) within a single scan, and hence contain no t_1 noise induced by the two-step cancellation technique, better quality data can be obtained, and usually in less time. This is especially useful for elucidating the structures of natural products. Because the structures are usually unknown and the sample sizes are often quite small, every improvement in the quality of HMBC data is welcomed.

PFG experiments can also suppress unwanted solvent resonances, often easily and without any extra setup effort by the operator. In addition, the quality of this suppression is much less dependent on the quality of the NMR lineshape than with other experiments. (Presaturation of the water resonance in an H_2O sample is a classic example in which the NMR spectral quality depends heavily on how well the lineshape of the water resonance can be shimmed to have a narrow base. The corresponding PFG experiments typically do not need such exacting shimming.) This attribute is important because of the large number of NMR studies performed on biomolecules dissolved in $H_2O:D_2O$ mixtures [65].

1. PFG Variations of Existing Experiments

The many beneficial attributes of using PFG experiments (listed above) have made PFG experiments quite popular. PFG versions of the indirect-detection experiments [66–68] are the most heavily used, but the PFG versions of many COSY-style experiments [69,70] are also popular. PFG-HMBC is a very striking example, and one that is very popular in natural-products programs [63,71]. Alternatives such as GHSMBC [72], ADEQUATE [73,74], EXSIDE [75], psge-HMBC [71], and ACCORD-HMBC [76] have also been developed. Most people would benefit by using PFG-COSY more routinely, as opposed to a non-PFG (phase-cycled) COSY [77]. PFG-HSQC [78] has become a standard experiment in biomolecular NMR (for rational drug design programs). PFG versions of the selective experiments 1D TOCSY and 1D NOESY experiments have also been developed [79].

2. New Experiments Made Possible by PFG

PFGs have also allowed new pulse sequences to be developed. The WATERGATE spin-echo sequence was developed for biomolecular water suppression [36]. A newer nonecho solvent suppression technique called WET [34], which combines PFG, shaped pulses, and SLP pulses, is now the standard for use in LC-NMR [80]—a technique that is becoming a popular tool for metabolism studies [81]. PFG-based WET suppression is also being used in the NMR analysis of combinatorial libraries dissolved in nondeuterated solvents [82]. Automated ^2H (and ^1H) gradient shimming, using gradients from both PFG coils as well as room-temperature shim coils, is becoming routine for the automated walkup NMR spectrometers used in medicinal chemistry programs [62]. Diffusion experiments [83], which rely heavily on PFG, are being used to study ligand binding and to evaluate library mixtures for compounds that bind to receptors in rational drug design programs [84,85]. Other PFG-based diffusion experiments are being used for solvent suppression [86].

III. SPECIALIZED NMR TOOLS

A. Biomolecular Structure Elucidation

Rational drug design programs are built on the idea that if the complete three-dimensional structure of a receptor could be determined, one could custom design a small molecule to bind into its receptor site. The challenge in this process is to determine the structure of the receptor (a protein). While three-dimensional protein structures can be determined using X-ray crystallography, it became apparent in the 1980s that this could also be done by using NMR spectroscopy, and NMR allows the solution-state structure of the protein to be determined.

Once the primary structure of a protein is known, the secondary and tertiary structure of the protein is determined with NMR by first making chemical shift assignments and then by measuring NOEs and coupling constants [87]. A ^1H-^1H NOE provides information about through-space distances. (If two protons show an NOE, and if they are located in different parts of the peptide chain, then this provides an intrastrand structural constraint that says these protons must reside close to each other in the final 3D structure of the protein.) Proton homonuclear or heteronuclear coupling constants provide information about the torsion angles of the bonds in the peptide backbone. Either of these methods can provide a 3D structure if enough structural constraints can be determined.

Structure determinations can be very difficult for proteins whose molecular weights are greater than 10 kDa (even if the primary structure is obtained by other means). First, the chemical shift assignments become more difficult as the spectral complexity increases, and second, the faster relaxation of larger molecules produces broader linewidths that make it harder to obtain coupling-constant information.

Biomolecular NMR became more important and grew significantly when three things happened. First, methods were developed for incorporating NMR-active isotopic labels (namely, ^{13}C and ^{15}N) into proteins. Second, indirect-detection techniques were developed that facilitated the chemical shift assignments of these labeled proteins [88,89]. Third, 3D and 4D NMR techniques were developed to simplify and sort the vast amount of information needed to determine the structure of these large molecule [90]. These three developments greatly simplified the interpretation of protein NMR data and made the determination of protein structures both more routine and more powerful. Although the techniques for acquiring indirect-detection NMR data on small molecules were well developed by the late 1980s, the requirements (and possibilities) of performing these experiments on proteins are a bit different. Much of this was worked out in the early 1990s, and the field of multiple-resonance protein NMR blossomed [6,39,87,91]. The resulting experiments (described below) are certainly powerful, and initially required new NMR hardware, but conceptually one can think of them as simply being composed of combinations of the fundamental techniques that had already been developed (and which have already been described above).

1. Multiple RF-Channel NMR

Because isotopically labeled proteins typically contain three kinds of NMR-active nuclei—^{1}H, ^{13}C, and ^{15}N—the one-step heteronuclear coherence transfers normally used in heteronuclear correlation experiments can be concatenated into a multiple-step transfer. An example of a multiple-step transfer would be magnetization transfer from ^{1}H to ^{13}C, then to ^{15}N where it evolves, back to ^{13}C, and then to ^{1}H for detection. Indirect-detection experiments allow any X nucleus to be examined, simply depending on where in the pulse sequence the t_1 evolution time is placed. Three- and four-dimensional experiments allow multiple evolution times to be used. Proteins exhibit a range of homonuclear and heteronuclear scalar coupling constants (J), and the $1/2J$ delays in a pulse sequence can be finely tuned so as to select between several different scalar coupling pathways in the molecule. These capabilities, combined with the ability to select either complete or partial isotopic labeling within a protein, allow experiments to be designed that can correlate almost any two kinds of spins. In practice, at least one of these spins is usually a proton bound to an amide-bonded nitrogen. The identity of the second or third spin depends on the structural data needed. It may even be one of several structurally different carbon nuclei, since NMR can easily distinguish carbonyl carbons from all other carbon resonances quite easily (using frequency-selective pulses). Figure 1 shows the intraresidue correlations that can be made using the HN(CA)CO experiment, as well as the interresidue correlations (to the previous adjacent carbonyl carbon) that can be made using the HNCO experiment. In HN(CA)CO, the magnetization starts on the NH proton, is transferred to the directly bonded ^{15}N (where there is an evolution time), is transferred to the C-α ^{13}C (no evolution), and then is transferred to the carbonyl ^{13}C where it has its second evolution. It then reverses its path (CO to CA to N to H) for detection of ^1H. The parentheses around the CA in HN(CA)CO indicates that the C-α nuclei are used in the transfer, but there is no evolution time and they are not actually detected. To make correlations to the C-α carbons (instead of the carbonyl carbons), the corresponding experiments would be HNCA (for intraresidue assignments) and HN(CO)CA (for interresidue assignments to the previous C-α carbon). In a similar manner, experiments like HN(COCA)NH, HCACO, HCA(CO)N, and HN(COCA)HA, as well as many more, can be constructed (Fig. 1).

Because proteins (and other biomolecules) are so large, their T_2 relaxation times are usually much shorter than those of small molecules. This causes their NMR resonances to have broader linewidths. Because most methods for determining accurate scalar coupling constants measure the separation of antiphase signals, and because this becomes less accurate as the linewidths increase, these experiments become less useful as the compound's molecular weight increases. As a consequence, DQFCOSY experiments are less useful for large proteins, and so the determination of the 3D structure via torsion-angle measurements becomes harder. Experiments have been designed in an attempt to overcome this limitation, principally through the use of combined hetero- and homonuclear scalar couplings [92,93].

2. Newer Biomolecular Experiments: TROSY, Hydrogen-Bond J Couplings, and Dipolar Couplings

Because large biomolecules have a faster T_2 relaxation than smaller molecules, their NMR signals will sometimes decay before they get through some pulse sequences. There are several schemes for addressing this problem. First, HSQC experiments can be used instead of HMQC experiments because transverse magnetization in a single-quantum state (HSQC) relaxes even more slowly than transverse magnetization in a multiple-quantum state (HMQC) [47]. Second, some pulse sequences now use a variety of heteronuclear and homonuclear decoupling schemes during evolution times to reduce T_2 decay rates. Third, some groups have resorted to perdeuteration of those large proteins that relax rapidly; this reduces

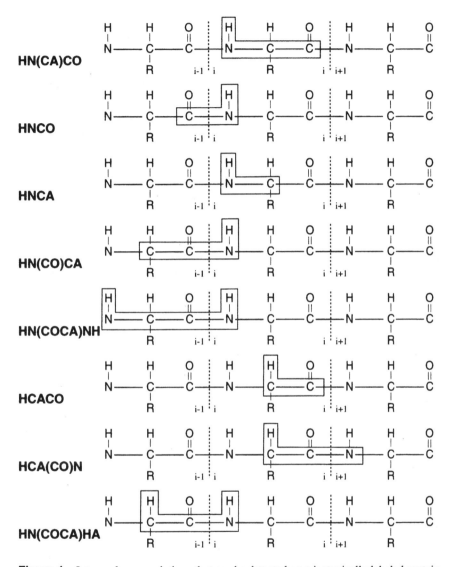

Figure 1 Internuclear correlations that can be detected on a isotopically labeled protein backbone using the listed triple-resonance experiments. Boxes with a solid outline designate the nuclei involved in each correlation experiment. Dotted vertical lines indicate the location of the peptide bonds.

the decay rate of signals in the transverse plane [94,95]. Fourth, the introduction of TROSY (transverse relaxation-optimized spectroscopy), which manipulates spins in a way that maintains those signals having longer relaxation times, is also allowing much larger proteins to be studied by NMR [96,97].

Another tool for structural elucidation became available with the recent discovery that NMR allows observation of correlations due to scalar couplings across hydrogen bonds. This indicates that hydrogen bonds can have a measurable amount of covalent character, so the phenomenon has been called "hydrogen-bond J couplings." Among the correlations observed are one-bond $^{1h}J_{HN}$ correlations [98], two-bond $^{2h}J_{NN}$ correlations [99], and three-bond $^{3h}J_{C'N}$ correlations [100,101], all of which have recently been explained theoretically [102]. Much like a long-range NOE correlation, these correlations add structural constraints to 3D structures (especially for nucleic acids).

There is a lot of interest in using NMR to study ligand–receptor binding. This is normally done by looking for intermolecular NOEs between the ligand and the receptor, but because the NMR spectrum of a protein–ligand complex can be complicated, small NOEs can be hard to detect. The problem is simplified if isotopically labeled ligands are mixed with unlabeled proteins and an isotope-filtered NMR experiment used to selectively observe the labeled resonances [103]. As more complex ligands and receptors are studied, techniques to do the opposite—selectively observe the resonances of just the unlabeled molecules—were developed (in part through the use of adiabatic pulses) [104].

The final trend in biomolecular NMR is to use the internuclear dipolar couplings of oriented molecules to determine structures [105]. When molecules are in solution and tumbling freely, these couplings are averaged to zero; however, if the molecules are aligned with the magnetic field even partially, these couplings will be nonzero and measurable. If one measures the one-bond ^{15}N-^{1}H and ^{13}C-^{1}H dipolar couplings, and knows the internuclear distances, then the orientation of the vectors of these bonds (with respect to the magnetic susceptibility tensor of the molecule) can be determined. This gives direct information about the torsion angles of the bonds and hence information about the structure of the biomolecule. This information also complements that which can be obtained from analyses of NOEs and J couplings.

Because many molecules naturally exhibit only weak alignments with the magnetic fields, a recent trend has been to use different kinds of liquid crystals and bicelles not only to create more alignment but to allow control over the degree of alignment [106]. Once aligned, measurement of the changes in the one-bond coupling constants (typically ^{1}JNH) or the ^{15}N chemical shifts, measured at a variety of magnetic field strengths, gives the dipolar couplings [107]. A recent alternative is to measure the differences in chemical shifts and coupling constants between data acquired with and without MAS (using solution-state samples and a nanoprobe; discussed below). The advantage of this technique is that only one set of measurements need be made.

B. Water (Solvent) Suppression

In all of these biomolecular experiments, the signals from the protons bound to the amide nitrogen are critical. Unfortunately, these amide protons also all readily exchange with water, so the samples cannot be dissolved in D_2O. To keep the samples in a predominately H_2O environment yet still supply a small amount of D_2O for a ^2H lock, they are usually dissolved in 90:10 or 95:5 $H_2O:D_2O$. Because that makes the H_2O signal 100,000 times larger than that of a single proton in a 1 mM protein, new techniques had to be developed for acquiring NMR data on these kinds of samples.

There are essentially three ways to deal with the problem. One is to suppress the water signal, the second is to not excite it in the first place, and the third is just to live with it. None of these strategies are perfect, and a wide range of techniques have been developed in an attempt to exploit at least the first two strategies. Many good reviews of water suppression techniques exist elsewhere [108,109]. It is of interest, however, to note two things. First, virtually all of the common water suppression techniques are combinations of shaped pulses, PFGs, and indirect-detection methods (all discussed above). Second, most techniques are designed only for water suppression, not for the more general concept of solvent suppression. Suppressing the NMR resonances of organic solvents is more difficult than water suppression because the ^1H signals contain ^{13}C satellites in addition to the central resonance. General solvent suppression is becoming important in several flow-NMR techniques and will be discussed later.

C. Hardware Developments

There are many examples of how developments in NMR techniques have required improvements in the hardware and software as well. The ever higher magnetic fields used to simplify complex spectra have required improvements in superconducting magnet materials and magnet designs. FT NMR required the development of pulsed rf, whereas 2D NMR required the development of rf hardware and pulse-sequence-control software that was capable of more flexible phase cycling and power level control. Indirect detection required the design of both more stable rf and of magnet antivibration hardware to improve the signal cancellation possible via rf phase cycling. Spinlock sequences (e.g., TOCSY) required phase-coherent rf to be developed. The complex pulse sequences of biomolecular multiple-resonance NMR required multiple rf channels (as many as five), each capable of delivering not only more but a wider variety of pulses per sequence. For example, any one rf channel may be called on to deliver high-power uniform-excitation broadband pulses, region-selective pulses, broadband or region-selective decoupling, broadband or region-selective spinlocks, or highly frequency-selective pulses. These rf requirements have driven the development of faster and more flexible rf control, including more powerful pulse-shaping hardware and software. In addition, because PFG pulses of a variety of amplitudes are also freely intermixed with rf pulses, stronger gradients with ever faster recoveries are always being sought.

1. Probe Developments

In addition to hardware developments in the spectrometer console and magnet, advanced NMR experiments have also driven improvements in probe designs. The emphasis on water (solvent) suppression has created an emphasis on lineshape specifications. NMR lineshape specifications—defined as the width of the NMR peak at 0.55% and 0.11% of the height of the peak (0.55%/0.11%)—are now half as wide as they were a decade ago. Proton NMR linewidths of 4/6 Hz have been obtained. Narrower lineshape specifications do not guarantee good water suppression but are often considered to be an essential element. The better specifications arise from improvements in probe designs, magnet designs, shim-set designs, and installation procedures. Although NMR resolution (the width of the NMR peak at 50% of the height of the peak) for spinning samples has not improved, most high-field NMR spectrometers are now capable of—and specified to have—much better nonspin resolution than in the past. Since most nD NMR experiments, and all water suppression experiments, are run nonspinning, this is also now considered an important specification.

The second-most important probe development has been ever increasing probe sensitivities. The ^{1}H sensitivity specifications of modern probes are several-fold better than they were a decade ago. Instrument time is always precious, and a 3.2-fold increase in signal-to-noise can reduce the total time of an NMR experiment by an order of magnitude.

The emphasis on multiple-pulse NMR experiments (such as HSQC and the triple/multiple-resonance experiments) has driven improvements in three other parameters of probe design: shorter pulse widths, better rf homogeneities, and improved "salt tolerance". The first parameter is important because spectral widths in higher field NMR—as measured in hertz—are wider. This requires the rf pulses to become shorter (in time) to maintain the same excitation bandwidth (as measured in ppm). One way to get shorter pulses is to use higher power rf amplifiers, but as magnetic fields continue to increase, not only must the corresponding probes be redesigned to handle the ever increasing powers, but unfortunately the components that can handle these increased voltages are also usually larger. The space inside a triple-resonance PFG probe is already crowded, so the demands of increased power handling create conflicts that cause 800-MHz probes to be more difficult to make than 500-MHz probes (assuming the probe diameter remains the same). This is also why the first few probes for a new magnetic field strength often do not produce as much signal-to-noise improvement as would be predicted by theory.

The second parameter—better rf homogeneities—arises because every probe produces rf pulses that are spatially nonuniform to different extents, so that different parts of the sample receive rf irradiation equivalent to slightly different pulse widths. The net effect of this is that every pulse in an NMR experiment can degrade the resulting sensitivity, with the degradation directly proportional to the nonuniformity (inhomogeneity) of the pulse. Five 90° pulses in a sequence may generate only 80–95% of the sensitivity of a single 90° pulse. The specification is often quoted as the ratio of signal intensities for a 450° versus a 90° pulse (the 450°/90° ratio) or, on better probes, as the 810°/90° ratio. The homogeneities of both the observe (inner) and decoupler (outer) coils must be taken into account for multiple-channel experiments.

The third probe design factor—better salt tolerance—is driven by the need to study biomolecular samples dissolved in aqueous ionic buffers. As the salt concentration increases and the sample become more conductive, two things happen. The first is that the NMR sensitivity drops. A sample dissolved in a 0.5 M buffer may have only 90% of the sensitivity of the same sample dissolved in plain water. This means that a probe optimized for high sensitivity for organic samples (e.g., ethylbenzene) is not necessarily optimized for samples dissolved in aqueous buffers. With salty samples, the signal-to-noise will decrease as the filling factor of the probe increases, as the probe volume increases, as the Q of the probe increases, and as the salt concentration increases. Large-volume (8 or 10 mm) ^1H probes, or superconducting probes, are particularly prone to this problem, and care must be taken when using them to study aqueous samples.

The second problem with acquiring NMR data on conductive samples is that they heat up as power is applied to the sample. For a given amount of power, the more conductive the sample is, the hotter it gets. Although this is a minor but measurable problem when running spinlock experiments (like TOCSY), it is a significant problem with indirect-detection experiments because the X-nucleus decoupling may use a relatively high power to increase its bandwidth. The resulting temperature increases change the chemical shifts of the solute (actually the frequency of water changes with temperature and this moves the ^2H lock frequency of D_2O) and can also change lineshapes and cause sample degradation. This has required probes to have better variable-temperature performance, partly to maintain more stable temperatures and partly to dissipate any heat generated within the sample by rf heating.

2. Probes for Larger and Smaller Volume Samples

Some samples do not allow acceptable signal-to-noise NMR data to be easily acquired with conventional NMR techniques. For solution-state samples, there are two solutions to this problem. One, if the sample solubility is the limiting factor, use a probe whose rf coil can hold a larger volume of the solution. Two, if the sample quantity is the limiting factor, dissolve it in a smaller volume of solvent and place it in a more efficient small-volume probe. Samples dissolved in a smaller volume of solvent and run in a smaller volume probe can exhibit higher NMR sensitivities and fewer interfering signals arising from excess solvent or solvent impurities.

The default probe geometry for solution-state NMR is normally a "5-mm" probe i.e., a probe with an rf coil optimized for 5-mm (OD) sample tubes (Fig. 2a). If higher NMR sensitivity is needed and enough sample exists, probes that handle 8- and 10-mm sample tubes can be used. (Probes that use sample tubes larger than 10 mm in diameter were more common in the past but are rarely used anymore.) Ten-millimeter-diameter X-observe probes have been available for years, whereas 8- and 10-mm diameter ^{1}H-observe probes (including indirect-detection probes) have been available only for the last few years. Although data can be acquired on samples in 5-mm tubes placed in larger diameter (8- or 10-mm) probes (Fig. 2b) (even though this decreases the net NMR sensitivity), the converse is not true; that is, 10-mm sample tubes cannot be placed in 5-mm probes.

Larger diameter sample tubes are useful if samples have limited solubility and if plenty of solute exists. This is classically encountered when acquiring X-observe NMR spectra on inorganic complexes of limited solubility, but some groups studying biomolecules (i.e., those doing rational drug design) often use dilute solutions to minimize problems caused by aggregation, and sometimes they try to compensate for the reduced signal-to-noise by using larger sample tubes. For the opposite situation, in which the amount of solute is limited but the solubility is not, better NMR sensitivity can be obtained by concentrating the sample. This is a common scenario in small-molecule pharmaceutical applications, especially when studying natural products or metabolites.

a. Microprobes and Microcells. Once the sample has been concentrated into a smaller volume of solution there are several options for obtaining NMR data. One option is to use a 5-mm-diameter sample tube with "susceptibility plugs" (or certain types of microcells)—of which a variety of types are available—to reduce the depth (length) of the sample (Fig. 2c). This gives higher sensitivity than Figure 2a, but the lineshape usually suffers a bit, and sample preparation can be significantly more difficult, largely because all air bubbles must be removed from the sample. A second option is to use a smaller diameter sample tube in a probe with a smaller diameter rf coil (Fig. 2d). This also gives higher sensitivity than Figure 2a, and the lineshape is as good or often better. The increased

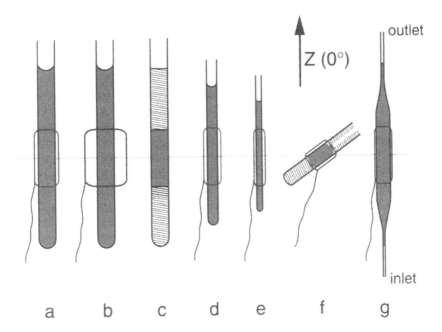

Figure 2 Representations of the various sample-tube geometries available for acquiring solution-state NMR data. Dark gray areas represent the sample solution. Outlines of the rf coils for each probe geometry are shown to illustrate the active volume of the rf coils. Shown from left to right in order are: (a) a sample in a standard 5-mm tube and the rf coil from a 5-mm probe; (b) a 5-mm tube in a 10-mm probe; (c) a 5-mm tube with susceptibility-matched restrictive inserts; (d) a 3-mm microprobe sample; (e) a 1.7-mm submicroprobe sample; (f) a Nanoprobe sample; (g) a flow probe. The Nanoprobe tube has a 40-μl total (and active) volume; the flow probe has a 60-μl active volume. All figures are drawn to the same scale.

sensitivity (in Figure 2d as compared to Figure 2a) is due in part to the ability to place a larger fraction of the sample volume in the active region of the rf coil without lineshape degradations. The better lineshape is due to the use of a smaller cross-section of the magnet. The sample volume depends on the diameter of the probe's rf coil (which itself ranges from 2.5 to 3 mm in diameter), but typically ranges from about 80 to 150 μl. Probes like this are now usually referred to as "microprobes" [53,110,111].

Probes designed for even smaller volumes now exist. The most conventional option is to use an even smaller diameter sample tube, typically with a diameter of 1.0 or 1.7 mm, in a probe with a matched-diameter rf coil (Fig. 2e). Probes like this were first made available in the 1970s [112] and might be making a comeback under the current moniker of "submicroprobe" [113]. Higher NMR sensitivities per amount of sample can often be achieved with submicroprobes, but the small size and fragility of the sample tubes has made sample handling difficult.

b. Nanoprobes. A totally different solution to the problem of obtaining NMR spectra on small-volume solution-state samples was introduced in the early 1990s. It uses a hybrid of MAS and traditional high-resolution probe technology. The resulting product, called a Nanoprobe, has had a large impact upon pharmaceutical research, as is covered in detail in two review articles [114,115].

All previous sample geometries for solution-state samples were approximations of an infinite cylinder (the sample is long relative to the rf coil) because this is a reliable and convenient way to obtain good lineshapes. This geometry moves all discontinuities of magnetic susceptibility (like liquid–air and liquid–glass interfaces) far away from the active region of the rf coil. The closer the discontinuities (interfaces) are to the rf coil, the more NMR line broadening they can introduce. Because perfectly cylindrical interfaces do not cause lineshape problems, the sample tubes themselves are made to be cylindrical. (Theory says that sample geometries that are spherical should also give good lineshapes; however, in practice the lineshape is usually substandard, presumably due to imperfections in the sphere such as the hole used to introduce the sample.)

Unfortunately, this "infinite cylinder approximation" sample geometry means that only a fraction of the sample can actually contribute to the NMR sensitivity. The available percentage that can be utilized depends on the diameter of the rf coil, but in a 5-mm probe the rf coil obtains most of its signal from the central 35% of the sample, and even a 3-mm probe uses only about 50% (Fig. 2). (For any given probe style, the percentage claimed can vary among different vendors and generations of probes, and for a 5-mm probe may even be as high as 45% or 50%; however, higher percentages always cause a performance trade-off such as a worse lineshape or a reduced rf homogeneity.) Susceptibility plugs can constrict the entire sample to within the active region of the rf coil, but as the percentage approaches 100% the lineshape usually degrades. (This is because the plugs can never be a perfect match to the magnetic susceptibility of the sample.) Sample handling also becomes more difficult when susceptibility plugs are used.

Nanoprobes, on the other hand, work on an entirely different principle [114–116]. To maximize sensitivity, 100% of the solution-state sample is placed the rf coil of the probe (Fig. 2f). Normally this would result in severe broadening of the NMR lines because of the various liquid–air and liquid–glass interfaces (magnetic-susceptibility discontinuities) close to the rf coil. To eliminate these magnetic-susceptibility line broadenings and regain a solution-state-quality lineshape, the samples are spun about the magic angle (54.7° relative to the z axis) [117,118]. This also allows samples that are smaller than the volume of the rf coil

(40 μl in the case of a standard Nanoprobe) to be properly studied by NMR. Smaller samples just leave a larger air bubble in the Nanoprobe sample cell, and MAS completely eliminates this line broadening. The author has obtained good NMR data on samples dissolved in less than 2 μl of solvent; linewidths and line-shapes are good, water suppression is outstanding, and even a stable ^{2}H lock can be maintained on this volume of solvent.

Nanoprobes were initially designed to allow NMR spectra to be obtained on small-volume (≤40 μl) solution-state samples [114,115]. This use is illustrated by five kinds of sample-limited applications. First, Nanoprobes capable of ^{1}H-only detection have solved the structures of several unknowns using the data from a variety of 1D and 2D ^{1}H NMR experiments (Fig. 3) [119,120]. Second, ^{13}C-observe Nanoprobes have used conventional 1D ^{13}C{^{1}H} NMR data to solve the structures of unknowns [121,122]. Third, ^{13}C-observe Nanoprobes have generated high-sensitivity INADEQUATE data that determined the complete carbon skele-

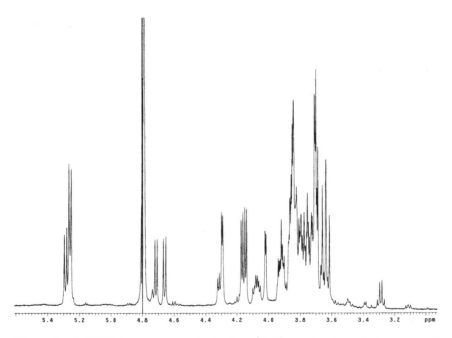

Figure 3 A ^{1}H NMR spectrum acquired using a ^{1}H Nanoprobe. Several micrograms of the unknown oligosaccharide were dissolved in an H_2O:D_2O mixture. The sample was spun about the magic angle at 1.8 kHz; the data were acquired in 1024 scans using presaturation to saturate the water resonance (at 4.8 ppm). The narrow water resonance is characteristic of Nanoprobe spectra, regardless of the sample volume. (Sample courtesy of A. Manzi, University of California, San Diego.)

ton of unknowns (in a more rigorous manner than an indirect-detection method like HMBC could) [123–125]. Fourth, Nanoprobes have been used to acquire solvent-suppressed ^1H NMR spectra on samples dissolved in 90:10 $H_2O:D_2O$ to solve structures using 1D and 2D NMR (homonuclear) techniques [126–129]. Fifth, Nanoprobes capable of generating indirect-detection and PFG data are now available as well [130]. These kinds of applications are primarily of benefit to natural product and metabolism chemists, both of which typically suffer from limited amounts of sample, but there is also an unrecognized potential to rational drug design programs (especially for the removal of dipolar couplings in large oriented molecules).

The advantages of the Nanoprobes are that they are the highest-sensitivity-per-nucleus NMR probes commercially available, they shim equally easily for 40- and 4-μl samples, and they have the unique capability of producing lineshapes for samples in H_2O that are very narrow at the base (which facilitates water suppression) (see Fig. 3). However, acquiring solution-state data while using MAS does have some experimental limitations. Because the sample is spinning during the entire experiment, spinning sidebands may be present in all spectra (even multidimensional spectra). The sample spinning also diminishes the signal stability and thus causes additional t_1 noise. This is a problem for experiments that utilize phase-cycled cancellation of large signals (like phase-cycled indirect detection), although the recent availability of Nanoprobes capable of running PFG experiments addresses this problem.

MAS is not a new invention. It has been in use since 1958 for narrowing linewidths in solid-state samples. It was never used before for fully solution-state samples for two reasons. First, MAS was initially designed to remove the much larger line broadenings that occur only in solid-state samples (i.e., those that arise from interactions such as dipolar coupling and chemical shift anisotropy). The capability of MAS to eliminate the much smaller line broadenings that arise from magnetic-susceptibility discontinuities was not considered nearly as important, although its utility was recognized early on by several groups [114,115,131,132]. Second, to obtain high-quality solution-state lineshapes (<1, 10, and 20 Hz at the 50%, 0.55%, and 0.11% levels, respectively) NMR probes also need to be built using materials and designs that are susceptibility matched. While this has long been a criteria in the design of vertical-spinning solution-state probes [133], it was never considered important in the design of solid-state MAS probes until recently [134]. The Nanoprobe was the first MAS probe designed to handle solution-state samples, and as such it was the first MAS probe to incorporate this magnetic-susceptibility-matched probe design technology. (Solid-state samples often have ^1H linewidths of 100 Hz or more, so that an additional line broadening of 5–20 Hz coming from the probe design was considered insignificant. This additional line broadening is large, however, for solution-state samples whose natural linewidths can be well under 1 Hz.) Conventional MAS probes are built to emphasize very high-speed spinning and the ability to handle high rf powers. These characteristics are needed for solid-state NMR but are unnecessary for (and often conflict with the requirements of) solution-state NMR.

After the (Varian) Nanoprobe demonstrated the virtues of using MAS on solution-state samples (and on a variety of semisolid samples, as discussed below), a variety of high-resolution MAS (HR-MAS) probes became available from several NMR probe vendors (including Bruker, Doty Scientific, and JEOL). The different probes exhibit a variety of performances caused by different balances of the contrasting needs of solution-state versus solid-state NMR. The biggest differences among the various HR-MAS probe designs are in the lineshape specifications and the filling factors (the sensitivity efficiencies). Less emphasized—but still important—differences include maximum spin rate, integrity of the sample container against leakage, cost of the sample container, cost and ease of automation, and ease of changing between MAS and non-MAS probes. The reliability of sample spinning is usually not an issue with liquid (or semisolid) samples.

There is one very big difference between MAS probes and microprobes (or other non-MAS probes). Non-MAS probes (those that orient samples along the vertical z axis of the magnet) use cylindrical (or spherical) sample geometries to eliminate line broadenings arising from those magnetic-susceptibility discontinuities surrounding the sample, but this has no effect on magnetic-susceptibility discontinuities within the sample itself. Only MAS can eliminate line broadenings that arise from these internal magnetic-susceptibility discontinuities (those within the sample). This is a crucial and critical difference. A homogeneous (filterable) solution-state sample has a uniform magnetic susceptibility only as long as there are no air bubbles in the sample. If any heterogeneity is introduced anywhere near the rf coil, either accidentally or purposefully—and this can be an air bubble, flocculent material, any amount of solid or liquid precipitate, or any form of emulsion, suspension, or slurry—the sample becomes physically heterogeneous to the NMR and only MAS can be used to regenerate narrow lineshapes. (The author has encountered a surprising number of situations in which spectroscopists thought their samples were physically homogeneous—because they were visually clear and produced reasonable NMR spectra—until it was found that the spectra acquired under HR-MAS were measurably different.) This means that cylindrical (or spherical) microcells must be filled completely, with no air bubbles, or the NMR resonances will be broadened, whereas an MAS microcell will generate the same lineshape regardless of how completely the microcell is filled. Note that MAS does not necessarily guarantee that all resonances will be narrow: although MAS removes some line broadening effects, it does not affect other parameters (such as rapid T_1 or T_2 relaxation) that can broaden linewidths.

Probes are a very important part of an NMR spectrometer, and as such there are other styles of probes yet to be discussed. In particular, flow probes will be discussed in Section III.E, and cryoprobes will be discussed in Section III.G. However, the next section covers an important application of HR-MAS NMR in more detail. This attention is justified because the author has found that an understanding of the physics involved in sample composition, sample preparation, and experimental parameters is necessary if optimal HR-MAS spectra are to be acquired. This contrasts with most other kinds of NMR spectroscopy, in which sample preparation, data acquisition, and data interpretation are usually more straightforward.

D. NMR of Solid-Phase Synthesis Resins

Techniques for obtaining NMR data on samples still bound to insoluble solid-phase synthesis (SPS) resins have been a topic of considerable importance during the last few years, especially to combinatorial chemists [114,115]. The typical chemist wants to obtain a solution-state style spectrum, which normally means obtaining spectra with narrow lineshapes. This requires a consideration of magnetic susceptibilities, molecular motions, and how the three main types of NMR probes behave for heterogeneous SPS-resin slurry samples [116,135].

The first thing a solid-phase resin chemist needs to do to obtain narrow NMR linewidths is to swell the resin to a slurry with an excess of solvent. This increases the mobility of the bound substrates, and mobile nuclei typically exhibit narrower resonances than do solid-state samples. (Solid-state samples exhibit broader resonances than solution-state samples because of several parameters, including faster relaxation, chemical shift anisotropy, sample heterogeneity, and homonuclear dipolar couplings.) (Although NMR data can be obtained on SPS resins in the solid state by using traditional solid-state tools like CP-MAS, this is of more interest to the fields of material science and polymer chemistry, and is not useful to organic or combinatorial chemists.)

1. The Observed Nucleus

The second parameter to consider is which nucleus will be observed (^{1}H, ^{13}C, etc.). Different nuclei are affected differently by the sample heterogeneity of an SPS-resin slurry. A slurry of SPS resin is a physically heterogeneous mixture that contains regions of free solvent, bound solvent, cross-linked polymer, bound samples, and possibly even long tethers, and each of these regions may possess its own unique magnetic susceptibility. This mix of magnetic-susceptibility discontinuities causes an NMR line broadening for nearby nuclei that scales with the frequency of NMR resonance. This means that ^{1}H spectra suffer four times as much magnetic-susceptibility line broadening as ^{13}C spectra because protons resonate at four times the frequency of ^{13}C nuclei. (For example, if ^{13}C nuclei resonate at 100 MHz, ^{1}H nuclei will resonate at 400 MHz.) This also means that resin spectra obtained on a 600-MHz NMR spectrometer will have linewidths twice as broad as those obtained on a 300-MHz system. Although this doubling of the linewidth may be completely offset by the corresponding doubling of the chemical shift dispersion (the number of hertz per ppm also doubles when going from 300 MHz to 600 MHz), this is only true if all the line broadenings observed in a given spectrum arise from magnetic-susceptibility discontinuities. This is certainly never the case for the resonances of the less mobile backbone of the cross-linked polymer, but it is a good approximation for the signals arising from the nuclei bound to the surface of the resin.

2. Choice of Resin and Solvent

The third and fourth parameters that control the NMR linewidths in an SPS resin slurry are the choice of the resin used and the solvent used to swell the resin [135,136]. The more mobility the nuclei of interest have, the narrower their resonances will be. Many resins used today for solid-phase organic synthesis contain long "tethers" that allow bound solutes to be located a significant distance away from the more rigid cross-linked polymer portion of the resin bead. Since the tethers are usually flexible straight chains, the bound solutes enjoy considerable freedom of motion. This is desirable for organic synthesis because it allows ready diffusion of reagents to the solute, and it is desirable for NMR because the additional freedom of motion decreases the efficiency of T_2 relaxation and hence produces narrower NMR resonances. This means that the NMR spectra of resins with either short or no tethers (like the original Merrifield resins) contain NMR linewidths that are broad compared to the linewidths obtained on resins with long tethers (like Tentagel or Argogel resins).

Then one must consider the solvent. Solvents that swell and properly solvate the resin (at least those portions of the resin that are around the bound solute) are more likely to produce narrow NMR linewidths. If parts of the resin are not properly solvated, the reduced molecular motion will increase the NMR linewidths. In summary, this means that to acquire an NMR spectrum with narrow linewidths, you need both a proper resin and a proper solvent; a poor choice of either will produce a low-quality NMR spectrum (i.e., one with only broad NMR resonances).

3. Choice of NMR Probe

The final parameter is the choice of which NMR probe is to be used: a conventional solution-state probe, an MAS probe, or a Nanoprobe or HR-MAS probe. The importance of this parameter depends on the previous four parameters. Conventional solution-state probes can generate high-resolution spectra for homogeneous liquids (because they use magnetic-susceptibility-matched probe design technology as discussed above) but they cannot eliminate magnetic-susceptibility line broadening caused by heterogeneous SPS resin slurries. Conventional MAS probes can remove magnetic-susceptibility line broadening caused by heterogeneous SPS resin slurries, but, because they do not use magnetic-susceptibility-matched probe design technology, the probe induces additional line broadening of its own (about 3–30 Hz depending on the resonance frequency). This is one reason why conventional MAS probes are inappropriate for acquiring NMR data on homogeneous liquids. Nanoprobes (and, to a lesser extent, other HR-MAS probes) use both MAS and magnetic-susceptibility-matched probe design technology, and so they can acquire high-quality narrow-linewidth NMR spectra on both homogeneous liquids and heterogeneous resin slurries.

Does this mean a Nanoprobe is required for all SPS resin spectra? No, it depends on what you need to do. A conventional solution-state probe produces acceptable ^{13}C NMR data; this technique is common enough to have acquired the name of "gel-phase NMR" [115,137,138], but ^{1}H NMR spectra acquired in this way are usually considered to exhibit unacceptably broad linewidths. A conventional MAS probe produces acceptable ^{13}C NMR data but poor-quality ^{1}H NMR data (although the data are better than they would be if a conventional solution-state probe was used). A Nanoprobe produces the best ^{1}H NMR data, and also produces the highest resolution ^{13}C NMR spectra, but often the additional resolution in the ^{13}C spectrum is not needed, and data from either of the other two probes would have been just fine [116]. Most people agree that a Nanoprobe (or other HR-MAS probe) is the only way to generate ^{1}H NMR data on SPS resins (Fig. 4) [114,115,139,140]. Nanoprobes were the first probes capable of acquiring high-resolution ^{1}H NMR spectra of compounds still bound to SPS resins [141] and they are responsible for starting the HR-MAS revolution. Nanoprobes are still the only probes capable of acquiring data on single 100-μm beads [142].

Note that if you are using a resin with no tether or have chosen a poor solvent, your spectra will contain broad lines regardless of which probe you use. (A Nanoprobe may allow the resonances to be narrower by 50 Hz, but if the lines are already 200 Hz wide it really won't help much.) All of these conclusions can also be extended to acquiring NMR data on any other kind of semisolid, slurry, emulsion, or membrane-bound compound; they are all examples of physically heterogeneous samples that contain enough localized mobility to allow NMR resonances to be narrow if the data are acquired properly. Biological tissues are another kind of semisolid; methods for using NMR to study them are an area of considerable interest to the pharmaceutical community [130], and investigations into the use of MAS and HR-MAS to acquire NMR spectra of tissues and intact cells are in progress [143–145]. This capability has the potential to have a big impact on both medical diagnostics and drug efficacy screening.

One final note about high-resolution MAS NMR: not all solution-state experiments translate directly into the realm of MAS. We have found, and the author has recently helped document, that spinlocked experiments like 2D TOCSY and ROESY do not always behave the same way as they do on conventional solution-state probes [145a]. The rf inhomogeneities of solenoidal coils, combined with sample spinning during the experiment, cause destructive interfer-

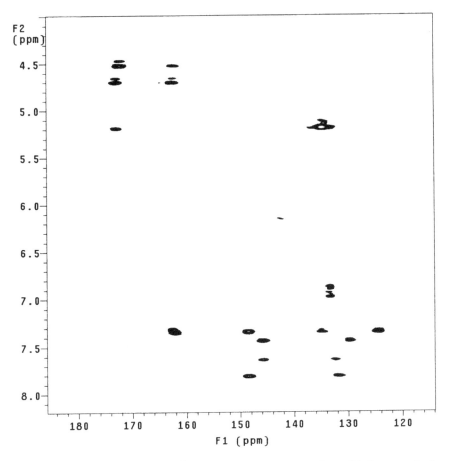

Figure 4 A multiple-bond ¹H-¹³C PFG HMBC spectrum of a solid-phase synthesis (SPS) resin acquired using a PFG indirect-detection Nanoprobe. The sample consisted of 0.5 mg of Fmoc-Asp(OtBu)-NovaSyn TGA (Calbiochem) slurried in 20 μl of CD_2Cl_2. The absolute-value HR-MAS dataset was acquired in 90 min using 32 scans for each of the 140 increments. The MAS spin rate was 2.1 kHz.

ences during the spinlocks that lead to signal intensities that are a function of the sample spinning rate. The solution is to use either different spinlocks [19] or different sample geometries (unpublished results).

E. Flow NMR

Some groups in the pharmaceutical industry are trying some entirely different approaches to introducing samples into the NMR spectrometer. All of these techniques can be grouped into a category called "flow NMR," and they all use "flow probes" (Fig. 2g), even though the samples may or may not be flowing at the time of NMR acquisition. The first example of this approach is HPLC-NMR, more commonly called just LC-NMR. More recently, direct-injection NMR (DI-NMR) and flow injection analysis NMR (FIA-NMR) have been developed as ways to acquire NMR data without the use of the traditional precision-glass sample tubes. By interfacing robotic autosamplers and liquid handlers to NMR spectrometers, samples in disposable vials and 96-well microtiter plates are now routinely being analyzed by NMR.

1. LC-NMR

The traditional way to separate a complex mixture and examine its individual components is to perform a chromatographic separation off-line, collect the individual fractions, evaporate them to dryness (to remove the mobile phase), redissolve them in a deuterated solvent, and examine them by conventional NMR using microcells and microprobes if needed. This off-line technique has its place but is inappropriate if the solutes are volatile, unstable, or air sensitive. LC-NMR offers a way to do an immediate analysis after an on-line separation, and as a technique it is becoming both more powerful and more popular.

Although LC-NMR was first developed in 1978, for the first 10–15 years it was regarded more as an academic curiosity rather than a robust analytical tool. Early reviews [146,147] and later reviews [148,149] of LC-NMR exist, but the technique has evolved rapidly as flow probes have become more common, as probe sensitivities have increased, and as techniques for working with nondeuterated solvents have been developed [34]. LC-NMR has now become almost a routine technique for metabolism groups [81,150] and is proving useful for drug production and quality control groups [151,152], combinatorial chemistry groups [153], and groups doing natural products research [154–156].

The unique advantage of LC-NMR over all other NMR techniques lies its is ability to separate components within a sample in situ. To many spectroscopists this may seem either obvious or nonessential (by thinking that the separation could always be performed off-line), but it has been shown that there are some analyses that do not lend themselves to off-line separations [157–161]. Whenever the analyzed component is unstable to light, air, time, or the environment, LC-NMR will probably be the preferred NMR technique.

The hardware for LC-NMR consists of an HPLC system connected to an NMR flow probe. The experiments can be run either in an on-flow mode, in which the mobile phase moves continuously (useful for preliminary or survey data acquisition), or in a stopped-flow mode, in which peaks of interest are stopped in the NMR flow probe for as long as needed for NMR data acquisition (useful for careful examination of individual components). In the stopped-flow mode, either 1D or 2D NMR data can be acquired, although the limited amounts of sample usually tolerated by HPLC columns sometimes makes the acquisition of extensive 2D heteronuclear correlation data difficult. The stopped-flow mode can employ any one of three different kinds of sample handling. First, the samples may be analyzed directly as they elute from the chromatography column, one chromatographic peak at a time. This is often the first, or default, mode of operation. Second, the LC pump may be programmed to "time-slice" through a chromatographic peak, stopping every few seconds to acquire a new spectrum. This is useful for resolving multiple components (by NMR) within a peak that are not fully resolved chromatographically or for verifying the purity of a chromatographic peak. (Alternatively, on-flow acquisition with a very slow flow rate has been used for similar purposes [162].) The third method is to collect the chromatographic peaks of interest into loops of tubing (off-line) and then flush the intact fractions into the NMR flow probe one at a time as needed. A variation of this technique is to trap the eluted peaks onto another chromatographic column, to allow concentration of the solute, and then re-elute them with a stronger solvent into the flow probe as a more concentrated slug [163].

There are several aspects of acquiring LC-NMR data that are challenging. The first is that all mobile phases in LC-NMR are mixtures, and the solvents are rarely fully deuterated, so that usually several solvent resonances need to be suppressed. Additionally, the resonances of the organic solvents contain ^{13}C satellites that need to be suppressed. Also, when the samples are flowing through the probe, solvent suppression sequences like presaturation take too much time and don't work well. All of these problems were solved when the WET solvent-suppression experiment was developed [34]. WET uses a combination of shaped-pulse selective excitation, multifrequency SLP pulses, PFG, and indirect-detection ^{13}C decoupling during the shaped pulses to quickly and efficiently suppress multiple resonances using only a simple two-channel spectrometer.

Another challenge in acquiring LC-NMR data is that, by definition, the solvent composition changes during the experiment. In reversed-phase LC-NMR one of the cosolvents is virtually always water, and unfortunately the chemical shift of water changes as the solvent composition changes. (The author has observed that this is also true to a much lesser extent for the resonances of several other solvents and modifiers.) In addition, if the mobile phase is fully protonated (nondeuterated) there will be no ^2H lock to keep the frequencies constant. (Also, D_2O serves as a poor lock signal because its chemical shift changes with solvent composition.) All of this means that the frequencies of solvent suppression are constantly changing. To allow this to be compensated for, and to allow the frequencies to be automatically optimized, the SCOUT scan technique was also developed [34]. This technique takes a single-scan, small-tip-angle, nonsuppressed ^1H spectrum, moves the transmitter to the constant resonance (serving as a ^1H lock), measures where the other peaks moved to, and creates an SLP pulse that suppresses these peaks. This whole process take only a few seconds. It can be used in an interleaved fashion during an on-flow solvent gradient run or as a precursor to the signal-averaged stopped-flow data acquisitions. We will see later how it forms an integral part of the DI-NMR and FIA-NMR techniques.

The presentation of the resulting LC-NMR data depends on the type of experiment being run. On-flow LC-NMR data are usually displayed as a contour map like a conventional 2D dataset, although the Fourier transform is only applied along one axis (the F_2 axis) to give a frequency versus elution time plot. The 1D data plotted along the "pseudo-t_1" axis may either be the LC detection output or a projection of the NMR data (Fig. 5). Stopped-flow LC-NMR data, on the other hand, are usually presented as a series of individual 1D spectra either one-spec-trum-per-page or as a stacked plot (Fig. 6).

LC-NMR is usually considered a very powerful (although usually not a fast) technique. Its power can be exploited by hyphenating it further with mass spectrometry to produce LC-NMR-MS. Usually a fraction of the chromatographic effluent prior to the NMR flow cell is diverted to the mass spectrometer. LC-NMR-MS is considered by some to be the ultimate tool for pharmaceutical analysis, and although it is still in its early days, it is proving its worth in one-injection analyses of compounds that are either sample limited or proving to be tough structural problems [80,81,164,165].

2. Flow Injection Analysis NMR (FIA-NMR) and Direct-Injection NMR (DI-NMR)

FIA-NMR and DI-NMR are essentially sample changers that exploit the speed and robustness of flow NMR. Neither technique uses chromatography, so they are not designed to analyze mixtures. DI-NMR is well suited for the analysis of combinatorial chemistry library samples, whereas FIA-NMR appears to be more useful as a tool for repetitive quality control style analyses.

The hardware for FIA-NMR is similar to that for LC-NMR except that there is no chromatography column, so it is sometimes referred to as "columnless LC-NMR" [114,115]. No additional detectors (other than the NMR) are needed, nor is a pump capable of running solvent gradient methods. FIA-NMR uses the mobile phase as a hydraulic push solvent, like a conveyer belt, to carry the injected plug of sample from the injector port to the NMR flow cell. After the pump stops, the spectrometer acquires the SCOUT scan, analyzes it, and acquires the signal-averaged data (again using WET solvent suppression). When finished, the NMR sends a start signal to the solvent pump so that it can flush the old sample from the NMR flow cell and bring in the next sample. In classic FIA-NMR, as in LC-NMR, the sample always flows in one direction, and enters and exits the NMR flow cell through different ports. The flow cell is always full of solvent.

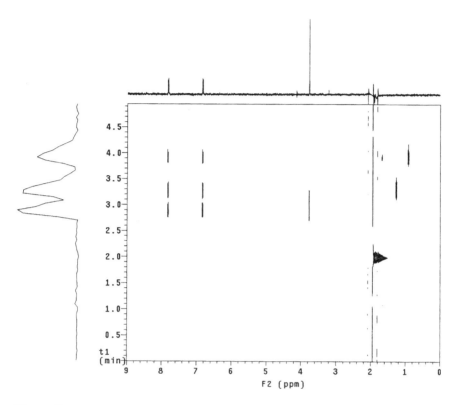

Figure 5 An on-flow LC-NMR spectrum. The three substituted benzoates were separated using a $CH_3CN:D_2O$ mobile phase. The ^1H chemical shift axis runs horizontally; the chromatographic time axis runs vertically. On the left is an "NMRgram" showing the summed ^1H signal intensity between 7.5 and 8 ppm; this display is analogous to a chromatogram. On the top is the ^1D spectrum (the "trace") of the methyl benzoate LC peak that eluted at 2.9 min. The data were acquired while the sample flowed continuously through the probe by using two-frequency WET solvent suppression (at 1.95 and 4.2 ppm); suppression frequencies were automatically determined using the SCOUT scan experiment. The small signals flanking the CH_3CN resonance are traces of its ^{13}C satellites.

DI-NMR, which was also first developed by our group [114,115], is significantly different. Rather than starting off with an NMR flow cell full of solvent and suffering the sensitivity losses caused by the ensuing dilution of the injected sample, the flow cell starts off empty in DI-NMR. A sample solution is injected directly into the NMR flow cell. The spectrometer then acquires the SCOUT scan, analyzes it, and acquires the signal-averaged data (with WET). When finished, the

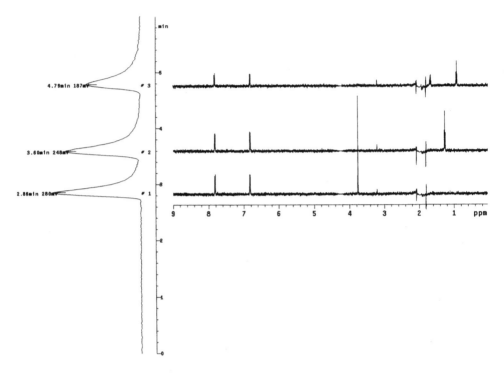

Figure 6 Stopped-flow LC-NMR data. The three substituted benzoates were separated using a $CH_3CN:D_2O$ mobile phase. The ^1H chemical shift axis runs horizontally; the chromatographic time axis runs vertically. On the left is the HPLC chromatogram; the corresponding ^1H NMR spectra are aligned with each peak. This is Varian's default (and automatic) output display for stopped-flow LC-NMR data. The data were acquired by using two-frequency WET solvent suppression (at 1.95 and 4.2 ppm) and a two-frequency DSP notch filters; suppression and filter frequencies were automatically determined using the SCOUT scan experiment. Each ^1H NMR spectrum was acquired in seven scans on a 25-µg on-column sample injection.

syringe pump pulls the sample back out of the NMR flow cell, in the reverse direction, and returns it to its original (or an alternate) sample container. Once the flow cell is emptied, clean solvent is injected and removed from the flow cell to rinse it. The solvents used for both the sample and the rinse must at least be miscible, and ideally should be identical, to avoid lineshape degradations caused by magnetic susceptibility discontinuities (due to liquid–liquid emulsions or precipitation of solutes in the flow cell) or any plugging of the transfer lines.

DI-NMR uses very different hardware than FIA-NMR. It uses the syringe pump in a standard Gilson 215 liquids handler to deliver samples to the NMR flow probe. Samples go directly into the NMR flow cell, through the bottom, via an unswitched Rheodyne injector port. The Gilson liquids handler is capable of accepting a wide variety of sample-container formats, including both vials and microtiter plates.

One of the justifications for the development of DI-NMR was to improve the robustness and speed of automated NMR. The improvement in robustness has occurred, partly through the elimination of techniques such as sample spinning, automatic gain adjustment, automatic locking, and simplex shimming (PFG gradient shimming is used instead). This has allowed 96 samples at a time (stored in 96-well microtiter plates) to be run without error, and some installations have run tens of thousands of samples in a highly automated fashion. Sample turnaround times are from 1 to 4 min per sample, but the speed at which it can be run depends quite heavily on the solvent being used. Although most solvents can be pumped in and out of the probe rapidly, DMSO, which is used commonly, is viscous enough that sample flow rates are decreased and the resulting analyses may not be much faster than traditional robotic sample changers.

In comparison, FIA-NMR and DI-NMR have different advantages and disadvantages, and are designed for different purposes. The advantages of DI-NMR are that it generates the highest signal-to-noise per sample and consumes less solvent. The disadvantages of DI-NMR are that it has a minimum sample volume (if the sample volume is smaller than the NMR flow cell the lineshape rapidly degrades) and no sample filtration is possible. The advantages of FIA-NMR are that is has no minimal sample volume (since the flow cell is always full) and can filter samples (with an in-line filter), and that it can rinse the NMR probe better in a shorter time (albeit by consuming more solvent). The disadvantages of FIA-NMR are that it generates a lower signal-to-noise (because of sample dilution) and it consumes more solvent. Both techniques will always have some degree of carryover (although it may be <0.1%) and be subject to blockages from solid particles. The only way to avoid these problems is to use a conventional robotic sample changer for glass tubes. In applications, FIA-NMR is more valuable for repetitive analyses or quality control functions, especially when there is plenty of sample and the samples are to be discarded. In contrast, DI-NMR is more valuable when there is a limited amount of sample and the samples must be recovered. DI-NMR, as implemented by Varian in the product called VAST, is becoming well regarded as a tool for the analysis of single-compound combinatorial chemistry libraries [82,130,166], biofluids, and for SAR-by-NMR studies (described below).

3. DI-NMR: Data Processing and Analysis

Now that DI-NMR (VAST) is becoming routine, the next big challenge is the presentation and analysis of the data. As an example, we can examine how to display the spectral data acquired on the samples in a 96-well microtiter plate. Because these are combinatorial chemistry samples, there will be relationships between samples located in each row and each column of the plate, and we may choose to examine each of those relationships separately.

The most conventional way to present the data is as a stack of 96 spectra, plotted one spectrum per page. After acquiring data on several plates worth of data, this option tends to prove less popular to the chemists responsible for interpreting all of the data. Another option is to display all 96 spectra (and/or their integrals) on one piece of paper (Fig. 7). This works best if only part of the chemical shift range is plotted, and serves better as a printed record of the data rather than as a means to analyze the data. An alternative, which is better for on-screen interactive analysis but is less useful as a printed record, is to display the data in a manner similar to that used to display LC-NMR data; namely, as a contour (or stacked) plot with the ^{1}H frequency axis along F_2 but in which the t_1 axis corresponds to individual wells (Fig. 8). A third option is to display the spectral data as a stacked plot, either from one row, one column, or from a discrete list of well locations (Fig. 9). The last option, which appeals to many, is to display integral information in one of three ways. First, one can extract integral intensities for different regions across the chemical shift range, for each of the 96 spectra, and list them serially in a text file. Second (and more usefully), one can take this text file and extract just one integral value per spectrum (all from the same region) and display it in a spreadsheet database. Third, one can display this same information as a color map, with color intensity representing integral intensity (or peak height or any other quantitative information). A more complete description of these various options appears elsewhere [82].

Obviously, the most desirable way to interpret the data is automatically with a computer. Although the technology does not yet exist to determine the structure of an unknown compound de novo from its 1D ^{1}H spectrum, it is currently possible for a computer to determine if a given NMR spectrum is consistent with a suspected structure. This is relatively routine with ^{13}C data but is harder for ^{1}H data because of the presence of homonuclear couplings (especially second-order couplings) and increased solvent effects, although software to accomplish this does exist [167]. This capability is expected to be of great interest in combinatorial chemistry since normally the expected structure already exists in an electronic database somewhere and can easily be submitted to the analysis software along with the experimental NMR spectral data.

4. Other Techniques, Applications, and Hardware: SAR-by-NMR

Rational drug design programs have also been using DI-NMR. Starting in 1996, a group at Abbott Laboratories published a series of articles about "SAR-by-NMR" [168]. SAR, or structure–activity relationship mapping, has been around for many

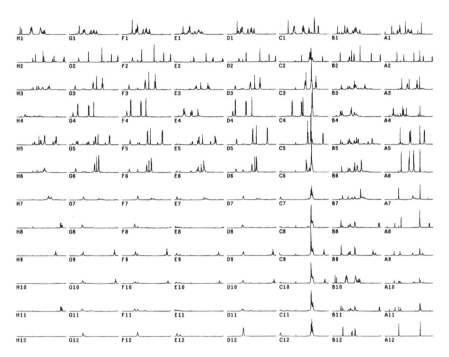

Figure 7 Direct-injection NMR (DI-NMR) data automatically acquired on samples stored in a 96-well microtiter plate using VAST. This is an 8 × 12 matrix plot of the 96 one-dimensional ^{1}H NMR spectra acquired on a plate of samples dissolved in DMSO-h_6. This represents one way to plot the data from an entire titer plate on one page. Each spectrum was acquired, processed, and plotted with identical parameters and is labeled with its alphanumeric position coordinates. For clarity, only an expansion of the proton spectrum (6–8 ppm) is displayed here. Data were acquired using WET solvent suppression as set up by the SCOUT scan experiment. Although the data presentation differs, there data are identical to these in Figure 8.

years, but the premise of SAR-by-NMR is to use changes in NMR chemical shifts to do the mapping. This is accomplished by first acquiring and assigning a ^{1}H{^{15}N} 2D correlation map (typically a PFG HSQC) of an ^{15}N-labeled receptor (a protein). Then ^{1}H{^{15}N} correlation maps are acquired on a series of samples made by adding different ligands (small molecules) to different aliquots of this receptor solution. If the ligand binds to the receptor, individual ^{1}H – ^{15}N correlations within the ^{1}H{^{15}N} HSQC spectrum will change positions, with the largest changes usually occurring for those nuclei that are closest to the active site of the receptor. (If the ligand does not bind to the receptor, the ^{1}H{^{15}N} HSQC spectrum will remain unchanged. The ligand itself is not ^{15}N labeled and will not appear in the HSQC

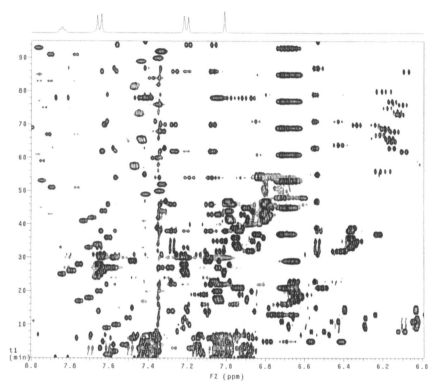

Figure 8 An contour plot of the 6- to 8-ppm region of the proton spectra of 96 one-dimensional ^{1}H NMR spectra acquired on the DMSO-$h_6$microtiter plate using VAST. Although the data presentation differs, these data are identical to those in Figure 7. This represents an alternative way to plot the data from an entire titer plate on one page. This style of data presentation is especially useful when it can be displayed on the computer screen in an interactive mode, and a user can select the one-dimensional spectra for individual wells at the top of the screen. Each spectrum was acquired, processed, and plotted with identical parameters.

spectrum.) By correlating the resonances that change position with the structures of the ligands, one can literally map the active site of the receptor. This technique has stimulated a flurry of interest in the primary literature [169,170]. One of the drawbacks to this technique is that, because a number of ligand–receptor complexes must be studied, a significant amount of purified ^{15}N-labeled protein is needed, which is not always easy to obtain.

Another issue is that, because a significant number of 2D NMR spectra must be acquired, automated techniques for handling the samples and acquiring the data

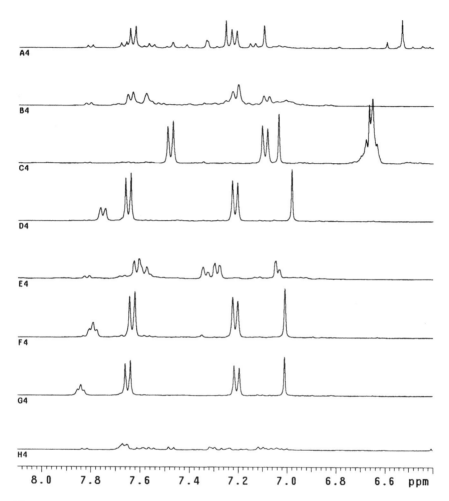

Figure 9 A stacked plot of the proton spectra (6.4–8.1 ppm) acquired on the "4" wells (wells A4 through H4—top to bottom) of the DMSO-h_6 microtiter plate using VAST. These data are a subset of those in Figures 7 and 8. This style of data presentation allows comparisons to be made between spectra acquired on different wells. Each spectrum was acquired, processed, and plotted with identical parameters.

are desirable. Although conventional automated NMR sample changers can be used, more recently DI-NMR systems have also proven useful. A DI-NMR system uses less sample than is required by a 5-mm tube, and the robotic liquids handler can be programmed to prepare the samples as well.

F. Mixture Analysis: Diffusion-Ordered and Relaxation-Ordered Experiments

One of the challenges of NMR is working with mixtures. In the past, NMR has always focused on the bulk properties of the solution, and—with the exception of LC-NMR—few attempts have been made to resolve the individual components of mixtures. The following three methods show that this is changing.

The most well-known method for analyzing mixtures by NMR is diffusion ordered spectroscopy (DOSY). It uses PFG to separate compounds based on their diffusion rates. PFG has been used since 1965 to measure diffusion rates [83]; but starting in 1992 it was shown how this technique could be used as a separations tool as well [171–173]. DOSY data are presented as a 2D contour (or stacked) plot where F_2 is the ^1H chemical shift axis and F_1 is the diffusion rate axis. Compounds having different diffusion rates are separated along F_1. Multiple components within a 5-mm tube have been separated [174]. The technique can also be combined with other experiments, and extended to multiple dimensions, to create COSY-DOSY, DOSY-TOCSY, DOSY-NOESY, ^{13}C-detected INEPT-DOSY and DEPT-DOSY, and DOSY-HMQC, among others [172].

In a related technique, Shapiro and coworkers combined PFG-based diffusion analysis with TOCSY to analyze mixtures in which the diffusion coefficients for each component are similar or in which there is extensive chemical shift overlap. Calling their version "diffusion-encoded spectroscopy" (DECODES) [84,85], they combined the standard longitudinal encode and decode (LED) sequence [175] with a 2D TOCSY sequence. Multiple 2D TOCSY datasets are acquired, each with a different diffusion delay. The TOCSY component resolves the chemical shift overlaps, and the peak intensities of resolved resonances are plotted against the diffusion delay to identify different chemical species in solution. (Each different chemical species in a mixture is likely to exhibit at least slightly different diffusion rates.) A variation of this technique, called "affinity NMR," was developed in which an unlabeled receptor was added to a mixture of ligands and a 1D or 2D DECODES spectrum was acquired [176]. If the diffusion delay is set long enough, only the resonances of the receptor and the bound ligands are visible. The TOCSY component then helps to resolve the chemical shifts of the detected (actively bound) individual components. A diffusion-filtered NOESY version of this technique has also been developed [177]. Unlike SAR-by-NMR, binding is detected by observing the ligand resonances and not by changes in the receptor resonances.

The third method for analyzing mixtures is relaxation-edited (or relaxation-resolved) spectroscopy. Large molecules have longer rotational correlation times than small molecules, and this results in shorter T_2 relaxation times (and larger NMR linewidths). These differences in T_2 relaxation can be used to edit the NMR spectrum of a mixture, based on the different relaxation rates of the individual components, in a manner analogous to diffusion ordering or diffusion editing [178–180]. A combination of diffusion and relaxation edited experiments (DIRE) was also reported and applied to the analysis of biofluids [179].

A big advantage of LC-NMR is that the chromatography column can take a mixture and separate it into individual chromatographic peaks. However, one disadvantage is that no single combination of mobile phase and column can completely resolve all compounds, and a single chromatographic peak may still contain multiple components. Often this can still be resolved by NMR because the individual components usually will have different chemical shifts, but this is only valid if the compounds and their chemical shifts assignments are already known in advance [162]. The hyphenated technique LC-DOSY-NMR (or DI-DOSY-NMR) would be a powerful way to analyze a mixture using as many as three different physical characteristics. Although this experiment has not yet been performed and the limited sample quantities used in LC-NMR may preclude its success, it remains an intriguing idea.

G. Other Probes: Superconducting Probes, Supercooled Probes, and Microcoils

Two other probe developments have also sprung from efforts to extract more signal-to-noise from a given sample. The first is the use of probes that use low-temperature rf coils to reduce the noise level. The rf coils are typically maintained at about 20°K while the samples are left at room temperature. Probes having coils made of either superconducting metal [181,182] or normal metal [183] have been made, although probes that have full PFG and indirect-detection capability have only recently become available. (The term *cryoprobe* is often loosely applied to both kinds of probes as a group.) The advantage of these probes is that they do exhibit higher sensitivities, and at a cost lower than that of the purchase of a higher field magnet (although without the increased dispersion). The current disadvantages are their significantly higher cost and limited availability. (They have also been associated with somewhat increased levels of t_1 noise because of their use of mechanical pumps.) The cost and delivery issues have precluded them from being widely used yet. Although that is changing rapidly, there are still a very limited number of published reports of their use [184,185]. One very good illustration of their usefulness was made by using an ^{19}F version of a superconducting probe to study the kinetics of protein folding [186]. Here, the higher sensitivity provided was critical because the reaction rate was too fast to allow signal averaging, so spectra acquired in only one scan each had to be used to follow the reaction.

The other probe development is the use of small-scale microcoils for data acquisition of very small samples. This work, done by Sweedler and Webb at the University of Illinois starting in 1994 [187], is allowing NMR data to be acquired on samples ranging in size from roughly 1 μl down to 1 nl [188,189]. The primary justification is to enable applications in flow NMR, i.e., to allow NMR data to be acquired on capillary HPLC and capillary electrophoresis effluents [190]. The biggest problem in using microcoils is dealing with the magnetic susceptibility interfaces [188]; however, probes have developed to the point that 2D indirect-detection data have recently been generated [191].

H. Combination Experiments

It is now routine in modern NMR spectroscopy to find that many of the above-mentioned techniques are combined in an ever-increasing number of combinations. Many such examples can be observed. The resolution and sensitivity of the HMBC experiment for poorly resolved multiplets was improved significantly by using semiselective pulses [192]. The 3D version of HMBC has been advocated for the elucidation of natural-product structures [193]. Selective excitation has been combined with a PFG version of a 3D triple-resonance experiment to make a 2D version (SELTRIP) for the study of small biomolecules [194].

PFGs and selective excitation have been combined into a powerful tool called the "double pulse field gradient spin echo" (DPFGSE), also known as "excitation sculpting" [28]. This tool offers a lot of flexibility in selecting desirable (or discriminating against undesirable) NMR signals to produce both cleaner and more sensitive NMR data. As such it has been used in a number of applications. One example is the DPFGSE-NOE experiment [28], which produces significantly cleaner data than the conventional 1D-difference NOE experiment. Another example is the HETGOESY indirect-detection experiment used for detecting heteronuclear NOEs [195]. DPFGSE sequences have been used to perform isotopic filtering to select only ^{13}C-bound protons [196] and for removing t_1 noise in 2D experiments [197]. It has also been used in band-selective homonuclear-decoupled (BASHD) TOCSY [198] and ROESY [199] experiments.

I. Software

Software tools to massage and analyze data are constantly becoming more powerful and more important. Digital signal processing (DSP) techniques that use low-pass filters are being used to enhance spectral signal-to-noise (through oversampling) and to reduce data size [200]. High-pass DSP filters, or notch filters, are being used to remove solvent resonances [32,201]. Linear prediction techniques are being used to flatten baselines and remove broad resonances [202]. Bayesian data analysis is providing more powerful and statistically meaningful spectral deconvolution, which can facilitate quantitative analysis [203]. FRED software is providing automated interpretation of INADEQUATE data [124,204] and is allowing complete carbon skeletons of unknown molecules to be determined both automatically and with higher effective signal-to-noise [123]. ACD software [205] is not only generating organic structures from 1D ^1H and ^{13}C data, but is also helping analyze NMR data acquired on combinatorial chemistry libraries [167]. The filter diagonalization method shows promise for very rapid 2D data acquisition and greatly reduced data storage requirements [206,207]. This too should prove useful for combinatorial chemistry.

J. Quantification

One of the big applications for NMR that seems to be on the verge of a growth spurt is in the area of quantitative analysis, especially in high-throughput techniques like combinatorial chemistry. Part of this seems to arise from the difficulty of performing accurate quantification with mass spectrometric techniques, especially for samples still bound to SPS resin beads [208]. NMR data can be highly quantitative, but certain precautions must be observed [209,210]. These include the need to use broadbanded excitation, generate flat baselines, minimize spectral overlap, minimize NOE interferences, and, in particular, ensure complete relaxation [211].

The other issue is the use of internal standards. Most internal standards have some drawbacks, such as too much volatility to be reliable (like TMS) or too little volatility for easy removal from the solute after measurement (like TSP). Some standards have also been shown to interact with glass sample containers [212]. To minimize spectral overlap the NMR resonance(s) of the standard should be sharp singlets (like TMS, TSP, HMDS, or $CHCl_3$), yet such resonances often exhibit very long T_1 relaxation rates (which complicates quantification). Recently, 2,5-dimethylfuran was proposed as an internal standard because the integrals of the two resonances can be compared to verify complete relaxation [213].

K. Automation

Of course, tools are needed to automate the acquisition and data analysis of all these experiments in a repetitive fashion. There are different levels and kinds of automation for NMR. The most primitive level lets a user change the sample manually but use software macros to automate the setup, acquisition, or processing of one or more datasets. The next level of automation entails the use of robotic devices to change samples automatically, and this is usually done in combination with software automation to acquire and plot (but not necessarily analyze) the data automatically. Some open-access NMR spectrometers run in this latter mode, although more open-access systems probably run in the former mode. Many service facilities operate in a highly manual mode.

Conventional tube-based NMR spectrometers equipped with robotic sample changers never run at 100% reliability. Estimates of reliability probably run from 75% to 99%, with autospin, autolock, and autoshim software failures being the most common hazards. The strengths of tube-based robotics is that the probe and spectrometer are always intact, and any failed sample is usually just ignored so that the spectrometer can move on to the next sample. Automation of sample preparation is often neglected.

The increased sample-throughput requirements of modern drug discovery programs are driving the development of more robust methods of NMR automation. Flow NMR techniques (the VAST DI-NMR system in particular) are being used to avoid failure-prone steps. This has pushed reliability up to 99.9% or higher, and this is important when thousands of samples are being analyzed. One advantage of DI-NMR is that sample preparation is minimal. One often forgotten limitation of DI-NMR is that dirty samples (those that contain precipitates, solids, emulsions, or immiscible mixtures) can clog up flow cells and degrade NMR lineshapes and solvent suppression performance. This suggests that DI-NMR is not ready for use in open-access environments and that tube-based NMR spectrometers are more appropriate for spectrometers seeing nonfiltered samples.

L. Research NMR vs. Analytical NMR

This brings up a final point about the dual nature of NMR spectroscopy. NMR started off as a tool for research. For the last several decades it continued to serve in that role, and to a large extent it still does (and will for the foreseeable future). However, eventually it will also become an analytical tool, serving to provide answers to repetitive questions. The current drive to develop automation and high-throughput techniques is a reflection of the beginning of this trend, which is expected to grow.

IV. CONCLUSION

The field of NMR spectroscopy has matured significantly, although this does not mean that the pace of development has slowed; rather, it means that this is a time of great opportunity. Many hardware and software tools have been developed to solve specific problems, and the key now is to apply these tools to new problems. One might even go so far as to say that the hardware and the pulse-sequence tools we have available are ahead of the potential applications, meaning that what remains are for users to find new ways to use the tools that have already been developed. Some of the most exciting possibilities undoubtedly lie at the boundaries of interdisciplinary problems; that is, scientists who are unfamiliar with NMR often have problems that could be solved with current technology if only these problems could be matched up with both people of vision and people with the correct technical expertise. As a result, it behooves all scientists in the field of drug discovery to—as much as possible—stay abreast of these many developments in NMR spectroscopy.

REFERENCES

1. Grant DM, Harris RK, eds. Encyclopedia of NMR. Volume 1. Historical Perspectives. West Sussex, England: John Wiley and Sons, Ltd., 1996.
2. Croasmun WR, Carlson RMK. Two-Dimensional NMR Spectroscopy. Applications for Chemists and Biochemists. 2nd ed. New York: VCH, 1994.
3. Martin GE, Zektzer AS. Two-Dimensional NMR Methods for Establishing Molecular Connectivity. New York: VCH, 1988.
4. Kessler H, Gehrke M, Griesinger C. Two-dimensional NMR spectroscopy: background and overview of the experiments. Angew Chem 1988;27:490–536.
5. Clore GM, Gronenborn AM. Applications of three- and four-dimensional heteronuclear NMR spectroscopy to protein structure determination. Prog Nucl Magn Reson Spectrosc 1991;23:43–92.
6. Oschkinat H, Mueller T, Dieckmann T. Protein structure determination with three- and four-dimensional NMR spectroscopy. Angew Chem Int Ed Engl 1994; 33:277–293.
7. Clore GM, Gronenborn AM. Structures of larger proteins in solution: three- and four-dimensional heteronuclear NMR spectroscopy. Science 1991;252:1390–1399.
8. Shaka AJ. Decoupling Methods. In: Grant DM, Harris RK, eds. Encyclopedia of Nuclear Magnetic Resonance. West Sussex, England: John Wiley and Sons, Ltd., 1996:1558–1564.
9. Shaka AJ, Keeler J. Broadband spin decoupling in isotropic liquids. Prog Nucl Magn Reson Spectrosc 1987;19:47–129.
10. Fujiwara T, Nagayama K. Composite inversion pulses with frequency switching and their application to broadband decoupling. J Magn Reson 1988;77:53–63.
11. Kupce E, Freeman R. Adiabatic pulses for wideband inversion and broadband decoupling. J Magn Reson A 1995;115:273–276.
12. Bendall MR. Broadband and narrow-band spin decoupling using adiabatic spin flips. J Magn Reson A 1995;112:126–129.
13. Silver MS, Joseph RI, Hoult DI. Highly selective pi/2 and pi pulse generation. J Magn Reson 1984;59:347–351.
14. Bothner-By AA, Stephens RL, Lee JM, Warren CD, Jeanloz RW. Structure determination of a tetrasaccharide: transient nuclear Overhauser effects in the rotating frame. J Am Chem Soc 1984;106:811–813.

15. Bax A, Davis DG. Practical aspects of two-dimensional transverse NOE spectroscopy. J Magn Reson 1985;63:207–213.

16. Kessler H, Griesinger C, Kerssebaum R, Wagner K, Ernst RR. Separation of cross-relaxation and J cross-peaks in 2D rotating-frame NMR spectroscopy. J Am Chem Soc 1987;109:607–609.

17. Braunschweiler L, Ernst RR. Coherence transfer by isotropic mixing: application to proton correlation spectroscopy. J Magn Reson 1983;53:521–528.

18. Bax A, Davis DG. MLEV-17-based two-dimensional homonuclear magnetization transfer spectroscopy. J Magn Reson 1985;65:355–360.

19. Kupce E, Schmidt P, Rance M, Wagner G. Adiabatic mixing in the liquid state. J Magn Reson 1998;135:361–367.

20. Messerle BA, Wider G, Otting G, Weber C, Wuethrich K. Solvent suppression using a spin lock in 2D and 3D NMR spectroscopy with aqueous solutions. J Magn Reson 1989;85:608–613.

21. Otting G, Wuethrich K. Efficient purging scheme for proton-detected heteronuclear two-dimensional NMR. J Magn Reson 1988;76:569–574.

22. Vold RL, Waugh JS, Klein MP, Phelps DE. Measurement of spin relaxation in complex systems. J Chem Phys 1968;48:3831–3832.

23. McDonald S, Warren WS. Uses of shaped pulses in NMR: a primer. Concepts Magn Reson 1991;3:55–81.

24. Bauer C, Freeman R, Frenkiel T, Keeler J, Shaka AJ. Gaussian pulses. J Magn Reson 1984;58:442–457.

25. Davis DG, Bax A. Simplification of proton NMR spectra by selective excitation of experimental subspectra. J Am Chem Soc 1985;107:7197–7198.

26. Anet FAL, Bourn AJR. Nuclear magnetic resonance spectral assignments from nuclear Overhauser effects. J Am Chem Soc 1965;87:5250–5251.

27. Stott K, Keeler J, Van QN, Shaka AJ. One-dimensional NOE experiments using pulsed field gradients. J Magn Reson 1997;125:302–324.

28. Stott K, Stonehouse J, Keeler J, Hwang T-L, Shaka AJ. Excitation sculpting in high-resolution nuclear magnetic resonance spectroscopy: application to selective NOE experiments. J Am Chem Soc 1995;117:4199–4200.

29. Berger S. Selective inverse correlation of ^{13}C and ^{1}H NMR signals, an alternative to 2D NMR. J Magn Reson 1989;81:561–564.

30. Crouch RC, Martin GE. Selective inverse multiple bond analysis: a simple 1D experiment for the measurement of long-range heteronuclear coupling constants. J Magn Reson 1991;92:189–194.

31. Berger S. Selective INADEQUATE. A farewell to 2D-NMR? Angew Chem 1988; 100:1198–1199.

32. Smallcombe SH. Solvent suppression with symmetrically-shifted pulses. J Am Chem Soc 1993;115:4776–4785.

33. Liu H, Weisz K, James TL. Tailored excitation by shaped RF pulses. Optimization and implementation of excitation containing a notch. J Magn Reson A 1993; 105:184–192.

34. Smallcombe SH, Patt SL, Keifer PA. WET solvent suppression and its applications to LC NMR and high-resolution NMR spectroscopy. J Magn Reson A 1995;117: 295–303.

35. Hore PJ. A new method for water suppression in the proton NMR spectra of aqueous solutions. J Magn Reson 1983;54:539–542.

36. Piotto M, Saudek V, Sklenar V. Gradient-tailored excitation for single-quantum NMR spectroscopy of aqueous solutions. J Biomol Nucl Magn Reson 1992; 2:661–665.

37. Morris GA, Freeman R. Selective excitation in Fourier transform nuclear magnetic resonance. J Magn Reson 1978;29:433–462.

38. Live DH, Greene K. Application of composite 180° pulses to selective inversion. J Magn Reson 1989;85:604–607.

39. Wang AC, Grzesiek S, Tschudin R, Lodi PJ, Bax A. Sequential backbone assignment of isotopically enriched proteins in D_2O by deuterium-decoupled HA(CA)N and HA(CACO)N. J Biomol Nucl Magn Reson 1995;5:376–382.

40. McCoy MA, Mueller L. Selective decoupling. J Magn Reson A 1993;101:122–130.

41. McCoy MA, Mueller L. Selective shaped pulse decoupling in NMR: homonuclear [carbon-13]carbonyl decoupling. J Am Chem Soc 1992;114:2108–2112.

42. Bendall MR. Heteronuclear J coupling precession during spin-lock and adiabatic pulses. Use of adiabatic inversion pulses in high-resolution NMR. J Magn Reson A 1995;116:46–58.

43. Hwang T-L, Van Zijl PCM, Garwood M. Asymmetric adiabatic pulses for NH selection. J Magn Reson 1999;138:173–177.

44. Hwang T-L, Van Zijl PCM, Garwood M. Fast broadband inversion by adiabatic pulses. J Magn Reson 1998;133:200–203.

45. Patt SL. Single- and multiple-frequency-shifted laminar pulses. J Magn Reson 1992; 96:94–102.

46. Mueller L. Sensitivity enhanced detection of weak nuclei using heteronuclear multiple quantum coherence. J Am Chem Soc 1979;101:4481–4484.

47. Bax A, Ikura M, Kay LE, Torchia DA, Tschudin R. Comparison of different modes of two-dimensional reverse-correlation NMR for the study of proteins. J Magn Reson 1990;86:304–318.

48. Reynolds WF, McLean S, Tay L-L, Yu M, Enriquez RG, Estwick DM, Pascoe KO. Comparison of ^{13}C resolution and sensitivity of HSQC and HMQC sequences and application of HSQC-based sequences to the total ^{1}H and ^{13}C spectral assignment of clionasterol. Magn Reson Chem 1997;35:455–462.

49. Rinehart KL, Holt TG, Fregeau NL, Stroh JG, Keifer PA, Sun F, Li LH, Martin DG. Ecteinascidins 729, 743, 745, 759A, 759B, and 770: potent antitumor agents from the Caribbean tunicate Ecteinascidia turbinata. J Org Chem 1990; 55:4512–4515.

50. Mukherjee R, Da Silva BA, Das BC, Keifer PA, Shoolery JN. Structure and stereochemistry of divaricine, a new bisindole alkaloid from Strychnos divaricans Ducke. Heterocycles 1991;32:985–990.

51. Mukherjee R, Das BC, Keifer PA, Shoolery JN. Structure and stereochemistry of divarine: another new bisindole alkaloid from Strychnos divaricans Ducke. Heterocycles 1994;38:1965–1970.

52. Crews P, Farias JJ, Emrich R, Keifer PA. Milnamide A, an unusual cytotoxic tripeptide from the marine sponge Auletta cf. constricta. J Org Chem 1994;59:2932–2934.

53. Vervoort HC, Fenical W, Keifer PA. A cyclized didemnimide alkaloid from the Caribbean ascidian Didemnum conchyliatum. J Nat Prod 1999;62:389–391.

54. Lauterbur PC. Image formation by induced local interactions: examples employing nuclear magnetic resonance. Nature 1973;242:190–191.

55. Barker P, Freeman R. Pulsed field gradients in NMR. An alternative to phase cycling. J Magn Reson 1985;64:334–338.

56. Vuister GW, Boelens R, Kaptein R, Hurd RE, John B, Van Zijl PCM. Gradient-enhanced HMQC and HSQC spectroscopy. Applications to ^{15}N-labeled Mnt repressor. J Am Chem Soc 1991;113:9688–9690.

57. Hurd RE, John BK. Gradient-enhanced proton-detected heteronuclear multiple-quantum coherence spectroscopy. J Magn Reson 1991;91:648–653.

58. Hurd RE. Field Gradients and Their Applications. In: Grant DM, Harris RK, eds. Encyclopedia of Nuclear Magnetic Resonance. West Sussex, England: John Wiley and Sons, Ltd., 1996:1990–2005.

59. Price WS. Gradient NMR. In: Webb GA, ed. Annual Reports on NMR Spectroscopy. Vol. 32. San Diego: Academic Press, 1996:51–142.

60. Sarkar SK, Kapadia RD. Magnetic resonance imaging in drug discovery research. In: Bluemich B, Kuhn W, eds. Magnetic Resonance Microscopy. Weinheim; VCH, 1992:513–531.

61. Sukumar S, Johnson MON, Hurd RE, Van Zijl PCM. Automated shimming for deuterated solvents using field profiling. J Magn Reson 1997;125:159–162.

62. Barjat H, Chilvers PB, Fetler BK, Horne TJ, Morris GA. A practical method for automated shimming with normal spectrometer hardware. J Magn Reson 1997;125:197–201.

63. Rinaldi PL, Keifer P. The utility of pulsed-field-gradient HMBC for organic structure determination. J Magn Reson 1994;108:259–262.

64. Rinaldi PL, Ray DG, Litman VE, Keifer PA. Utility of pulsed-field gradient-HMBC indirect detection NMR experiments for polymer structure determination. Polym Int 1995;36:177–185.

65. Altieri AS, Miller KE, Byrd RA. A comparison of water suppression techniques using pulsed field gradients for high-resolution NMR of biomolecules. Magn Reson Rev 1996;17:27–81.

66. Ruiz-Cabello J, Vuister GW, Moonen CTW, Van Zijl PCM. Gradient-enhanced heteronuclear correlation spectroscopy. Theory and experimental aspects. J Magn Reson 1992;100:282–302.

67. Tolman JR, Chung J, Prestegard JH. Pure-phase heteronuclear multiple-quantum spectroscopy using field gradient selection. J Magn Reson 1992;98:462–467.

68. Davis AL, Keeler J, Laue ED, Moskau D. Experiments for recording pure-absorption heteronuclear correlation spectra using pulsed field gradients. J Magn Reson 1992;98:207–216.

69. Shaw AA, Salaun C, Dauphin J-F, Ancian B. Artifact-free PFG-enhanced double-quantum-filtered COSY experiments. J Magn Reson A 1996;120:110–115.

70. Hurd RE. Gradient-enhanced spectroscopy. J Magn Reson 1990;87:422–428.

71. Sheng S, Van Halbeek H. Accurate and precise measurement of heteronuclear long-range couplings by a gradient-enhanced two-dimensional multiple-bond correlation experiment. J Magn Reson 1998;130:296–299.

72. Marek R, Kralik L, Sklenar V. Gradient-enhanced HSQC experiments for phase-sensitive detection of multiple bond interactions. Tetrahedron Lett 1997;38:665–668.

73. Reif B, Koeck M, Kerssebaum R, Schleucher J, Griesinger C. Determination of 1J, 2J, and 3J carbon–carbon coupling constants at natural abundance. J Magn Reson 1996;112:295–301.

74. Reif B, Kock M, Kerssebaum R, Kang H, Fenical W, Griesinger C. ADEQUATE, a new set of experiments to determine the constitution of small molecules at natural abundance. J Magn Reson 1996;118:282–285.

75. Krishnamurthy VV. Excitation-sculptured indirect-detection experiment (EXSIDE) for long-range CH coupling-constant measurement. J Magn Reson 1996;121:33–41.

76. Wagner R, Berger S. ACCORD-HMBC: a superior technique for structural elucidation. Magn Reson Chem 1998;36:S44–S46.

77. Von Kienlin M, Moonen CTW, Van der Toorn A, Van Zijl PCM. Rapid recording of solvent suppressed 2D COSY spectra with inherent quadrature detection using pulsed field gradients. J Magn Reson 1991;93:423–429.

78. Kay L, Keifer P, Saarinen T. Pure absorption gradient enhanced heteronuclear single quantum correlation spectroscopy with improved sensitivity. J Am Chem Soc 1992;114:10663–10665.

79. Uhrin D, Barlow PN. Gradient-enhanced one-dimensional proton chemical-shift correlation with full sensitivity. J Magn Reson 1997;126:248–255.

80. Holt RM, Newman MJ, Pullen FS, Richards DS, Swanson AG. High-performance liquid chromatography/NMR spectrometry/mass spectrometry: further advances in hyphenated technology. J Mass Spectrom 1997;32:64–70.

81. Ehlhardt WJ, Woodland JM, Baughman TM, Vandenbranden M, Wrighton SA, Kroin JS, Norman BH, Maple SR. Liquid chromatography/nuclear magnetic resonance spectroscopy and liquid chromatography/mass spectrometry identification of novel metabolites of the multidrug resistance modulator LY335979 in rat bile and human liver microsomal incubations. Drug Metab Dispos 1998;26:42–51.

82. Keifer PA, Smallcombe SH, Williams EH, Salomon KE, Mendez G, Belletire JL, Moore CD. Direct-injection NMR (DI-NMR): a flow NMR technique for the analysis of combinatorial chemistry libraries. J Comb Chem 2000;2:151–171.

83. Stejskal EO, Tanner JE. Spin diffusion measurements: spin echoes in the presence of a time-dependent field gradient. J Chem Phys 1965;42:288–292.

84. Lin M, Shapiro MJ, Wareing JR. Diffusion-edited NMR—affinity NMR for direct observation of molecular interactions. J Am Chem Soc 1997;119:5249–5250.

85. Lin M, Shapiro MJ, Wareing JR. Screening mixtures by affinity NMR. J Org Chem 1997;62:8930–8931.

86. Van Zijl PCM, Moonen CTW. Complete water suppression for solutions of large molecules based on diffusional differences between solute and solvent (DRYCLEAN). J Magn Reson 1990;87:18–25.

87. Cavanagh J, Fairbrother WJ, Palmer AG, III., Skelton NJ. Protein NMR spectroscopy—principles and practice. San Diego: Academic Press, 1996.

88. Kay LE, Ikura M, Tschudin R, Bax A. Three-dimensional triple-resonance NMR spectroscopy of isotopically enriched proteins. J Magn Reson 1990;89:496–514.

89. Ikura M, Kay LE, Bax A. A novel approach for sequential assignment of proton, carbon-13, and nitrogen-15 spectra of larger proteins: heteronuclear triple-resonance three-dimensional NMR spectroscopy. Application to calmodulin. Biochemistry 1990;29:4659–4667.

90. Marion D, Kay LE, Sparks SW, Torchia DA, Bax A. Three-dimensional heteronuclear NMR of nitrogen-15 labeled proteins. J Am Chem Soc 1989;111:1515–1517.

91. Wider G. Technical aspects of NMR spectroscopy with biological macromolecules and studies of hydration in solution. Prog Nucl Magn Reson Spectrosc 1998; 32:193–275.

92. Biamonti C, Rios CB, Lyons BA, Montelione GT. Multidimensional NMR experiments and analysis techniques for determining homo- and heteronuclear scalar coupling constants in proteins and nucleic acids. Adv Biophys Chem 1994;4:51–120.

93. Montelione GT, Emerson SD, Lyons BA. A general approach for determining scalar coupling constants in polypeptides and proteins. Biopolymers 1992;32:327–334.

94. Zwahlen C, Gardner KH, Sarma SP, Horita DA, Byrd RA, Kay LE. An NMR experiment for measuring methyl-methyl NOEs in ^{13}C-labeled proteins with high resolution. J Am Chem Soc 1998;120:7617–7625.

95. Venters RA, Huang C-C, Farmer BTI, Trolard R, Spicer LD, Fierke CA. High-level ^{2}H/^{13}C/^{15}N labeling of proteins for NMR studies. J Biomol Nucl Magn Reson 1995;5:339–344.

96. Pervushin K, Riek R, Wider G, Wuthrich K. Attenuated T2 relaxation by mutual cancellation of dipole–dipole coupling and chemical shift anisotropy indicates an avenue to NMR structures of very large biological macromolecules in solution. Proc Natl Acad Sci USA 1997;94:12366–12371.

97. Wuthrich K. The second decade—into the third millenium. Nat Struct Biol 1998; 5:492–495.

98. Pervushin K, Ono A, Fernandez C, Szyperski T, Lainosho M, Wuthrich K. NMR scalar couplings across Watson–Crick base pair hydrogen bonds in DNA observed by transverse relaxation-optimized spectroscopy. Proc Natl Acad Sci USA 1998;95: 14147–14151.

99. Dingley AJ, Grzesiek S. Direct observation of hydrogen bonds in nucleic acid base pairs by internucleotide 2JNN couplings. J Am Chem Soc 1998;120:8293–8297.

100. Cordier F, Grzesiek S. Direct observation of hydrogen bonds in proteins by interresidue 3hJNC' scalar couplings. J Am Chem Soc 1999;121:1601–1602.

101. Cornilescu G, Hu J-S, Bax A. Identification of the hydrogen bonding network in a protein by scalar couplings. J Am Chem Soc 1999;121:2949–2950.

102. Dingley AJ, Masse JE, Peterson RD, Barfield M, Feigon J, Grzesiek S. Internucleotide scalar couplings across hydrogen bonds in Watson–Crick and Hoogsteen base pairs of a DNA triplex. J Am Chem Soc 1999;121:6019–6027.

103. Ikura M, Bax A. Isotope-filtered 2D NMR of a protein–peptide complex: study of a skeletal muscle myosin light chain kinase fragment bound to calmodulin. J Am Chem Soc 1992;114:2433–2440.

104. Zwahlen C, Legault P, Vincent SJF, Greenblatt J, Konrat R, Kay LE. Methods for measurement of intermolecular NOEs by multinuclear NMR spectroscopy: application to a bacteriophage lamba N-peptide/boxB RNA complex. J Am Chem Soc 1997;119:6711–6721.

105. Tjandra N, Omichinski JG, Gronenborn AM, Clore GM, Bax A. Use of dipolar ^{1}H-^{15}N and ^{1}H-^{13}C couplings in the structure determination of magnetically oriented macromolecules in solution. Nat Struct Biol 1997;4:732–738.

106. Tjandra N, Bax A. Direct measurement of distances and angles in biomolecules by NMR in a dilute liquid crystalline medium. Science 1997;278:1111–1114.

107. Tjandra N, Grzesiek S, Bax A. Magnetic field dependence of nitrogen-proton J splittings in ^{15}N-enriched human ubiquitin resulting from relaxation interference and residual dipolar coupling. J Am Chem Soc 1996;118:6264–6272.

108. Gueron M, Plateau P, Decorps M. Solvent signal suppression in NMR. Prog Nucl Magn Reson Spectrosc 1991;23:135–209.

109. Gueron M, Plateau P. Water signal suppression in NMR of biomolecules. In: Grant DM, Harris RK, eds. Encyclopedia of Nuclear Magnetic Resonance. West Sussex, England: John Wiley and Sons, Ltd., 1996:4931–4942.

110. Crouch RC, Martin GE. Micro inverse-detection: a powerful technique for natural product structure elucidation. J Nat Prod 1992;55:1343–1347.

111. Crouch RC, Martin GE. Comparative evaluation of conventional 5 mm inverse and micro inverse detection probes at 500 MHz. Magn Reson Chem 1992;30:S66–S70.

112. Shoolery JN. Small coils for NMR microsamples. Top Carbon-13 NMR Spectrosc 1979;3:28–38.

113. Martin GE, Guido JE, Robins RH, Sharaf MHM, Schiff PL Jr, Tackie AN. Submicro inverse-detection gradient NMR: a powerful new way of conducting structure elucidation studies with <0.05 μ mol samples. J Nat Prod 1998;61:555–559.

114. Keifer PA. High-resolution NMR techniques for solid-phase synthesis and combinatorial chemistry. Drug Disc Today 1997;2:468–478.

115. Keifer PA. New methods for obtaining high-resolution NMR spectra of solid-phase synthesis resins, natural products, and solution-state combinatorial chemistry libraries. Drugs Future 1998;23:301–317.

116. Keifer PA, Baltusis L, Rice DM, Tymiak AA, Shoolery JN. A comparison of NMR spectra obtained for solid-phase-synthesis resins using conventional high-resolution, magic-angle-spinning, and high-resolution magic-angle-spinning probes. J Magn Reson A 1996;119:65–75.

117. Springer CS, Jr.. Physiochemical principles influencing magnetopharmaceuticals. In: Gillies RJ, ed. NMR in Physiology and Biomedicine. San Diego: Academic Press, 1994:75–99.

118. Barbara TM. Cylindrical demagnetization fields and microprobe design in high-resolution NMR. J Magn Reson A 1994;109:265–269.

119. Manzi A, Salimath PV, Spiro RC, Keifer PA, Freeze HH. Identification of a novel glycosaminoglycan core-like molecule I. 500 MHz ^{1}H NMR analysis using a nano-NMR probe indicates the presence of a terminal α-GalNAc residue capping 4-methylumbelliferyl-β-D-xylosides. J Biol Chem 1995;270:9154–9163.

120. Manzi AE, Keifer PA. New frontiers in nuclear magnetic resonance spectroscopy. Use of a nanoNMR probe for the analysis of microgram quantities of complex carbohydrates. In: Townsend RR, Hotchkiss AT Jr, eds. Techniques in Glycobiology. New York: Marcel Dekker, 1997:1–16.

121. Klein D, Braekman JC, Daloze D, Hoffman L, Demoulin V. Laingolide, a novel 15-membered macrolide from Lyngbya bouillonii (Cyanophyceae). Tetrahedron Lett 1996;37:7519–7520.

122. Klein D, Braekman JC, Daloze D, Hoffman L, Castillo G, Demoulin V. Lyng-

byapeptin A, a modified tetrapeptide from Lyngbya bouillonii (Cyanophyceae). Tetrahedron Lett 1999;40:695–696.

123. Chauret DC, Durst T, Arnason JT, Sanchez-Vindas P, Roman LS, Poveda L, Keifer PA. Novel Steroids from Trichilia hirta as Identified by Nanoprobe INADEQUATE 2D-NMR Spectroscopy. Tetrahedron Lett 1996;37:7875–7878.

124. Harper JK, Dunkel R, Wood SG, Owen NL, Li D, Cates RG, Grant DM. NMR characterization of obscurinervine and obscurinervidine using novel computerized analysis techniques. J Chem Soc, Perkin Trans 2 1996;1:91–100.

125. MacKinnon SL, Keifer P, Ayer WA. Components from the phytotoxic extract of Alternaria brassicicola, a black spot pathogen of canola. Phytochemistry 1999; 51:215–221.

126 Delepierre M, Prochnicka-Chalufour A, Possani LD. A novel potassium channel blocking toxin from the scorpion Pandinus imperator: a ^{1}H NMR analysis using a nano-NMR probe. Biochemistry 1997;36:2649–2658.

127. Roux P, Delepierre M, Goldberg ME, Chaffotte AF. Kinetics of secondary structure recovery during the refolding of reduced hen egg white lysozyme. J Biol Chem 1997;272:24843–24849.

128. Delepierre M, Roux P, Chaffotte AF, Goldberg ME. 1H NMR Characterization of renatured lysozyme obtained from fully reduced lysozyme under folding/oxidation conditions: a high-resolution liquid NMR study at magic angle spinning. Magn Reson Chem 1998;36:645–650.

129. Delepierre M, Porchnicka-Chalufour A, Boisbouvier J, Possani LD. Pi7, an orphan peptide isolated from the scorpion Pandinus imperator: ^{1}H NMR analysis using a nano-nmr probe. Biochemistry 1999;38:16756–16765.

130. Keifer PA. NMR tools for biotechnology. Curr Opin Biotechnol 1999;10(1):34–41.

131. Doskocilová D, Schneider B. Narrowing of proton NMR lines by magic angle rotation. Chem Phys Lett 1970;6:381–384.

132. Doskocilová D, Dang DT, Schneider B. Effects of macroscopic spinning upon line width of NMR signals of liquid in magnetically inhomogeneous systems. Czech J Phys 1975;B25:202–209.

133. Fuks LF, Huang FSC, Carter CM, Edelstein WA, Roemer PB. Susceptibility, lineshape, and shimming in high-resolution NMR. J Magn Reson 1992;100:229–242.

134. Doty FD, Entzminger G, Yang YA. Magnetism in high-resolution NMR probe design. II: HR MAS. Concepts Magn Reson 1998;10(4):239–260.

135. Keifer PA. Influence of resin structure, tether length, and solvent upon the high-resolution ^{1}H NMR spectra of solid-phase-synthesis resins. J Org Chem 1996; 61:1558–1559.

136. Keifer PA, Sehrt B. A catalog of ^{1}H NMR spectra of different SPS resins with varying solvents and experimental techniques—an exploration of nano-nmr probe technology. Palo Alto, CA: Varian NMR Instruments, 1996.

137. Giralt E, Rizo J, Pedroso E. Application of gel-phase carbon-13 NMR to monitor solid phase peptide synthesis. Tetrahedron 1984;40:4141–4152.

138. Epton R, Goddard P, Ivin KJ. Gel phase carbon-13 NMR spectroscopy as an analytical method in solid (gel) phase peptide synthesis. Polymer 1980;21:1367–1371.

139. Hochlowski JE, Whittern DN, Sowin TJ. Encoding of combinatorial chemistry libraries by fluorine-19 NMR. J Comb Chem 1999;1:291–293.

140. Wehler T, Westman J. Magic angle spinning NMR: a valuable tool for monitoring the progress of reactions in solid phase synthesis. Tetrahedron Lett 1996;37:4771–4774.

141. Fitch WL, Detre G, Holmes CP, Shoolery JN, Keifer PA. High-resolution ^{1}H NMR in solid-phase organic synthesis. J Org Chem 1994;59:7955–7956.

142. Sarkar SK, Garigipati RS, Adams JL, Keifer PA. An NMR method to identify non-destructively chemical compounds bound to a single solid-phase-synthesis bead for combinatorial chemistry applications. J Am Chem Soc 1996;118:2305–2306.

143. Cheng LL, Chang IW, Louis DA, Gonzalez RG. Correlation of high resolution magic angle spinning proton MR spectroscopy with histopathology of intact human brain tumor specimens. Cancer Res 1998;58:1825–1832.

144. Moka D, Vorreuther R, Schicha H, Spraul M, Humpfer E, Lipinski M, Foxall PJD, Nicholson JK, Lindon JC. Biochemical classification of kidney carcinoma biopsy samples using magic-angle-spinning ^{1}H nuclear magnetic resonance spectroscopy. J Pharm Biomed Anal 1998;17:125–132.

145. Weybright P, Millis K, Campbell N, Cory DG, Singer S. Gradient, high-resolution magic-angle spinning ^{1}H nuclear magnetic resonance spectroscopy of intact cells. Magn Reson Med 1998;39:337–344.

145a. Kupce E, Keifer PA, Delepierre M. Adiabatic TOCSY MAS in liquids. J Magn Reson 2001;148:115–120.

146. Dorn HC. Proton-NMR: a new detector for liquid chromatography. Anal Chem 1984;56:747A–758A.

147. Albert K, Bayer E. High-performance liquid chromatography–nuclear magnetic resonance online coupling. Trends Anal Chem 1988;7:288–293.

148. Albert K. Online use of NMR detection in separation chemistry. J Chromatogr 1995;703:123–147.

149. Lindon JC, Nicholson JK, Wilson ID. Direct coupling of chromatographic separations to NMR spectroscopy. Prog Nucl Magn Reson Spectrosc 1996;29:1–49.

150. Lindon JC, Nicholson JK, Sidelmann UG, Wilson ID. Directly coupled HPLC-NMR and its application to drug metabolism. Drug Metab Rev 1997;29:705–746.

151. Mistry N, Ismail IM, Smith MS, Nicholson JK, Lindon JC. Characterization of impurities in bulk drug batches of fluticasone propionate using directly coupled HPLC-NMR spectroscopy and HPLC-MS. J Pharm Biomed Anal 1997;16:697–705.

152. Roberts JK, Smith RJ. Use of liquid chromatography–nuclear magnetic resonance spectroscopy for the identification of impurities in drug substances. J Chromatogr 1994;677:385–389.

153. Chin J, Fell JB, Jarosinski M, Shapiro MJ, Wareing JR. HPLC/NMR in combinatorial chemistry. J Org Chem 1998;63:386–390.

154. Wolfender J-L, Rodriguez S, Hostettmann K. Liquid chromatography coupled to mass spectrometry and nuclear magnetic resonance spectroscopy for the screening of plant constituents. J Chromatogr 1998;794:299–316.

155. Spring O, Heil N, Vogler B. Sesquiterpene lactones and flavanones in Scalesia species. Phytochemistry 1997;46:1369–1373.

156. Wolfender J-L, Rodriguez S, Hostettmann K, Hiller W. Liquid chromatography/ultraviolet/mass spectrometric and liquid chromatography/nuclear magnetic resonance spectroscopic analysis of crude extracts of Gentianaceae species. Phytochem Anal 1997;8:97–104.

157. Strohschein S, Rentel C, Lacker T, Bayer E, Albert K. Separation and identification of tocotrienol isomers by HPLC-MS and HPLC-NMR coupling. Anal Chem 1999;71:1780–1785.

158. Strohschein S, Schlotterbeck G, Richter J, Pursch M, Tseng L-H, Haendel H, Albert K. Comparison of the separation of cis/trans isomers of tretinoin with different stationary phases by liquid chromatography–nuclear magnetic resonance coupling. J Chromatogr 1997;765:207–214.

159. Strohschein S, Pursch M, Handel H, Albert K. Structure elucidation of β-carotene isomers by HPLC-NMR coupling using a C30-bound phase. Fresenius J Anal Chem 1997;357:498–502.

160. Schlotterbeck G, Tseng L-H, Haendel H, Braumann U, Albert K. Direct online coupling of capillary HPLC with ^{1}H NMR spectroscopy for the structural determination of retinyl acetate dimers: 2D NMR spectroscopy in the nanoliter scale. Anal Chem 1997;69:1421–1425.

161. Sidelmann UG, Lenz EM, Spraul M, Hoffmann M, Troke J, Sanderson PN, Lindon JC, Wilson ID, Nicholson JK. 750 MHz HPLC-NMR spectroscopic studies on the separation and characterization of the positional isomers of the glucuronides of 6,11-dihydro-11-oxodibenz[b,e]oxepin-2-acetic acid. Anal Chem 1996;68:106–110.

162. Albert K, Schlotterbeck G, Braumann U, Haendel H, Spraul M, Krack G. Structure determination of vitamin A acetate isomers through coupled HPLC and ^{1}H NMR spectroscopy. Angew Chem 1995;34:1014–1016.

163. Griffiths L, Horton R. Optimization of LC-NMR. III. Increased signal-to-noise ratio through column trapping. Magn Reson Chem 1998;36:104–109.

164. Pullen FS, Swanson AG, Newman MJ, Richards DS. "Online" liquid chromatography/nuclear magnetic resonance mass spectrometry—a powerful spectroscopic tool for the analysis of mixtures of pharmaceutical interest. Rapid Commun Mass Spectrom 1995;9:1003–1006.

165. Burton KI, Everett JR, Newman MJ, Pullen FS, Richards DS, Swanson AG. Online liquid chromatography coupled with high field NMR and mass spectrometry (LC-NMR-MS): a new technique for drug metabolite structure elucidation. J Pharm Biomed Anal 1997;15:1903–1912.

166. Hamper BC, Synderman DM, Owen TJ, Scates AM, Owsley DC, Kesselring AS, Chott RC. High-throughput ^{1}H NMR and HPLC characterization of a 96-member substituted methylene malonamic acid library. J Comb Chem 1999;1:140–150.

167. Williams A, Bakulin S, Golotvin S. NMR prediction software and tubeless NMR—an analytical tool for screening of combinatorial libraries. Poster #2. First Annual SMASH Small Molecule NMR Conference, Argonne, IL, Aug 15–18, 1999.

168. Shuker SB, Hajduk PJ, Meadows RP, Fesik SW. Discovering high-affinity ligands for proteins: SAR by NMR. Science 1996;274:1531–1534.

169. Hajduk PJ, Dinges J, Miknis GF, Merlock M, Middleton T, Kempf DJ, Egan DA, Walter KA, Robins TS, Shuker SB, Holzman TF, Fesik SW. NMR-based discovery of lead inhibitors that block DNA binding of the human papillomavirus E2 protein. J Med Chem 1997;40:3144–3150.

170. Hajduk PJ, Sheppard G, Nettesheim DG, Olejniczak ET, Shuker SB, Meadows RP, Steinman DH, Carrera GM, Jr., Marcotte PA, Severin J, Walter K, Smith H, Gubbins E, Simmer R, Holzman TF, Morgan DW, Davidsen SK, Summers JB, Fesik SW. Dis-

covery of potent nonpeptide inhibitors of stromelysin using SAR by NMR. J Am Chem Soc 1997;119:5818–5827.

171. Morris KF, Johnson CS Jr. Mobility ordered 2D-NMR spectroscopy. J Am Chem Soc 1992;114:776–777.

172. Johnson CS Jr. Diffusion ordered nuclear magnetic resonance spectroscopy: principles and applications. Prog Nucl Magn Reson Spectrosc 1999;34:203–256.

173. Morris GA, Barjat H. High resolution diffusion ordered spectroscopy. In: Koever K, Batta G, Szantay C Jr, eds. Methods for Structure Elucidation by High Resolution NMR. Amsterdam: Elsevier, 1997:209–226.

174. Barjat H, Morris GA, Smart S, Swanson AG, Williams SCR. High-resolution diffusion-ordered 2D spectroscopy (HR-DOSY)—a new tool for the analysis of complex mixtures. J Magn Reson B 1995;108:170–172.

175. Gibbs SJ, Johnson CS Jr. A PFG NMR experiment for accurate diffusion and flow studies in the presence of eddy currents. J Magn Reson 1991;93:395–402.

176. Anderson RC, Lin M, Shapiro MJ. Affinity NMR: decoding DNA binding. J Comb Chem 1999;1:69–72.

177. Ponstingl H, Otting G. Detection of protein-ligand NOEs with small, weakly binding ligands by combined relaxation and diffusion filtering. J Biomol NMR 1997;9:441–444.

178. Rabenstein DL, Millis KK, Strauss EJ. Proton NMR Spectroscopy of human blood plasma. Anal Chem 1988;60:1380A–1392A.

179. Liu M, Nicholson JK, Lindon JC. High-resolution diffusion and relaxation edited one- and two-dimensional ^{1}H NMR spectroscopy of biological fluids. Anal Chem 1996;68:3370–3376.

180. Hajduk PJ, Olejniczak ET, Fesik SW. One-dimensional relaxation- and diffusion-edited NMR methods for screening compounds that bind to macromolecules. J Am Chem Soc 1997;119:12257–12261.

181. Hill HDW. Improved sensitivity of NMR spectroscopy probes by use of high-temperature superconductive detection coils. Trans Appl Supercond 1997;7:3750–3756.

182. Anderson WA, Brey WW, Brooke AL, Cole B, Delin KA, Fuks LF, Hill HDW, Johanson ME, Kotsubo VY, Nast R, Withers RS, Wong WH. High-sensitivity NMR spectroscopy probe using superconductive coils. Bull Magn Reson 1995;17:98–102.

183. Styles P, Soffe NF, Scott CA, Cragg DA, Row F, White DJ, White PCJ. A high-resolution NMR probe in which the coil and preamplifier are cooled with liquid helium. J Magn Reson 1984;60:397–404.

184. Logan TA, Murali N, Wang G, Jolivet C. Application of a high-resolution superconducting NMR probe in natural product structure determination. Magn Reson Chem 1999;37:512–515.

185. Flynn PF, Mattiello DL, Hill HDW, Wand AJ. Optimal use of cryogenic probe technology in NMR studies of proteins. J Am Chem Soc 2000;122:4823–4824.

186. Hoeltzli SD, Frieden C. Refolding of [$^{6-19}$F]tryptophan-labeled Escherichia coli dihydrofolate reductase in the presence of ligand: a stopped-flow NMR spectroscopy study. Biochemistry 1998;37:387–398.

187. Wu N, Peck TL, Webb AG, Magin RL, Sweedler JV. ^{1}H-NMR spectroscopy on

the nanoliter scale for static and online measurements. Anal Chem 1994;66:3849–3857.

188. Webb AG. Radiofrequency microcoils in magnetic resonance. Prog Nucl Magn Reson Spectrosc 1997;31:1–42.

189. Olson DL, Lacey ME, Sweedler JV. The nanoliter niche. Anal Chem 1998;70:257A–264A.

190. Wu N, Peck TL, Webb AG, Magin RL, Sweedler JV. Nanoliter volume sample cells for ^{1}H NMR: application to online detection in capillary electrophoresis. J Am Chem Soc 1994;116:7929–7930.

191. Subramanian R, Sweedler JV, Webb AG. Rapid two-dimensional inverse detected heteronuclear correlation experiments with <100 nmol samples with solenoidal microcoil NMR probes. J Am Chem Soc 1999;121:2333–2334.

192. Bax A, Farley KA, Walker GS. Increased HMBC sensitivity for correlating poorly resolved proton multiplets to carbon-13 using selective or semi-selective pulses. J Magn Reson 1996;119:134–138.

193. Furihata K, Seto H. ^{3}D-HMBC, a new NMR technique useful for structural studies of complicated molecules. Tetrahedron Lett 1996;37:8901–8902.

194. Wagner R, Berger S. gs-SELTRIP (SELective TRIPle resonance), an improved proton detection of X, Y heteronuclear connectivity. J Magn Reson 1996;120:258–260.

195. Stott K, Keeler J. Gradient-enhanced one-dimensional heteronuclear NOE experiment with ^{1}H detection. Magn Reson Chem 1996;34:554–558.

196. Emetarom C, Hwang T-L, Mackin G, Shaka AJ. Isotope editing of NMR spectra. Excitation sculpting using BIRD pulses. J Magn Reson 1995;115:137–140.

197. Van QN, Shaka AJ. Improved cross peak detection in two-dimensional proton NMR spectra using excitation sculpting. J Magn Reson 1998;132:154–158.

198. Krishnamurthy VV. Application of semi-selective excitation sculpting for homonuclear decoupling during evolution in multi-dimensional NMR. Magn Reson Chem 1997;35:9–12.

199. Kaerner A, Rabenstein DL. An ω 1-band-selective, ω 1-homonuclear decoupled ROESY experiment: application to the assignment of ^{1}H NMR spectra of difficult-to-assign peptide sequences. Magn Reson Chem 1998;36:601–607.

200. Rosen ME. Selective detection in NMR by time-domain digital filtering. J Magn Reson A 1994;107:119–125.

201. Marion D, Ikura M, Bax A. Improved solvent suppression in one- and two-dimensional NMR spectra by convolution of time-domain data. J Magn Reson 1989;84:425–430.

202. Reynolds WF, Yu M, Enriquez RG, Leon I. Investigation of the advantages and limitations of forward linear prediction for processing 2D data sets. Magn Reson Chem 1997;35:505–519.

203. Kotyk JJ, Hoffman NG, Hutton WC, Bretthorst GL, Ackerman JJH. Comparison of Fourier and Bayesian analysis of NMR signals. II. Examination of truncated free induction decay NMR data. J Magn Reson 1995;116:1–9.

204. Foster MP, Mayne CL, Dunkel R, Pugmire RJ, Grant DM, Kornprobst JM, Verbist JF, Biard JF, Ireland CM. Revised structure of bistramide A (bistratene A): application of a new program for the automated analysis of 2D INADEQUATE spectra. J Am Chem Soc 1992;114:1110–1111.

205. ACD Labs, 133 Richmond St. West, Suite 605, Toronto, Ontario, M5H 2L3, Canada (www.acdlabs.com).

206. Mandelshtam VA, Van QN, Shaka AJ. Obtaining proton chemical shifts and multiplets from several ^{1}D NMR signals. J Am Chem Soc 1998;120:12161–12162.

207. Hu H, Van QN, Mandelshtam VA, Shaka AJ. Reference deconvolution, phase correction, and line listing of NMR spectra by the 1D filter diagonalization method. J Magn Reson 1998;134:76–87.

208. Czarnik AW, Dewitt SH. A practical guide to combinatorial chemistry. Washington, DC: American Chemical Society, 1997.

209. Rabenstein DL, Keire DA. Quantitative chemical analysis by NMR. Pract Spectrosc 1991;11:323–369.

210. Holzgrabe U, Diehl BW, Wawer I. NMR spectroscopy in pharmacy. J Pharm Biomed Anal 1998;17:557–616.

211. Traficante DD, Steward LR. The relationship between sensitivity and integral accuracy. Further comments on optimum tip angle and relaxation delay for quantitative analysis. Concepts Magn Reson 1994;6:131–135.

212. Larive CK, Jayawickrama D, Orfi L. Quantitative analysis of peptides with NMR spectroscopy. Appl Spectrosc 1997;51:1531–1536.

213. Gerritz SW, Sefler AM. 2,5-Dimethylfuran (DMFu): an internal standard for the "traceless" quantitation of unknown samples via ^{1}H NMR. J Comb Chem 2000;2: 39–41.

20
Materials Management

David A. Kniaz
SciQuest Inc.
Newton Square, Pennsylvania

I. INTRODUCTION

During the rational drug design phase of the 1980s, effective materials management was an important, but not crucial, aspect of the drug discovery process. However, during the 1990s, as drug discovery methods became increasingly automated and probabilistic, efficient management of materials became a critical component of the drug discovery process.

This chapter will define materials management, describe its current role in drug discovery, and discuss future trends in the field. With a focus on the management of chemical reagents, natural products, and proprietary compounds, the chapter will explore both *automation technology,* which is used for management of the physical materials, and materials management *information technology,* which is central to an overall drug discovery informatics environment.

II. MATERIALS MANAGEMENT: A DEFINITION

Materials management refers to the systems, work processes, facilities, and technology involved in selecting, acquiring, receiving, storing, tracking, controlling, safely handling, distributing, and disposing of the materials defined below.

- *Reagents.* Materials, usually commercially available from a chemical supplier that are used throughout the performance of an experimental method. Within this chapter, the term *reagents* refers to the specialty organic chemicals used by chemists as starting materials (including catalysts and solvents) in the synthesis of novel compounds.

543

- *Compounds.* Proprietary chemicals synthesized or acquired for the purpose of testing for biological activity. A compound may be synthesized by an in-house medicinal chemist through manual or combinatorial methods or may be acquired from an external organization, such as a university or a government agency, or from an alliance partner. The term *compound* may refer to one known chemical structure or to a mixture of multiple chemical structures.
- *Natural products.* Naturally occurring materials that a drug discovery organization acquires and screens for biological activity.

Materials management processes are designed to:

- Maximize the throughput of chemical synthesis by streamlining the process of selecting, acquiring, and managing reagents
- Minimize costs involved in managing reagents by identifying duplicate inventory and excessive carrying and disposal costs
- Maximize screening throughput by streamlining the process of preparing proprietary samples for screening
- Reduce the risk of materials handling errors by creating an integrated informatics environment that obviates the collection and entry of incorrect data
- Improve safety and regulatory compliance by providing tools for environmental, health, and safety personnel to monitor hazardous material usage and support preparation of regulatory reports

In summary, materials management processes are designed to reduce cycle times, maximize productivity and efficiency, control costs, and enhance environmental health and safety.

III. ROLE OF MATERIALS MANAGEMENT IN DRUG DISCOVERY

Figure 1 shows how materials management fits into the drug discovery process. Reagents are selected and acquired by medicinal chemists to support synthesis processes during both lead generation and lead optimization. To support screening processes, compounds are received, stored, and distributed for screening. Following results analysis, leads are requested for follow-up. Central to the overall materials management process is a materials management system that provides the foundation of a drug discovery informatics environment.

Figure 2 shows how SciQuest's Enterprise Substance Manager (ESM) solution integrates the overall discovery informatics environment. The informatics environment shown in the figure breaks down as follows:

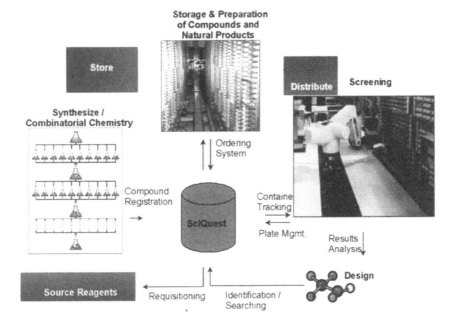

Figure 1   Materials management in drug discovery.

- Supply-chain data, which includes such information from reagent suppliers as product description, package quantity, and pricing information.
- Enterprise resource planning systems, which provide purchasing and payment of reagents acquired from reagent suppliers.
- Cheminformatics and bioinformatics systems, which provide chemical, physical property, and biological activity data associated with materials. Compound registration systems and biological activity management systems are all integrated through a centralized inventory or materials management system.
- Process automation, such as robotic liquid-handling equipment and automated sample storage and retrieval systems.

After establishing the physical sample as the primary object with which all components of an informatics framework are integrated, a materials management system matches the attributes of materials with the attributes of containers to provide an underlying data structure that integrates all of the components. As described by Frank Brown, "Using the sample object allows for simple change and additions to the description of the sample without a complete rewrite of the data structures. The hub of the chemical information system is the inventory system. The registration number should be considered a name and not a primary key for

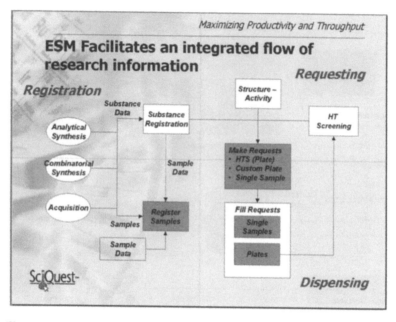

Figure 2   Materials management system.

building relationship given the complexity of parsing needed to break the registration number into its pieces."

IV.   JOB FUNCTIONS INVOLVED IN MATERIALS MANAGEMENT

Now that we have discussed how materials management fits into the drug discovery process and the informatics environment, it is important to discuss the way various job functions are involved in the materials management processes. Following is a description of these job functions.

- *Medicinal chemists.* Select, order, track, and dispose of reagents as well as synthesize, register, and distribute proprietary compounds.
- *Purchasing personnel.* Place orders for reagents, interact with suppliers on pricing and availability, and provide status updates to requesters of materials.
- *Receiving/stockroom personnel.* Receive reagents at the facility, label containers of reagents, maintain and replenish stock, and provide delivery services to scientists for requested reagents.

- *Waste management personnel.* Collect waste, prepare waste manifests for waste haulers, and provide reports of what material has been removed from a facility by what mechanism.
- *Compound management personnel.* Receive, store, and track proprietary compounds and prepare samples for screening.
- *Registrar* Ensure data integrity of chemical and physical property data entered into the corporate compound registration database. May or may not be part of the compound management group.
- *High-throughput screening scientists.* Request samples for screening and perform plate management functions—including plate replication and combination—to support high-throughput screening activities.
- *Therapeutic area biologists.* Select compounds of interest and place requests for samples for follow-up screening.
- *Information technology personnel* Assist with design, development, integration, maintenance, and support of materials management systems.
- *Environmental health and safety personnel.* Maintain lists of materials that require monitoring; track training requirements of personnel handling hazardous materials; and monitor and provide reports for regulatory purpose on acquisition, usage, and disposal of hazardous materials. They are responsible for the chemical assessment and clearance procedures.

V. MATERIALS MANAGEMENT WORK PROCESSES

Figure 3 provides a summary of the key work processes—by job function—involved in materials management. The five primary work processes are (1) reagent sourcing; (2) reagent receiving and tracking; (3) new compound registration and sample submission; (4) master plate preparation and distribution for high-throughput screening; and (5) follow-up screening. Each is discussed in detail below.

A. Reagent Sourcing

Reagent sourcing refers to the selection and sourcing of reagents to support synthesis processes. The steps in the process are as follows:

1. A medicinal chemist will establish a synthesis plan and design a virtual library of chemical structures.
2. The chemist conducts a search for commercially available reagents that can be used as starting materials for synthesis of the library. The "hit list" may be further refined using chemical structure analysis tools to eliminate undesirable functional groups and maximize structural diver-

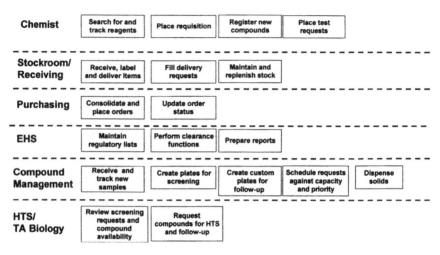

Figure 3   Materials management work processes.

sity; it ensures that the molecular weights of the desired products are within acceptable ranges.

3. The chemist conducts an inventory search for reagents on his on her list that are already available in-house and researches paper and/or electronic catalogs for products that can be purchased. For desired reagents that are not available, the chemist may consider custom synthesis. In some organizations, environmental health and safety personnel are part of the approval process for orders of hazardous materials but not part of the order approval process; they passively monitor orders, prepare reports of hazardous material usage, and identify any regulatory issues.

4. For items available in-house, the chemist will retrieve the item from another lab or place an internal requisition to a stockroom. For items not available in-house, the chemist will submit a purchase requisition for the other items on the list. Depending on the organization, the purchase order is placed by routing a paper requisition, through integration with a purchasing system or directly to suppliers via the Internet or electronic data interchange (EDI) mechanisms. Some companies have preferred relationships with suppliers and allow chemists to place orders directly, using credit cards. In other cases, the purchasing department or a third-party purchasing agent may be responsible for placing orders with suppliers and communicating the order status from the suppliers back to the original requester; this process can be automated as part of a business-to-business e-commerce application.

B. Reagent Receiving and Tracking

Once reagents are received by a facility they are delivered to the requester, tracked, and disposed of. The steps of the process are as follows:

1. The supplier delivers ordered items to the loading dock.
2. Receiving personnel unpack the box and match the packing slip to the original order and note any discrepancies. In some organizations, all orders for chemicals are processed by a chemical stockroom and are delivered directly by receiving personnel to the stockroom. When the item is unpacked, the purchasing system is updated to note receipt and process payment. Most organizations then update an internal tracking system to generate bar code labels and start tracking individual containers.
3. Receiving personnel deliver the item to the original requester.
4. The original requester uses the reagent and then places the remainder in a disposal bin, stores it in the lab, or returns the item to a centralized storeroom for reuse. The storeroom may update quantity-available information.
5. When items are ready to be disposed of, the individual responsible for waste management removes the material and prepares a manifest in conjunction with the waste hauler.

C. New Compound Registration and Sample Submission

Once the chemist completes synthesis of a new compound or library of compounds, the compound has to be registered and the physical sample submitted for storage and distribution. The steps in the process are as follows:

1. Once the chemist synthesizes new proprietary compounds (or compounds are received from outside), he or she enters the chemical and physical attributes of the compounds into the corporate database or registration system. In some organizations the processes of registering the compound and submitting it for analytical testing are integrated. In some cases, the chemist does the registering; in others, a centralized registration group handles the registration process. At a minimum, the centralized registration group will have final quality control to ensure that the compound's chemical structure is consistently entered into the corporate database for consistent data retrieval. Following registration of the compound(s), a company code number is assigned to provide an internal naming convention. The registration database is then used as the chemical structure/information source in support of structure and biological activity database searches. In some companies, registration

of the physical sample precedes compound registration. This happens more and more often in high-throughput processes where the structure characterization of the compound is done following completion of biological screening activities. Furthermore, as part of collaboration agreements, some companies might do "blind" screening of plates without knowing the structures of the screened compounds.

2. In conjunction with registration of both the chemical and physical attributes of the new compound, the physical sample is usually distributed to a centralized compound management group for storage, distribution, and inventory management.

3. Along with logging the new sample into the materials management system and placing the sample in storage, the compound management group may be responsible for the initial registration of the compounds and natural products received from external sources.

D. Master Plate Preparation and Distribution for High-Throughput Screening

Once compounds are synthesized, they are plated and distributed for screening. The steps of the process are as follows:

1. On receiving the compounds from the chemist, the compound management group will create master plates from the source compounds at standardized concentrations and volumes. This may be an automated process, using liquid-handling automation equipment and robotic weighing equipment, or it may be a semiautomated process, with technicians manually flicking small amounts of material to support plate preparation.

2. Once the master plates are prepared, they are replicated and stored, usually in cold storage.

3. Replicates are distributed for screening, either on demand or as part of a standard work process. Usually when plates are distributed for screening, the contents of the plates are also entered into the biological activity database for future association with screening results. There may be manual population of plate data from the biological database or automated population via integration between the materials management system and the biological screening database.

E. Follow-up Screening

Once hits are identified, samples must be prepared for follow-up screening. The steps of the process are as follows:

1. When screening is completed, the results are entered into the biological activity database.

2.   After the hits are identified via searches against the biological activity database, a request for samples is submitted to the materials management system based on the hit list.

3.   The materials management system logs the request and identifies source containers that can be used to fill the request. Frequently, custom plates are prepared by "cherry picking," or removing materials from individual wells across multiple source plates. Often, serial dilutions are performed to generate dose–response results.

4.   When follow-up screening yields positive results, additional follow-up screens and solid samples are requested from the materials management system and obtained from solid storage.

VI. MATERIALS MANAGEMENT TECHNOLOGIES

A variety of technologies are in use to support the above work processes. Following is a description of available technologies.

A. Chemical Structure–Based Reagent Selection Tools and Products

Chemists select reagents via chemical structure criteria. A variety of chemical structure–based software tools are available on the market to search chemical databases by chemical structure, substructure, structural similarity, and other mechanisms. Numerous tools are also available to provide chemical structure searching capabilities. Among these tools are MDL's ISIS products, Oxford Molecular's RS3 product, Daylight, Tripos tools, MSI's tools, CAS, Scifinder, and CambridgeSoft's tools.

In the realm of materials management, these tools are at their most powerful when incorporated into an overall materials management system. SciQuest has incorporated chemical structure searching tools into their reagent manager materials management product line, just as MDL has incorporated chemical structure searching tools into their product. Another example of how chemical structure searching information technology is applied to materials management is MDL's Reagent Selector. Both SciQuest and MDL products evaluate result sets of reagent-product chemical structures, based on criteria such as molecular weight and structure diversity, and easily allows for the elimination of structures with undesirable functional groups or elements.

B. ERP Systems, Supplier Catalogs, and Electronic Commerce

Chemical structure searching tools are only as good as the content data they are searching against—which in turn are only as good as the level of integration with purchasing applications. The most widely used electronic catalog of reagents is MDL's *Available Chemicals Directory (ACD)*. This product is a compilation of several catalogs providing chemical structures, as well as packaging and pricing information. Periodically, MDL provides these data to their customers in the form of a database that can be searched by chemical structure tools. Other vendors, such as CAS, provide similar products. Suppliers such as Sigma-Aldrich provide product information either through CD or directly through their web site. Some suppliers (e.g., Sigma-Aldrich) also provide detailed chemical information and safety information through their web site.

Whereas chemists will search through electronic catalogs to select reagents, enterprise resource planning systems, such as SAP, are used to place orders to suppliers. Technology is also available to place orders directly through with suppliers by electronic data interchange mechanisms or via placement of orders directly into suppliers' web sites. Companies such as SciQuest provide third-party mechanisms to aggregate catalogs of available materials and support sourcing and procurement functions.

C. Robotic Weighing and Liquid Handling Workstations

Plate preparation processes involve a number of repetitive steps in weighing samples and transferring liquids to solubilize samples, as well as preparing plates at desired concentrations and volumes. A number of robotics weighing systems, such as those provided by Zymark, are on the market to tare-weigh empty vials and gross-weigh vials full of solid material. The robotic workstations are integrated with laboratory balances to collect weight information and transfer data to formatted files.

Similarly, liquid-handling systems automate repetitive plate-preparation tasks, including solubilizing samples, transferring liquid samples from a source container to a plate, adding top-off volumes to achieve desired concentrations, creating replicate plates for distribution for screening, and combining multiple plates into single plates. Examples of liquid-handling systems are the workstations provided by TECAN and Hamilton. Both robotic weighing and liquid transfer workstations exchange data to and from materials management systems, usually via formatted file transfers.

D. Materials Management Systems

As mentioned earlier, materials management systems provide the foundation for an integrated discovery research informatics architecture. The physical sample is the key data element that integrates supplier data, process-automation systems, and chemical and bioinformatics systems. A robust materials management system supports such functions as:

- Selecting reagents by chemical structure
- Placing orders, either directly with suppliers or via enterprise resource-planning systems
- Receiving items from suppliers
- Tracking container usage
- Submitting sample proprietary materials
- Submitting and fulfilling requests for samples in support of screening
- Preparing, replicating, and combining plates

Such a system requires integration with supplier catalogs, purchasing systems, compound registration systems, biological results databases, robotic plate-preparation equipment, laboratory balances, and automated sample storage and retrieval systems.

SciQuest's product line is one such materials management system currently on the market. SciQuest refers to its offerings as research supply chain solutions, given its foundation level within the informatics environment and given its focus on logistics functions. MDL's SMART product also provides some materials management capabilities across tracking containers of reagents and supporting capabilities to track proprietary samples. Some organizations have also built their own materials management systems, with Affymax being an example of one that is reported in the literature.

E. Automated Sample Storage and Retrieval Systems

As their quantity of samples begin to stretch into the millions, the larger drug discovery organizations are procuring sample storage and retrieval systems that will automate their materials management functions. Such systems integrate a wide variety of functions including submitting samples for storage, solubilizing and replicating plates, retrieving samples from storage, and weighing out and dispensing solid samples—all within an environmentally controlled secure, usually cold storage area. Usually provided by systems integration firms, these systems encompass both the equipment and the technology to handle robotic weighing and liquid-handling equipment, laboratory balances, storage units (such as Kardex's Lektriever), and software to integrate all of these components. Usually such systems integrate tightly with an external materials management system or have scaled-down versions of these systems as part of the overall solution. Examples of these solutions include TAP's Haystack system as well as systems provided by RTS Thurnall, REMP, and Aurora.

VII. FUTURE DIRECTIONS

The future in drug discovery materials management technology is all about miniaturization, factory automation, leveraging the Internet, and object-oriented information technology. As screening technology gets smaller, sample sizes and plate formats also continue to get smaller—meaning the use of 1536 well plates and microfluidic technology for management of samples in chip format.

Automation technology will improve throughput, further automating the discovery process and resulting in the application of factory automation principles to the discovery research process. Discreet automated components will be integrated, leading to tighter integration of automated storage and retrieval systems and ultrahigh-throughput screening technology. Materials management systems will extend to provide production management and work scheduling functions to support automation processes. This high degree of automation and the unimaginable volumes of data that will be generated will introduce even more downstream bottlenecks.

The Internet will be leveraged to integrate drug discovery organizations more tightly with their suppliers and their partners. Chemists will be able to obtain real-time product, pricing, and availability information from their suppliers, minimizing out-of-date information and reducing bottlenecks. Furthermore, as drug discovery organizations continue to partner with other companies, the Internet will support the establishment of virtual-project-based organizations to seamlessly share, track, and handle materials management information.

With the increase in throughput, the need for seamless informatics integration will continue. The migration to object-oriented systems using standards such as CORBA will allow discrete systems to integrate tightly, provided that an overall data architecture is established by information management professionals.

REFERENCES

1. Wedin R. Taming the monster haystack. The challenge of compound management. Mo Drug Disc January/February 1999; 47–53.
2. Brown F. Cheminformatics: what is it and how does it impact drug discovery. Annu Rep Med Chem 1998; 35:375–383.
3. Ausman D. Virtual stockroom tracks chemical building blocks. R&D Magazine April 1998; S10–S12.
4. Drews J. In Quest of Tomorrow's Medicines. New York: Springer-Verlag, 1999.
5. Thayer A. E-commerce connects chemical businesses. Chem Eng News July 12, 1999; 13–18.

Index